21st Edition

The Reference Manual of the

Official Documents

of the American Occupational Therapy Association, Inc.

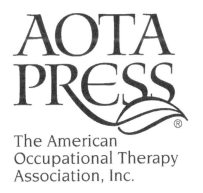

AOTA PRESS

The American
Occupational Therapy
Association, Inc.

AOTA *Vision 2025*

Occupational therapy maximizes health, well-being, and quality of life for all people, populations, and communities through effective solutions that facilitate participation in everyday living.

AOTA Mission Statement

The American Occupational Therapy Association advances the quality, availability, use, and support of occupational therapy through standard-setting, advocacy, education, and research on behalf of its members and the public.

AOTA Staff

Frederick P. Somers, *Executive Director*
Christopher M. Bluhm, *Chief Operating Officer*

Chris Davis, *Director, AOTA Press*
Caroline Polk, *Digital Manager and Managing Editor,* AJOT
Ashley Hofmann, *Development/Acquisitions Editor*
Barbara Dickson, *Production Editor*

Rebecca Rutberg, *Director, Marketing*
Amanda Goldman, *Marketing Manager*
Jennifer Folden, *Marketing Specialist*

The American Occupational Therapy Association, Inc.
4720 Montgomery Lane
Bethesda, MD 20814
Phone: 301-652-AOTA (2682)
TDD: 800-377-8555
Fax: 301-652-7711
http://www.aota.org

Disclaimers

This publication is designed to provide accurate and authoritative information in regard to the subject matter covered. It is sold or distributed with the understanding that the publisher is not engaged in rendering legal, accounting, or other professional services. If legal advice or other expert assistance is required, the services of a competent professional person should be sought.
—*From the Declaration of Principles jointly adopted by the American Bar Association and a Committee of Publishers and Associations*

ISBN-13: 978-1-56900-395-4

Library of Congress Control Number: 2016945485

Printing by Sheridan Books, Inc., Chelsea, MI

Reference citation: American Occupational Therapy Association. (2016). *The reference manual of the official documents of the American Occupational Therapy Association, Inc.* (21st ed.). Bethesda, MD: Author.

However, the preferred citation for individual chapters is their original citation from the *American Journal of Occupational Therapy.*

For permissions inquiries, visit http://www.copyright.com.

Contents

*Articles in **bold** are new to this edition. Dates indicate the year the document was approved.*

Introduction

The Reference Manual of the Official Documents of the American Occupational Therapy Association, Inc. (AOTA) was first published in 1980 and had been fully revised biennially in even-numbered years, with an addendum produced in alternating years. In 2006, AOTA Press began publishing a fully revised edition of the *Reference Manual* annually.

The 21st edition of this important work contains the following material:

- Part I contains AOTA's current official documents, which are "those approved by the membership or other official body of the Association in conformance with applicable law, the Articles of Incorporation, or the Bylaws for the use of the Association and its membership" (AOTA, 2015a).

- Part II contains Societal Statements.

- Part III contains historical information on past official documents.

Official documents of the Association may be classified as governance and professional:

- *Governance:* Documents evidencing the corporate status of the Association and required by law for carrying out the activities of the Association. Examples are the Articles of Incorporation, Bylaws, Policies and Procedures, official minutes of Assembly and Board meetings, and official minutes of the Annual Business Meeting.

- *Professional:* Documents related to practice and professional standards of the occupational therapy profession. Examples are *Standards of Practice, Standards of Continuing Competence,* and the *Occupational Therapy Code of Ethics* (AOTA, 2015b).

Types of official and other documents (AOTA, 2014) include the following:

I. **Types of Official Documents**

   A. **Guidelines**—Provide descriptions, examples, or recommendations of procedures pertaining to the education of occupational therapy practitioners and the practice of occupational therapy. (*Note:* The AOTA Occupational Therapy Practice Guidelines series are not included in the official document development or adoption process. AOTA's Practice Guidelines are a product of the Evidence-Based Practice Project and therefore follow a process of development as determined by the Institute of Medicine and National Guideline Clearinghouse.)

   B. **Position Papers**—Present the official stance of the Association on a substantive issue or subject. They are developed in response to a particular issue, concern, or need of the Association and may be written for internal or external use.

   C. **Standards**—Include a general description of the topic and define the minimum requirements for performance and quality.

D. **Statements**—Describe and clarify (vs. present an official stance on) an aspect or issue related to education or practice and are linked to the fundamental concepts of occupational therapy. They are developed in response to a particular issue, concern, or need of the Association and may be written for internal or external use.

II. Other Types of Documents

Other association documents that are included in this publication are **Societal Statements.** Written in the form of public announcements, these statements identify a societal issue of concern; state how the issue affects the participation of individuals, families, groups, or communities in society; and may offer action to be taken by individuals, groups, or communities.

The documents contained in this manual have been developed by the combined efforts of many AOTA volunteers and staff. Authorship and citations for where these documents have been published in the *American Journal of Occupational Therapy* can be found at the end of each document. For additional information, visit http://www.aota.org and http://otjournal.net. Official documents are also included in the ECRI Institute Online Directory (http://www.ecri.org), and Practice Guidelines are abstracted in the National Guideline Clearinghouse (http://www.guideline.gov).

References

American Occupational Therapy Association. (2014). *RACC standard operating procedures—Official documents (Attachment A).* (Available from the American Occupational Therapy Association, 4720 Montgomery Lane, Bethesda, MD 20824-1220)

American Occupational Therapy Association. (2015a, November). Policy A.17. Official documents of the Association. In *Policy manual* (2015 ed., p. 19). Bethesda, MD: Author.

American Occupational Therapy Association. (2015b). Occupational therapy code of ethics (2015). *American Journal of Occupational Therapy, 69*(Suppl. 3), 6913410030. http://dx.doi.org/10.5014/ajot.2015.696S03

Categories of Occupational Therapy Personnel

Code: RA Motion 4/95, 4/96, 1998M22, 1999M29, 2001C41, 2006C379
Effective: 7/94
Revised: 4/95, 4/96, 4/98, 4/99, 4/01, 4/06
BPPC Reviewed: 10/01, 1/02, 1/03, 1/06, 1/11, 7/15
Rescinded:

PURPOSE: To establish policy assuring that Association documents use consistent terminology when referring to individuals who provide or support the delivery of occupational therapy services.

It Shall Be the Policy of the Association That

The following terms are used as defined herein in all Association documents and publications:

1. **Occupational Therapist (OT):** Any individual initially certified to practice as an OT or licensed or regulated by a state, commonwealth, district, or territory of the United States to practice as an OT and who has not had that certification, license, or regulation revoked due to disciplinary action.

2. **Occupational Therapy Assistant (OTA):** Any individual initially certified to practice as an OTA or licensed or regulated by a state, commonwealth, district, or territory of the United States to practice as an OTA and who has not had that certification, license, or regulation revoked due to disciplinary action.

3. **Occupational Therapy Student (OTS):** Any individual who is enrolled in an occupational therapy educational program that is accredited, approved, or pending approval or accreditation by ACOTE®.

4. **Occupational Therapy Assistant Student (OTAS):** An individual who is enrolled in an OTA educational program that is accredited, approved, or pending approval or accreditation by ACOTE®.

5. **Occupational Therapy Practitioner:** An individual initially certified to practice as an OT or OTA or licensed or regulated by a state, district, commonwealth, or territory of the United States to practice as an OT or OTA and who has not had that certification, license, or regulation revoked due to disciplinary action.

6. **Aide:** A person who is not licensed or regulated and who provides supportive services to OTs and OTAs. An aide shall function under the guidance and responsibility of the licensed or regulated OT and may be supervised by the OT or an OTA for specifically selected routine tasks for which the aide has been trained and has demonstrated competence. The aide is not a primary service provider of occupational therapy in a practice setting and does not provide skilled occupational therapy services.

Reference

American Occupational Therapy Association. (2015). Policy A.23. Categories of occupational therapy personnel. In *Policy Manual* (pp. 25–26). Bethesda, MD: Author.

PART I

Official Documents

Incorporation Papers and Bylaws

The

Articles of Incorporation
of
The American Occupational Therapy
Association

******

Composite Articles of Incorporation of The American Occupational Therapy Association as amended*

We, The Undersigned, All being persons of full age, and all being citizens of the United States desiring to form a corporation, pursuant to Sub-Chapter 3, of Chapter 18, of the Code of Law for the District of Columbia, do hereby make, sign and acknowledge this Certificate as follows:

FIRST: The name of the corporation is to be "The American Occupational Therapy Association."**

SECOND: The term of existence of the corporation shall be perpetual.

THIRD: The purpose or purposes which it will hereafter pursue are to *advance the therapeutic value of occupation; to research the effects of occupation upon human beings and to disseminate that research;* to promote the use of occupational therapy and to advance the standards of education and training in this field; *to educate consumers about the effect of occupation upon their well-being;* and to engage in such other activities as may be considered to be advantageous to the profession, its members, and the consumers of occupational therapy services. [Italicized portions adopted by Executive Board 1/16/76.]

FOURTH: *The Corporation is to have members.*

FIFTH: *The Corporation is to be divided into classes of members. The designation of each class of members, the qualifications, rights, and limitations of the members of each class and conferring, limiting, or denying the right to vote are as follows:*

a. Members: The classes of members are (1) occupational therapist, (2) occupational therapy assistant, (3) occupational therapy student, (4) organizational, and (5) associate. The Bylaws may designate other classes of members.

b. Qualifications, Rights, and Limitations: The qualifications, rights, and limitations of the members of each class shall be provided in the Bylaws

c. Voting: Members are entitled to vote for Association officers and bylaw changes; members shall have such other voting rights as are provided in the Bylaws. Associate members and Organizational members shall not be entitled to vote for Association Officers and bylaw changes.

SIXTH: All corporate powers shall be exercised by and under the authority of the board of directors except as provided in this Sixth Article. The number of trustees, directors, or managers of the corporation shall be not less than five (5) or more than fifty (50), and shall be known as the Board of Directors. The manner of election or appointment of such directors shall be provided in the Bylaws. There shall be a designated body of the board known as the Representative Assembly which shall be directly responsible for the establishment of professional standards and policies.

SEVENTH: The territory in which its operations are principally to be conducted is the United States of America, the territories, possessions, and dependencies thereof and the District of Columbia, but the operations of the corporation shall not be limited to such territory.

EIGHTH: The location of the principal office of the corporation shall be fixed by the Bylaws of the corporation.

NINTH: The time for holding its annual meeting shall be fixed by the Bylaws of the corporation.

TENTH: *In the event this corporation shall be dissolved for any reason, any remaining assets shall be distributed for purposes within the scope of Internal Revenue code 501(c) (6) or any amendment thereto, and in accordance with the corporate statutes of the District of Columbia.*

ELEVENTH: The address, including street and number, of its registered office in the District of Columbia is 918-16th St N.W., Washington, DC 20006, and the name of its registered agent at such address is C.T. Corporation System.

TWELFTH: The names and places of residence of the persons to be its directors until its first annual meeting are as follows:

William R. Dunton, Jr., MD, of Sheppard and Enoch Pratt Hospital of Towson, Maryland; Susan C. Johnson, of 350 West 85th Street, New York City, New York; Eleanor Clarke Slagle, of the Hotel Alexandria, Chicago, Illinois; Susan E. Tracy, of Jamaica Plain, Massachusetts; and George Edward Barton, of Consolation House, Clifton Springs, New York.

IN WITNESS WHEREOF: We have made signed and acknowledged this certificate in duplicate.
Date, Clifton Springs, Ontario County, New York, this fifteenth day of March, A.D. 1917.
William R. Dunton, Jr.
Susan C. Johnson
Eleanor Clarke Slagle
George Edward Barton
Isabel G. Newton
T.B. Kidner

STATE OF NEW YORK
COUNTY OF ONTARIO: SS
On the fifteenth day of March, 1917, before me personally came William R. Dunton, Jr., Susan C. Johnson, Eleanor Clarke Slagle, George Edward Barton, Isabel G. Newton, and T.B. Kidner, to me known and known to me to be the same persons described in and who executed the foregoing certificate the same.
James A. Rolfe,
Notary Public.

(NOTARIAL SEAL)

* A resolution recommending that the corporation accept the jurisdiction of the District of Columbia Nonprofit Corporation Act (29 D.C. Code Chapter 10 then) was adopted at a meeting of the Executive Board on January 16, 1976. The formal Statement of Election to Accept was filed and certified on August 30, 1976. Italicized items were filed as part of that Statement to amend existing article number three, and to add new provisions with information required to be included in the Articles under Chapter 10 (now Chapter 5).

The 1981 amendment added the organizational category of membership without vote in Article 5, and corrected the word "The" in Article one.
The 1990 amendment added the Associate category of membership without vote in Article 5 and provides for other classes of membership to be designated in the Bylaws.
This compilation represents a re-numbered composite of all official amendments or documents affecting incorporation from March 1917 through May 1990.
The 2003 amendments removed "registered" and "certified" in Members in Article 5 and changed from "Executive Board" to "Board of Directors" in Article 6.
The 2013 amendments add by name the Representative Assembly as a designated body of the board, responsible for the establishment of professional standards and policies. This change was made to incorporate AOTA's then existing organizational structure into the framework of the 2012 changes in the DC nonprofit corporate law.

** Name changed from National Society for the Promotion of Occupational Therapy, Inc. Jan. 27, 1923

CERTIFICATE OF INCORPORATION

OF THE

NATIONAL SOCIETY FOR THE PROMOTION OF OCCUPATIONAL THERAPY, INC.

We, The Undersigned, All being persons of full age, and all being citizens of the United States, desiring to form a corporation, pursuant to Sub-Chapter 3 of Chapter 18, of the Code of Law for the District of Columbia, do hereby make, sign and acknowledge this Certificate as follows:

FIRST: The name of the Corporation is to be "THE NATIONAL SOCIETY FOR THE PROMOTION OF OCCUPATIONAL THERAPY, INC."

SECOND: The particular objects for which the corporation is formed are as follows: The advancement of occupation as a therapeutic measure; for the study of the effect of occupation upon the human being; and for the scientific dispensation of this knowledge.

THIRD: The territory in which its operations are to be principally conducted is the United States of America.

FOURTH: Its principal business office is to be located in the Village of Clifton Springs, County of Ontario and State of New York.

FIFTH: The number of its directors is to be five.

SIXTH: The names and places of residence of the persons to be its directors until its first annual meeting are as follows:

William R. Dunton, Jr., M.D. of Sheppard and Enoch Pratt Hospital of Towson, Maryland.

Susan C. Johnson, of 350 West 85th Street, New York City, New York.

Eleanor Clarke Slagle, of the Hotel Alexandria, Chicago, Illinois.

George Edward Barton, of Consolation House, Clifton Springs, New York.

SEVENTH: The time for holding its annual meeting is on the first Monday of September in each year.

IN WITNESS WHEREOF: We have made, signed and acknowledged this certificate in duplicate.

Dated, Clifton Springs, Ontario County, New York, this fifteenth day of March, A.D. 1917.

> William R. Dunton, Jr.
> Susan C. Johnson
> Eleanor Clarke Slagle
> George Edward Barton
> Isabel G. Newton
> T. B. Kidner

STATE OF NEW YORK

COUNTY OF ONTARIO: SS

On this fifteenth day of March, 1917, before me personally came William R. Dunton, Jr., Susan C. Johnson, Eleanor Clarke Siagle, George Edward Barton, Isabel G. Newton and T. B. Kidner, to me known and known to me to be the same persons described in and who executed the foregoing certificate and they severally duly acknowledged to me that they executed the same.

James A. Rolfe,

Notary Public

(NOTARIAL SEAL)

The

Official Bylaws
of
The American Occupational
Therapy Association, Inc.

2016

******

The American Occupational Therapy Association, Inc.

Bylaws
Table of Contents

i

ii

ARTICLE I.

Name

Section 1.   Name

The name of the organization shall be The American Occupational Therapy Association, Inc., hereinafter referred to as the Association.

Section 2.   Purpose

The Association is organized under the District of Columbia (D.C.) Nonprofit Corporation Act.

ARTICLE II.

Noninurement

Section 1.   Noninurement

No part of the net earnings of the Association shall inure to the use or benefit of any individual. The Association shall not engage in any activities that are prohibited by the Internal Revenue Code, Section 501(c)(6).

ARTICLE III.

Members

Section 1.   Membership Classes

There shall be six (6) classes of membership.

A.   Occupational Therapist (OT): Any individual initially certified to practice as an OT or licensed or regulated by a state, commonwealth, district, or territory of the United States to practice as an occupational therapist and who has not had that certification, license, or regulation revoked due to disciplinary action shall be eligible to be an Occupational Therapist Member.

B.   Occupational Therapist New Practitioner and Occupational Therapy Assistant New Practitioner: Any individual who has graduated with an occupational therapy degree from an occupational therapy or occupational therapy assistant entry level educational program that is accredited by the Accreditation Council for Occupational Therapy Education (ACOTE®) and that is located in the United States, or in a state, commonwealth, district, or territory of the United States in the past 24 months.

1

C. Occupational Therapy Assistant (OTA): Any individual initially certified to practice as an OTA or licensed or regulated by a state, commonwealth, district, or territory of the United States to practice as an occupational therapy assistant and who has not had that certification, license, or regulation revoked due to disciplinary action shall be eligible to be an Occupational Therapy Assistant Member.

D. Occupational Therapy Student (OTS) and Occupational Therapy Assistant Student (OTAS): Any individual enrolled in an entry level occupational therapy educational program that is accredited, or pending accreditation by the Accreditation Council for Occupational Therapy Education (ACOTE®) and that is located in the United States, or in a state, commonwealth, district, or territory of the United States, shall be eligible to be a Student Member.

E. Organizational: An organization, institution, or agency interested in occupational therapy may be an Organizational Member.

F. Associate: An individual interested in occupational therapy that does not satisfy the requirements of subsections A, B, C, or D of this section may be an Associate Member.

Section 2. **Voting Rights and Privileges of Members**

A. Occupational Therapist, Occupational Therapy Assistant, and OT/OTA New Practitioner Members:

 1. Shall be entitled to vote

  a. for Officers of the Association, Board Directors, and Delegate and Alternate Delegate to the World Federation of Occupational Therapists (WFOT);

  b. for Representative(s);

  c. for Chairpersons-Elect of the Commission on Education (COE), Commission on Practice (COP), Ethics Commission (EC), Commission on Continuing Competence and Professional Development (CCCPD), Special Interest Sections Council (SISC), Chairperson of the Volunteer Leadership Development Committee (VLDC), and for the OTA Representative and OTA Representative-Elect to the Assembly;

  d. at Annual Business Meetings and special meetings of the Association; and

2

e.   for Association Bylaws.

2.   May submit motions to the Agenda Committee of the Assembly.

3.   May serve on Association commissions/committees and run for offices of the Association.

4.   Shall be eligible to receive other privileges as designated by the Board.

5.   May have voice in all appropriate forums in accordance with established practice.

6.   May seek review of the Associations actions pursuant to the procedures set forth in Article XV.

7.   May inspect and copy records of the Association upon delivering a signed notice to the Secretary of the Association at the Association headquarters at least 21 calendar days before the date a member wishes to inspect the records during reasonable business hours at the office of the Association. The Association shall keep and members shall have the right to inspect and copy the records required by and under the terms of the D.C. law applicable to nonprofit corporations.

B.   Student Members:

1.   Shall be entitled to vote

a.   for Officers of the Association, Board Directors, and Delegate and Alternate Delegate to the WFOT;

b.   at Annual Business Meetings or special meetings of the Association;

c.   for Chairpersons-Elect of the COE, COP, EC, CCCPD, SISC, Chairperson of the VLDC and for Representatives, the OTA Representative and OTA Representative-Elect to the Assembly;

d.   for Chairperson and Officers of the ASD and Student Member Representative to the Assembly; and

e.   for Association Bylaws.

2.   May submit motions to the Agenda Committee of the Assembly.

3.   May serve on Association commissions/committees.

3

4.   Shall be eligible to be an officer or member of ASD.

5.   Shall be entitled to receive other privileges as designated by the Board.

6.   May seek review of the Associations actions pursuant to the procedures set forth in Article XV.

7.   May inspect and copy records of the Association upon delivering a signed notice to the secretary of the Association at least 21 days before the date a member wishes to inspect the records during reasonable business hours at office of the Association. The Association shall keep and members shall have the right to inspect and copy the records required by and under the terms of the D.C. law applicable to nonprofit corporations.

C.   Organizational and Associate Members:

Shall be entitled to receive privileges as designated by the Board.

Section 3.   Dues and Good Standing

A.   Dues and fees, if any, for all classes of membership shall be established by the Board.

B.   A member shall be in good standing if he or she currently meets the qualifications for the class of membership, has paid all applicable dues, and membership has not been terminated pursuant to Section 4.

Section 4.   Termination of Membership

A.   Any member whose dues are still in arrears 30 days after payment is due shall automatically be removed from membership. Membership shall automatically be reinstated by payment of dues in arrears.

B.   Members of any classification may have their membership revoked or suspended for cause. Cause may include violation of the AOTA *Code of Ethics*.

C.   For any cause other than nonpayment of dues, a vote for revocation or suspension shall occur only after the member has been notified of the complaint for revocation and has been given reasonable opportunity for defense. Cause shall mean; (1) any violation of any Association policy, procedures, or terms of use which reflects negatively on one's professional role, the profession or the reputation of the Association; or (2) any persistent course of conduct which detracts from the Association's mission or reflects negatively on the profession.

4

D.   Any member may submit a complaint to the Board requesting that another member be removed for cause.

ARTICLE IV.

Meetings of the Membership of the Association

Section 1.   **Meeting Location**

A.   Annual or special meetings of the membership need not be held in a geographic location. Alternatively, the meeting may be held by means of the internet or other electronic communications technology in a fashion such that the members have the opportunity to read or hear the proceedings substantially concurrently (although not necessarily simultaneous) with their occurrence, vote on matters submitted to the members, and pose questions and make comments.

B.   The President shall be the chairperson at all membership meetings, and in the absence of the President it shall be the Vice President.

Section 2.   **Annual Business Meeting**

A.   The regular meeting of the membership, the Annual Business Meeting, shall be held within each calendar year.

B.   An official publication of the Association shall list the place, day, and hour of the Annual Business Meeting at least 90 days before the meeting date.

C.   The record date for determining members entitled to notice of and to vote at an annual meeting shall be 30 days prior to the meeting or action requiring a determination by the members.

Section 3.   **Special Meetings**

A.   The President, a majority of voting members of the Board, two thirds of the Assembly with respect to a matter within the scope of its Purpose as set forth in Article VII, Section 1, or 10% of the members of the Association may call a special meeting.

B.   Members shall be notified by mail, electronic, or telephonic transmission of the place, day, hour, and purpose of the special meeting at least 21 days before the meeting.

C.   At a special meeting, the only business conducted shall be the matters stated in the meeting notification.

5

D.   The record date for determining members entitled to demand a special meeting shall be the date the first member signs a demand for the special meeting.

E.   The record date for determining members entitled to give notice of and to vote at a special meeting is the day the first notice is given to members, and the record date shall not be more than 30 days before the meeting or action requiring a determination by the members.

Section 4.   **Quorum for Annual and Special Meetings**

A quorum shall be 100 members. Once a quorum is established, it shall remain established for the duration of the meeting in conformance with the law applicable to non-profit corporations in D.C.

Section 5.   **Voting**

A.   Mail, electronic, or telephonic transmission may be used by OT, OTA, and student members for voting.

B.   At any annual or special meeting of the members, there shall be no voting by proxy.

C.   The Board in conformance with the law applicable to non-profit corporations in D.C. shall determine the process for counting and recording the vote except as otherwise provided in Article IX of these Bylaws.

D.   Any action that may be taken at any annual, special, or regular meeting of the members may be taken without a meeting by ballot in accordance with D.C. Law. Elections by ballots shall be conducted by ballot in accordance with Article IX.

E.   An action is approved by the membership if the votes cast favoring the action exceed the votes cast opposing the action, unless the Articles, Bylaws, or D.C. law requires a greater or lesser number of affirmative votes for the specific matter that is the subject of the vote.

ARTICLE V.

Board of Directors

Section 1.   **Purpose**

The Board of Directors, herein called the Board, shall govern the affairs of the

6

Association in accordance with all duly vested statutory, corporate, and Bylaws powers. Each member of the Board shall have a fiduciary duty when discharging duties as a director to act in good faith and in a manner reasonably believed to be in the best interest of the Association and otherwise in accordance with standards of conduct under D.C. law for directors in non-profit associations.

Section 2.   **Composition**

A.   Voting Members

    1.   Officers of the Association: President, Vice President, Secretary, and Treasurer

    2.   Six Directors (at least one of whom must be an OTA and at least one of whom must be an OT)

    3.   Speaker of the Assembly

B.   Nonvoting Members

    1.   President-Elect

    2.   Public Advisor

    3.   Consumer Advisor

    4.   Association Executive Director

    5.   President, American Occupational Therapy Foundation (AOTF)

    6.   An additional person designated by AOTF from their Board

Section 3.   **Term and Qualifications of Board Directors**

A.   Term of Office

    1.   A Director shall serve a 3-year term, or until a successor has been elected but in no event shall a Director serve in excess of 5 consecutive years without being appointed or elected to a new term.

    2.   A Director shall only be eligible to serve another elected term after the expiration of 2 intervening years.

    3.   A vacancy on the Board may be filled until the next scheduled election by a vote of a majority of the Directors remaining in office, even if they constitute less than a quorum.

7

4. Directors may only be removed for cause by the members of the Board as provided in Article XII or by a vote of the membership. Notice of a meeting at which removal of a Director is being considered shall state that the purpose, or one of the purposes, of the meeting is removal of the Director(s).

B. Qualifications

1. A Director shall have been initially certified with at least 5 years of experience as an OT or OTA at the time of nomination.

2. A Director shall have the qualifications necessary to execute the duties of the office held as outlined by the Volunteer Leadership Development Committee (VLDC).

Section 4. **Appointment, Term, and Qualifications of Appointed Participants**

A. Appointment

The Consumer Advisor and Public Advisor are appointed by the President.

B. Term of Office

The Consumer Advisor and Public Advisor shall serve a 3-year term that coincides with the term of the President.

C. Qualifications

1. Consumer Advisor

a. Knowledge of the profession of occupational therapy through personal experience.

b. Experience serving on boards, committees, or other bodies.

2. Public Advisor

a. Knowledge of the profession of occupational therapy through professional experience in health care reimbursement, regulatory, or policy arenas.

b. Experience serving on boards, committees, or other bodies.

Section 5. **Functions**

The Board shall perform such functions as are necessary to fulfill the purpose of the Board

8

of Directors set forth in this Article at Section 1, including the functions set forth below.

A.   Establish the policies and procedures of the Board and the Association with the exception of the procedures that govern the Assembly.

B.   Develop and approve the strategic plan of the Association.

C.   Review and approve the Association budget for each fiscal year.

D.   Manage the Association headquarters through appointment of the Executive Director as Chief Executive Officer of the Association.

E.   Approve investment policies of the Association and review compliance therewith.

F.   Unless otherwise provided, act as, or appoint, the appeal body of the Association for matters for which such appeals are provided under these Bylaws.

G.   Determine location of the principal office of the Association.

H.   Declare and take action during an emergency.

I.   Create committees of the Board and advisory committees and entities.

Section 6.   Meetings

A.   Regular Meetings

    1.   The Board shall have at least one regular meeting a year.

    2.   The time and place of a regular meeting shall be designated at least 30 days before the meeting date by mail, electronic, or telephonic transmission to Board members.

    3.   The Board may invite any person to a Board meeting to advance the business of the Board.

    4.   The Board may permit any or all Directors to participate in regular or special meetings by, or conduct the meetings through, the use of any means of communication by which all Directors participating may simultaneously hear each other during the meeting.

B.   Special Meetings

    1.   Special meetings of the Board may be called by the President or any three members to address specific issues.

9

2. Board members shall be notified by mail, electronic, or telephonic transmission of the date, time, place, and purpose of the meeting at least 1 week before the date.

3. Only business as stated in the call may be transacted at the special meeting.

4. Urgent business may be transacted by voting members of the Board via conference call on notice that is appropriate under the circumstances.

C. Conduct of the Meeting

All meetings are open to Association members consistent with Association Policy A.6.

D. Quorum

A majority of all voting members, including at least two officers, shall constitute a quorum.

E. Voting

1. If a quorum is present when a vote is taken, the affirmative vote of a majority of the Directors present shall be an act of the Directors unless a greater vote is required by the Articles of Incorporation, Bylaws, or law for the specific matter before the Board.

2. Action may be taken without a meeting if each Director signs consent in the form of a record describing the action to be taken.

3. Actions taken at a Board meeting approving a transaction and contract where a board member or officer has an actual or potential conflict of interest shall be valid if the interested Director disclosed the conflict to the Board prior to the vote and if the transaction or contract would not be void or voidable under D.C. Code § 29-406.70(a) (1) or (a) (2). That a contract or transaction meets the fairness requirement of D.C. Code § 29-406.70(a) (3) shall not be sufficient basis to validate a Board action in which a board member had a conflict of interest.

Section 7.   Committees of the Board

The Board shall have the authority to establish committees consisting of board members as necessary to carry out the purposes of the Association provided that the Board may not delegate overall responsibility for conduct of the business of the Association. The Board shall also have authority to establish advisory committees that may consist of Board and/or non-Board members. Advisory committees cannot exercise any power of the

10

Board.

Section 8.   Organizational Advisors

The following shall act in an advisory capacity to the Board to provide information regarding strategic planning and budgeting with respect to matters within the expertise of the specific Organizational Advisor: Accreditation Council for Occupational Therapy Education (ACOTE®) Chairperson, American Occupational Therapy Political Action Committee (AOTPAC®) Chairperson, Affiliated State Association Presidents (ASAP) Chairperson, World Federation of Occupational Therapists (WFOT) Delegate, OT Academic Leadership Council (OT-ALC) Chairperson, and OTA Academic Leadership Council (OTA-ALC) Chairperson.

Section 9.   Standing Advisory Committees

The following committees shall be standing advisory committees of the Board.

A.   Finance and Audit Committee

Purpose: To assist the Board in its oversight of
   a. Integrity in financial statements;
   b. Compliance with legal and regulatory requirements as well as Association conflict of interest policies; and
   c. Selection of a qualified independent auditor.

The Treasurer shall serve as the Chairperson of the Finance and Audit Committee for a 3-year term.

B.   Bylaws, Policies, and Procedures Committee (BPPC)

Purpose: To review Association governance documents and recommend changes to appropriate body(ies) for consideration. The Board shall appoint the Chairperson of BPPC for a 3-year term.

C.   Volunteer Leadership Development Committee (VLDC)

Purpose: To promote member participation and engagement, volunteer leadership development, and participation initiatives of the Association. The VLDC will identify and recruit diverse and qualified candidates for service to the Association through routine elections and appointments, recipients of awards, and other leadership activities. The Chairperson of VLDC shall be elected by the membership for a 3-year term.

D.   Special Interest Sections Council (SISC)

Purpose: To coordinate and facilitate activities of the Special Interest Sections with standing and advisory commissions and committees of the

11

Association. The Chairperson shall be elected by the membership for a 3-year term.

E.   Assembly of Student Delegates (ASD)

Purpose: To provide an opportunity for student members to have input into decision making and actions of the Association; to promote participation, professional growth, and leadership development of students; and to enhance students' knowledge of the structure of the Association. The ASD Chairperson shall be elected for a 2-year term.

The Board may set forth in standard operating procedures (SOPs) the procedures for selection and approval of the members of the standing advisory committee, the term of the members, and any other matters relating to operation of the committees.

Section 10.   Associated Advisory Council of the Board

ACOTE®

Purpose: To accredit occupational therapy educational programs and occupational therapy assistant educational programs. ACOTE® establishes, approves, and administers educational standards to evaluate occupational therapy and occupational therapy assistant educational programs. ACOTE® shall have complete autonomy in establishing standards for educational programs; developing and implementing policies, rules, and procedures for conducting accreditation reviews; and making accreditation decisions.

ARTICLE VI.

Officers of the Association

Section 1.   Officers

The Officers shall be the President, Vice President, Secretary, and Treasurer.

Section 2.   Officer Qualifications

A.   Officers shall have been initially certified with at least 10 years of experience as an OT or OTA at the time of nomination.

B.   An officer shall have the qualifications necessary to execute duties of the office held as stated in Association documents.

C.   An officer shall be a member in good standing of the Association and of a state affiliate at the time of nomination and throughout the term of office.

Section 3.   Duties

12

A.   President

    1.   Shall be the chief elected officer of the Association and represent the Association to the public.

    2.   Shall be an ex officio member of all committees of the Association except the VLDC and the EC.

    3.   Shall preside at all meetings of the Association membership.

    4.   Shall preside at Board meetings as Chairperson of the Board.

    5.   Shall appoint ad hoc committee chairpersons.

    6.   Shall appoint a member of the Board to serve as liaison to ASD.

    7.   Shall appoint liaisons to external national organizations.

    8.   Shall perform all other duties incident to the office of President.

B.   Vice President

    1.   Shall fulfill presidential duties in the absence of the President.

    2.   Shall perform all other duties incident to the office of Vice President.

C.   Secretary

    1.   Shall record minutes of the Annual Business Meeting, special meetings of the Association, minutes of Board meetings, and be the custodian of such records.

    2.   Shall serve as a member of the BPPC.

    3.   Shall call to order an Annual Business Meeting or special meeting of the Association in the absence of the President and Vice President and shall preside over an election by the members present of a chairperson pro tempore.

    4.   Shall perform all other duties incident to the office of Secretary.

D.   Treasurer

    1.   Shall oversee financial affairs of the Association.

    2.   Shall serve as chairperson of the Board's Finance and Audit

13

Committee.

3.   Shall be bonded at the expense of the Association.

4.   Shall have accounts of the Association audited annually by an independent auditor.

5.   Shall perform all other duties incident to the office of Treasurer.

ARTICLE VII.

Representative Assembly

Section 1.   Purpose

The Representative Assembly, herein called the Assembly, shall be a designated body of the Board directly responsible for the establishment of professional standards and policies. With respect to matters within the scope of its purpose, each member of the Assembly shall have a fiduciary duty when discharging responsibilities as a member of the Assembly to act in good faith and in a manner reasonably believed to be in the best interest of the Association and otherwise in accordance with standards of conduct under the D.C. law for fiduciaries in non-profit associations.

Section 2.   Composition

A.   Voting Members

1.   Elected Representative(s), as determined by proportional representation of the election area(s).

2.   A Representative for Internationally Based Practitioners

3.   Officials of the Assembly: Speaker, Vice Speaker, and Recorder

4.   Officers of the Association: President, Vice President, Secretary, and Treasurer

5.   Student Member Representative

6.   OTA Representative

7.   Chairpersons of the COE, COP, CCCPD, and EC

8.   ASAP Representative

9.   Consumer Member

14

B.   Nonvoting Members

    1.   President-Elect

    2.   AOTA Executive Director

    3.   Chairpersons-Elect of the COE, COP, CCCPD, and EC, and OTA Representative-Elect

    4.   Chairpersons of the Agenda and Credentials Review and Accountability Committee (CRAC)

Section 3.   **Election, Term, and Qualifications of Elected Members**

A.   Election

    1.   Representatives of an election area are elected by OT, OTA, and student members within that election area. The election will be conducted by the Association. An election area is defined by state, district, commonwealth, or territory boundaries and there shall be only one election area within the boundaries of each state, district, commonwealth, or territory.

    2.   VLDC shall conduct the ASD election for Student Member Representative to the Assembly.

B.   Term of Office

    1.   Representatives shall serve a 3-year term or until successors have been elected.

    2.   Representatives shall not be eligible to serve more than two consecutive terms in the same position.

    3.   The Student Member Representative shall serve a 2-year term.

    4.   The OTA Representative shall serve a 3-year term.

    5.   Vacancies in the position of Representative of an election area may be filled by appointment until the end of the unexpired term for the vacancy by a majority vote of the Representative Assembly Leadership Committee (RALC).

    6.   Vacancies in the positions other than Representatives of an election area will be handled as outlined in Article XII, Section 5: Vacancies.

C.   Qualifications

15

1.   Representatives shall have the qualifications necessary to execute duties of the office held as stated in Association documents.

2.   Representatives shall be members in good standing of the Association, and of his/her state election area at the time of nomination and throughout the term of office.

3.   The OTA Representative and OTA Representative-Elect shall be members in good standing of the Association, and of a state affiliate at the time of nomination and throughout the term of office.

4.   Representatives, the OTA Representative, and the OTA Representative-Elect shall maintain any election area regulatory requirements necessary to identify themselves as an OT or OTA throughout the term of office.

5.   The Student Representative shall be a voting member in good standing of the Association, and of his/her state election area and must be enrolled in an accredited occupational therapy educational program with at least 6 months remaining in his/her program (coursework, fieldwork, and thesis) following induction into office.

Section 4.   **Appointment, Term, and Qualifications of Consumer Member**

A.   Appointment

The Consumer Member is appointed by the Speaker.

B.   Term of Office

The Consumer Member shall serve a 3-year term that coincides with the term of the Speaker.

C.   Qualifications

1.   Knowledge of the profession of occupational therapy through personal experience.

2.   Experience serving on boards, committees, or other bodies.

Section 5.   **Functions**

A.   Formulate and approve Association policies relating to the specific purposes of the Assembly as set forth in Section 1 above.

B.   Exercise powers and functions necessary to carry out duties of the

16

Assembly's associated advisory commissions and committees.

C.   Elect a Chairperson for each of the following Committees: Agenda and CRAC.

Section 6.   **Meetings**

A.   Regular Meetings

      1.   At least one meeting of the Assembly shall be held annually.

      2.   The time and place of the meeting shall be designated by mail, electronic, or telephonic transmission to Representatives at least 30 days before the meeting date and shall be published in an official publication of the Association.

      3.   The Assembly may invite any person to an Assembly meeting to advance business of the Assembly.

B.   Special Meetings

      1.   Special meetings may be called by one third of the Assembly members, the Speaker of the Assembly, the Board, or the President of the Association.

      2.   Special meetings of the Assembly may be held by electronic means including, but not limited to, electronic or other Internet communication systems, telephone, or video conferences.

      3.   The time, place, and purpose of the meeting shall be designated by mail, electronic, or telephonic transmission to Representatives at least 21 days before the meeting date and shall be published in an official publication of the Association.

      4.   Only business stated in the notice may be transacted at the special meeting.

C.   Conduct of the Meeting

All meetings are open to Association members consistent with Association Policy A.6.

D.   Quorum

A majority of voting members shall constitute a quorum at any meeting of the Assembly. Once a quorum is established, it shall remain established for the duration of the meeting in conformance with the law applicable to

17

non-profit corporations in D.C.

E. Voting

1. If a quorum is present when a vote is taken, the affirmative vote of a majority of the Representatives present shall be an act of the Assembly unless a greater vote is required by the Articles of Incorporation, Bylaws, or by law for the specific matter before the Assembly.

2. The Assembly meetings need not be held in a geographic location. Alternatively, the meeting may be held by means of the internet or other electronic communications technology in a fashion such that Representatives have the opportunity to read or hear the proceedings substantially concurrently (although not necessarily simultaneous) with their occurrence, vote on matters submitted to the Representatives, and pose questions and make comments.

Section 7.   Advisory Commissions and Committees of the Assembly

The Assembly shall have the authority to establish advisory commissions and committees as necessary to carry out the purposes of the Assembly. The Assembly shall establish membership criteria for all such commissions and committees. The Assembly shall have the following:

A. Commission on Education (COE)

Purpose: To promote the quality of education for OTs and OTAs relative to educator, student, and consumer needs.

B. Commission on Practice (COP)

Purpose: To promote and guide best practice in, and standards for, occupational therapy relative to practitioner and consumer needs.

C. Ethics Commission (EC)

Purpose: To serve Association members and the public through development, review, interpretation, and education of the Code and Ethics Standards and to provide the process whereby they are enforced.

D. Commission on Continuing Competence and Professional Development (CCCPD)

Purpose: To promote continuing competence and professional development of practitioners in accordance with the Association's

18

standards.

E.   Agenda Committee

Purpose: To facilitate business of the Assembly.

F.   Credentials Review and Accountability Committee (CRAC)

Purpose: To ensure that Representatives from each election area, committee/commission chairpersons and chairpersons-elect, officers, officials, Representative for Internationally Based Practitioners, ASAP Representative, ASD Representative, OTA Representative and Representative-Elect, and Agenda and CRAC Chairpersons meet the qualifications to be members of the Assembly.

G.   Representative Assembly Coordinating Committee (RACC)

Purpose: To coordinate activities and manage integrated projects of the COE, COP, EC, and CCCPD.

Members of the RACC shall be the chairpersons of the COE, COP, EC and CCCPD; and the Speaker as Ex Officio. The Vice Speaker shall be the Chairperson of the RACC.

H.   Representative Assembly Leadership Committee (RALC)

Purpose: To plan, manage, and expedite work of the Assembly.

Members of the RALC shall be the Speaker, Vice Speaker, Agenda Chairperson, CRAC Chairperson, and Recorder. The Speaker shall be the Chairperson of the RALC.

Unless otherwise stated above, Chairpersons of the Advisory Commissions and Committees of the Assembly shall be elected by the membership for a 3-year term and shall hold only one position in the Association at a time.

The Chairpersons of the Agenda Committee and CRAC are elected by members of the Assembly, as conducted by the VLDC, for a 3-year term and shall hold only one position in the Association at a time.

ARTICLE VIII.

Officials of the Representative Assembly

Section 1.   **Officials**

19

The officials shall be the Speaker, Vice Speaker, and Recorder.

Section 2.   **Election**

A.   The officials shall be elected by voting members of the Assembly.

B.   The VLDC shall prepare a slate, preferably of at least two qualified candidates, for each position and shall conduct the election.

C.   When a Representative is elected as an official, the person shall vacate the position of Representative.

Section 3.   **Qualifications**

A.   A candidate shall have the qualifications necessary to execute duties of the position held as stated in Association documents.

B.   A candidate shall be a member in good standing of the Association, and an election area affiliate at the time of nomination and throughout the term of office.

C.   A candidate shall be or have been a duly elected Representative, current commission or committee chairperson, or a current official seeking election.

D.   A candidate shall have served at least 2 full years in the Assembly within 5 years of the election.

Section 4.   **Duties**

A.   Speaker

1.   Shall preside at Assembly meetings.

2.   Shall have the same voting rights as other voting members of the Assembly but may abstain from voting to maintain impartiality as the presiding officer unless it would affect the outcome.

3.   Shall be an ex officio member of all committees of the Assembly except those associated with the EC.

4.   Shall appoint ad hoc chairpersons and members of ad hoc committees of the Assembly.

5.   Shall perform all other duties incident to the office of Speaker.

6.   Shall serve as a member of the Board.

20

B.   Vice Speaker

      1.   Shall fulfill duties of the Speaker in the absence of the Speaker.

      2.   Shall serve as Chairperson to the RACC.

C.   Recorder

      1.   Shall take minutes of the meetings of the Assembly.

      2.   Shall be the custodian of such records.

ARTICLE IX.

Nominations and Elections of the Association

Section 1.   **Nominations**

A.   Any member of the Association may submit nominations to the VLDC for:

      1.   Officers and Officers-Elect of the Association,

      2.   Board Directors,

      3.   Delegate and Alternate Delegate to the WFOT,

      4.   Representative of an election area in which the individual member is a voting member,

      5.   OTA Representative-Elect,

      6.   Chairpersons-Elect of COE, COP, CCCPD, SISC, and EC, and Chairperson of VLDC.

B.   Any member of ASD may submit nominations to the VLDC for ASD officers.

C.   Any member of the Assembly may submit nominations to the VLDC for Officials of the Assembly.

D.   The call for nominations for the positions provided for in this Section shall be placed in an official publication of the Association 45 days before preparation of the ballot.

Section 2.   **Eligibility**

All candidates for elected and appointed positions must be members of AOTA with the

21

exception of public and consumer members of the Board and Assembly. An individual elected or appointed to a position may not serve in any other position at the same time unless designated in an SOP or job description (JD) or appointed to a smaller group of the body to which he or she was elected.

Section 3.   Slate

The VLDC shall prepare a slate, preferably of at least two qualified candidates, for all elected positions to be filled.

Section 4.   Ballot for Elections of the Association

A.   Preparation

      1.   The VLDC shall prepare a ballot for the election of positions listed in Section 1.A of this Article.

      2.   The Ballot: shall:
        a.   set forth the name of the candidates,
        b.   provide the opportunity to vote for, or withhold a vote for each candidate for election, and
        c.   indicate the number of responses needed to meet quorum requirements.

      3.   Ballots shall be delivered by mail, electronic, telephonic, or facsimile transmission to each member of the Association entitled to vote in the election.

      4.   Ballots shall state the deadline date for receipt of the ballot and the address or location to which the ballot shall be returned.

      5.   Ballots must have a method of authenticating the eligibility of each voter (e.g., a member number).

B.   Deadline

      1.   The deadline for receipt of all marked ballots by the agent authorized to receive and count ballots shall be at least 45 days before the Annual Business Meeting.

      2.   The election shall be closed on the deadline date and no ballots received thereafter shall be counted.

C.   Vote

      1.   The election of a candidate shall be by plurality vote of those ballots cast by members entitled to vote in the election at a

22

meeting at which a quorum is present.

2.   Approval by ballot in an election is valid only when the number of votes cast by ballot equals or exceeds the quorum required to be present at a meeting where the election voting would take place.

D.   Tie Vote

1.   In the event of a tie vote the ballots shall be recounted.

2.   In the event that the result is still tied, the election for that position shall be conducted again.

E.   Contested Vote

1.   In the event that a vote is contested and the vote tally is separated by no more than 5% of ballots counted, the ballots shall be recounted.

2.   Results of the recount shall be binding.

F.   Invalid Election

The VLDC shall have the authority to determine grounds for declaring an invalid election subject to approval of the Board.

ARTICLE X.

Affiliates

Section 1.   Boundaries

An Affiliate represents members located within an individual state, commonwealth, the District of Columbia, or Puerto Rico.

Section 2.   Purpose

An Affiliate is a professional organization of OTs, OTAs, and students that has been recognized by the Association. The purpose of the affiliation is to foster communication and collaboration between the Association and Affiliates.

Section 3.   Recognition

An organization becomes an Affiliate of the Association through the process described in the *Affiliation Principles for AOTA and State Associations*. Continued recognition is

23

dependent on compliance with the *Affiliation Principles for AOTA and State Associations.*

Section 4.   Termination

Termination (disaffiliation) of an Affiliate can occur for the reasons and through the process described in the *Affiliation Principles for AOTA and State Associations.*

Section 5.   Appeal Process

The Affiliate shall have notice and opportunity to appeal.

Section 6.   Affiliated State Association Presidents (ASAP)

The Presidents of the Affiliates will be the voice and resource representing state affiliate members to the Association; advising the Board and the Assembly; and providing a forum for communicating, networking, training, and mentoring state affiliate leadership.

ARTICLE XI.

World Federation of Occupational Therapists—Delegates

Section 1.   Delegates

The Association shall have a Delegate and an Alternate Delegate as representatives to the World Federation of Occupational Therapists, hereinafter referred to as WFOT.

Section 2.   Election and Term of Office

A.   The Delegate and Alternate Delegate to WFOT shall be elected by OT, OTA, and student members of the Association.

B.   The Delegate and Alternate Delegate shall serve an initial term of 4 years or until successors are elected. The Delegate and Alternate Delegate shall be eligible for reelection to successive terms of 2 years for a maximum of 8 years served.

Section 3.   Qualifications

A.   Shall be an OT member of the Association with a minimum of 5 years of experience.

B.   Shall be an individual member of WFOT for at least 3 years immediately prior to running for office.

Section 4.   Duties

24

A.   Delegate

1.   Shall be instructed by the Board on the agenda to come before the WFOT council and shall represent the Association to WFOT.

2.   Shall represent WFOT to the Association.

3.   Shall serve as an Organizational Advisor to the Board.

B.   Alternate Delegate

1.   Shall serve in the Assembly with voice and vote as the Internationally Based Practitioners' Representative.

2.   Shall assume duties of the Delegate in the absence of the Delegate.

ARTICLE XII.

Administrative Procedures for All Elected or Appointed Positions

Section 1.   Resignation

A.   Elected or appointed officials of the Association shall submit a written resignation to the appropriate Association official as provided in the Administrative SOP.

B.   The Association shall act upon such requests, including notifying appropriate committees concerning the vacancy.

Section 2.   Censure

Elected and appointed officials may be subject to censure as the term is defined in Policy A.7 of the Association's Policy Manual. Motions for censure of an elected or appointed official may be made by any member of the committee, body or other entity in which the elected or appointed official holds a position. The determination of such motion shall be made by the committee, body or other entity in which the elected or appointed official holds a position in accordance with a fundamentally fair process set forth in the disciplinary procedures in the Administrative SOP.

Section 3.   Removal

Elected and appointed officials shall only be removed for cause. Grounds for removal for cause of an elected or appointed official are: (1) those set forth in Policy A.8 of the of the Association's Policy Manual, and/or (2) violation of the Code and Ethics Standards. Motions for removal of an elected or appointed official may be made by any member of the committee, body, or other entity in which the elected or appointed official holds a position. The determination of such motion shall be made by the committee, body, or

25

other entity in which the elected or appointed official holds a position in accordance with a fundamentally fair process set forth in the disciplinary procedures in the Administrative SOP.

Section 4.   Appeal

The decision to remove an elected or appointed official may be appealed in accordance with due process as set forth in the Administrative SOP.

Section 5.   Vacancies

Unless otherwise provided, in the case of vacancy in any office, except the President, the vacancy shall be filled by appointment by the presiding officer of the Board or Assembly until the next regular election. In the case of a vacancy in the office of the President, the Vice President shall serve. The procedures for handling vacancies in elected positions are outlined in the Administrative SOP.

Section 6.   Assumption of Office

All elected and appointed officers and officials assume office on July 1.

ARTICLE XIII.

Fiscal Year

The fiscal year of the Association shall be determined by the Board.

ARTICLE XIV.

Dissolution Clause

Should the corporation be dissolved for any reason, the remaining assets shall be distributed for purposes within the scope of the Internal Revenue Code, Section 501(c)(6), or any amendment thereto, and in accordance with the corporate statutes of the District of Columbia (D.C.).

ARTICLE XV.

Petition to Challenge Association Action

Members shall have the right to submit a written objection to an action of the Association taken by the membership, Board, or Assembly to the extent that the member is or may be affected by such action.

Any member seeking to challenge Association action shall do so in conformance with the procedure set forth in this Article, unless there is another designated procedure set forth in the official documents of the Association that specifically addresses the action which

26

the member seeks to challenge. Any challenge to Association action covered by this Article shall be in the form of a written Petition addressed to the Board setting forth the specific action challenged, the grounds for the challenge, and requested action. The Petition must be filed within 90 days of the action challenged and shall be delivered to the Secretary at the Association's headquarters. The Board shall submit the Petition to an ad hoc committee of the Board to investigate the matter, to determine the merits of the Petition, and to make a recommendation to the President as to the appropriate disposition. The President shall provide the Association's response to the Petition in writing to the Petitioner in not more than 90 days from the date the Petition was received by the Secretary and shall include a concise statement of the reasons for the disposition. The ad hoc committee of the Board shall process the Petition in accordance with the procedure set forth in the Administrative SOP specifically designated for Challenges to Association Action.

ARTICLE XVI.

Amendments to Bylaws

Section 1. **Procedure**

A.   BPPC shall announce a call for amendments in an official publication to all OT, OTA, and student members.

B.   OT, OTA, and student members shall have 60 days from the date of publication to submit suggestions to the BPPC.

C.   BPPC shall present to the Board a report containing proposed Amendments to and comments on the Bylaws.

D.   The Board shall consider, approve or disapprove at its regular meetings any proposed Bylaws amendments.

E.   Proposed Bylaws amendments which have been previously approved by the Board shall be presented to voting members at the Annual Business Meeting for adoption.

Section 2. **Technical Corrections**

The BPPC is authorized to correct Article and Section designations, punctuation, and cross-references and to make such other technical and conforming changes to the Bylaws and other governing documents of the Association as may be necessary to reflect the intent of vote of the membership in approving the Bylaws and amendments.

Section 3. **Effective Date**

Amendments to the Bylaws shall become effective immediately upon adoption by vote of the membership or at such other time designated by the membership in connection with

27

the adoption of the Bylaws.

ARTICLE XVII.

Indemnification

Any present or former Board member, officer, employee, official, or agent of the Association, or other such persons so designated at the discretion of the Board, or the legal representative of such person, shall be indemnified (including advances against expenses) by the Association against all judgments, fines, settlements, and other reasonable costs, expenses, and counsel fees paid or incurred in connection with any action, suit, or proceeding to which any person or his or her legal representative may be made a party by reason of his or her being or having been such a Board member, officer, employee, official, or agent, to the greatest extent permitted by law. No indemnification or advance against expenses shall be approved by the Board or paid by the Association until after receipt from legal counsel of an opinion concerning the legality of the proposed indemnification or advance.

28

The
Glossary
of the
American Occupational Therapy
Association

******

Absence

Failure to attend or appear when expected; the state of being away or not present (e.g., the Treasurer is not present for the Association Annual Business Meeting)

Accreditation

The process by which an agency or organization evaluates and recognizes a program of study or an institution as meeting certain predetermined qualifications or standards. It applies only to institutions and their programs of study or their services.

ACOTE®

Accreditation Council for Occupational Therapy Education®

Ad Hoc

A special body (e.g., committee, task force, task group, body) not established by the Bylaws. An ad hoc body is appointed for a specific purpose and assigned a specific task that is not an ongoing function in the Association.

Advisory

Having the function of giving advice, usually with the implication that the advice given need not be followed

Affiliate

A professional organization that represents OTs, OTAs, and students in a state and that is recognized by the Association

Agenda (plural of Agendum)

A list of things to be done, especially the program for a meeting (e.g., the order of business of the Assembly meeting)

Amendments

Changes to the Bylaws that are neither revisions nor technical corrections

Annual Business Meeting

The scheduled gathering of Association members that must occur at least one time per year

Annual Conference

A meeting of persons from across the country to discuss or consult on various topics or issues (e.g., the Annual Conference of the Association)

AOTF®

American Occupational Therapy Foundation®

AOTPAC®

American Occupational Therapy Political Action Committee®

Articles of Incorporation

The original statements that provided the framework for the development and organization of the Association

ASAP

Affiliated State Association Presidents

ASD

Assembly of Student Delegates

Associate Member
A category of AOTA membership for individuals who are interested in the profession of occupational therapy but are not an OT practitioner or student

Board
The AOTA Board of Directors

Body
An organized group of individuals that has an official function

BPPC
Bylaws, Policies, and Procedures Committee

CCCPD
Commission on Continuing Competence and Professional Development

Censure
A formal expression of strong disapproval that is public

Certification
The process by which a nongovernmental agency or association grants recognition to an individual who has met certain predetermined qualifications specified by that agency or association

Chairperson
The presiding officer

Code of Ethics
An official document that serves as a "public statement of principles used to promote and maintain high standards of conduct with the profession." (Preamble to the AOTA *Occupational Therapy Code of Ethics 2010)*

COE
Commission on Education

Commission
A group of people authorized or directed to carry out a duty or task. A commission is responsible for a broad area of information relevant to the Association.

COP
Commission on Practice

Council
An appointed or elected body of people with an administrative, advisory, or representative function

CRAC
Credentials Review and Accountability Committee

Credential
Evidence of authority, status, rights, entitlement, or privileges, usually in written form (e.g., written notice of election of a person as a representative from an election area)

EC
Ethics Commission

Election Area
A geographic area that is defined as eligible for representation in the Representative Assembly

Emergency, Association

An emergency that would alter the Association's ability to effectively conduct business and that may be declared by the Executive Director, President, or Vice President

Emergency, National

An emergency declared by the President of the United States or Congress that results in restriction of travel, expenditures or collections, or personal activity and that requires a temporary policy or procedure to meet the situation

Executive Director

The person selected by the Board of Directors to occupy the position of executive director

Executive Session

A meeting or portion of a meeting at which the proceedings are private and only members, special invitees, and designated staff may be present. In the Association, Executive Session is used primarily to discuss information and issues that involve proprietary information, privileged information affecting individual member and personnel matters of the Association, or matters that may be the subject of litigation and/or are subject to attorney–client privilege. The purpose is to protect confidentiality, not to deprive members of their right to know.

Fee

A sum paid or charged for a privilege (e.g., the fee for membership in the Association)

Fiduciary Duty

Responsibility of members in elected and appointed positions to act in good faith and in a manner reasonably believed to be in the best interest of the Association in accordance with the duty of care and duty of loyalty

Internationally Based Practitioners

OT, OTA, or student members of the Association who live outside the United States

NBCOT®

National Board for Certification in Occupational Therapy®

Occupational Therapist

Any individual initially certified to practice as an OT or licensed or regulated by a state, commonwealth, district, or territory of the United States to practice as an OT

Occupational Therapy Assistant

Any individual initially certified to practice as an OTA or licensed or regulated by a state, commonwealth, district, or territory of the United States to practice as an OTA

Official Documents

Those documents constructed and approved by the Association for the use of the Association and its members

OT

Occupational therapist

OTA

Occupational therapy assistant

OTAS
Occupational therapy assistant student

OTS
Occupational therapy student

Organizational Advisors
Critical governance bodies within the organization that advise the Board and promote active collaboration and effective dialogue among the Board, appropriate bodies of the Board, the Representative Assembly, and AOTA

Organizational Member
A category of AOTA membership for institutions or agencies that are interested in the profession or practice of occupational therapy (e.g., another professional health care organization)

Parliamentary Procedure
The rules contained in the current edition of *Modern Parliamentary Procedure* that govern the Association in all cases in which they are applicable and in which they are not inconsistent with the Bylaws and any special rules of order the Association may adopt

Postprofessional Program
An educational curriculum in occupational therapy that offers courses designed to enhance knowledge and skills beyond the basic entry level for persons who are already OTs

Pro Tem (Pro Tempore)
Temporarily; for the time being (e.g., a person who acts as a Chairperson for a group for a meeting)

RA
Representative Assembly

RACC
Representative Assembly Coordinating Committee

RALC
Representative Assembly Leadership Committee

Recorder
A person who sets down something in writing or other permanent form (e.g., the person who prepares and keeps the minutes of the Representative Assembly)

Representative
A member of the AOTA Representative Assembly

Representative Assembly
The body composed of representatives from identified constituencies (election areas) whose function is to legislate and establish professional policies and standards for the Association

SCB
Specialty Certification Board

Seated
In a position from which authority is exercised; also, the approval a person receives from the group authorizing participation in the conduct of business

SISs
Special Interest Sections

SISC
Special Interest Sections Council

Slate
A list of candidates, officers, and so forth to be considered for nomination, appointment, election, and the like

Special Interest Section
A group of members recognized by the Representative Assembly as having a mutual interest in an area of practice in occupational therapy

Standard Operating Procedure
Regular procedures or actions that are taken by a group to accomplish an activity, charge, or item of business. Standard operating procedures are recorded in written form and are referred to as SOPs.

Standing Advisory Committee
A permanent committee established in the Bylaws dealing with a designated function (e.g., elections, recognitions, finance). A committee is responsible for a specific area of information relevant to the Association and the Board.

Steering Committee
A selected group of persons charged to function as an organizing unit to conduct certain business for a larger group. The function of the Steering Committee is to expedite the work of a larger group.

Vacancy
An unoccupied position or office (e.g., the Presidency is vacant if the President resigns)

VLDC
Volunteer Leadership Development Committee

WFOT
World Federation of Occupational Therapists

WFOT Alternate Delegate
Representative of Internationally Based Practitioners in the Representative Assembly who may also serve in the position of WFOT Delegate in the event of an absence, resignation, removal, death, or disabling condition

WFOT Delegate
Representative from AOTA to the World Federation of Occupational Therapists

BPPC Reviewed: 9/7/03, 1/05, 1/07, 1/08, 9/10, 9/14
Adopted RA: 11/03, 5/05, 4/07, 11/10
Adopted BOD: 10/14

SECTION I.B.

Accreditation

2011 Accreditation Council for Occupational Therapy Education (ACOTE®) Standards

(Adopted December 4, 2011; effective July 31, 2013)

Standard Number	Accreditation Standards for a Doctoral-Degree-Level Educational Program for the Occupational Therapist	Accreditation Standards for a Master's-Degree-Level Educational Program for the Occupational Therapist	Accreditation Standards for an Associate-Degree-Level Educational Program for the Occupational Therapy Assistant
PREAMBLE			
	The rapidly changing and dynamic nature of contemporary health and human services delivery systems provides challenging opportunities for the occupational therapist to use knowledge and skills in a practice area as a direct care provider, consultant, educator, manager, leader, researcher, and advocate for the profession and the consumer.	The rapidly changing and dynamic nature of contemporary health and human services delivery systems requires the occupational therapist to possess basic skills as a direct care provider, consultant, educator, manager, researcher, and advocate for the profession and the consumer.	The rapidly changing and dynamic nature of contemporary health and human services delivery systems requires the occupational therapy assistant to possess basic skills as a direct care provider, educator, and advocate for the profession and the consumer.
	A graduate from an ACOTE-accredited doctoral-degree-level occupational therapy program must • Have acquired, as a foundation for professional study, a breadth and depth of knowledge in the liberal arts and sciences and an understanding of issues related to diversity. • Be educated as a generalist with a broad exposure to the delivery models and systems used in settings where occupational therapy is currently practiced and where it is emerging as a service.	A graduate from an ACOTE-accredited master's-degree-level occupational therapy program must • Have acquired, as a foundation for professional study, a breadth and depth of knowledge in the liberal arts and sciences and an understanding of issues related to diversity. • Be educated as a generalist with a broad exposure to the delivery models and systems used in settings where occupational therapy is currently practiced and where it is emerging as a service.	A graduate from an ACOTE-accredited associate-degree-level occupational therapy assistant program must • Have acquired an educational foundation in the liberal arts and sciences, including a focus on issues related to diversity. • Be educated as a generalist with a broad exposure to the delivery models and systems used in settings where occupational therapy is currently practiced and where it is emerging as a service.

(Continued)

Standard Number	Accreditation Standards for a Doctoral-Degree-Level Educational Program for the Occupational Therapist	Accreditation Standards for a Master's-Degree-Level Educational Program for the Occupational Therapist	Accreditation Standards for an Associate-Degree-Level Educational Program for the Occupational Therapy Assistant
	• Have achieved entry-level competence through a combination of academic and field-work education. • Be prepared to articulate and apply occupational therapy theory and evidence-based evaluations and interventions to achieve expected outcomes as related to occupation. • Be prepared to articulate and apply therapeutic use of occupations with individuals or groups for the purpose of participation in roles and situations in home, school, workplace, community, and other settings. • Be able to plan and apply occupational therapy interventions to address the physical, cognitive, psychosocial, sensory, and other aspects of performance in a variety of contexts and environments to support engagement in everyday life activities that affect health, well-being, and quality of life. • Be prepared to be a lifelong learner and keep current with evidence-based professional practice. • Uphold the ethical standards, values, and attitudes of the occupational therapy profession. • Understand the distinct roles and responsibilities of the occupational therapist and occupational therapy assistant in the supervisory process.	• Have achieved entry-level competence through a combination of academic and field-work education. • Be prepared to articulate and apply occupational therapy theory and evidence-based evaluations and interventions to achieve expected outcomes as related to occupation. • Be prepared to articulate and apply therapeutic use of occupations with individuals or groups for the purpose of participation in roles and situations in home, school, workplace, community, and other settings. • Be able to plan and apply occupational therapy interventions to address the physical, cognitive, psychosocial, sensory, and other aspects of performance in a variety of contexts and environments to support engagement in everyday life activities that affect health, well-being, and quality of life. • Be prepared to be a lifelong learner and keep current with evidence-based professional practice. • Uphold the ethical standards, values, and attitudes of the occupational therapy profession. • Understand the distinct roles and responsibilities of the occupational therapist and occupational therapy assistant in the supervisory process.	• Have achieved entry-level competence through a combination of academic and field-work education. • Be prepared to articulate and apply occupational therapy principles and intervention tools to achieve expected outcomes as related to occupation. • Be prepared to articulate and apply therapeutic use of occupations with individuals or groups for the purpose of participation in roles and situations in home, school, workplace, community, and other settings. • Be able to apply occupational therapy interventions to address the physical, cognitive, psychosocial, sensory, and other aspects of performance in a variety of contexts and environments to support engagement in everyday life activities that affect health, well-being, and quality of life. • Be prepared to be a lifelong learner and keep current with the best practice. • Uphold the ethical standards, values, and attitudes of the occupational therapy profession. • Understand the distinct roles and responsibilities of the occupational therapist and occupational therapy assistant in the supervisory process.

(Continued)

Standard Number	Accreditation Standards for a Doctoral-Degree-Level Educational Program for the Occupational Therapist	Accreditation Standards for a Master's-Degree-Level Educational Program for the Occupational Therapist	Accreditation Standards for an Associate-Degree-Level Educational Program for the Occupational Therapy Assistant
	• Be prepared to effectively communicate and work interprofessionally with those who provide care for individuals and/or populations in order to clarify each member's responsibility in executing components of an intervention plan.	• Be prepared to effectively communicate and work interprofessionally with those who provide care for individuals and/or populations in order to clarify each member's responsibility in executing components of an intervention plan.	• Be prepared to effectively communicate and work interprofessionally with those who provide care for individuals and/or populations in order to clarify each member's responsibility in executing components of an intervention plan.
	• Be prepared to advocate as a professional for the occupational therapy services offered and for the recipients of those services.	• Be prepared to advocate as a professional for the occupational therapy services offered and for the recipients of those services.	• Be prepared to advocate as a professional for the occupational therapy services offered and for the recipients of those services.
	• Be prepared to be an effective consumer of the latest research and knowledge bases that support practice and contribute to the growth and dissemination of research and knowledge.	• Be prepared to be an effective consumer of the latest research and knowledge bases that support practice and contribute to the growth and dissemination of research and knowledge.	
	• Demonstrate in-depth knowledge of delivery models, policies, and systems related to the area of practice in settings where occupational therapy is currently practiced and where it is emerging as a service.		
	• Demonstrate thorough knowledge of evidence-based practice.		
	• Demonstrate active involvement in professional development, leadership, and advocacy.		
	• Relate theory to practice and demonstrate synthesis of advanced knowledge in a practice area through completion of a culminating project.		

(Continued)

51

Standard Number	Accreditation Standards for a Doctoral-Degree-Level Educational Program for the Occupational Therapist	Accreditation Standards for a Master's-Degree-Level Educational Program for the Occupational Therapist	Accreditation Standards for an Associate-Degree-Level Educational Program for the Occupational Therapy Assistant
	• Develop in-depth experience in one or more of the following areas through completion of a doctoral experiential component: clinical practice skills, research skills, administration, leadership, program and policy development, advocacy, education, and theory development.		
SECTION A: GENERAL REQUIREMENTS			
A.1.0.	**SPONSORSHIP AND ACCREDITATION**		
A.1.1.	The sponsoring institution(s) and affiliates, if any, must be accredited by the recognized regional accrediting authority. For programs in countries other than the United States, ACOTE will determine an alternative and equivalent external review process.	The sponsoring institution(s) and affiliates, if any, must be accredited by the recognized regional accrediting authority. For programs in countries other than the United States, ACOTE will determine an alternative and equivalent external review process.	The sponsoring institution(s) and affiliates, if any, must be accredited by a recognized regional or national accrediting authority.
A.1.2.	Sponsoring institution(s) must be authorized under applicable law or other acceptable authority to provide a program of postsecondary education and have appropriate doctoral degree-granting authority.	Sponsoring institution(s) must be authorized under applicable law or other acceptable authority to provide a program of postsecondary education and have appropriate degree-granting authority.	Sponsoring institution(s) must be authorized under applicable law or other acceptable authority to provide a program of postsecondary education and have appropriate degree-granting authority, or the institution must be a program offered within the military services.

(Continued)

Standard Number	Accreditation Standards for a Doctoral-Degree-Level Educational Program for the Occupational Therapist	Accreditation Standards for a Master's-Degree-Level Educational Program for the Occupational Therapist	Accreditation Standards for an Associate-Degree-Level Educational Program for the Occupational Therapy Assistant
A.1.3.	Accredited occupational therapy educational programs may be established only in senior colleges, universities, or medical schools.	Accredited occupational therapy educational programs may be established only in senior colleges, universities, or medical schools.	Accredited occupational therapy assistant educational programs may be established only in community, technical, junior, and senior colleges; universities; medical schools; vocational schools or institutions; or military services.
A.1.4.	The sponsoring institution(s) must assume primary responsibility for appointment of faculty, admission of students, and curriculum planning at all locations where the program is offered. This would include course content, satisfactory completion of the educational program, and granting of the degree. The sponsoring institution(s) must also be responsible for the coordination of classroom teaching and supervised fieldwork practice and for providing assurance that the practice activities assigned to students in a fieldwork setting are appropriate to the program.	The sponsoring institution(s) must assume primary responsibility for appointment of faculty, admission of students, and curriculum planning at all locations where the program is offered. This would include course content, satisfactory completion of the educational program, and granting of the degree. The sponsoring institution(s) must also be responsible for the coordination of classroom teaching and supervised fieldwork practice and for providing assurance that the practice activities assigned to students in a fieldwork setting are appropriate to the program.	The sponsoring institution(s) must assume primary responsibility for appointment of faculty, admission of students, and curriculum planning at all locations where the program is offered. This would include course content, satisfactory completion of the educational program, and granting of the degree. The sponsoring institution(s) must also be responsible for the coordination of classroom teaching and supervised fieldwork practice and for providing assurance that the practice activities assigned to students in a fieldwork setting are appropriate to the program.
A.1.5.	The program must • Inform ACOTE of the transfer of program sponsorship or change of the institution's name within 30 days of the transfer or change.	The program must • Inform ACOTE of the transfer of program sponsorship or change of the institution's name within 30 days of the transfer or change.	The program must • Inform ACOTE of the transfer of program sponsorship or change of the institution's name within 30 days of the transfer or change.

(Continued)

Standard Number	Accreditation Standards for a Doctoral-Degree-Level Educational Program for the Occupational Therapist	Accreditation Standards for a Master's-Degree-Level Educational Program for the Occupational Therapist	Accreditation Standards for an Associate-Degree-Level Educational Program for the Occupational Therapy Assistant
	• Inform ACOTE within 30 days of the date of notification of any adverse accreditation action taken to change the sponsoring institution's accreditation status to probation or withdrawal of accreditation. • Notify and receive ACOTE approval for any significant program changes prior to the admission of students into the new/changed program. • Inform ACOTE within 30 days of the resignation of the program director or appointment of a new or interim program director. • Pay accreditation fees within 90 days of the invoice date. • Submit a Report of Self-Study and other required reports (e.g., Interim Report, Plan of Correction, Progress Report) within the period of time designated by ACOTE. All reports must be complete and contain all requested information. • Agree to a site visit date before the end of the period for which accreditation was previously awarded. • Demonstrate honesty and integrity in all interactions with ACOTE.	• Inform ACOTE within 30 days of the date of notification of any adverse accreditation action taken to change the sponsoring institution's accreditation status to probation or withdrawal of accreditation. • Notify and receive ACOTE approval for any significant program changes prior to the admission of students into the new/changed program. • Inform ACOTE within 30 days of the resignation of the program director or appointment of a new or interim program director. • Pay accreditation fees within 90 days of the invoice date. • Submit a Report of Self-Study and other required reports (e.g., Interim Report, Plan of Correction, Progress Report) within the period of time designated by ACOTE. All reports must be complete and contain all requested information. • Agree to a site visit date before the end of the period for which accreditation was previously awarded. • Demonstrate honesty and integrity in all interactions with ACOTE.	• Inform ACOTE within 30 days of the date of notification of any adverse accreditation action taken to change the sponsoring institution's accreditation status to probation or withdrawal of accreditation. • Notify and receive ACOTE approval for any significant program changes prior to the admission of students into the new/changed program. • Inform ACOTE within 30 days of the resignation of the program director or appointment of a new or interim program director. • Pay accreditation fees within 90 days of the invoice date. • Submit a Report of Self-Study and other required reports (e.g., Interim Report, Plan of Correction, Progress Report) within the period of time designated by ACOTE. All reports must be complete and contain all requested information. • Agree to a site visit date before the end of the period for which accreditation was previously awarded. • Demonstrate honesty and integrity in all interactions with ACOTE.

(Continued)

Standard Number	Accreditation Standards for a Doctoral-Degree-Level Educational Program for the Occupational Therapist	Accreditation Standards for a Master's-Degree-Level Educational Program for the Occupational Therapist	Accreditation Standards for an Associate-Degree-Level Educational Program for the Occupational Therapy Assistant
A.2.0.	**ACADEMIC RESOURCES**		
A.2.1.	The program must identify an individual as the program director who is assigned to the occupational therapy educational program on a full-time basis. The director may be assigned other institutional duties that do not interfere with the management and administration of the program. The institution must document that the program director has sufficient release time to ensure that the needs of the program are being met.	The program must identify an individual as the program director who is assigned to the occupational therapy educational program on a full-time basis. The director may be assigned other institutional duties that do not interfere with the management and administration of the program. The institution must document that the program director has sufficient release time to ensure that the needs of the program are being met.	The program must identify an individual as the program director who is assigned to the occupational therapy educational program on a full-time basis. The director may be assigned other institutional duties that do not interfere with the management and administration of the program. The institution must document that the program director has sufficient release time to ensure that the needs of the program are being met.
A.2.2.	The program director must be an initially certified occupational therapist who is licensed or otherwise regulated according to regulations in the state(s) or jurisdiction(s) in which the program is located. The program director must hold a doctoral degree awarded by an institution that is accredited by a regional accrediting body recognized by the U.S. Department of Education (USDE). The doctoral degree is not limited to a doctorate in occupational therapy.	The program director must be an initially certified occupational therapist who is licensed or otherwise regulated according to regulations in the state(s) or jurisdiction(s) in which the program is located. The program director must hold a doctoral degree awarded by an institution that is accredited by a regional accrediting body recognized by the U.S. Department of Education (USDE). The doctoral degree is not limited to a doctorate in occupational therapy.	The program director must be an initially certified occupational therapist or occupational therapy assistant who is licensed or otherwise regulated according to regulations in the state(s) or jurisdiction(s) in which the program is located. The program director must hold a minimum of a master's degree awarded by an institution that is accredited by a regional or national accrediting body recognized by the U.S. Department of Education (USDE). The master's degree is not limited to a master's degree in occupational therapy.

(Continued)

Standard Number	Accreditation Standards for a Doctoral-Degree-Level Educational Program for the Occupational Therapist	Accreditation Standards for a Master's-Degree-Level Educational Program for the Occupational Therapist	Accreditation Standards for an Associate-Degree-Level Educational Program for the Occupational Therapy Assistant
A.2.3.	The program director must have a minimum of 8 years of documented experience in the field of occupational therapy. This experience must include • Clinical practice as an occupational therapist; • Administrative experience including, but not limited to, program planning and implementation, personnel management, evaluation, and budgeting; • Scholarship (e.g., scholarship of application, scholarship of teaching and learning); and • At least 3 years of experience in a full-time academic appointment with teaching responsibilities at the postbaccalaureate level.	The program director must have a minimum of 8 years of documented experience in the field of occupational therapy. This experience must include • Clinical practice as an occupational therapist; • Administrative experience including, but not limited to, program planning and implementation, personnel management, evaluation, and budgeting; • Scholarship (e.g., scholarship of application, scholarship of teaching and learning); and • At least 3 years of experience in a full-time academic appointment with teaching responsibilities at the postsecondary level.	The program director must have a minimum of 5 years of documented experience in the field of occupational therapy. This experience must include • Clinical practice as an occupational therapist or occupational therapy assistant; • Administrative experience including, but not limited to, program planning and implementation, personnel management, evaluation, and budgeting; • Understanding of and experience with occupational therapy assistants; and • At least 1 year of experience in a full-time academic appointment with teaching responsibilities at the postsecondary level.
A.2.4.	The program director must be responsible for the management and administration of the program, including planning, evaluation, budgeting, selection of faculty and staff, maintenance of accreditation, and commitment to strategies for professional development.	The program director must be responsible for the management and administration of the program, including planning, evaluation, budgeting, selection of faculty and staff, maintenance of accreditation, and commitment to strategies for professional development.	The program director must be responsible for the management and administration of the program, including planning, evaluation, budgeting, selection of faculty and staff, maintenance of accreditation, and commitment to strategies for professional development.

(Continued)

56

Standard Number	Accreditation Standards for a Doctoral-Degree-Level Educational Program for the Occupational Therapist	Accreditation Standards for a Master's-Degree-Level Educational Program for the Occupational Therapist	Accreditation Standards for an Associate-Degree-Level Educational Program for the Occupational Therapy Assistant
A.2.5.	*(No related Standard)*	*(No related Standard)*	In addition to the program director, the program must have at least one full-time equivalent (FTE) faculty position at each accredited location where the program is offered. This position may be shared by up to three individuals who teach as adjunct faculty. These individuals must have one or more additional responsibilities related to student advisement, supervision, committee work, program planning, evaluation, recruitment, and marketing activities.
A.2.6.	The program director and faculty must possess the academic and experiential qualifications and backgrounds (identified in documented descriptions of roles and responsibilities) that are necessary to meet program objectives and the mission of the institution.	The program director and faculty must possess the academic and experiential qualifications and backgrounds (identified in documented descriptions of roles and responsibilities) that are necessary to meet program objectives and the mission of the institution.	The program director and faculty must possess the academic and experiential qualifications and backgrounds (identified in documented descriptions of roles and responsibilities) that are necessary to meet program objectives and the mission of the institution.
A.2.7.	The program must identify an individual for the role of academic fieldwork coordinator who is specifically responsible for the program's compliance with the fieldwork requirements of Standards Section C.1.0 and is assigned to the occupational therapy educational program as a full-time faculty member as defined by ACOTE. The academic fieldwork coordinator may be assigned other institutional duties that do not interfere with the management and administration	The program must identify an individual for the role of academic fieldwork coordinator who is specifically responsible for the program's compliance with the fieldwork requirements of Standards Section C.1.0 and is assigned to the occupational therapy educational program as a full-time faculty member as defined by ACOTE. The academic fieldwork coordinator may be assigned other institutional duties that do not interfere with the management and administration	The program must identify an individual for the role of academic fieldwork coordinator who is specifically responsible for the program's compliance with the fieldwork requirements of Standards Section C.1.0 and is assigned to the occupational therapy educational program as a full-time faculty member as defined by ACOTE. The academic fieldwork coordinator may be assigned other institutional duties that do not interfere with the management and administration

(Continued)

Standard Number	Accreditation Standards for a Doctoral-Degree-Level Educational Program for the Occupational Therapist	Accreditation Standards for a Master's-Degree-Level Educational Program for the Occupational Therapist	Accreditation Standards for an Associate-Degree-Level Educational Program for the Occupational Therapy Assistant
	of the fieldwork program. The institution must document that the academic fieldwork coordinator has sufficient release time to ensure that the needs of the fieldwork program are being met.	of the fieldwork program. The institution must document that the academic fieldwork coordinator has sufficient release time to ensure that the needs of the fieldwork program are being met.	of the fieldwork program. The institution must document that the academic fieldwork coordinator has sufficient release time to ensure that the needs of the fieldwork program are being met.
	This individual must be a licensed or otherwise regulated occupational therapist. Coordinators must hold a doctoral degree awarded by an institution that is accredited by a USDE-recognized regional accrediting body.	This individual must be a licensed or otherwise regulated occupational therapist. Coordinators must hold a minimum of a master's degree awarded by an institution that is accredited by a USDE-recognized regional accrediting body.	This individual must be a licensed or otherwise regulated occupational therapist or occupational therapy assistant. Coordinators must hold a minimum of a baccalaureate degree awarded by an institution that is accredited by a USDE-recognized regional or national accrediting body.
A.2.8.	Core faculty who are occupational therapists or occupational therapy assistants must be currently licensed or otherwise regulated according to regulations in the state or jurisdiction in which the program is located.	Core faculty who are occupational therapists or occupational therapy assistants must be currently licensed or otherwise regulated according to regulations in the state or jurisdiction in which the program is located.	Core faculty who are occupational therapists or occupational therapy assistants must be currently licensed or otherwise regulated according to regulations in the state or jurisdiction in which the program is located.
	Faculty in residence and teaching at additional locations must be currently licensed or otherwise regulated according to regulations in the state or jurisdiction in which the additional location is located.	Faculty in residence and teaching at additional locations must be currently licensed or otherwise regulated according to regulations in the state or jurisdiction in which the additional location is located.	Faculty in residence and teaching at additional locations must be currently licensed or otherwise regulated according to regulations in the state or jurisdiction in which the additional location is located.

(Continued)

Standard Number	Accreditation Standards for a Doctoral-Degree-Level Educational Program for the Occupational Therapist	Accreditation Standards for a Master's-Degree-Level Educational Program for the Occupational Therapist	Accreditation Standards for an Associate-Degree-Level Educational Program for the Occupational Therapy Assistant
A.2.9.	*(No related Standard)*	*(No related Standard)*	In programs where the program director is an occupational therapy assistant, an occupational therapist must be included on faculty and contribute to the functioning of the program through a variety of mechanisms including, but not limited to, teaching, advising, and committee work. In a program where there are only occupational therapists on faculty who have never practiced as an occupational therapy assistant, the program must demonstrate that an individual who is an occupational therapy assistant or an occupational therapist who has previously practiced as an occupational therapy assistant is involved in the program as an adjunct faculty or teaching assistant.
A.2.10.	All full-time faculty teaching in the program must hold a doctoral degree awarded by an institution that is accredited by a USDE-recognized regional accrediting body. The doctoral degree is not limited to a doctorate in occupational therapy.	The majority of full-time faculty who are occupational therapists or occupational therapy assistants must hold a doctoral degree. All full-time faculty must hold a minimum of a master's degree. All degrees must be awarded by an institution that is accredited by a USDE-recognized regional accrediting body. The degrees are not limited to occupational therapy. For an even number of full-time faculty, at least half must hold doctorates. The program director is counted as a faculty member.	All occupational therapy assistant faculty who are full-time must hold a minimum of a baccalaureate degree awarded by an institution that is accredited by a USDE-recognized regional or national accrediting body.

(Continued)

59

Standard Number	Accreditation Standards for a Doctoral-Degree-Level Educational Program for the Occupational Therapist	Accreditation Standards for a Master's-Degree-Level Educational Program for the Occupational Therapist	Accreditation Standards for an Associate-Degree-Level Educational Program for the Occupational Therapy Assistant
A.2.11.	The faculty must have documented expertise in their area(s) of teaching responsibility and knowledge of the content delivery method (e.g., distance learning).	The faculty must have documented expertise in their area(s) of teaching responsibility and knowledge of the content delivery method (e.g., distance learning).	The faculty must have documented expertise in their area(s) of teaching responsibility and knowledge of the content delivery method (e.g., distance learning).
A.2.12.	For programs with additional accredited location(s), the program must identify a faculty member who is an occupational therapist as site coordinator at each location who is responsible for ensuring uniform implementation of the program and ongoing communication with the program director.	For programs with additional accredited location(s), the program must identify a faculty member who is an occupational therapist as site coordinator at each location who is responsible for ensuring uniform implementation of the program and ongoing communication with the program director.	For programs with additional accredited location(s), the program must identify a faculty member who is an occupational therapist or occupational therapy assistant as site coordinator at each location who is responsible for ensuring uniform implementation of the program and ongoing communication with the program director.
A.2.13.	The occupational therapy faculty at each accredited location where the program is offered must be sufficient in number and must possess the expertise necessary to ensure appropriate curriculum design, content delivery, and program evaluation. The faculty must include individuals competent to ensure delivery of the broad scope of occupational therapy practice. Multiple adjuncts, part-time faculty, or full-time faculty may be configured to meet this goal. Each accredited additional location must have at least one full-time equivalent (FTE) faculty member.	The occupational therapy faculty at each accredited location where the program is offered must be sufficient in number and must possess the expertise necessary to ensure appropriate curriculum design, content delivery, and program evaluation. The faculty must include individuals competent to ensure delivery of the broad scope of occupational therapy practice. Multiple adjuncts, part-time faculty, or full-time faculty may be configured to meet this goal. Each accredited additional location must have at least one full-time equivalent (FTE) faculty member.	The occupational therapy assistant faculty at each accredited location where the program is offered must be sufficient in number and must possess the expertise necessary to ensure appropriate curriculum design, content delivery, and program evaluation. The faculty must include individuals competent to ensure delivery of the broad scope of occupational therapy practice. Multiple adjuncts, part-time faculty, or full-time faculty may be configured to meet this goal. Each accredited additional location must have at least one full-time equivalent (FTE) faculty member.

(Continued)

Standard Number	Accreditation Standards for a Doctoral-Degree-Level Educational Program for the Occupational Therapist	Accreditation Standards for a Master's-Degree-Level Educational Program for the Occupational Therapist	Accreditation Standards for an Associate-Degree-Level Educational Program for the Occupational Therapy Assistant
A.2.14.	Faculty responsibilities must be consistent with and supportive of the mission of the institution.	Faculty responsibilities must be consistent with and supportive of the mission of the institution.	Faculty responsibilities must be consistent with and supportive of the mission of the institution.
A.2.15.	The faculty–student ratio must permit the achievement of the purpose and stated objectives for laboratory and lecture courses, be compatible with accepted practices of the institution for similar programs, and ensure student and consumer safety.	The faculty–student ratio must permit the achievement of the purpose and stated objectives for laboratory and lecture courses, be compatible with accepted practices of the institution for similar programs, and ensure student and consumer safety.	The faculty–student ratio must permit the achievement of the purpose and stated objectives for laboratory and lecture courses, be compatible with accepted practices of the institution for similar programs, and ensure student and consumer safety.
A.2.16.	Clerical and support staff must be provided to the program, consistent with institutional practice, to meet programmatic and administrative requirements, including support for any portion of the program offered by distance education.	Clerical and support staff must be provided to the program, consistent with institutional practice, to meet programmatic and administrative requirements, including support for any portion of the program offered by distance education.	Clerical and support staff must be provided to the program, consistent with institutional practice, to meet programmatic and administrative requirements, including support for any portion of the program offered by distance education.
A.2.17.	The program must be allocated a budget of regular institutional funds, not including grants, gifts, and other restricted sources, sufficient to implement and maintain the objectives of the program and to fulfill the program's obligation to matriculated and entering students.	The program must be allocated a budget of regular institutional funds, not including grants, gifts, and other restricted sources, sufficient to implement and maintain the objectives of the program and to fulfill the program's obligation to matriculated and entering students.	The program must be allocated a budget of regular institutional funds, not including grants, gifts, and other restricted sources, sufficient to implement and maintain the objectives of the program and to fulfill the program's obligation to matriculated and entering students.
A.2.18.	Classrooms and laboratories must be provided that are consistent with the program's educational objectives, teaching methods, number of students, and safety and health standards of the	Classrooms and laboratories must be provided that are consistent with the program's educational objectives, teaching methods, number of students, and safety and health standards of the	Classrooms and laboratories must be provided that are consistent with the program's educational objectives, teaching methods, number of students, and safety and health standards of

(Continued)

Standard Number	Accreditation Standards for a Doctoral-Degree-Level Educational Program for the Occupational Therapist	Accreditation Standards for a Master's-Degree-Level Educational Program for the Occupational Therapist	Accreditation Standards for an Associate-Degree-Level Educational Program for the Occupational Therapy Assistant
	institution, and they must allow for efficient operation of the program.	institution, and they must allow for efficient operation of the program.	the institution, and they must allow for efficient operation of the program.
A.2.19.	If the program offers distance education, it must include • A process through which the program establishes that the student who registers in a distance education course or program is the same student who participates in and completes the program and receives academic credit, • Technology and resources that are adequate to support a distance-learning environment, and • A process to ensure that faculty are adequately trained and skilled to use distance education methodologies.	If the program offers distance education, it must include • A process through which the program establishes that the student who registers in a distance education course or program is the same student who participates in and completes the program and receives academic credit, • Technology and resources that are adequate to support a distance-learning environment, and • A process to ensure that faculty are adequately trained and skilled to use distance education methodologies.	If the program offers distance education, it must include • A process through which the program establishes that the student who registers in a distance education course or program is the same student who participates in and completes the program and receives academic credit, • Technology and resources that are adequate to support a distance-learning environment, and • A process to ensure that faculty are adequately trained and skilled to use distance education methodologies.
A.2.20.	Laboratory space provided by the institution must be assigned to the occupational therapy program on a priority basis. If laboratory space for occupational therapy lab classes is provided by another institution or agency, there must be a written and signed agreement to ensure assignment of space for program use.	Laboratory space provided by the institution must be assigned to the occupational therapy program on a priority basis. If laboratory space for occupational therapy lab classes is provided by another institution or agency, there must be a written and signed agreement to ensure assignment of space for program use.	Laboratory space provided by the institution must be assigned to the occupational therapy assistant program on a priority basis. If laboratory space for occupational therapy assistant lab classes is provided by another institution or agency, there must be a written and signed agreement to ensure assignment of space for program use.
A.2.21.	Adequate space must be provided to store and secure equipment and supplies.	Adequate space must be provided to store and secure equipment and supplies.	Adequate space must be provided to store and secure equipment and supplies.

(Continued)

62

Standard Number	Accreditation Standards for a Doctoral-Degree-Level Educational Program for the Occupational Therapist	Accreditation Standards for a Master's-Degree-Level Educational Program for the Occupational Therapist	Accreditation Standards for an Associate-Degree-Level Educational Program for the Occupational Therapy Assistant
A.2.22.	The program director and faculty must have office space consistent with institutional practice.	The program director and faculty must have office space consistent with institutional practice.	The program director and faculty must have office space consistent with institutional practice.
A.2.23.	Adequate space must be provided for the private advising of students.	Adequate space must be provided for the private advising of students.	Adequate space must be provided for the private advising of students.
A.2.24.	Appropriate and sufficient equipment and supplies must be provided by the institution for student use and for the didactic, supervised fieldwork, and experiential components of the curriculum.	Appropriate and sufficient equipment and supplies must be provided by the institution for student use and for the didactic and supervised fieldwork components of the curriculum.	Appropriate and sufficient equipment and supplies must be provided by the institution for student use and for the didactic and supervised fieldwork components of the curriculum.
A.2.25.	Students must be given access to and have the opportunity to use the evaluative and treatment methodologies that reflect both current practice and practice in the geographic area served by the program.	Students must be given access to and have the opportunity to use the evaluative and treatment methodologies that reflect both current practice and practice in the geographic area served by the program.	Students must be given access to and have the opportunity to use the evaluative and treatment methodologies that reflect both current practice and practice in the geographic area served by the program.
A.2.26.	Students must have ready access to a supply of current and relevant books, journals, periodicals, computers, software, and other reference materials needed for the practice areas and to meet the requirements of the curriculum. This may include, but is not limited to, libraries, online services, interlibrary loan, and resource centers.	Students must have ready access to a supply of current and relevant books, journals, periodicals, computers, software, and other reference materials needed to meet the requirements of the curriculum. This may include, but is not limited to, libraries, online services, interlibrary loan, and resource centers.	Students must have ready access to a supply of current and relevant books, journals, periodicals, computers, software, and other reference materials needed to meet the requirements of the curriculum. This may include, but is not limited to, libraries, online services, interlibrary loan, and resource centers.

(Continued)

63

Standard Number	Accreditation Standards for a Doctoral-Degree-Level Educational Program for the Occupational Therapist	Accreditation Standards for a Master's-Degree-Level Educational Program for the Occupational Therapist	Accreditation Standards for an Associate-Degree-Level Educational Program for the Occupational Therapy Assistant
A.2.27.	Instructional aids and technology must be available in sufficient quantity and quality to be consistent with the program objectives and teaching methods.	Instructional aids and technology must be available in sufficient quantity and quality to be consistent with the program objectives and teaching methods.	Instructional aids and technology must be available in sufficient quantity and quality to be consistent with the program objectives and teaching methods.
A.3.0.	**STUDENTS**		
A.3.1.	Admission of students to the occupational therapy program must be made in accordance with the practices of the institution. There must be stated admission criteria that are clearly defined and published and reflective of the demands of the program.	Admission of students to the occupational therapy program must be made in accordance with the practices of the institution. There must be stated admission criteria that are clearly defined and published and reflective of the demands of the program.	Admission of students to the occupational therapy assistant program must be made in accordance with the practices of the institution. There must be stated admission criteria that are clearly defined and published and reflective of the demands of the program.
A.3.2.	Institutions must require that program applicants hold a baccalaureate degree or higher prior to admission to the program.	*(No related Standard)*	*(No related Standard)*
A.3.3.	Policies pertaining to standards for admission, advanced placement, transfer of credit, credit for experiential learning (if applicable), and prerequisite educational or work experience requirements must be readily accessible to prospective students and the public.	Policies pertaining to standards for admission, advanced placement, transfer of credit, credit for experiential learning (if applicable), and prerequisite educational or work experience requirements must be readily accessible to prospective students and the public.	Policies pertaining to standards for admission, advanced placement, transfer of credit, credit for experiential learning (if applicable), and prerequisite educational or work experience requirements must be readily accessible to prospective students and the public.
A.3.4.	Programs must document implementation of a mechanism to ensure that students receiving	Programs must document implementation of a mechanism to ensure that students receiving	Programs must document implementation of a mechanism to ensure that students receiving

(Continued)

Standard Number	Accreditation Standards for a Doctoral-Degree-Level Educational Program for the Occupational Therapist	Accreditation Standards for a Master's-Degree-Level Educational Program for the Occupational Therapist	Accreditation Standards for an Associate-Degree-Level Educational Program for the Occupational Therapy Assistant
	credit for previous courses and/or work experience have met the content requirements of the appropriate doctoral Standards.	credit for previous courses and/or work experience have met the content requirements of the appropriate master's Standards.	credit for previous courses and/or work experience have met the content requirements of the appropriate occupational therapy assistant Standards.
A.3.5.	Criteria for successful completion of each segment of the educational program and for graduation must be given in advance to each student.	Criteria for successful completion of each segment of the educational program and for graduation must be given in advance to each student.	Criteria for successful completion of each segment of the educational program and for graduation must be given in advance to each student.
A.3.6.	Evaluation content and methods must be consistent with the curriculum design; objectives; and competencies of the didactic, fieldwork, and experiential components of the program.	Evaluation content and methods must be consistent with the curriculum design, objectives, and competencies of the didactic and fieldwork components of the program.	Evaluation content and methods must be consistent with the curriculum design, objectives, and competencies of the didactic and fieldwork components of the program.
A.3.7.	Evaluation must be conducted on a regular basis to provide students and program officials with timely indications of the students' progress and academic standing.	Evaluation must be conducted on a regular basis to provide students and program officials with timely indications of the students' progress and academic standing.	Evaluation must be conducted on a regular basis to provide students and program officials with timely indications of the students' progress and academic standing.
A.3.8.	Students must be informed of and have access to the student support services that are provided to other students in the institution.	Students must be informed of and have access to the student support services that are provided to other students in the institution.	Students must be informed of and have access to the student support services that are provided to other students in the institution.
A.3.9.	Advising related to professional coursework, fieldwork education, and the experiential component of the program must be the responsibility of the occupational therapy faculty.	Advising related to professional coursework and fieldwork education must be the responsibility of the occupational therapy faculty.	Advising related to coursework in the occupational therapy assistant program and fieldwork education must be the responsibility of the occupational therapy assistant faculty.

(Continued)

65

Standard Number	Accreditation Standards for a Doctoral-Degree-Level Educational Program for the Occupational Therapist	Accreditation Standards for a Master's-Degree-Level Educational Program for the Occupational Therapist	Accreditation Standards for an Associate-Degree-Level Educational Program for the Occupational Therapy Assistant
A.4.0.	**OPERATIONAL POLICIES**		
A.4.1.	All program publications and advertising—including, but not limited to, academic calendars, announcements, catalogs, handbooks, and Web sites—must accurately reflect the program offered.	All program publications and advertising—including, but not limited to, academic calendars, announcements, catalogs, handbooks, and Web sites—must accurately reflect the program offered.	All program publications and advertising—including, but not limited to, academic calendars, announcements, catalogs, handbooks, and Web sites—must accurately reflect the program offered.
A.4.2.	Accurate and current information regarding student and program outcomes must be readily available to the public on the program's Web page. At a minimum, the following data must be reported for the previous 3 years: • Total number of program graduates • Graduation rates. The program must provide the direct link to the National Board for Certification in Occupational Therapy (NBCOT) program data results on the program's home page.	Accurate and current information regarding student and program outcomes must be readily available to the public on the program's Web page. At a minimum, the following data must be reported for the previous 3 years: • Total number of program graduates • Graduation rates. The program must provide the direct link to the National Board for Certification in Occupational Therapy (NBCOT) program data results on the program's home page.	Accurate and current information regarding student and program outcomes must be readily available to the public on the program's Web page. At a minimum, the following data must be reported for the previous 3 years: • Total number of program graduates, • Graduation rates. The program must provide the direct link to the National Board for Certification in Occupational Therapy (NBCOT) program data results on the program's home page.
A.4.3.	The program's accreditation status and the name, address, and telephone number of ACOTE must be published in all of the following materials used by the institution: catalog, Web site, and program-related brochures or flyers available to prospective students. A link to www.acoteonline.org must be provided on the program's home page.	The program's accreditation status and the name, address, and telephone number of ACOTE must be published in all of the following materials used by the institution: catalog, Web site, and program-related brochures or flyers available to prospective students. A link to www.acoteonline.org must be provided on the program's home page.	The program's accreditation status and the name, address, and telephone number of ACOTE must be published in all of the following materials used by the institution: catalog, Web site, and program-related brochures or flyers available to prospective students. A link to www.acoteonline.org must be provided on the program's home page.

(Continued)

Standard Number	Accreditation Standards for a Doctoral-Degree-Level Educational Program for the Occupational Therapist	Accreditation Standards for a Master's-Degree-Level Educational Program for the Occupational Therapist	Accreditation Standards for an Associate-Degree-Level Educational Program for the Occupational Therapy Assistant
A.4.4.	All practices within the institution related to faculty, staff, applicants, and students must be nondiscriminatory.	All practices within the institution related to faculty, staff, applicants, and students must be nondiscriminatory.	All practices within the institution related to faculty, staff, applicants, and students must be nondiscriminatory.
A.4.5.	Graduation requirements, tuition, and fees must be accurately stated, published, and made known to all applicants. When published fees are subject to change, a statement to that effect must be included.	Graduation requirements, tuition, and fees must be accurately stated, published, and made known to all applicants. When published fees are subject to change, a statement to that effect must be included.	Graduation requirements, tuition, and fees must be accurately stated, published, and made known to all applicants. When published fees are subject to change, a statement to that effect must be included.
A.4.6.	The program or sponsoring institution must have a defined and published policy and procedure for processing student and faculty grievances.	The program or sponsoring institution must have a defined and published policy and procedure for processing student and faculty grievances.	The program or sponsoring institution must have a defined and published policy and procedure for processing student and faculty grievances.
A.4.7.	Policies and procedures for handling complaints against the program must be published and made known. The program must maintain a record of student complaints that includes the nature and disposition of each complaint.	Policies and procedures for handling complaints against the program must be published and made known. The program must maintain a record of student complaints that includes the nature and disposition of each complaint.	Policies and procedures for handling complaints against the program must be published and made known. The program must maintain a record of student complaints that includes the nature and disposition of each complaint.
A.4.8.	Policies and processes for student withdrawal and for refunds of tuition and fees must be published and made known to all applicants.	Policies and processes for student withdrawal and for refunds of tuition and fees must be published and made known to all applicants.	Policies and processes for student withdrawal and for refunds of tuition and fees must be published and made known to all applicants.
A.4.9.	Policies and procedures for student probation, suspension, and dismissal must be published and made known.	Policies and procedures for student probation, suspension, and dismissal must be published and made known.	Policies and procedures for student probation, suspension, and dismissal must be published and made known.

(Continued)

Standard Number	Accreditation Standards for a Doctoral-Degree-Level Educational Program for the Occupational Therapist	Accreditation Standards for a Master's-Degree-Level Educational Program for the Occupational Therapist	Accreditation Standards for an Associate-Degree-Level Educational Program for the Occupational Therapy Assistant
A.4.10.	Policies and procedures for human-subject research protocol must be published and made known.	Policies and procedures for human-subject research protocol must be published and made known.	Policies and procedures for human-subject research protocol must be published and made known (if applicable to the program).
A.4.11.	Programs must make available to students written policies and procedures regarding appropriate use of equipment and supplies and for all educational activities that have implications for the health and safety of clients, students, and faculty (including infection control and evacuation procedures).	Programs must make available to students written policies and procedures regarding appropriate use of equipment and supplies and for all educational activities that have implications for the health and safety of clients, students, and faculty (including infection control and evacuation procedures).	Programs must make available to students written policies and procedures regarding appropriate use of equipment and supplies and for all educational activities that have implications for the health and safety of clients, students, and faculty (including infection control and evacuation procedures).
A.4.12.	A program admitting students on the basis of ability to benefit (defined by the USDE as admitting students who do not have either a high school diploma or its equivalent) must publicize its objectives, assessment measures, and means of evaluating the student's ability to benefit.	A program admitting students on the basis of ability to benefit (defined by the USDE as admitting students who do not have either a high school diploma or its equivalent) must publicize its objectives, assessment measures, and means of evaluating the student's ability to benefit.	A program admitting students on the basis of ability to benefit (defined by the USDE as admitting students who do not have either a high school diploma or its equivalent) must publicize its objectives, assessment measures, and means of evaluating the student's ability to benefit.
A.4.13.	Documentation of all progression, retention, graduation, certification, and credentialing requirements must be published and made known to applicants. A statement on the program's Web site about the potential impact of a felony conviction on a graduate's eligibility for certification and credentialing must be provided.	Documentation of all progression, retention, graduation, certification, and credentialing requirements must be published and made known to applicants. A statement on the program's Web site about the potential impact of a felony conviction on a graduate's eligibility for certification and credentialing must be provided.	Documentation of all progression, retention, graduation, certification, and credentialing requirements must be published and made known to applicants. A statement on the program's Web site about the potential impact of a felony conviction on a graduate's eligibility for certification and credentialing must be provided.
A.4.14.	The program must have a documented and published policy to ensure that students complete	The program must have a documented and published policy to ensure that students com-	The program must have a documented and published policy to ensure that students complete

(Continued)

68

Standard Number	Accreditation Standards for a Doctoral-Degree-Level Educational Program for the Occupational Therapist	Accreditation Standards for a Master's-Degree-Level Educational Program for the Occupational Therapist	Accreditation Standards for an Associate-Degree-Level Educational Program for the Occupational Therapy Assistant
	all graduation, fieldwork, and experiential component requirements in a timely manner. This policy must include a statement that all Level II fieldwork and the experiential component of the program must be completed within a time frame established by the program.	plete all graduation and fieldwork requirements in a timely manner. This policy must include a statement that all Level II fieldwork must be completed within a time frame established by the program.	all graduation and fieldwork requirements in a timely manner. This policy must include a statement that all Level II fieldwork must be completed within a time frame established by the program.
A.4.15.	Records regarding student admission, enrollment, fieldwork, and achievement must be maintained and kept in a secure setting. Grades and credits for courses must be recorded on students' transcripts and permanently maintained by the sponsoring institution.	Records regarding student admission, enrollment, fieldwork, and achievement must be maintained and kept in a secure setting. Grades and credits for courses must be recorded on students' transcripts and permanently maintained by the sponsoring institution.	Records regarding student admission, enrollment, fieldwork, and achievement must be maintained and kept in a secure setting. Grades and credits for courses must be recorded on students' transcripts and permanently maintained by the sponsoring institution.

A.5.0. STRATEGIC PLAN AND PROGRAM ASSESSMENT

For programs that are offered at more than one location, the program's strategic plan, evaluation plan, and results of ongoing evaluation must address each program location as a component of the overall plan.

A.5.1.	The program must document a current strategic plan that articulates the program's future vision and guides the program development (e.g., faculty recruitment and professional growth, scholarship, changes in the curriculum design, priorities in academic resources, procurement of fieldwork and experiential component sites). A program strategic plan must be for a minimum	The program must document a current strategic plan that articulates the program's future vision and guides the program development (e.g., faculty recruitment and professional growth, scholarship, changes in the curriculum design, priorities in academic resources, procurement of fieldwork sites). A program strategic plan must be for a minimum of a	The program must document a current strategic plan that articulates the program's future vision and guides the program development (e.g., faculty recruitment and professional growth, scholarship, changes in the curriculum design, priorities in academic resources, procurement of fieldwork sites). A program strategic plan must be for a minimum of a

(Continued)

Standard Number	Accreditation Standards for a Doctoral-Degree-Level Educational Program for the Occupational Therapist	Accreditation Standards for a Master's-Degree-Level Educational Program for the Occupational Therapist	Accreditation Standards for an Associate-Degree-Level Educational Program for the Occupational Therapy Assistant
	of a 3-year period and include, but need not be limited to, • Evidence that the plan is based on program evaluation and an analysis of external and internal environments. • Long-term goals that address the vision and mission of both the institution and the program, as well as specific needs of the program. • Specific measurable action steps with expected timelines by which the program will reach its long-term goals. • Person(s) responsible for action steps. • Evidence of periodic updating of action steps and long-term goals as they are met or as circumstances change.	3-year period and include, but need not be limited to, • Evidence that the plan is based on program evaluation and an analysis of external and internal environments. • Long-term goals that address the vision and mission of both the institution and the program, as well as specific needs of the program. • Specific measurable action steps with expected timelines by which the program will reach its long-term goals. • Person(s) responsible for action steps. • Evidence of periodic updating of action steps and long-term goals as they are met or as circumstances change.	3-year period and include, but need not be limited to, • Evidence that the plan is based on program evaluation and an analysis of external and internal environments. • Long-term goals that address the vision and mission of both the institution and the program, as well as specific needs of the program. • Specific measurable action steps with expected timelines by which the program will reach its long-term goals. • Person(s) responsible for action steps. • Evidence of periodic updating of action steps and long-term goals as they are met or as circumstances change.
A.5.2.	The program director and each faculty member who teaches two or more courses must have a current written professional growth and development plan. Each plan must contain the signature of the faculty member and supervisor. At a minimum, the plan must include, but need not be limited to, • Goals to enhance the faculty member's ability to fulfill designated responsibilities (e.g., goals related to currency in areas of teaching responsibility, teaching effectiveness, research, scholarly activity).	The program director and each faculty member who teaches two or more courses must have a current written professional growth and development plan. Each plan must contain the signature of the faculty member and supervisor. At a minimum, the plan must include, but need not be limited to, • Goals to enhance the faculty member's ability to fulfill designated responsibilities (e.g., goals related to currency in areas of teaching responsibility, teaching effectiveness, research, scholarly activity).	The program director and each faculty member who teaches two or more courses must have a current written professional growth and development plan. Each plan must contain the signature of the faculty member and supervisor. At a minimum, the plan must include, but need not be limited to, • Goals to enhance the faculty member's ability to fulfill designated responsibilities (e.g., goals related to currency in areas of teaching responsibility, teaching effectiveness, research, scholarly activity).

(Continued)

Standard Number	Accreditation Standards for a Doctoral-Degree-Level Educational Program for the Occupational Therapist	Accreditation Standards for a Master's-Degree-Level Educational Program for the Occupational Therapist	Accreditation Standards for an Associate-Degree-Level Educational Program for the Occupational Therapy Assistant
	• Specific measurable action steps with expected timelines by which the faculty member will achieve the goals. • Evidence of annual updates of action steps and goals as they are met or as circumstances change. • Identification of the ways in which the faculty member's professional development plan will contribute to attaining the program's strategic goals.	• Specific measurable action steps with expected timelines by which the faculty member will achieve the goals. • Evidence of annual updates of action steps and goals as they are met or as circumstances change. • Identification of the ways in which the faculty member's professional development plan will contribute to attaining the program's strategic goals.	• Specific measurable action steps with expected timelines by which the faculty member will achieve the goals. • Evidence of annual updates of action steps and goals as they are met or as circumstances change. • Identification of the ways in which the faculty member's professional development plan will contribute to attaining the program's strategic goals.
A.5.3.	Programs must routinely secure and document sufficient qualitative and quantitative information to allow for meaningful analysis about the extent to which the program is meeting its stated goals and objectives. This must include, but need not be limited to, • Faculty effectiveness in their assigned teaching responsibilities. • Students' progression through the program. • Student retention rates. • Fieldwork and experiential component performance evaluation. • Student evaluation of fieldwork and the experiential component experience. • Student satisfaction with the program. • Graduates' performance on the NBCOT certification exam.	Programs must routinely secure and document sufficient qualitative and quantitative information to allow for meaningful analysis about the extent to which the program is meeting its stated goals and objectives. This must include, but need not be limited to, • Faculty effectiveness in their assigned teaching responsibilities. • Students' progression through the program. • Student retention rates. • Fieldwork performance evaluation. • Student evaluation of fieldwork experience. • Student satisfaction with the program. • Graduates' performance on the NBCOT certification exam. • Graduates' job placement and performance as determined by employer satisfaction.	Programs must routinely secure and document sufficient qualitative and quantitative information to allow for meaningful analysis about the extent to which the program is meeting its stated goals and objectives. This must include, but need not be limited to, • Faculty effectiveness in their assigned teaching responsibilities. • Students' progression through the program. • Student retention rates. • Fieldwork performance evaluation. • Student evaluation of fieldwork experience. • Student satisfaction with the program. • Graduates' performance on the NBCOT certification exam. • Graduates' job placement and performance as determined by employer satisfaction.

(Continued)

Standard Number	Accreditation Standards for a Doctoral-Degree-Level Educational Program for the Occupational Therapist	Accreditation Standards for a Master's-Degree-Level Educational Program for the Occupational Therapist	Accreditation Standards for an Associate-Degree-Level Educational Program for the Occupational Therapy Assistant
	• Graduates' job placement and performance as determined by employer satisfaction. • Graduates' scholarly activity (e.g., presentations, publications, grants obtained, state and national leadership positions, awards).		
A.5.4.	Programs must routinely and systematically analyze data to determine the extent to which the program is meeting its stated goals and objectives. An annual report summarizing analysis of data and planned action responses must be maintained.	Programs must routinely and systematically analyze data to determine the extent to which the program is meeting its stated goals and objectives. An annual report summarizing analysis of data and planned action responses must be maintained.	Programs must routinely and systematically analyze data to determine the extent to which the program is meeting its stated goals and objectives. An annual report summarizing analysis of data and planned action responses must be maintained.
A.5.5.	The results of ongoing evaluation must be appropriately reflected in the program's strategic plan, curriculum, and other dimensions of the program.	The results of ongoing evaluation must be appropriately reflected in the program's strategic plan, curriculum, and other dimensions of the program.	The results of ongoing evaluation must be appropriately reflected in the program's strategic plan, curriculum, and other dimensions of the program.
A.5.6.	The average pass rate over the 3 most recent calendar years for graduates attempting the national certification exam within 12 months of graduation from the program must be 80% or higher (regardless of the number of attempts). If a program has less than 25 test takers in the 3 most recent calendar years, the program may include test takers from additional years until it reaches 25 or until the 5 most recent calendar years are included in the total.	The average pass rate over the 3 most recent calendar years for graduates attempting the national certification exam within 12 months of graduation from the program must be 80% or higher (regardless of the number of attempts). If a program has less than 25 test takers in the 3 most recent calendar years, the program may include test takers from additional years until it reaches 25 or until the 5 most recent calendar years are included in the total.	The average pass rate over the 3 most recent calendar years for graduates attempting the national certification exam within 12 months of graduation from the program must be 80% or higher (regardless of the number of attempts). If a program has less than 25 test takers in the 3 most recent calendar years, the program may include test takers from additional years until it reaches 25 or until the 5 most recent calendar years are included in the total.

(Continued)

Standard Number	Accreditation Standards for a Doctoral-Degree-Level Educational Program for the Occupational Therapist	Accreditation Standards for a Master's-Degree-Level Educational Program for the Occupational Therapist	Accreditation Standards for an Associate-Degree-Level Educational Program for the Occupational Therapy Assistant
A.6.0. CURRICULUM FRAMEWORK The curriculum framework is a description of the program that includes the program's mission, philosophy, and curriculum design.			
A.6.1.	The curriculum must ensure preparation to practice as a generalist with a broad exposure to current practice settings (e.g., school, hospital, community, long-term care) and emerging practice areas (as defined by the program). The curriculum must prepare students to work with a variety of populations including, but not limited to, children, adolescents, adults, and elderly persons in areas of physical and mental health.	The curriculum must include preparation for practice as a generalist with a broad exposure to current practice settings (e.g., school, hospital, community, long-term care) and emerging practice areas (as defined by the program). The curriculum must prepare students to work with a variety of populations including, but not limited to, children, adolescents, adults, and elderly persons in areas of physical and mental health.	The curriculum must include preparation for practice as a generalist with a broad exposure to current practice settings (e.g., school, hospital, community, long-term care) and emerging practice areas (as defined by the program). The curriculum must prepare students to work with a variety of populations including, but not limited to, children, adolescents, adults, and elderly persons in areas of physical and mental health.
A.6.2.	The curriculum must include course objectives and learning activities demonstrating preparation beyond a generalist level in, but not limited to, practice skills, research skills, administration, professional development, leadership, advocacy, and theory.	*(No related Standard)*	*(No related Standard)*
A.6.3.	The occupational therapy doctoral degree must be awarded after a period of study such that the total time to the degree, including both preprofessional and professional preparation, equals at least 6 FTE academic years. The program must document a system and rationale for ensuring that the length of study of the program is appropriate to the expected learning and competence of the graduate.	The program must document a system and rationale for ensuring that the length of study of the program is appropriate to the expected learning and competence of the graduate.	The program must document a system and rationale for ensuring that the length of study of the program is appropriate to the expected learning and competence of the graduate.

(Continued)

Standard Number	Accreditation Standards for a Doctoral-Degree-Level Educational Program for the Occupational Therapist	Accreditation Standards for a Master's-Degree-Level Educational Program for the Occupational Therapist	Accreditation Standards for an Associate-Degree-Level Educational Program for the Occupational Therapy Assistant
A.6.4.	The curriculum must include application of advanced knowledge to practice through a combination of experiential activities and a culminating project.	*(No related Standard)*	*(No related Standard)*
A.6.5.	The statement of philosophy of the occupational therapy program must reflect the current published philosophy of the profession and must include a statement of the program's fundamental beliefs about human beings and how they learn.	The statement of philosophy of the occupational therapy program must reflect the current published philosophy of the profession and must include a statement of the program's fundamental beliefs about human beings and how they learn.	The statement of philosophy of the occupational therapy assistant program must reflect the current published philosophy of the profession and must include a statement of the program's fundamental beliefs about human beings and how they learn.
A.6.6.	The statement of the mission of the occupational therapy program must be consistent with and supportive of the mission of the sponsoring institution. The program's mission statement should explain the unique nature of the program and how it helps fulfill or advance the mission of the sponsoring institution, including religious missions.	The statement of the mission of the occupational therapy program must be consistent with and supportive of the mission of the sponsoring institution. The program's mission statement should explain the unique nature of the program and how it helps fulfill or advance the mission of the sponsoring institution, including religious missions.	The statement of the mission of the occupational therapy assistant program must be consistent with and supportive of the mission of the sponsoring institution. The program's mission statement should explain the unique nature of the program and how it helps fulfill or advance the mission of the sponsoring institution, including religious missions.
A.6.7.	The curriculum design must reflect the mission and philosophy of both the occupational therapy program and the institution and must provide the basis for program planning, implementation, and evaluation. The design must identify curricular threads and educational goals and describe the selection of the content, scope, and sequencing of coursework.	The curriculum design must reflect the mission and philosophy of both the occupational therapy program and the institution and must provide the basis for program planning, implementation, and evaluation. The design must identify curricular threads and educational goals and describe the selection of the content, scope, and sequencing of coursework.	The curriculum design must reflect the mission and philosophy of both the occupational therapy assistant program and the institution and must provide the basis for program planning, implementation, and evaluation. The design must identify curricular threads and educational goals and describe the selection of the content, scope, and sequencing of coursework.

(Continued)

Standard Number	Accreditation Standards for a Doctoral-Degree-Level Educational Program for the Occupational Therapist	Accreditation Standards for a Master's-Degree-Level Educational Program for the Occupational Therapist	Accreditation Standards for an Associate-Degree-Level Educational Program for the Occupational Therapy Assistant
A.6.8.	The program must have clearly documented assessment measures by which students are regularly evaluated on their acquisition of knowledge, skills, attitudes, and competencies required for graduation.	The program must have clearly documented assessment measures by which students are regularly evaluated on their acquisition of knowledge, skills, attitudes, and competencies required for graduation.	The program must have clearly documented assessment measures by which students are regularly evaluated on their acquisition of knowledge, skills, attitudes, and competencies required for graduation.
A.6.9.	The program must have written syllabi for each course that include course objectives and learning activities that, in total, reflect all course content required by the Standards. Instructional methods (e.g., presentations, demonstrations, discussion) and materials used to accomplish course objectives must be documented. Programs must also demonstrate the consistency between course syllabi and the curriculum design.	The program must have written syllabi for each course that include course objectives and learning activities that, in total, reflect all course content required by the Standards. Instructional methods (e.g., presentations, demonstrations, discussion) and materials used to accomplish course objectives must be documented. Programs must also demonstrate the consistency between course syllabi and the curriculum design.	The program must have written syllabi for each course that include course objectives and learning activities that, in total, reflect all course content required by the Standards. Instructional methods (e.g., presentations, demonstrations, discussion) and materials used to accomplish course objectives must be documented. Programs must also demonstrate the consistency between course syllabi and the curriculum design.

Section B: CONTENT REQUIREMENTS

The content requirements are written as expected student outcomes. Faculty are responsible for developing learning activities and evaluation methods to document that students meet these outcomes.

B.1.0.	FOUNDATIONAL CONTENT REQUIREMENTS		FOUNDATIONAL CONTENT REQUIREMENTS
	Program content must be based on a broad foundation in the liberal arts and sciences. A strong foundation in the biological, physical, social, and behavioral sciences supports an understanding of occupation across the lifespan. If the content of the Standard is met through prerequisite coursework, the application of foundational content in sciences must also be evident in professional coursework. The student will be able to		**Program content must be based on a broad foundation in the liberal arts and sciences. A strong foundation in the biological, physical, social, and behavioral sciences supports an understanding of occupation across the**

(Continued)

Standard Number	Accreditation Standards for a Doctoral-Degree-Level Educational Program for the Occupational Therapist	Accreditation Standards for a Master's-Degree-Level Educational Program for the Occupational Therapist	Accreditation Standards for an Associate-Degree-Level Educational Program for the Occupational Therapy Assistant
			lifespan. If the content of the Standard is met through prerequisite coursework, the application of foundational content in sciences must also be evident in professional coursework. The student will be able to
B.1.1.	Demonstrate knowledge and understanding of the structure and function of the human body to include the biological and physical sciences. Course content must include, but is not limited to, biology, anatomy, physiology, neuroscience, and kinesiology or biomechanics.	Demonstrate knowledge and understanding of the structure and function of the human body to include the biological and physical sciences. Course content must include, but is not limited to, biology, anatomy, physiology, neuroscience, and kinesiology or biomechanics.	Demonstrate knowledge and understanding of the structure and function of the human body to include the biological and physical sciences. Course content must include, but is not limited to, anatomy, physiology, and biomechanics.
B.1.2.	Demonstrate knowledge and understanding of human development throughout the lifespan (infants, children, adolescents, adults, and older adults). Course content must include, but is not limited to, developmental psychology.	Demonstrate knowledge and understanding of human development throughout the lifespan (infants, children, adolescents, adults, and older adults). Course content must include, but is not limited to, developmental psychology.	Demonstrate knowledge and understanding of human development throughout the lifespan (infants, children, adolescents, adults, and older adults). Course content must include, but is not limited to, developmental psychology.
B.1.3.	Demonstrate knowledge and understanding of the concepts of human behavior to include the behavioral sciences, social sciences, and occupational science. Course content must include, but is not limited to, introductory psychology, abnormal psychology, and introductory sociology or introductory anthropology.	Demonstrate knowledge and understanding of the concepts of human behavior to include the behavioral sciences, social sciences, and occupational science. Course content must include, but is not limited to, introductory psychology, abnormal psychology, and introductory sociology or introductory anthropology.	Demonstrate knowledge and understanding of the concepts of human behavior to include the behavioral and social sciences (e.g., principles of psychology, sociology, abnormal psychology) and occupational science.

(Continued)

(Continued)

Standard Number	Accreditation Standards for a Doctoral-Degree-Level Educational Program for the Occupational Therapist	Accreditation Standards for a Master's-Degree-Level Educational Program for the Occupational Therapist	Accreditation Standards for an Associate-Degree-Level Educational Program for the Occupational Therapy Assistant
B.1.4.	Apply knowledge of the role of sociocultural, socioeconomic, and diversity factors and lifestyle choices in contemporary society to meet the needs of individuals and communities. Course content must include, but is not limited to, introductory psychology, abnormal psychology, and introductory sociology or introductory anthropology.	Demonstrate knowledge and appreciation of the role of sociocultural, socioeconomic, and diversity factors and lifestyle choices in contemporary society. Course content must include, but is not limited to, introductory psychology, abnormal psychology, and introductory sociology or introductory anthropology.	Demonstrate knowledge and appreciation of the role of sociocultural, socioeconomic, and diversity factors and lifestyle choices in contemporary society (e.g., principles of psychology, sociology, and abnormal psychology)
B.1.5.	Demonstrate an understanding of the ethical and practical considerations that affect the health and wellness needs of those who are experiencing or are at risk for social injustice, occupational deprivation, and disparity in the receipt of services.	Demonstrate an understanding of the ethical and practical considerations that affect the health and wellness needs of those who are experiencing or are at risk for social injustice, occupational deprivation, and disparity in the receipt of services.	Articulate the ethical and practical considerations that affect the health and wellness needs of those who are experiencing or are at risk for social injustice, occupational deprivation, and disparity in the receipt of services.
B.1.6.	Demonstrate knowledge of global social issues and prevailing health and welfare needs of populations with or at risk for disabilities and chronic health conditions.	Demonstrate knowledge of global social issues and prevailing health and welfare needs of populations with or at risk for disabilities and chronic health conditions.	Demonstrate knowledge of global social issues and prevailing health and welfare needs of populations with or at risk for disabilities and chronic health conditions.
B.1.7.	Apply quantitative statistics and qualitative analysis to interpret tests, measurements, and other data for the purpose of establishing and/or delivering evidence-based practice.	Demonstrate the ability to use statistics to interpret tests and measurements for the purpose of delivering evidence-based practice.	Articulate the importance of using statistics, tests, and measurements for the purpose of delivering evidence-based practice.
B.1.8.	Demonstrate an understanding of the use of technology to support performance, participation, health and well-being. This technology may	Demonstrate an understanding of the use of technology to support performance, participation, health and well-being. This technology may	Demonstrate an understanding of the use of technology to support performance, participation, health and well-being. This technology may

Standard Number	Accreditation Standards for a Doctoral-Degree-Level Educational Program for the Occupational Therapist	Accreditation Standards for a Master's-Degree-Level Educational Program for the Occupational Therapist	Accreditation Standards for an Associate-Degree-Level Educational Program for the Occupational Therapy Assistant
	include, but is not limited to, electronic documentation systems, distance communication, virtual environments, and telehealth technology.	include, but is not limited to, electronic documentation systems, distance communication, virtual environments, and telehealth technology.	include, but is not limited to, electronic documentation systems, distance communication, virtual environments, and telehealth technology.
B.2.0. BASIC TENETS OF OCCUPATIONAL THERAPY Coursework must facilitate development of the performance criteria listed below. The student will be able to			
B.2.1.	Explain the history and philosophical base of the profession of occupational therapy and its importance in meeting society's current and future occupational needs.	Articulate an understanding of the importance of the history and philosophical base of the profession of occupational therapy.	Articulate an understanding of the importance of the history and philosophical base of the profession of occupational therapy.
B.2.2.	Explain the meaning and dynamics of occupation and activity, including the interaction of areas of occupation, performance skills, performance patterns, activity demands, context(s) and environments, and client factors.	Explain the meaning and dynamics of occupation and activity, including the interaction of areas of occupation, performance skills, performance patterns, activity demands, context(s) and environments, and client factors.	Describe the meaning and dynamics of occupation and activity, including the interaction of areas of occupation, performance skills, performance patterns, activity demands, context(s) and environments, and client factors.
B.2.3.	Articulate to consumers, potential employers, colleagues, third-party payers, regulatory boards, policymakers, other audiences, and the general public both the unique nature of occupation as viewed by the profession of occupational therapy and the value of occupation to support performance, participation, health, and well-being.	Articulate to consumers, potential employers, colleagues, third-party payers, regulatory boards, policymakers, other audiences, and the general public both the unique nature of occupation as viewed by the profession of occupational therapy and the value of occupation to support performance, participation, health, and well-being.	Articulate to consumers, potential employers, colleagues, third-party payers, regulatory boards, policymakers, other audiences, and the general public both the unique nature of occupation as viewed by the profession of occupational therapy and the value of occupation support performance, participation, health, and well-being.

(Continued)

(Continued)

Standard Number	Accreditation Standards for a Doctoral-Degree-Level Educational Program for the Occupational Therapist	Accreditation Standards for a Master's-Degree-Level Educational Program for the Occupational Therapist	Accreditation Standards for an Associate-Degree-Level Educational Program for the Occupational Therapy Assistant
B.2.4.	Articulate the importance of balancing areas of occupation with the achievement of health and wellness for the clients.	Articulate the importance of balancing areas of occupation with the achievement of health and wellness for the clients.	Articulate the importance of balancing areas of occupation with the achievement of health and wellness for the clients.
B.2.5.	Explain the role of occupation in the promotion of health and the prevention of disease and disability for the individual, family, and society.	Explain the role of occupation in the promotion of health and the prevention of disease and disability for the individual, family, and society.	Explain the role of occupation in the promotion of health and the prevention of disease and disability for the individual, family, and society.
B.2.6.	Analyze the effects of heritable diseases, genetic conditions, disability, trauma, and injury to the physical and mental health and occupational performance of the individual.	Analyze the effects of heritable diseases, genetic conditions, disability, trauma, and injury to the physical and mental health and occupational performance of the individual.	Understand the effects of heritable diseases, genetic conditions, disability, trauma, and injury to the physical and mental health and occupational performance of the individual.
B.2.7.	Demonstrate task analysis in areas of occupation, performance skills, performance patterns, activity demands, context(s) and environments, and client factors to formulate an intervention plan.	Demonstrate task analysis in areas of occupation, performance skills, performance patterns, activity demands, context(s) and environments, and client factors to formulate an intervention plan.	Demonstrate task analysis in areas of occupation, performance skills, performance patterns, activity demands, context(s) and environments, and client factors to implement the intervention plan.
B.2.8.	Use sound judgment in regard to safety of self and others and adhere to safety regulations throughout the occupational therapy process as appropriate to the setting and scope of practice.	Use sound judgment in regard to safety of self and others and adhere to safety regulations throughout the occupational therapy process as appropriate to the setting and scope of practice.	Use sound judgment in regard to safety of self and others and adhere to safety regulations throughout the occupational therapy process as appropriate to the setting and scope of practice.
B.2.9.	Express support for the quality of life, well-being, and occupation of the individual, group, or population to promote physical and mental health and	Express support for the quality of life, well-being, and occupation of the individual, group, or population to promote physical and mental health and	Express support for the quality of life, well-being, and occupation of the individual, group, or population to promote physical and mental health

Standard Number	Accreditation Standards for a Doctoral-Degree-Level Educational Program for the Occupational Therapist	Accreditation Standards for a Master's-Degree-Level Educational Program for the Occupational Therapist	Accreditation Standards for an Associate-Degree-Level Educational Program for the Occupational Therapy Assistant
	prevention of injury and disease considering the context (e.g., cultural, personal, temporal, virtual) and environment.	prevention of injury and disease considering the context (e.g., cultural, personal, temporal, virtual) and environment.	and prevention of injury and disease considering the context (e.g., cultural, personal, temporal, virtual) and environment.
B.2.10.	Use clinical reasoning to explain the rationale for and use of compensatory strategies when desired life tasks cannot be performed.	Use clinical reasoning to explain the rationale for and use of compensatory strategies when desired life tasks cannot be performed.	Explain the need for and use of compensatory strategies when desired life tasks cannot be performed.
B.2.11.	Analyze, synthesize, evaluate, and apply models of occupational performance.	Analyze, synthesize, and apply models of occupational performance.	Identify interventions consistent with models of occupational performance.

B.3.0.   OCCUPATIONAL THERAPY THEORETICAL PERSPECTIVES
The program must facilitate the development of the performance criteria listed below. The student will be able to

Standard Number	Accreditation Standards for a Doctoral-Degree-Level Educational Program for the Occupational Therapist	Accreditation Standards for a Master's-Degree-Level Educational Program for the Occupational Therapist	Accreditation Standards for an Associate-Degree-Level Educational Program for the Occupational Therapy Assistant
B.3.1.	Evaluate and apply theories that underlie the practice of occupational therapy.	Apply theories that underlie the practice of occupational therapy.	Describe basic features of the theories that underlie the practice of occupational therapy.
B.3.2.	Compare, contrast, and integrate a variety of models of practice and frames of reference that are used in occupational therapy.	Compare and contrast models of practice and frames of reference that are used in occupational therapy.	Describe basic features of models of practice and frames of reference that are used in occupational therapy.
B.3.3.	Use theories, models of practice, and frames of reference to guide and inform evaluation and intervention.	Use theories, models of practice, and frames of reference to guide and inform evaluation and intervention.	(No related Standard)

(Continued)

Standard Number	Accreditation Standards for a Doctoral-Degree-Level Educational Program for the Occupational Therapist	Accreditation Standards for a Master's-Degree-Level Educational Program for the Occupational Therapist	Accreditation Standards for an Associate-Degree-Level Educational Program for the Occupational Therapy Assistant
B.3.4.	Analyze and discuss how occupational therapy history, occupational therapy theory, and the sociopolitical climate influence and are influenced by practice.	Analyze and discuss how occupational therapy history, occupational therapy theory, and the sociopolitical climate influence practice.	Discuss how occupational therapy history and occupational therapy theory, and the sociopolitical climate influence practice.
B.3.5.	Apply theoretical constructs to evaluation and intervention with various types of clients in a variety of practice contexts and environments, including population-based approaches, to analyze and effect meaningful occupation outcomes.	Apply theoretical constructs to evaluation and intervention with various types of clients in a variety of practice contexts and environments to analyze and effect meaningful occupation outcomes.	*(No related Standard)*
B.3.6.	Articulate the process of theory development in occupational therapy and its desired impact and influence on society.	Discuss the process of theory development and its importance to occupational therapy.	*(No related Standard)*
B.4.0.	**SCREENING, EVALUATION, AND REFERRAL** The process of screening, evaluation, referral, and diagnosis as related to occupational performance and participation must be culturally relevant and based on theoretical perspectives, models of practice, frames of reference, and available evidence. In addition, this process must consider the continuum of need from individuals to populations. The program must facilitate development of the performance criteria listed below. The student will be able to	**SCREENING, EVALUATION, AND REFERRAL** The process of screening, evaluation, and referral as related to occupational performance and participation must be culturally relevant and based on theoretical perspectives, models of practice, frames of reference, and available evidence. In addition, this process must consider the continuum of need from individuals to populations. The program must facilitate development of the performance criteria listed below. The student will be able to	**SCREENING AND EVALUATION** The process of screening and evaluation as related to occupational performance and participation must be conducted under the supervision of and in cooperation with the occupational therapist and must be culturally relevant and based on theoretical perspectives, models of practice, frames of reference, and available evidence. The program must facilitate development of the performance criteria listed below. The student will be able to

(Continued)

81

Standard Number	Accreditation Standards for a Doctoral-Degree-Level Educational Program for the Occupational Therapist	Accreditation Standards for a Master's-Degree-Level Educational Program for the Occupational Therapist	Accreditation Standards for an Associate-Degree-Level Educational Program for the Occupational Therapy Assistant
B.4.1.	Use standardized and nonstandardized screening and assessment tools to determine the need for occupational therapy intervention. These tools include, but are not limited to, specified screening tools; assessments; skilled observations; occupational histories; consultations with other professionals; and interviews with the client, family, significant others, and community.	Use standardized and nonstandardized screening and assessment tools to determine the need for occupational therapy intervention. These tools include, but are not limited to, specified screening tools; assessments; skilled observations; occupational histories; consultations with other professionals; and interviews with the client, family, significant others, and community.	Gather and share data for the purpose of screening and evaluation using methods including, but not limited to: specified screening tools; assessments; skilled observations; occupational histories; consultations with other professionals; and interviews with the client, family, and significant others.
B.4.2.	Select appropriate assessment tools on the basis of client needs, contextual factors, and psychometric properties of tests. These must be culturally relevant, based on available evidence, and incorporate use of occupation in the assessment process.	Select appropriate assessment tools on the basis of client needs, contextual factors, and psychometric properties of tests. These must be culturally relevant, based on available evidence, and incorporate use of occupation in the assessment process.	Administer selected assessments using appropriate procedures and protocols (including standardized formats) and use occupation for the purpose of assessment.
B.4.3.	Use appropriate procedures and protocols (including standardized formats) when administering assessments.	Use appropriate procedures and protocols (including standardized formats) when administering assessments.	*(No related Standard)*
B.4.4.	Evaluate client(s)' occupational performance in activities of daily living (ADLs), instrumental activities of daily living (IADLs), education, work, play, rest, sleep, leisure, and social participation. Evaluation of occupational performance using	Evaluate client(s)' occupational performance in activities of daily living (ADLs), instrumental activities of daily living (IADLs), education, work, play, rest, sleep, leisure, and social participation. Evaluation of occupational performance using	Gather and share data for the purpose of evaluating client(s)' occupational performance in activities of daily living (ADLs), instrumental activities of daily living (IADLs), education, work, play, rest, sleep, leisure, and social

(Continued)

82

Standard Number	Accreditation Standards for a Doctoral-Degree-Level Educational Program for the Occupational Therapist	Accreditation Standards for a Master's-Degree-Level Educational Program for the Occupational Therapist	Accreditation Standards for an Associate-Degree-Level Educational Program for the Occupational Therapy Assistant
	standardized and nonstandardized assessment tools includes • The occupational profile, including participation in activities that are meaningful and necessary for the client to carry out roles in home, work, and community environments. • Client factors, including values, beliefs, spirituality, body functions (e.g., neuromuscular, sensory and pain, visual, perceptual, cognitive, mental) and body structures (e.g., cardiovascular, digestive, nervous, genitourinary, integumentary systems). • Performance patterns (e.g., habits, routines, rituals, roles). • Context (e.g., cultural, personal, temporal, virtual) and environment (e.g., physical, social). • Performance skills, including motor and praxis skills, sensory–perceptual skills, emotional regulation skills, cognitive skills, and communication and social skills.	standardized and nonstandardized assessment tools includes • The occupational profile, including participation in activities that are meaningful and necessary for the client to carry out roles in home, work, and community environments. • Client factors, including values, beliefs, spirituality, body functions (e.g., neuromuscular, sensory and pain, visual, perceptual, cognitive, mental) and body structures (e.g., cardiovascular, digestive, nervous, genitourinary, integumentary systems). • Performance patterns (e.g., habits, routines, rituals, roles). • Context (e.g., cultural, personal, temporal, virtual) and environment (e.g., physical, social). • Performance skills, including motor and praxis skills, sensory–perceptual skills, emotional regulation skills, cognitive skills, and communication and social skills.	participation. Evaluation of occupational performance includes • The occupational profile, including participation in activities that are meaningful and necessary for the client to carry out roles in home, work, and community environments. • Client factors, including values, beliefs, spirituality, body functions (e.g., neuromuscular, sensory and pain, visual, perceptual, cognitive, mental) and body structures (e.g., cardiovascular, digestive, nervous, genitourinary, integumentary systems). • Performance patterns (e.g., habits, routines, rituals, roles). • Context (e.g., cultural, personal, temporal, virtual) and environment (e.g., physical, social). • Performance skills, including motor and praxis skills, sensory–perceptual skills, emotional regulation skills, cognitive skills, and communication and social skills.
B.4.5	Compare and contrast the role of the occupational therapist and occupational therapy assistant in the screening and evaluation process along with the importance of and rationale for supervision and collaborative work between the occupational therapist and occupational therapy assistant in that process.	Compare and contrast the role of the occupational therapist and occupational therapy assistant in the screening and evaluation process along with the importance of and rationale for supervision and collaborative work between the occupational therapist and occupational therapy assistant in that process.	Articulate the role of the occupational therapy assistant and occupational therapist in the screening and evaluation process along with the importance of and rationale for supervision and collaborative work between the occupational therapy assistant and occupational therapist in that process.

(Continued)

Standard Number	Accreditation Standards for a Doctoral-Degree-Level Educational Program for the Occupational Therapist	Accreditation Standards for a Master's-Degree-Level Educational Program for the Occupational Therapist	Accreditation Standards for an Associate-Degree-Level Educational Program for the Occupational Therapy Assistant
B.4.6.	Interpret criterion-referenced and norm-referenced standardized test scores on the basis of an understanding of sampling, normative data, standard and criterion scores, reliability, and validity.	Interpret criterion-referenced and norm-referenced standardized test scores on the basis of an understanding of sampling, normative data, standard and criterion scores, reliability, and validity.	*(No related Standard)*
B.4.7.	Consider factors that might bias assessment results, such as culture, disability status, and situational variables related to the individual and context.	Consider factors that might bias assessment results, such as culture, disability status, and situational variables related to the individual and context.	*(No related Standard)*
B.4.8.	Interpret the evaluation data in relation to accepted terminology of the profession, relevant theoretical frameworks, and interdisciplinary knowledge.	Interpret the evaluation data in relation to accepted terminology of the profession and relevant theoretical frameworks.	*(No related Standard)*
B.4.9.	Evaluate appropriateness and discuss mechanisms for referring clients for additional evaluation to specialists who are internal and external to the profession.	Evaluate appropriateness and discuss mechanisms for referring clients for additional evaluation to specialists who are internal and external to the profession.	Identify when to recommend to the occupational therapist the need for referring clients for additional evaluation.
B.4.10.	Document occupational therapy services to ensure accountability of service provision and to meet standards for reimbursement of services, adhering to the requirements of applicable facility, local, state, federal, and reimbursement agencies. Documentation must effectively communicate the need and rationale for occupational therapy services.	Document occupational therapy services to ensure accountability of service provision and to meet standards for reimbursement of services, adhering to the requirements of applicable facility, local, state, federal, and reimbursement agencies. Documentation must effectively communicate the need and rationale for occupational therapy services.	Document occupational therapy services to ensure accountability of service provision and to meet standards for reimbursement of services, adhering to the requirements of applicable facility, local, state, federal, and reimbursement agencies. Documentation must effectively communicate the need and rationale for occupational therapy services.

(Continued)

Standard Number	Accreditation Standards for a Doctoral-Degree-Level Educational Program for the Occupational Therapist	Accreditation Standards for a Master's-Degree-Level Educational Program for the Occupational Therapist	Accreditation Standards for an Associate-Degree-Level Educational Program for the Occupational Therapy Assistant
B.4.11.	Articulate screening and evaluation processes for all practice areas. Use evidence-based reasoning to analyze, synthesize, evaluate, and diagnose problems related to occupational performance and participation.	*(No related Standard)*	*(No related Standard)*
B.5.0.	**INTERVENTION PLAN: FORMULATION AND IMPLEMENTATION** The process of formulation and implementation of the therapeutic intervention plan to facilitate occupational performance and participation must be culturally relevant; reflective of current and emerging occupational therapy practice; based on available evidence; and based on theoretical perspectives, models of practice, and frames of reference. In addition, this process must consider the continuum of need from individual- to population-based interventions. The program must facilitate development of the performance criteria listed below. The student will be able to	**INTERVENTION PLAN: FORMULATION AND IMPLEMENTATION** The process of formulation and implementation of the therapeutic intervention plan to facilitate occupational performance and participation must be culturally relevant; reflective of current occupational therapy practice; based on available evidence; and based on theoretical perspectives, models of practice, and frames of reference. The program must facilitate development of the performance criteria listed below. The student will be able to	**INTERVENTION AND IMPLEMENTATION** The process of intervention to facilitate occupational performance and participation must be done under the supervision of and in cooperation with the occupational therapist and must be culturally relevant, reflective of current occupational therapy practice, and based on available evidence. The program must facilitate development of the performance criteria listed below. The student will be able to
B.5.1.	Use evaluation findings to diagnose occupational performance and participation based on appropriate theoretical approaches, models of practice, frames of reference, and interdisciplinary knowledge. Develop occupation-based intervention	Use evaluation findings based on appropriate theoretical approaches, models of practice, and frames of reference to develop occupation-based intervention plans and strategies (including goals and methods to achieve them)	Assist with the development of occupation-based intervention plans and strategies (including goals and methods to achieve them) on the basis of the stated needs of the client as well as data gathered during the evaluation

(Continued)

Standard Number	Accreditation Standards for a Doctoral-Degree-Level Educational Program for the Occupational Therapist	Accreditation Standards for a Master's-Degree-Level Educational Program for the Occupational Therapist	Accreditation Standards for an Associate-Degree-Level Educational Program for the Occupational Therapy Assistant
	plans and strategies (including goals and methods to achieve them) on the basis of the stated needs of the client as well as data gathered during the evaluation process in collaboration with the client and others. Intervention plans and strategies must be culturally relevant, reflective of current occupational therapy practice, and based on available evidence. Interventions address the following components: • The occupational profile, including participation in activities that are meaningful and necessary for the client to carry out roles in home, work, and community environments. • Client factors, including values, beliefs, spirituality, body functions (e.g., neuromuscular, sensory and pain, visual, perceptual, cognitive, mental) and body structures (e.g., cardiovascular, digestive, nervous, genitourinary, integumentary systems). • Performance patterns (e.g., habits, routines, rituals, roles). • Context (e.g., cultural, personal, temporal, virtual) and environment (e.g., physical, social). • Performance skills, including motor and praxis skills, sensory–perceptual skills, emotional regulation skills, cognitive skills, and communication and social skills.	on the basis of the stated needs of the client as well as data gathered during the evaluation process in collaboration with the client and others. Intervention plans and strategies must be culturally relevant, reflective of current occupational therapy practice, and based on available evidence. Interventions address the following components: • The occupational profile, including participation in activities that are meaningful and necessary for the client to carry out roles in home, work, and community environments. • Client factors, including values, beliefs, spirituality, body functions (e.g., neuromuscular, sensory and pain, visual, perceptual, cognitive, mental) and body structures (e.g., cardiovascular, digestive, nervous, genitourinary, integumentary systems). • Performance patterns (e.g., habits, routines, rituals, roles). • Context (e.g., cultural, personal, temporal, virtual) and environment (e.g., physical, social). • Performance skills, including motor and praxis skills, sensory–perceptual skills, emotional regulation skills, cognitive skills, and communication and social skills.	process in collaboration with the client and others. Intervention plans and strategies must be culturally relevant, reflective of current occupational therapy practice, and based on available evidence. Interventions address the following components: • The occupational profile, including participation in activities that are meaningful and necessary for the client to carry out roles in home, work, and community environments. • Client factors, including values, beliefs, spirituality, body functions (e.g., neuromuscular, sensory and pain, visual, perceptual, cognitive, mental) and body structures (e.g., cardiovascular, digestive, nervous, genitourinary, integumentary systems). • Performance patterns (e.g., habits, routines, rituals, roles). • Context (e.g., cultural, personal, temporal, virtual) and environment (e.g., physical, social). • Performance skills, including motor and praxis skills, sensory–perceptual skills, emotional regulation skills, cognitive skills, and communication and social skills.

(Continued)

86

(Continued)

Standard Number	Accreditation Standards for a Doctoral-Degree-Level Educational Program for the Occupational Therapist	Accreditation Standards for a Master's-Degree-Level Educational Program for the Occupational Therapist	Accreditation Standards for an Associate-Degree-Level Educational Program for the Occupational Therapy Assistant
B.5.2.	Select and provide direct occupational therapy interventions and procedures to enhance safety, health and wellness, and performance in ADLs, IADLs, education, work, play, rest, sleep, leisure, and social participation.	Select and provide direct occupational therapy interventions and procedures to enhance safety, health and wellness, and performance in ADLs, IADLs, education, work, play, rest, sleep, leisure, and social participation.	Select and provide direct occupational therapy interventions and procedures to enhance safety, health and wellness, and performance in ADLs, IADLs, education, work, play, rest, sleep, leisure, and social participation.
B.5.3.	Provide therapeutic use of occupation, exercises, and activities (e.g., occupation-based intervention, purposeful activity, preparatory methods).	Provide therapeutic use of occupation, exercises, and activities (e.g., occupation-based intervention, purposeful activity, preparatory methods).	Provide therapeutic use of occupation, exercises, and activities (e.g., occupation-based intervention, purposeful activity, preparatory methods).
B.5.4.	Design and implement group interventions based on principles of group development and group dynamics across the lifespan.	Design and implement group interventions based on principles of group development and group dynamics across the lifespan.	Implement group interventions based on principles of group development and group dynamics across the lifespan.
B.5.5.	Provide training in self-care, self-management, health management and maintenance, home management, and community and work integration.	Provide training in self-care, self-management, health management and maintenance, home management, and community and work integration.	Provide training in self-care, self-management, health management and maintenance, home management, and community and work integration.
B.5.6.	Provide development, remediation, and compensation for physical, mental, cognitive, perceptual, neuromuscular, behavioral skills, and sensory functions (e.g., vision, tactile, auditory, gustatory, olfactory, pain, temperature, pressure, vestibular, proprioception).	Provide development, remediation, and compensation for physical, mental, cognitive, perceptual, neuromuscular, behavioral skills, and sensory functions (e.g., vision, tactile, auditory, gustatory, olfactory, pain, temperature, pressure, vestibular, proprioception).	Provide development, remediation, and compensation for physical, mental, cognitive, perceptual, neuromuscular, behavioral skills, and sensory functions (e.g., vision, tactile, auditory, gustatory, olfactory, pain, temperature, pressure, vestibular, proprioception).

Standard Number	Accreditation Standards for a Doctoral-Degree-Level Educational Program for the Occupational Therapist	Accreditation Standards for a Master's-Degree-Level Educational Program for the Occupational Therapist	Accreditation Standards for an Associate-Degree-Level Educational Program for the Occupational Therapy Assistant
B.5.7.	Demonstrate therapeutic use of self, including one's personality, insights, perceptions, and judgments, as part of the therapeutic process in both individual and group interaction.	Demonstrate therapeutic use of self, including one's personality, insights, perceptions, and judgments, as part of the therapeutic process in both individual and group interaction.	Demonstrate therapeutic use of self, including one's personality, insights, perceptions, and judgments, as part of the therapeutic process in both individual and group interaction.
B.5.8.	Develop and implement intervention strategies to remediate and/or compensate for cognitive deficits that affect occupational performance.	Develop and implement intervention strategies to remediate and/or compensate for cognitive deficits that affect occupational performance.	Implement intervention strategies to remediate and/or compensate for cognitive deficits that affect occupational performance.
B.5.9.	Evaluate and adapt processes or environments (e.g., home, work, school, community) applying ergonomic principles and principles of environmental modification.	Evaluate and adapt processes or environments (e.g., home, work, school, community) applying ergonomic principles and principles of environmental modification.	Adapt environments (e.g., home, work, school, community) and processes, including the application of ergonomic principles.
B.5.10.	Articulate principles of and be able to design, fabricate, apply, fit, and train in assistive technologies and devices (e.g., electronic aids to daily living, seating and positioning systems) used to enhance occupational performance and foster participation and well-being.	Articulate principles of and be able to design, fabricate, apply, fit, and train in assistive technologies and devices (e.g., electronic aids to daily living, seating and positioning systems) used to enhance occupational performance and foster participation and well-being.	Articulate principles of and demonstrate strategies with assistive technologies and devices (e.g., electronic aids to daily living, seating and positioning systems) used to enhance occupational performance and foster participation and well-being.
B.5.11.	Provide design, fabrication, application, fitting, and training in orthotic devices used to enhance occupational performance and participation. Train in the use of prosthetic devices, based on scientific principles of kinesiology, biomechanics, and physics.	Provide design, fabrication, application, fitting, and training in orthotic devices used to enhance occupational performance and participation. Train in the use of prosthetic devices, based on scientific principles of kinesiology, biomechanics, and physics.	Provide fabrication, application, fitting, and training in orthotic devices used to enhance occupational performance and participation, and training in the use of prosthetic devices.

(Continued)

Standard Number	Accreditation Standards for a Doctoral-Degree-Level Educational Program for the Occupational Therapist	Accreditation Standards for a Master's-Degree-Level Educational Program for the Occupational Therapist	Accreditation Standards for an Associate-Degree-Level Educational Program for the Occupational Therapy Assistant
B.5.12.	Provide recommendations and training in techniques to enhance functional mobility, including physical transfers, wheelchair management, and mobility devices.	Provide recommendations and training in techniques to enhance functional mobility, including physical transfers, wheelchair management, and mobility devices.	Provide training in techniques to enhance functional mobility, including physical transfers, wheelchair management, and mobility devices.
B.5.13.	Provide recommendations and training in techniques to enhance community mobility, including public transportation, community access, and issues related to driver rehabilitation.	Provide recommendations and training in techniques to enhance community mobility, including public transportation, community access, and issues related to driver rehabilitation.	Provide training in techniques to enhance community mobility, including public transportation, community access, and issues related to driver rehabilitation.
B.5.14.	Provide management of feeding, eating, and swallowing to enable performance (including the process of bringing food or fluids from the plate or cup to the mouth, the ability to keep and manipulate food or fluid in the mouth, and swallowing assessment and management) and train others in precautions and techniques while considering client and contextual factors.	Provide management of feeding, eating, and swallowing to enable performance (including the process of bringing food or fluids from the plate or cup to the mouth, the ability to keep and manipulate food or fluid in the mouth, and swallowing assessment and management) and train others in precautions and techniques while considering client and contextual factors.	Enable feeding and eating performance (including the process of bringing food or fluids from the plate or cup to the mouth, the ability to keep and manipulate food or fluid in the mouth, and the initiation of swallowing) and train others in precautions and techniques while considering client and contextual factors.
B.5.15.	Demonstrate safe and effective application of superficial thermal and mechanical modalities as a preparatory measure to manage pain and improve occupational performance, including foundational knowledge, underlying principles, indications, contraindications, and precautions.	Demonstrate safe and effective application of superficial thermal and mechanical modalities as a preparatory measure to manage pain and improve occupational performance, including foundational knowledge, underlying principles, indications, contraindications, and precautions.	Recognize the use of superficial thermal and mechanical modalities as a preparatory measure to improve occupational performance. On the basis of the intervention plan, demonstrate safe and effective administration of superficial thermal and mechanical modalities to achieve established goals while adhering to contraindications and precautions.

(Continued)

89

Standard Number	Accreditation Standards for a Doctoral-Degree-Level Educational Program for the Occupational Therapist	Accreditation Standards for a Master's-Degree-Level Educational Program for the Occupational Therapist	Accreditation Standards for an Associate-Degree-Level Educational Program for the Occupational Therapy Assistant
B.5.16.	Explain the use of deep thermal and electrotherapeutic modalities as a preparatory measure to improve occupational performance, including indications, contraindications, and precautions.	Explain the use of deep thermal and electrotherapeutic modalities as a preparatory measure to improve occupational performance, including indications, contraindications, and precautions.	(No related Standard)
B.5.17.	Develop and promote the use of appropriate home and community programming to support performance in the client's natural environment and participation in all contexts relevant to the client.	Develop and promote the use of appropriate home and community programming to support performance in the client's natural environment and participation in all contexts relevant to the client.	Promote the use of appropriate home and community programming to support performance in the client's natural environment and participation in all contexts relevant to the client.
B.5.18.	Demonstrate an understanding of health literacy and the ability to educate and train the client, caregiver, family and significant others, and communities to facilitate skills in areas of occupation as well as prevention, health maintenance, health promotion, and safety.	Demonstrate an understanding of health literacy and the ability to educate and train the client, caregiver, family and significant others, and communities to facilitate skills in areas of occupation as well as prevention, health maintenance, health promotion, and safety.	Demonstrate an understanding of health literacy and the ability to educate and train the client, caregiver, and family and significant others to facilitate skills in areas of occupation as well as prevention, health maintenance, health promotion, and safety.
B.5.19.	Apply the principles of the teaching–learning process using educational methods to design experiences to address the needs of the client, family, significant others, communities, colleagues, other health providers, and the public.	Apply the principles of the teaching–learning process using educational methods to design experiences to address the needs of the client, family, significant others, colleagues, other health providers, and the public.	Use the teaching–learning process with the client, family, significant others, colleagues, other health providers, and the public. Collaborate with the occupational therapist and learner to identify appropriate educational methods.
B.5.20.	Effectively interact through written, oral, and nonverbal communication with the client, family, significant others, communities, colleagues, other health providers, and the public in a professionally acceptable manner.	Effectively interact through written, oral, and nonverbal communication with the client, family, significant others, colleagues, other health providers, and the public in a professionally acceptable manner.	Effectively interact through written, oral, and nonverbal communication with the client, family, significant others, colleagues, other health providers, and the public in a professionally acceptable manner.

(Continued)

90

Standard Number	Accreditation Standards for a Doctoral-Degree-Level Educational Program for the Occupational Therapist	Accreditation Standards for a Master's-Degree-Level Educational Program for the Occupational Therapist	Accreditation Standards for an Associate-Degree-Level Educational Program for the Occupational Therapy Assistant
B.5.21.	Effectively communicate, coordinate, and work interprofessionally with those who provide services to individuals, organizations, and/or populations in order to clarify each member's responsibility in executing components of an intervention plan.	Effectively communicate and work interprofessionally with those who provide services to individuals, organizations, and/or populations in order to clarify each member's responsibility in executing an intervention plan.	Effectively communicate and work interprofessionally with those who provide services to individuals and groups in order to clarify each member's responsibility in executing an intervention plan.
B.5.22.	Refer to specialists (both internal and external to the profession) for consultation and intervention.	Refer to specialists (both internal and external to the profession) for consultation and intervention.	Recognize and communicate the need to refer to specialists (both internal and external to the profession) for consultation and intervention.
B.5.23.	Grade and adapt the environment, tools, materials, occupations, and interventions to reflect the changing needs of the client, the sociocultural context, and technological advances.	Grade and adapt the environment, tools, materials, occupations, and interventions to reflect the changing needs of the client, the sociocultural context, and technological advances.	Grade and adapt the environment, tools, materials, occupations, and interventions to reflect the changing needs of the client and the sociocultural context.
B.5.24.	Select and teach compensatory strategies, such as use of technology and adaptations to the environment, that support performance, participation, and well-being.	Select and teach compensatory strategies, such as use of technology and adaptations to the environment, that support performance, participation, and well-being.	Teach compensatory strategies, such as use of technology and adaptations to the environment, that support performance, participation, and well-being.
B.5.25.	Identify and demonstrate techniques in skills of supervision and collaboration with occupational therapy assistants and other professionals on therapeutic interventions.	Identify and demonstrate techniques in skills of supervision and collaboration with occupational therapy assistants and other professionals on therapeutic interventions.	Demonstrate skills of collaboration with occupational therapists and other professionals on therapeutic interventions.

(Continued)

Standard Number	Accreditation Standards for a Doctoral-Degree-Level Educational Program for the Occupational Therapist	Accreditation Standards for a Master's-Degree-Level Educational Program for the Occupational Therapist	Accreditation Standards for an Associate-Degree-Level Educational Program for the Occupational Therapy Assistant
B.5.26.	Demonstrate use of the consultative process with groups, programs, organizations, or communities.	Understand when and how to use the consultative process with groups, programs, organizations, or communities.	Understand when and how to use the consultative process with specific consumers or consumer groups as directed by an occupational therapist.
B.5.27.	Demonstrate care coordination, case management, and transition services in traditional and emerging practice environments.	Describe the role of the occupational therapist in care coordination, case management, and transition services in traditional and emerging practice environments.	Describe the role of the occupational therapy assistant in care coordination, case management, and transition services in traditional and emerging practice environments.
B.5.28.	Monitor and reassess, in collaboration with the client, caregiver, family, and significant others, the effect of occupational therapy intervention and the need for continued or modified intervention.	Monitor and reassess, in collaboration with the client, caregiver, family, and significant others, the effect of occupational therapy intervention and the need for continued or modified intervention.	Monitor and reassess, in collaboration with the client, caregiver, family, and significant others, the effect of occupational therapy intervention and the need for continued or modified intervention, and communicate the identified needs to the occupational therapist.
B.5.29.	Plan for discharge, in collaboration with the client, by reviewing the needs of the client, caregiver, family, and significant others; available resources; and discharge environment. This process includes, but is not limited to, identification of client's current status within the continuum of care; identification of community, human, and fiscal resources; recommendations for environmental adaptations; and home programming to facilitate the client's progression along the continuum toward outcome goals.	Plan for discharge, in collaboration with the client, by reviewing the needs of the client, caregiver, family, and significant others; available resources; and discharge environment. This process includes, but is not limited to, identification of client's current status within the continuum of care; identification of community, human, and fiscal resources; recommendations for environmental adaptations; and home programming to facilitate the client's progression along the continuum toward outcome goals.	Facilitate discharge planning by reviewing the needs of the client, caregiver, family, and significant others; available resources; and discharge environment, and identify those needs to the occupational therapist, client, and others involved in discharge planning. This process includes, but is not limited to, identification of community, human, and fiscal resources; recommendations for environmental adaptations; and home programming.

(Continued)

92

(Continued)

Standard Number	Accreditation Standards for a Doctoral-Degree-Level Educational Program for the Occupational Therapist	Accreditation Standards for a Master's-Degree-Level Educational Program for the Occupational Therapist	Accreditation Standards for an Associate-Degree-Level Educational Program for the Occupational Therapy Assistant
B.5.30.	Organize, collect, and analyze data in a systematic manner for evaluation of practice outcomes. Report evaluation results and modify practice as needed to improve client outcomes.	Organize, collect, and analyze data in a systematic manner for evaluation of practice outcomes. Report evaluation results and modify practice as needed to improve client outcomes.	Under the direction of an administrator, manager, or occupational therapist, collect, organize, and report on data for evaluation of client outcomes.
B.5.31.	Terminate occupational therapy services when stated outcomes have been achieved or it has been determined that they cannot be achieved. This process includes developing a summary of occupational therapy outcomes, appropriate recommendations, and referrals and discussion of postdischarge needs with the client and with appropriate others.	Terminate occupational therapy services when stated outcomes have been achieved or it has been determined that they cannot be achieved. This process includes developing a summary of occupational therapy outcomes, appropriate recommendations, and referrals and discussion of post-discharge needs with the client and with appropriate others.	Recommend to the occupational therapist the need for termination of occupational therapy services when stated outcomes have been achieved or it has been determined that they cannot be achieved. Assist with developing a summary of occupational therapy outcomes, recommendations, and referrals.
B.5.32.	Document occupational therapy services to ensure accountability of service provision and to meet standards for reimbursement of services. Documentation must effectively communicate the need and rationale for occupational therapy services and must be appropriate to the context in which the service is delivered.	Document occupational therapy services to ensure accountability of service provision and to meet standards for reimbursement of services. Documentation must effectively communicate the need and rationale for occupational therapy services and must be appropriate to the context in which the service is delivered.	Document occupational therapy services to ensure accountability of service provision and to meet standards for reimbursement of services. Documentation must effectively communicate the need and rationale for occupational therapy services and must be appropriate to the context in which the service is delivered.
B.5.33.	Provide population-based occupational therapy intervention that addresses occupational needs as identified by a community.	*(No related Standard)*	*(No related Standard)*

Standard Number	Accreditation Standards for a Doctoral-Degree-Level Educational Program for the Occupational Therapist	Accreditation Standards for a Master's-Degree-Level Educational Program for the Occupational Therapist	Accreditation Standards for an Associate-Degree-Level Educational Program for the Occupational Therapy Assistant
B.6.0. CONTEXT OF SERVICE DELIVERY Context of service delivery includes the knowledge and understanding of the various contexts, such as professional, social, cultural, political, economic, and ecological, in which occupational therapy services are provided. The program must facilitate development of the performance criteria listed below. The student will be able to			
B.6.1.	Evaluate and address the various contexts of health care, education, community, political, and social systems as they relate to the practice of occupational therapy.	Evaluate and address the various contexts of health care, education, community, political, and social systems as they relate to the practice of occupational therapy.	Describe the contexts of health care, education, community, and social systems as they relate to the practice of occupational therapy.
B.6.2.	Analyze the current policy issues and the social, economic, political, geographic, and demographic factors that influence the various contexts for practice of occupational therapy.	Analyze the current policy issues and the social, economic, political, geographic, and demographic factors that influence the various contexts for practice of occupational therapy.	Identify the potential impact of current policy issues and the social, economic, political, geographic, or demographic factors on the practice of occupational therapy.
B.6.3.	Integrate current social, economic, political, geographic, and demographic factors to promote policy development and the provision of occupational therapy services.	Integrate current social, economic, political, geographic, and demographic factors to promote policy development and the provision of occupational therapy services.	*(No related Standard)*
B.6.4.	Advocate for changes in service delivery policies, effect changes in the system, and identify opportunities to address societal needs.	Articulate the role and responsibility of the practitioner to advocate for changes in service delivery policies, to effect changes in the system, and to identify opportunities in emerging practice areas.	Identify the role and responsibility of the practitioner to advocate for changes in service delivery policies, to effect changes in the system, and to recognize opportunities in emerging practice areas.

(Continued)

Standard Number	Accreditation Standards for a Doctoral-Degree-Level Educational Program for the Occupational Therapist	Accreditation Standards for a Master's-Degree-Level Educational Program for the Occupational Therapist	Accreditation Standards for an Associate-Degree-Level Educational Program for the Occupational Therapy Assistant
B.6.5.	Analyze the trends in models of service delivery, including, but not limited to, medical, educational, community, and social models, and their potential effect on the practice of occupational therapy.	Analyze the trends in models of service delivery, including, but not limited to, medical, educational, community, and social models, and their potential effect on the practice of occupational therapy.	*(No related Standard)*
B.6.6.	Integrate national and international resources in education, research, practice, and policy development.	Utilize national and international resources in making assessment or intervention choices and appreciate the influence of international occupational therapy contributions to education, research, and practice.	*(No related Standard)*
B.7.0.	**LEADERSHIP AND MANAGEMENT** Leadership and management skills include principles and applications of leadership and management theory. The program must facilitate development of the performance criteria listed below. The student will be able to	**MANAGEMENT OF OCCUPATIONAL THERAPY SERVICES** Management of occupational therapy services includes the application of principles of management and systems in the provision of occupational therapy services to individuals and organizations. The program must facilitate development of the performance criteria listed below. The student will be able to	**ASSISTANCE WITH MANAGEMENT OF OCCUPATIONAL THERAPY SERVICES** Assistance with management of occupational therapy services includes the application of principles of management and systems in the provision of occupational therapy services to individuals and organizations. The program must facilitate development of the performance criteria listed below. The student will be able to
B.7.1.	Identify and evaluate the impact of contextual factors on the management and delivery of occupational therapy services for individuals and populations.	Describe and discuss the impact of contextual factors on the management and delivery of occupational therapy services.	Identify the impact of contextual factors on the management and delivery of occupational therapy services.

(Continued)

Standard Number	Accreditation Standards for a Doctoral-Degree-Level Educational Program for the Occupational Therapist	Accreditation Standards for a Master's-Degree-Level Educational Program for the Occupational Therapist	Accreditation Standards for an Associate-Degree-Level Educational Program for the Occupational Therapy Assistant
B.7.2.	Identify and evaluate the systems and structures that create federal and state legislation and regulations and their implications and effects on practice and policy.	Describe the systems and structures that create federal and state legislation and regulations and their implications and effects on practice.	Identify the systems and structures that create federal and state legislation and regulations and their implications and effects on practice.
B.7.3.	Demonstrate knowledge of applicable national requirements for credentialing and requirements for licensure, certification, or registration under state laws.	Demonstrate knowledge of applicable national requirements for credentialing and requirements for licensure, certification, or registration under state laws.	Demonstrate knowledge of applicable national requirements for credentialing and requirements for licensure, certification, or registration under state laws.
B.7.4.	Demonstrate knowledge of various reimbursement systems (e.g., federal, state, third party, private payer), appeals mechanisms, and documentation requirements that affect society and the practice of occupational therapy.	Demonstrate knowledge of various reimbursement systems (e.g., federal, state, third party, private payer), appeals mechanisms, and documentation requirements that affect the practice of occupational therapy.	Demonstrate knowledge of various reimbursement systems (e.g., federal, state, third party, private payer) and documentation requirements that affect the practice of occupational therapy.
B.7.5.	Demonstrate leadership skills in the ability to plan, develop, organize, and market the delivery of services to include the determination of programmatic needs and service delivery options and formulation and management of staffing for effective service provision.	Demonstrate the ability to plan, develop, organize, and market the delivery of services to include the determination of programmatic needs and service delivery options and formulation and management of staffing for effective service provision.	Demonstrate the ability to participate in the development, marketing, and management of service delivery options.
B.7.6.	Demonstrate leadership skills in the ability to design ongoing processes for quality improvement (e.g., outcome studies analysis) and develop program changes as needed to ensure quality of services and to direct administrative changes.	Demonstrate the ability to design ongoing processes for quality improvement (e.g., outcome studies analysis) and develop program changes as needed to ensure quality of services and to direct administrative changes.	Participate in the documentation of ongoing processes for quality improvement and implement program changes as needed to ensure quality of services.

(Continued)

(Continued)

Standard Number	Accreditation Standards for a Doctoral-Degree-Level Educational Program for the Occupational Therapist	Accreditation Standards for a Master's-Degree-Level Educational Program for the Occupational Therapist	Accreditation Standards for an Associate-Degree-Level Educational Program for the Occupational Therapy Assistant
B.7.7.	Develop strategies for effective, competency-based legal and ethical supervision of occupational therapy and non–occupational therapy personnel.	Develop strategies for effective, competency-based legal and ethical supervision of occupational therapy and non–occupational therapy personnel.	Identify strategies for effective, competency-based legal and ethical supervision of nonprofessional personnel.
B.7.8.	Describe the ongoing professional responsibility for providing fieldwork education and the criteria for becoming a fieldwork educator.	Describe the ongoing professional responsibility for providing fieldwork education and the criteria for becoming a fieldwork educator.	Describe the ongoing professional responsibility for providing fieldwork education and the criteria for becoming a fieldwork educator.
B.7.9.	Demonstrate knowledge of and the ability to write program development plans for provision of occupational therapy services to individuals and populations.	*(No related Standard)*	*(No related Standard)*
B.7.10.	Identify and adapt existing models or develop new service provision models to respond to policy, regulatory agencies, and reimbursement and compliance standards.	*(No related Standard)*	*(No related Standard)*
B.7.11.	Identify and develop strategies to enable occupational therapy to respond to society's changing needs.	*(No related Standard)*	*(No related Standard)*
B.7.12.	Identify and implement strategies to promote staff development that are based on evaluation of the personal and professional abilities and competencies of supervised staff as they relate to job responsibilities.	*(No related Standard)*	*(No related Standard)*

Standard Number	Accreditation Standards for a Doctoral-Degree-Level Educational Program for the Occupational Therapist	Accreditation Standards for a Master's-Degree-Level Educational Program for the Occupational Therapist	Accreditation Standards for an Associate-Degree-Level Educational Program for the Occupational Therapy Assistant
B.8.0. SCHOLARSHIP Promotion of scholarly endeavors will serve to describe and interpret the scope of the profession, establish new knowledge, and interpret and apply this knowledge to practice. The program must facilitate development of the performance criteria listed below. The student will be able to			
B.8.1.	Articulate the importance of how scholarly activities contribute to the development of a body of knowledge relevant to the profession of occupational therapy.	Articulate the importance of how scholarly activities contribute to the development of a body of knowledge relevant to the profession of occupational therapy.	Articulate the importance of how scholarly activities and literature contribute to the development of the profession.
B.8.2.	Effectively locate, understand, critique, and evaluate information, including the quality of evidence.	Effectively locate, understand, critique, and evaluate information, including the quality of evidence.	Effectively locate and understand information, including the quality of the source of information.
B.8.3.	Use scholarly literature to make evidence-based decisions.	Use scholarly literature to make evidence-based decisions.	Use professional literature to make evidence-based practice decisions in collaboration with the occupational therapist.
B.8.4.	Select, apply, and interpret basic descriptive, correlational, and inferential quantitative statistics and code, analyze, and synthesize qualitative data.	Understand and use basic descriptive, correlational, and inferential quantitative statistics and code, analyze, and synthesize qualitative data.	*(No related Standard)*
B.8.5.	Understand and critique the validity of research studies, including their design (both quantitative and qualitative) and methodology.	Understand and critique the validity of research studies, including their design (both quantitative and qualitative) and methodology.	*(No related Standard)*

(Continued)

Standard Number	Accreditation Standards for a Doctoral-Degree-Level Educational Program for the Occupational Therapist	Accreditation Standards for a Master's-Degree-Level Educational Program for the Occupational Therapist	Accreditation Standards for an Associate-Degree-Level Educational Program for the Occupational Therapy Assistant
B.8.6.	Design a scholarly proposal that includes the research question, relevant literature, sample, design, measurement, and data analysis.	Demonstrate the skills necessary to design a scholarly proposal that includes the research question, relevant literature, sample, design, measurement, and data analysis.	*(No related Standard)*
B.8.7.	Implement a scholarly study that evaluates professional practice, service delivery, and/or professional issues (e.g., Scholarship of Integration, Scholarship of Application, Scholarship of Teaching and Learning).	Participate in scholarly activities that evaluate professional practice, service delivery, and/or professional issues (e.g., Scholarship of Integration, Scholarship of Application, Scholarship of Teaching and Learning).	Identify how scholarly activities can be used to evaluate professional practice, service delivery, and/or professional issues (e.g., Schclarship of Integration, Scholarship of Application, Scholarship of Teaching and Learning).
B.8.8.	Write scholarly reports appropriate for presentation or for publication in a peer-reviewed journal. Examples of scholarly reports would include position papers, white papers, and persuasive discussion papers.	Demonstrate skills necessary to write a scholarly report in a format for presentation or publication.	Demonstrate the skills to read and understand a scholarly report.
B.8.9.	Demonstrate an understanding of the process of locating and securing grants and how grants can serve as a fiscal resource for scholarly activities.	Demonstrate an understanding of the process of locating and securing grants and how grants can serve as a fiscal resource for scholarly activities.	*(No related Standard)*
B.8.10.	Complete a culminating project that relates theory to practice and demonstrates synthesis of advanced knowledge in a practice area.	*(No related Standard)*	*(No related Standard)*

(Continued)

Standard Number	Accreditation Standards for a Doctoral-Degree-Level Educational Program for the Occupational Therapist	Accreditation Standards for a Master's-Degree-Level Educational Program for the Occupational Therapist	Accreditation Standards for an Associate-Degree-Level Educational Program for the Occupational Therapy Assistant
B.9.0.	**PROFESSIONAL ETHICS, VALUES, AND RESPONSIBILITIES** Professional ethics, values, and responsibilities include an understanding and appreciation of ethics and values of the profession of occupational therapy. The program must facilitate development of the performance criteria listed below. The student will be able to		
B.9.1.	Demonstrate knowledge and understanding of the American Occupational Therapy Association (AOTA) *Occupational Therapy Code of Ethics and Ethics Standards* and AOTA *Standards of Practice* and use them as a guide for ethical decision making in professional interactions, client interventions, and employment settings.	Demonstrate knowledge and understanding of the American Occupational Therapy Association (AOTA) *Occupational Therapy Code of Ethics and Ethics Standards* and AOTA *Standards of Practice* and use them as a guide for ethical decision making in professional interactions, client interventions, and employment settings.	Demonstrate knowledge and understanding of the American Occupational Therapy Association (AOTA) *Occupational Therapy Code of Ethics and Ethics Standards* and AOTA *Standards of Practice* and use them as a guide for ethical decision making in professional interactions, client interventions, and employment settings.
B.9.2.	Discuss and justify how the role of a professional is enhanced by knowledge of and involvement in international, national, state, and local occupational therapy associations and related professional associations.	Discuss and justify how the role of a professional is enhanced by knowledge of and involvement in international, national, state, and local occupational therapy associations and related professional associations.	Explain and give examples of how the role of a professional is enhanced by knowledge of and involvement in international, national, state, and local occupational therapy associations and related professional associations.
B.9.3.	Promote occupational therapy by educating other professionals, service providers, consumers, third-party payers, regulatory bodies, and the public.	Promote occupational therapy by educating other professionals, service providers, consumers, third-party payers, regulatory bodies, and the public.	Promote occupational therapy by educating other professionals, service providers, consumers, third-party payers, regulatory bodies, and the public.
B.9.4.	Identify and develop strategies for ongoing professional development to ensure that practice is consistent with current and accepted standards.	Discuss strategies for ongoing professional development to ensure that practice is consistent with current and accepted standards.	Discuss strategies for ongoing professional development to ensure that practice is consistent with current and accepted standards.

(Continued)

Standard Number	Accreditation Standards for a Doctoral-Degree-Level Educational Program for the Occupational Therapist	Accreditation Standards for a Master's-Degree-Level Educational Program for the Occupational Therapist	Accreditation Standards for an Associate-Degree-Level Educational Program for the Occupational Therapy Assistant
B.9.5.	Discuss professional responsibilities related to liability issues under current models of service provision.	Discuss professional responsibilities related to liability issues under current models of service provision.	Identify professional responsibilities related to liability issues under current models of service provision.
B.9.6.	Discuss and evaluate personal and professional abilities and competencies as they relate to job responsibilities.	Discuss and evaluate personal and professional abilities and competencies as they relate to job responsibilities.	Identify personal and professional abilities and competencies as they relate to job responsibilities.
B.9.7.	Discuss and justify the varied roles of the occupational therapist as a practitioner, educator, researcher, policy developer, program developer, advocate, administrator, consultant, and entrepreneur.	Discuss and justify the varied roles of the occupational therapist as a practitioner, educator, researcher, consultant, and entrepreneur.	Identify and appreciate the varied roles of the occupational therapy assistant as a practitioner, educator, and research assistant.
B.9.8.	Explain and justify the importance of supervisory roles, responsibilities, and collaborative professional relationships between the occupational therapist and the occupational therapy assistant.	Explain and justify the importance of supervisory roles, responsibilities, and collaborative professional relationships between the occupational therapist and the occupational therapy assistant.	Identify and explain the need for supervisory roles, responsibilities, and collaborative professional relationships between the occupational therapist and the occupational therapy assistant.
B.9.9.	Describe and discuss professional responsibilities and issues when providing service on a contractual basis.	Describe and discuss professional responsibilities and issues when providing service on a contractual basis.	Identify professional responsibilities and issues when providing service on a contractual basis.
B.9.10.	Demonstrate strategies for analyzing issues and making decisions to resolve personal and organizational ethical conflicts.	Demonstrate strategies for analyzing issues and making decisions to resolve personal and organizational ethical conflicts.	Identify strategies for analyzing issues and making decisions to resolve personal and organizational ethical conflicts.

(Continued)

Standard Number	Accreditation Standards for a Doctoral-Degree-Level Educational Program for the Occupational Therapist	Accreditation Standards for a Master's-Degree-Level Educational Program for the Occupational Therapist	Accreditation Standards for an Associate-Degree-Level Educational Program for the Occupational Therapy Assistant
B.9.11.	Demonstrate a variety of informal and formal strategies for resolving ethics disputes in varying practice areas.	Explain the variety of informal and formal systems for resolving ethics disputes that have jurisdiction over occupational therapy practice.	Identify the variety of informal and formal systems for resolving ethics disputes that have jurisdiction over occupational therapy practice.
B.9.12.	Describe and implement strategies to assist the consumer in gaining access to occupational therapy and other health and social services.	Describe and discuss strategies to assist the consumer in gaining access to occupational therapy services.	Identify strategies to assist the consumer in gaining access to occupational therapy services.
B.9.13.	Demonstrate advocacy by participating in and exploring leadership positions in organizations or agencies promoting the profession (e.g., AOTA, World Federation of Occupational Therapists, advocacy organizations), consumer access and services, and the welfare of the community.	Demonstrate professional advocacy by participating in organizations or agencies promoting the profession (e.g., AOTA, state occupational therapy associations, advocacy organizations).	Demonstrate professional advocacy by participating in organizations or agencies promoting the profession (e.g., AOTA, state occupational therapy associations, advocacy organizations).

SECTION C: FIELDWORK EDUCATION AND DOCTORAL EXPERIENTIAL COMPONENT

C.1.0. FIELDWORK EDUCATION

Fieldwork education is a crucial part of professional preparation and is best integrated as a component of the curriculum design. Fieldwork experiences should be implemented and evaluated for their effectiveness by the educational institution. The experience should provide the student with the opportunity to carry out professional responsibilities under supervision of a qualified occupational therapy practitioner serving as a role model. The academic fieldwork coordinator is responsible for the program's compliance with fieldwork education requirements. The academic fieldwork coordinator will

| C.1.1. | Ensure that the fieldwork program reflects the sequence and scope of content in the curriculum design in collaboration with faculty so | Ensure that the fieldwork program reflects the sequence and scope of content in the curriculum design in collaboration with faculty so | Ensure that the fieldwork program reflects the sequence and scope of content in the curriculum design in collaboration with faculty so |

(Continued)

(Continued)

Standard Number	Accreditation Standards for a Doctoral-Degree-Level Educational Program for the Occupational Therapist	Accreditation Standards for a Master's-Degree-Level Educational Program for the Occupational Therapist	Accreditation Standards for an Associate-Degree-Level Educational Program for the Occupational Therapy Assistant
	that fieldwork experiences strengthen the ties between didactic and fieldwork education.	that fieldwork experiences strengthen the ties between didactic and fieldwork education.	that fieldwork experiences strengthen the ties between didactic and fieldwork education.
C.1.2.	Document the criteria and process for selecting fieldwork sites, to include maintaining memoranda of understanding, complying with all site requirements, maintaining site objectives and site data, and communicating this information to students.	Document the criteria and process for selecting fieldwork sites, to include maintaining memoranda of understanding, complying with all site requirements, maintaining site objectives and site data, and communicating this information to students.	Document the criteria and process for selecting fieldwork sites, to include maintaining memoranda of understanding, complying with all site requirements, maintaining site objectives and site data, and communicating this information to students.
C.1.3.	Demonstrate that academic and fieldwork educators collaborate in establishing fieldwork objectives and communicate with the student and fieldwork educator about progress and performance during fieldwork.	Demonstrate that academic and fieldwork educators collaborate in establishing fieldwork objectives and communicate with the student and fieldwork educator about progress and performance during fieldwork.	Demonstrate that academic and fieldwork educators collaborate in establishing fieldwork objectives and communicate with the student and fieldwork educator about progress and performance during fieldwork.
C.1.4.	Ensure that the ratio of fieldwork educators to students enables proper supervision and the ability to provide frequent assessment of student progress in achieving stated fieldwork objectives.	Ensure that the ratio of fieldwork educators to students enables proper supervision and the ability to provide frequent assessment of student progress in achieving stated fieldwork objectives.	Ensure that the ratio of fieldwork educators to students enables proper supervision and the ability to provide frequent assessment of student progress in achieving stated fieldwork objectives.
C.1.5.	Ensure that fieldwork agreements are sufficient in scope and number to allow completion of graduation requirements in a timely manner in accordance with the policy adopted by the program as required by Standard A.4.14.	Ensure that fieldwork agreements are sufficient in scope and number to allow completion of graduation requirements in a timely manner in accordance with the policy adopted by the program as required by Standard A.4.14.	Ensure that fieldwork agreements are sufficient in scope and number to allow completion of graduation requirements in a timely manner in accordance with the policy adopted by the program as required by Standard A.4.14.

Standard Number	Accreditation Standards for a Doctoral-Degree-Level Educational Program for the Occupational Therapist	Accreditation Standards for a Master's-Degree-Level Educational Program for the Occupational Therapist	Accreditation Standards for an Associate-Degree-Level Educational Program for the Occupational Therapy Assistant
C.1.6.	The program must have evidence of valid memoranda of understanding in effect and signed by both parties at the time the student is completing the Level I or Level II fieldwork experience. (Electronic memoranda of understanding and signatures are acceptable.) Responsibilities of the sponsoring institution(s) and each fieldwork site must be clearly documented in the memorandum of understanding.	The program must have evidence of valid memoranda of understanding in effect and signed by both parties at the time the student is completing the Level I or Level II fieldwork experience. (Electronic memoranda of understanding and signatures are acceptable.) Responsibilities of the sponsoring institution(s) and each fieldwork site must be clearly documented in the memorandum of understanding.	The program must have evidence of valid memoranda of understanding in effect and signed by both parties at the time the student is completing the Level I or Level II fieldwork experience. (Electronic memoranda of understanding and signatures are acceptable.) Responsibilities of the sponsoring institution(s) and each fieldwork site must be clearly documented in the memorandum of understanding.
C.1.7.	Ensure that at least one fieldwork experience (either Level I or Level II) has as its focus psychological and social factors that influence engagement in occupation.	Ensure that at least one fieldwork experience (either Level I or Level II) has as its focus psychological and social factors that influence engagement in occupation.	Ensure that at least one fieldwork experience (either Level I or Level II) has as its focus psychological and social factors that influence engagement in occupation.
The goal of Level I fieldwork is to introduce students to the fieldwork experience, to apply knowledge to practice, and to develop understanding of the needs of clients. The program will			
C.1.8.	Ensure that Level I fieldwork is integral to the program's curriculum design and include experiences designed to enrich didactic coursework through directed observation and participation in selected aspects of the occupational therapy process.	Ensure that Level I fieldwork is integral to the program's curriculum design and include experiences designed to enrich didactic coursework through directed observation and participation in selected aspects of the occupational therapy process.	Ensure that Level I fieldwork is integral to the program's curriculum design and include experiences designed to enrich didactic coursework through directed observation and participation in selected aspects of the occupational therapy process.
C.1.9.	Ensure that qualified personnel supervise Level I fieldwork. Examples may include, but are not limited to, currently licensed or otherwise	Ensure that qualified personnel supervise Level I fieldwork. Examples may include, but are not limited to, currently licensed or otherwise	Ensure that qualified personnel supervise Level I fieldwork. Examples may include, but are not limited to, currently licensed or oth-

(Continued)

104

Standard Number	Accreditation Standards for a Doctoral-Degree-Level Educational Program for the Occupational Therapist	Accreditation Standards for a Master's-Degree-Level Educational Program for the Occupational Therapist	Accreditation Standards for an Associate-Degree-Level Educational Program for the Occupational Therapy Assistant
	regulated occupational therapists and occupational therapy assistants, psychologists, physician assistants, teachers, social workers, nurses, and physical therapists.	regulated occupational therapists and occupational therapy assistants, psychologists, physician assistants, teachers, social workers, nurses, and physical therapists.	erwise regulated occupational therapists and occupational therapy assistants, psychologists, physician assistants, teachers, social workers, nurses, and physical therapists.
C.1.10.	Document all Level I fieldwork experiences that are provided to students, including mechanisms for formal evaluation of student performance. Ensure that Level I fieldwork is not substituted for any part of Level II fieldwork.	Document all Level I fieldwork experiences that are provided to students, including mechanisms for formal evaluation of student performance. Ensure that Level I fieldwork is not substituted for any part of Level II fieldwork.	Document all Level I fieldwork experiences that are provided to students, including mechanisms for formal evaluation of student performance. Ensure that Level I fieldwork is not substituted for any part of Level II fieldwork.
The goal of Level II fieldwork is to develop competent, entry-level, generalist occupational therapists. Level II fieldwork must be integral to the program's curriculum design and must include an in-depth experience in delivering occupational therapy services to clients, focusing on the application of purposeful and meaningful occupation and research, administration, and management of occupational therapy services. It is recommended that the student be exposed to a variety of clients across the lifespan and to a variety of settings. The program will			**The goal of Level II fieldwork is to develop competent, entry-level, generalist occupational therapy assistants. Level II fieldwork must be integral to the program's curriculum design and must include an in-depth experience in delivering occupational therapy services to clients, focusing on the application of purposeful and meaningful occupation. It is recommended that the student be exposed to a variety of clients across the lifespan and to a variety of settings. The program will**
C.1.11.	Ensure that the fieldwork experience is designed to promote clinical reasoning and reflective practice, to transmit the values and beliefs that enable	Ensure that the fieldwork experience is designed to promote clinical reasoning and reflective practice, to transmit the values and beliefs that enable	Ensure that the fieldwork experience is designed to promote clinical reasoning appropriate to the occupational therapy assistant role,

(Continued)

Standard Number	Accreditation Standards for a Doctoral-Degree-Level Educational Program for the Occupational Therapist	Accreditation Standards for a Master's-Degree-Level Educational Program for the Occupational Therapist	Accreditation Standards for an Associate-Degree-Level Educational Program for the Occupational Therapy Assistant
	ethical practice, and to develop professionalism and competence in career responsibilities.	ethical practice, and to develop professionalism and competence in career responsibilities.	to transmit the values and beliefs that enable ethical practice, and to develop professionalism and competence in career responsibilities.
C.1.12.	Provide Level II fieldwork in traditional and/ or emerging settings, consistent with the curriculum design. In all settings, psychosocial factors influencing engagement in occupation must be understood and integrated for the development of client-centered, meaningful, occupation-based outcomes. The student can complete Level II fieldwork in a minimum of one setting if it is reflective of more than one practice area, or in a maximum of four different settings.	Provide Level II fieldwork in traditional and/or emerging settings, consistent with the curriculum design. In all settings, psychosocial factors influencing engagement in occupation must be understood and integrated for the development of client-centered, meaningful, occupation-based outcomes. The student can complete Level II fieldwork in a minimum of one setting if it is reflective of more than one practice area, or in a maximum of four different settings.	Provide Level II fieldwork in traditional and/or emerging settings, consistent with the curriculum design. In all settings, psychosocial factors influencing engagement in occupation must be understood and integrated for the development of client-centered, meaningful, occupation-based outcomes. The student can complete Level II fieldwork in a minimum of one setting if it is reflective of more than one practice area, or in a maximum of three different settings.
C.1.13.	Require a minimum of 24 weeks' full-time Level II fieldwork. This may be completed on a part-time basis, as defined by the fieldwork placement in accordance with the fieldwork placement's usual and customary personnel policies, as long as it is at least 50% of an FTE at that site.	Require a minimum of 24 weeks' full-time Level II fieldwork. This may be completed on a part-time basis, as defined by the fieldwork placement in accordance with the fieldwork placement's usual and customary personnel policies, as long as it is at least 50% of an FTE at that site.	Require a minimum of 16 weeks' full-time Level II fieldwork. This may be completed on a part-time basis, as defined by the fieldwork placement in accordance with the fieldwork placement's usual and customary personnel policies, as long as it is at least 50% of an FTE at that site.
C.1.14.	Ensure that the student is supervised by a currently licensed or otherwise regulated occupational therapist who has a minimum of 1 year full-time (or its equivalent) of practice experience subsequent to initial certification and who is adequately prepared to serve as a fieldwork	Ensure that the student is supervised by a currently licensed or otherwise regulated occupational therapist who has a minimum of 1 year full-time (or its equivalent) of practice experience subsequent to initial certification and who is adequately prepared to serve as a fieldwork	Ensure that the student is supervised by a currently licensed or otherwise regulated occupational therapist or occupational therapy assistant (under the supervision of an occupational therapist) who has a minimum of 1 year full-time (or its equivalent) of practice experience subsequent

(Continued)

Standard Number	Accreditation Standards for a Doctoral-Degree-Level Educational Program for the Occupational Therapist	Accreditation Standards for a Master's-Degree-Level Educational Program for the Occupational Therapist	Accreditation Standards for an Associate-Degree-Level Educational Program for the Occupational Therapy Assistant
	educator. The supervising therapist may be engaged by the fieldwork site or by the educational program.	educator. The supervising therapist may be engaged by the fieldwork site or by the educational program.	to initial certification and who is adequately prepared to serve as a fieldwork educator. The supervising therapist may be engaged by the fieldwork site or by the educational program.
C.1.15.	Document a mechanism for evaluating the effectiveness of supervision (e.g., student evaluation of fieldwork) and for providing resources for enhancing supervision (e.g., materials on supervisory skills, continuing education opportunities, articles on theory and practice).	Document a mechanism for evaluating the effectiveness of supervision (e.g., student evaluation of fieldwork) and for providing resources for enhancing supervision (e.g., materials on supervisory skills, continuing education opportunities, articles on theory and practice).	Document a mechanism for evaluating the effectiveness of supervision (e.g., student evaluation of fieldwork) and for providing resources for enhancing supervision (e.g., materials on supervisory skills, continuing education opportunities, articles on theory and practice).
C.1.16.	Ensure that supervision provides protection of consumers and opportunities for appropriate role modeling of occupational therapy practice. Initially, supervision should be direct and then decrease to less direct supervision as appropriate for the setting, the severity of the client's condition, and the ability of the student.	Ensure that supervision provides protection of consumers and opportunities for appropriate role modeling of occupational therapy practice. Initially, supervision should be direct and then decrease to less direct supervision as appropriate for the setting, the severity of the client's condition, and the ability of the student.	Ensure that supervision provides protection of consumers and opportunities for appropriate role modeling of occupational therapy practice. Initially, supervision should be direct and then decrease to less direct supervision as appropriate for the setting, the severity of the client's condition, and the ability of the student.
C.1.17.	Ensure that supervision provided in a setting where no occupational therapy services exist includes a documented plan for provision of occupational therapy services and supervision by a currently licensed or otherwise regulated occupational therapist with at least 3 years' full-time or its equivalent of professional experience. Supervision must include a minimum of 8 hours	Ensure that supervision provided in a setting where no occupational therapy services exist includes a documented plan for provision of occupational therapy services and supervision by a currently licensed or otherwise regulated occupational therapist with at least 3 years' full-time or its equivalent of professional experience. Supervision must include a minimum of 8 hours	Ensure that supervision provided in a setting where no occupational therapy services exist includes a documented plan for provision of occupational therapy assistant services and supervision by a currently licensed or otherwise regulated occupational therapist or occupational therapy assistant (under the direction of an occupational therapist) with at least 3 years'

(Continued)

Standard Number	Accreditation Standards for a Doctoral-Degree-Level Educational Program for the Occupational Therapist	Accreditation Standards for a Master's-Degree-Level Educational Program for the Occupational Therapist	Accreditation Standards for an Associate-Degree-Level Educational Program for the Occupational Therapy Assistant
	of direct supervision each week of the fieldwork experience. An occupational therapy supervisor must be available, via a variety of contact measures, to the student during all working hours. An on-site supervisor designee of another profession must be assigned while the occupational therapy supervisor is off site.	of direct supervision each week of the fieldwork experience. An occupational therapy supervisor must be available, via a variety of contact measures, to the student during all working hours. An on-site supervisor designee of another profession must be assigned while the occupational therapy supervisor is off site.	full-time or its equivalent of professional experience. Supervision must include a minimum of 8 hours of direct supervision each week of the fieldwork experience. An occupational therapy supervisor must be available, via a variety of contact measures, to the student during all working hours. An on-site supervisor designee of another profession must be assigned while the occupational therapy supervisor is off site.
C.1.18.	Document mechanisms for requiring formal evaluation of student performance on Level II fieldwork (e.g., the AOTA *Fieldwork Performance Evaluation for the Occupational Therapy Student* or equivalent).	Document mechanisms for requiring formal evaluation of student performance on Level II fieldwork (e.g., the AOTA *Fieldwork Performance Evaluation for the Occupational Therapy Student* or equivalent).	Document mechanisms for requiring formal evaluation of student performance on Level II fieldwork (e.g., the AOTA *Fieldwork Performance Evaluation for the Occupational Therapy Assistant Student* or equivalent).
C.1.19.	Ensure that students attending Level II fieldwork outside the United States are supervised by an occupational therapist who graduated from a program approved by the World Federation of Occupational Therapists and has 1 year of experience in practice.	Ensure that students attending Level II fieldwork outside the United States are supervised by an occupational therapist who graduated from a program approved by the World Federation of Occupational Therapists and has 1 year of experience in practice.	Ensure that students attending Level II fieldwork outside the United States are supervised by an occupational therapist who graduated from a program approved by the World Federation of Occupational Therapists and has 1 year of experience in practice.
C.2.0. DOCTORAL EXPERIENTIAL COMPONENT **The goal of the doctoral experiential component is to develop occupational therapists with advanced skills (those that are beyond a generalist level). The doctoral experiential component shall be an integral part of the**			

(Continued)

108

Standard Number	Accreditation Standards for a Doctoral-Degree-Level Educational Program for the Occupational Therapist	Accreditation Standards for a Master's-Degree-Level Educational Program for the Occupational Therapist	Accreditation Standards for an Associate-Degree-Level Educational Program for the Occupational Therapy Assistant
	program's curriculum design and shall include an in-depth experience in one or more of the following: clinical practice skills, research skills, administration, leadership, program and policy development, advocacy, education, or theory development.		
	The student must successfully complete all coursework and Level II fieldwork and pass a competency requirement prior to the commencement of the doctoral experiential component. The specific content and format of the competency requirement is determined by the program. Examples include a written comprehensive exam, oral exam, NBCOT certification exam readiness tool, and the NBCOT practice exams.		
C.2.1.	Ensure that the doctoral experiential component is designed and administered by faculty and provided in setting(s) consistent with the program's curriculum design, including individualized specific objectives and plans for supervision.	*(No related Standard)*	*(No related Standard)*
C.2.2.	Ensure that there is a memorandum of understanding that, at a minimum, includes individualized specific objectives, plans for supervision or mentoring, and responsibilities of all parties.	*(No related Standard)*	*(No related Standard)*
C.2.3.	Require that the length of this doctoral experiential component be a minimum of 16 weeks (640 hours). This may be completed on a part-	*(No related Standard)*	*(No related Standard)*

(Continued)

Standard Number	Accreditation Standards for a Doctoral-Degree-Level Educational Program for the Occupational Therapist	Accreditation Standards for a Master's-Degree-Level Educational Program for the Occupational Therapist	Accreditation Standards for an Associate-Degree-Level Educational Program for the Occupational Therapy Assistant
	time basis and must be consistent with the individualized specific objectives and culminating project. No more than 20% of the 640 hours can be completed outside of the mentored practice setting(s). Prior fieldwork or work experience may not be substituted for this experiential component.		
C.2.4.	Ensure that the student is mentored by an individual with expertise consistent with the student's area of focus. The mentor does not have to be an occupational therapist.	(No related Standard)	(No related Standard)
C.2.5.	Document a formal evaluation mechanism for objective assessment of the student's performance during and at the completion of the doctoral experiential component.	(No related Standard)	(No related Standard)

Glossary

Definitions given below are for the purposes of these documents.

ability to benefit—A phrase that refers to a student who does not have a high school diploma or its recognized equivalent but is eligible to receive funds under the Title IV Higher Education Act programs after taking an independently administered examination and achieving a score, specified by the Secretary of the U.S. Department of Education (USDE), indicating that the student has the ability to benefit from the education being offered.

academic calendar—The official institutional document that lists registration dates, semester/quarter stop and start dates, holidays, graduation dates, and other pertinent events. Generally, the academic year is divided into two major semesters, each approximately 14 to 16 weeks long. A smaller number of institutions have quarters rather than semesters. Quarters are approximately 10 weeks long; there are three major quarters and the summer session.

activity—A term that describes a class of human actions that are goal directed (AOTA, 2008b).

advanced—The stage of being beyond the elementary or introductory.

affiliate—An entity that formally cooperates with a sponsoring institution in implementing the occupational therapy educational program.

areas of occupation—Activities in which people engage: activities of daily living, instrumental activities of daily living, rest and sleep, education, work, play, leisure, and social participation.

assist—To aid, help, or hold an auxiliary position.

body functions—The physiological functions of body systems (including psychological functions).

body structures—Anatomical parts of the body, such as organs, limbs, and their components.

care coordination—The process that links clients with appropriate services and resources.

case management—A system to ensure that individuals receive appropriate health care services.

client—The term used to name the entity that receives occupational therapy services. Clients may include (1) individuals and other persons relevant to the client's life, including family, caregivers, teachers, employers, and others who may also help or be served indirectly; (2) organizations, such as businesses, industries, or agencies; and (3) populations within a community (AOTA, 2008b).

client-centered service delivery—An orientation that honors the desires and priorities of clients in designing and implementing interventions.

client factors—Factors that reside within the client and that may affect performance in areas of occupation. Client factors include body functions and body structures.

clinical reasoning—Complex multifaceted cognitive process used by practitioners to plan, direct, perform, and reflect on intervention.

collaborate—To work together with a mutual sharing of thoughts and ideas.

competent—To have the requisite abilities/qualities and capacity to function in a professional environment.

consumer—The direct and/or indirect recipient of educational and/or practitioner services offered.

context/contextual factors and environment:

> **context**—The variety of interrelated conditions within and surrounding the client that influence performance. Contexts include cultural, personal, temporal, and virtual aspects.

> **environment**—The external physical and social environment that surrounds the client and in which the client's daily life occupations occur.

context of service delivery—The knowledge and understanding of the various contexts in which occupational therapy services are provided.

criterion-referenced—Tests that compare the performance of an individual with that of another group, known as the *norm group.*

culminating project—A project that is completed by a doctoral student that demonstrates the student's ability to relate theory to practice and to synthesize advanced knowledge in a practice area.

curriculum design—An overarching set of assumptions that explains how the curriculum is planned, implemented, and evaluated. Typically, a curriculum design includes educational goals and curriculum threads and provides a clear rationale for the selection of content, the determination of scope of content, and the sequence of the content. A curriculum design is expected to be consistent with the mission and philosophy of the sponsoring institution and the program.

curriculum threads—Curriculum threads, or *themes,* are identified by the program as areas of study and development that follow a path through the curriculum and represent the unique qualities of the program, as demonstrated by the program's graduates. Curriculum threads are typically based on the profession's and program's vision, mission, and philosophy (e.g., occupational needs of society, critical thinking/professional reasoning, diversity/globalization; AOTA, 2008a).

diagnosis—The process of analyzing the cause or nature of a condition, situation, or problem. Diagnosis as stated in Standard B.4.0. refers to the occupational therapist's ability to analyze a problem associated with occupational performance and participation.

distance education—Education that uses one or more of the technologies listed below to deliver instruction to students who are separated from the instructor and to support regular and substantive interaction between the students and the instructor, either synchronously or asynchronously. The technologies may include

- The Internet;
- One-way and two-way transmissions through open broadcast, closed circuit, cable, microwave, broadband lines, fiber optics, satellite, or wireless communications devices;
- Audio conferencing; or
- Video cassettes, DVDs, and CD-ROMs, if the cassettes, DVDs, or CD-ROMs are used in a course.

driver rehabilitation—Specialized evaluation and training to develop mastery of specific skills and techniques to effectively drive a motor vehicle independently and in accordance with state department of motor vehicles regulations.

entry-level occupational therapist—The outcome of the occupational therapy educational and certification process; an individual prepared to begin generalist practice as an occupational therapist with less than 1 year of experience.

entry-level occupational therapy assistant—The outcome of the occupational therapy educational and certification process; an individual prepared to begin generalist practice as an occupational therapy assistant with less than 1 year of experience.

faculty:

> **faculty, core**—Persons who are resident faculty, including the program director, appointed to and employed primarily in the occupational therapy educational program.

> **faculty, full time**—Core faculty members who hold an appointment that is full time, as defined by the institution, and whose job responsibilities include teaching and/or contributing to the delivery of the designed curriculum regardless of the position title (e.g., full-time instructional staff and clinical instructors would be considered faculty).

> **faculty, part time**—Core faculty members who hold an appointment that is considered by that institution to constitute less than full-time service and whose job responsibilities include teaching and/or contributing to the delivery of the designed curriculum regardless of the position title.

> **faculty, adjunct**—Persons who are responsible for teaching at least 50% of a course and are part-time, nonsalaried, non-tenure-track faculty members who are paid for each class they teach.

fieldwork coordinator—Faculty member who is responsible for the development, implementation, management, and evaluation of fieldwork education.

frame of reference—A set of interrelated, internally consistent concepts, definitions, postulates, and principles that provide a systematic description of a practitioner's interaction with clients. A frame of reference is intended to link theory to practice.

full-time equivalent (FTE)—An equivalent position for a full-time faculty member (as defined by the institution). An FTE can be made up of no more than three individuals.

graduation rate—The total number of students who graduated from a program within 150% of the published length of the program, divided by the number of students on the roster who started in the program.

habits—"Automatic behavior that is integrated into more complex patterns that enable people to function on a day-to-day basis" (Neidstadt & Crepeau, 1998).

health literacy—Degree to which individuals have the capacity to obtain, process, and understand basic health information and services needed to make appropriate health decisions (National Network of Libraries of Medicine, 2011).

interprofessional collaborative practice—"Multiple health workers from different professional backgrounds working together with patients, families, careers, and communities to deliver the highest quality of care" (World Health Organization, 2010).

memorandum of understanding (MOU)—A document outlining the terms and details of an agreement between parties, including each parties' requirements and responsibilities. A memorandum of understanding may be signed by any individual who is authorized by the institution to sign fieldwork memoranda of understanding on behalf of the institution.

mentoring—A relationship between two people in which one person (the mentor) is dedicated to the personal and professional growth of the other (the mentee). A mentor has more experience and knowledge than the mentee.

mission—A statement that explains the unique nature of a program or institution and how it helps fulfill or advance the goals of the sponsoring institution, including religious missions.

modalities—Application of a therapeutic agent, usually a physical agent modality.

deep thermal modalities—Modalities such as therapeutic ultrasound and phonophoresis.

electrotherapeutic modalities—Modalities such as biofeedback, neuromuscular electrical stimulation, functional electrical stimulation, transcutaneous electrical nerve stimulation, electrical stimulations for tissue repair, high-voltage galvanic stimulation, and iontophoresis.

mechanical modalities—Modalities such as vasopneumatic devices and continuous passive motion.

superficial thermal—Modalities such as hydrotherapy, whirlpool, cryotherapy, fluidotherapy, hot packs, paraffin, water, and infrared.

model of practice—The set of theories and philosophies that defines the views, beliefs, assumptions, values, and domain of concern of a particular profession or discipline. Models of practice delimit the boundaries of a profession.

occupation—"Activities . . . of everyday life, named, organized and given value and meaning by individuals and a culture. Occupation is everything that people do to occupy themselves, including looking after themselves . . . enjoying life . . . and contributing to the social and economic fabric of their communities" (Law, Polatajko, Baptiste, & Townsend, 1997).

occupational profile—An analysis of a client's occupational history, routines, interests, values, and needs to engage in occupations and occupational roles.

occupational therapy—The art and science of applying occupation as a means to effect positive, measurable change in the health status and functional outcomes of a client by a qualified occupational therapist and/or occupational therapy assistant (as appropriate).

occupational therapy practitioner—An individual who is initially credentialed as an occupational therapist or an occupational therapy assistant.

participation—Active engagement in occupations.

performance patterns—Patterns of behavior related to daily life activities that are habitual or routine. Performance patterns include habits, routines, rituals, and roles.

performance skills—Features of what one does, not what one has, related to observable elements of action that have implicit functional purposes. Performance skills include motor and praxis, sensory–perceptual, emotional regulation, cognitive, and communication and social skills.

philosophy—The underlying belief and value structure for a program that is consistent with the sponsoring institution and which permeates the curriculum and the teaching learning process.

population-based interventions—Interventions focused on promoting the overall health status of the community by preventing disease, injury, disability, and premature death. A population-based health intervention can include assessment of the community's needs, health promotion and public education, disease and disability prevention, monitoring of services, and media interventions. Most interventions are tailored to reach a subset of a population, although some may be targeted toward the population at large. Populations and subsets may be defined by geography, culture, race and ethnicity, socioeconomic status, age, or other characteristics. Many of these characteristics relate to the health of the described population (Keller, Schaffer, Lia-Hoagberg, & Strohschein, 2002).

preparatory methods—Intervention techniques focused on client factors to help a client's function in specific activities.

program director (associate-degree-level occupational therapy assistant)—An initially certified occupational therapist or occupational therapy assistant who is licensed or credentialed according to regulations in the state or jurisdiction in which the program is located. The program director must hold a minimum of a master's degree.

program director (master's-degree-level occupational therapist)—An initially certified occupational therapist who is licensed or credentialed according to regulations in the state or jurisdiction in which the program is located. The program director must hold a doctoral degree.

program director (doctoral-degree-level occupational therapist)—An initially certified occupational therapist who is licensed or credentialed according to regulations in the state or jurisdiction in which the program is located. The program director must hold a doctoral degree.

program evaluation—A continuing system for routinely and systematically analyzing data to determine the extent to which the program is meeting its stated goals and objectives.

purposeful activity—"An activity used in treatment that is goal directed and that the [client] sees as meaningful or purposeful" (Low, 2002).

recognized regional or national accrediting authority—Regional and national accrediting agencies recognized by the USDE and/or the Council for Higher Education Accreditation (CHEA) to accredit postsecondary educational programs/institutions. The purpose of recognition is to ensure that the accrediting agencies are reliable authorities for evaluating quality education or training programs in the institutions they accredit.

Regional accrediting bodies recognized by USDE:

- Accrediting Commission for Community and Junior Colleges, Western Association of Schools and Colleges (ACCJC/WASC)

- Accrediting Commission for Senior Colleges and Universities, Western Association of Schools and Colleges (ACSCU/WASC)

- Commission on Colleges, Southern Association of Colleges and Schools (SACS)

- Commission on Institutions of Higher Education, New England Association of Schools and Colleges (CIHE/NEASC)

- Higher Learning Commission, North Central Association of Colleges and Schools (HLC)

- Middle States Commission on Higher Education, Middle States Association of Colleges and Schools (MSCHE)

- Northwest Commission on Colleges and Universities (NWCCU)

National accrediting bodies recognized by USDE:

- Accrediting Bureau of Health Education Schools (ABHES)

- Accrediting Commission of Career Schools and Colleges (ACCSC)

- Accrediting Council for Continuing Education and Training (ACCET)

- Accrediting Council for Independent Colleges and Schools (ACICS)

- Council on Occupational Education (COE)

- Distance Education and Training Council Accrediting Commission (DETC)

reflective practice—Thoughtful consideration of one's experiences and knowledge when applying such knowledge to practice. Reflective practice includes being coached by professionals.

release time—Period when a person is freed from regular duties, especially teaching, to allow time for other tasks or activities.

retention rate—A measure of the rate at which students persist in their educational program, calculated as the percentage of students on the roster, after the add period, from the beginning of the previous academic year who are again enrolled in the beginning of the subsequent academic year.

scholarship—"A systematic investigation . . . designed to develop or to contribute to generalizable knowledge" (45 CFR § 46). Scholarship is made public, subject to review, and part of the discipline or professional knowledge base (Glassick, Huber, & Macroff, 1997). It allows others to build on it and further advance the field (AOTA, 2009).

scholarship of discovery: Engagement in activity that leads to the development of "knowledge for its own sake." The Scholarship of Discovery encompasses original research that contributes to expanding the knowledge base of a discipline (Boyer, 1990).

scholarship of integration: Investigations making creative connections both within and across disciplines to integrate, synthesize, interpret, and create new perspectives and theories (Boyer, 1990).

scholarship of application: Practitioners apply the knowledge generated by scholarship of discovery or integration to address real problems at all levels of society (Boyer, 1990). In occupational therapy, an example would be the application of theoretical knowledge to practice interventions or to teaching in the classroom.

scholarship of teaching and learning: "Involves the systematic study of teaching and/or learning and the public sharing and review of such work through presentations, publications, and performances" (McKinney, 2007, p. 10).

skill—The ability to use one's knowledge effectively and readily in execution or performance.

sponsoring institution—The identified legal entity that assumes total responsibility for meeting the minimal standards for ACOTE accreditation.

strategic plan—A comprehensive plan that articulates the program's future vision and guides the program development (e.g., faculty recruitment and professional growth, changes in the curriculum design, priorities in academic resources, procurement of fieldwork sites). A program's strategic plan must include, but need not be limited to,

- Evidence that the plan is based on program evaluation and an analysis of external and internal environments,
- Long-term goals that address the vision and mission of both the institution and program as well as specific needs of the program,
- Specific measurable action steps with expected timelines by which the program will reach its long-term goals,
- Person(s) responsible for action steps, and
- Evidence of periodic updating of action steps and long-term goals as they are met or as circumstances change.

supervise—To direct and inspect the performance of workers or work.

supervision, direct—Supervision that occurs in real time and offers both audio and visual capabilities to ensure opportunities for timely feedback.

supervisor—One who ensures that tasks assigned to others are performed correctly and efficiently.

theory—A set of interrelated concepts used to describe, explain, or predict phenomena.

transfer of credit—A term used in higher education to award a student credit for courses earned in another institution prior to admission to the occupational therapy or occupational therapy assistant program.

References

American Occupational Therapy Association. (2008a). *Occupational therapy model curriculum.* Bethesda MD: Author. Retrieved from www.aota.org/Educate/EdRes/COE/Other-Education-Documents/OT-Model-Curriculum.aspx

American Occupational Therapy Association. (2008b). Occupational therapy practice framework: Domain and process (2nd ed.). *American Journal of Occupational Therapy, 62,* 625–683.

American Occupational Therapy Association. (2009). Scholarship in occupational therapy. *American Journal of Occupational Therapy, 63,* 790–796. http://dx.doi.org/10.5014/ajot.63.6.790

Boyer, E. L. (1990). *Scholarship reconsidered: Priorities of the professoriate.* San Francisco: Jossey-Bass.

Crepeau, E. B., Cohn, E., & Schell, B. (Eds.). (2008). *Willard and Spackman's occupational therapy* (11th ed.). Philadelphia: Lippincott Williams & Wilkins.

Glassick, C. E., Huber, M. T., & Maeroff, G. I. (1997). *Scholarship assessed: Evaluation of the professoriate.* San Francisco: Jossey-Bass.

Interprofessional Education Collaborative Expert Panel. (2011). *Core competencies for interprofessional collaborative practice: Report of an expert panel.* Washington, DC: Interprofessional Education Collaborative.

Keller, L., Schaffer, M., Lia-Hoagberg, B., & Strohschein S. (2002). Assessment, program planning and evaluation in population-based public health practice. *Journal of Public Health Management and Practice, 8*(5), 30–44.

Law, M., Polatajko, H., Baptiste, W., & Townsend, E. (1997). Core concepts of occupational therapy. In E. Townsend (Ed.), *Enabling occupation: An occupational therapy perspective* (pp. 29–56). Ottawa, ON: Canadian Association of Occupational Therapists.

Low, J. (2002). Historical and social foundations for practice. In C. A. Trombly & M. V. Radomski (Eds.), *Occupational therapy for physical dysfunction* (5th ed., pp. 17–30). Philadelphia: Lippincott Williams & Wilkins.

McKinney, K. (2007). *Enhancing learning through the scholarship of teaching and learning.* San Francisco: Jossey-Bass.

National Network of Libraries of Medicine. (2011). *Health literacy.* Retrieved February 3, 2012, from http://nnlm.gov/outreach/consumer/hlthlit.html

Schon, D. A. (1987). *Educating the reflective practitioner.* San Francisco: Jossey-Bass.

Public welfare: Protection of human subjects, 45 CFR § 46 (2005).

U.S. Department of Education (2011). *Funding your education: The guide to federal student aid, 2012–13.* Retrieved February 3, 2012, from http://studentaid.ed.gov/students/attachments/siteresources/12–13_Guide.pdf

World Health Organization. (2010). *Framework for action on interprofessional education and collaborative practice.* Geneva: Author. Retrieved from http://whqlibdoc.who.int/hq/2010/WHO_HRH_HPN_10.3_eng.pdf

Concept Papers

A Descriptive Review of Occupational Therapy Education

Introduction

In August 2002, the Commission on Education developed *A Guide to Occupational Therapy Education.* With the advent and passing of Resolution J—which became Resolution 670–99 at the 1999 Representative Assembly meeting of the American Occupational Therapy Association (AOTA; Accreditation Council for Occupational Therapy Education® [ACOTE®], 1999)—and new degree structures within the profession (i.e., professional/clinical doctorate), a new guide to occupational therapy education was warranted. This resultant guide, retitled *A Descriptive Review of Occupational Therapy Education,* is intended for practitioners, academicians, and potential occupational therapy program applicants to augment their understanding of current occupational therapy education.

Organization of Review

The Review is organized into several sections. The introductory section describes the process of developing the Descriptive Review. The second section distinguishes between professional and graduate education and provides the background and foundational groundwork for the Review. The next section describes levels of education in the United States used by most colleges and universities. It is the common language used in all degree majors and programs and should be the guide for occupational therapy so that degrees in occupational therapy can be recognized and understood by other fields. The Review then delineates the levels of education in occupational therapy in the United States from the technical level of education to the doctoral level. Finally, the Review describes types of accreditation for occupational therapy programs and lists factors that should be considered when choosing an occupational therapy program.

The Review was written to describe the present state of occupational therapy education within the American educational system and is limited to this perspective only. It does not intend to promote one occupational therapy degree over any other, nor is it intended to resolve the multiple issues regarding the various degree levels or entry-level competencies.

Levels of Education in the United States

One of the hallmarks of higher education in the United States is the diversity of institutions, degrees, and programs available. A prospective student may choose to pursue higher education at a research university, comprehensive university, 4-year college, community college, or technical school. Institutions may be public or private, for profit or nonprofit (Bok, 2013). One well-known classification system for American higher education institutions is the Carnegie Classification (Indiana University Center for Postsecondary Research, n.d.).

Common Carnegie Classifications for institutions offering occupational therapy programs include Research Universities (very high research activity), Research Universities (high research activity), Doctoral/Research Universities, Master's Colleges and Universities, Baccalaureate Colleges—Diverse Fields, Baccalaureate/Associate's Colleges, and Special Focus Institutions. Common Carnegie Classifications for institutions offering occupational therapy assistant programs include Master's Colleges and Universities, Baccalaureate Colleges, Baccalaureate/Associate's Colleges, Special Focus Institutions, Associates—Public Rural-serving, Associate's—Public Suburban-serving, Associate's—Public Urban-serving, Associate's—

Private Not-for-Profit, and Associate's—Private For-Profit. Although this is not a complete list of Carnegie Classifications, it represents the range of types of institutions that house occupational therapy and occupational therapy assistant programs. Each type of institution has a different focus or emphasis in terms of research, student body, curriculum, and funding formula. Further description of Carnegie Classifications can be found at http://carnegieclassifications.iu.edu/descriptions/basic.php.

Levels of education are represented by the academic degree conferred to graduates. A *degree* is a credential or title "conferred by a college or university as official recognition for the completion of a program of studies" (Shafritz, Koeppe, & Soper, 1988, p. 145). Academic degree levels include associate, baccalaureate, master's, and doctoral.

Associate Degree

The associate degree is recognized among higher education degrees. According to the National Center for Education Statistics, an *associate degree* is defined as

> an award that requires completion of an organized program of study of at least 2 but less than 4 years of full-time academic study or more than 60, but less than 120 semester credit hours. . . . Most associate degrees earned in academic programs are associate of arts (AA) or science (AS) degrees. Associate degrees earned in professional, technical or terminal programs are frequently called associate of applied science (AAS) degrees, but will sometimes carry the name of the program of study in the title. (U.S. Department of Education [USDE], 2008a, p. 1)

Baccalaureate

A *baccalaureate degree* is an award requiring completion of 4 to 5 full-time equivalent academic years of college-level work in an academic or occupationally specific field of study and that satisfies institutional standards of the requirement of the degree level (USDE, 2008b). Two common baccalaureate degrees are the bachelor of arts (BA or AB, for the Latin *atrium baccalaureus*) for programs in the humanities and the bachelor of science (BS) for programs in the sciences. Some institutions offer baccalaureate degrees in specialized areas, for example, bachelor of music (BMus) or bachelor of education (BEd; Unger, 1996).

Master's

The *master's degree* is the first graduate-level degree awarded in the United States and typically requires 2 years of postbaccalaureate education to complete. The value of the master's degree varies, depending on the field. The master's degree may serve as the entry into an area of study, as the terminal degree, or as a step toward the doctoral degree. Recent years have seen more doctoral programs admitting students at the baccalaureate level, eliminating the need for the master's degree in these programs (USDE, 2008c).

Research Master's

The *research master's degree* typically involves advanced study in the field, a comprehensive examination, and preparation and defense of either a master's thesis or a major project. The most commonly awarded master's degrees are the master of arts (MA) and the master of science (MS; USDE, 2008c).

Professional Master's

Professional education has been part of higher education in the United States for more than a century, and today most students enrolled in institutions of higher education are in professional or preprofessional programs (Sullivan, 2012). The professional master's degree structure can vary, depending upon the profession. Some *professional master's degree* programs are similar to research master's in that they involve advanced study in the field combined with a thesis or other major project. Other professional degrees are intended to prepare students to work in the field and typically do not include a thesis, although they often require a professional internship under supervision (USDE, 2008c).

Doctorate: Research and Professional

A *doctoral degree* is the highest degree conferred by an institution of higher education. Most doctoral degrees require the equivalent of 3 years of full-time postbaccalaureate study (Kapel, Gifford, & Kapel, 1991). Commonly, universities require a minimum of 72 hours of postbaccalaureate study plus a residence requirement. "Doctorate entitles bearers to be addressed as 'Doctor' and to append their names with the appropriate letters of their degrees—that is, PhD (doctor of philosophy) or MD (doctor of medicine)" (Unger, 1996, p. 305). There are two types of doctoral degrees: the research doctorate and the professional doctorate (Shafritz et al., 1988; Unger, 1996). The professional doctorate is also referred to as a *clinical doctorate* in many health professions (Pierce & Peyton, 1999).

Research Doctorate

The *research doctorate* (also called the *academic doctorate*), or PhD, was originally awarded for the study of philosophy in the mid-to-late 19th century. However, the degree was extended to include many disciplines of the humanities and sciences, with each PhD simply modified to indicate the field of study; for example, PhD in engineering, PhD in history, or PhD in chemistry. The purpose of the PhD degree is to develop graduates who are independent researchers and are knowledgeable in a specific area of study. Requirements for the PhD degree usually include a course of didactic study, followed by written or oral comprehensive examinations (upon passing, one applies for candidacy) and the completion of a dissertation in an area of new knowledge as deemed appropriate by a committee of senior faculty after an oral defense of the research (Shafritz et al., 1988).

The *doctor of science* (ScD) is an alternative doctoral degree similar to the PhD. Its curriculum is focused on the study of an applied science, such as audiology, occupational therapy, and so forth. ScD degree programs commonly include didactic coursework focused on the study of an applied science, an advanced clinical practicum, and a supervised clinical research project (Kidd, Cox, & Matthies, 2003).

Professional Doctorate

The *professional doctorate* reflects academic attainment and seldom requires a master's degree or dissertation (Unger, 1996). Unlike the PhD's focus on developing independent researchers, "sophisticated practice competencies" (Pierce & Peyton, 1999, p. 64) are emphasized in the professional doctorate degree. A person with a professional doctorate, such as an MD or doctor of jurisprudence (JD), must pass state or national qualifying examinations to obtain a license to practice (Unger, 1996). In the health sciences, the term *clinical doctorate* is synonymous with the term *professional doctorate,* and the program of study typically requires "mentored advanced clinical experiences for autonomous practice competencies" (Pierce & Peyton, 1999, p. 65; see also Edens & Labadie, 1987; Faut-Callahan, 1992; Hummer, Hunt, & Figuers, 1994; Watson, 1988).

Postdoctoral Education

As a result of globalization and the increased pace and complexity of knowledge, postdoctoral education has emerged to meet the growing need for scholars trained in both basic and translational science (Nerad, 2011). The adjective *postdoctoral* is frequently used to describe the variety of postdoctoral educational experiences. For example, terms such as *postdoctoral fellow, postdoctoral research associate,* and *postdoctoral trainee* are typically used. The competencies expected from postdoctoral education now require skills such as project management, which are well beyond those typically found in academia (Manathunga & Pitt, 2009).

Residencies

Residencies are a form of postprofessional education that are becoming more common in occupational therapy. "The purpose of post professional residency education is to advance the resident's preparation as a provider of patient care services in a defined (specialized) area of clinical practice" (Di Fabio, 1999,

p. 81). Residencies are focused on advancing knowledge, performance and interpersonal skills, and critical and ethical reasoning of practitioners in a focused area of practice (AOTA, 2014). Residency programs are between 9 and 12 months in length and may be situated in hospitals, schools, organizations, or community sites. As of mid-2015, there were four approved occupational therapy residency sites and one additional candidate residency site (AOTA, n.d.).

Levels of Education in Occupational Therapy

Occupational Therapy Assistant

Associate Degree–Level OTA

Occupational therapy assistant (OTA) programs are commonly offered at community colleges, private junior colleges, and some 4-year colleges and universities. OTA programs obtain accreditation from ACOTE and must adhere to the *Standards for an Accredited Educational Program for the Occupational Therapy Assistant* (ACOTE, 2016). As articulated in the Preamble of the Standards, a graduate from an ACOTE-accredited associate degree–level OTA program must

- Have acquired an educational foundation in the liberal arts and sciences, including a focus on issues related to diversity;

- Be educated as a generalist with a broad exposure to the delivery models and systems used in settings where occupational therapy is currently practiced and where it is emerging as a service;

- Have achieved entry-level competence through a combination of academic and fieldwork education;

- Be prepared to articulate and apply occupational therapy principles and intervention tools to achieve expected outcomes as related to occupation;

- Be prepared to articulate and apply therapeutic use of occupations with individuals or groups for the purpose of participation in roles and situations in home, school, workplace, community, and other settings;

- Be able to apply occupational therapy interventions to address the physical, cognitive, psychosocial, sensory, and other aspects of performance in a variety of contexts and environments to support engagement in everyday life activities that affect health, well-being, and quality of life;

- Be prepared to be a lifelong learner and keep current with best practice;

- Uphold the ethical standards, values, and attitudes of the occupational therapy profession;

- Understand the distinct roles and responsibilities of the occupational therapist and the occupational therapy assistant in the supervisory process;

- Be prepared to effectively communicate and work interprofessionally with those who provide care for individuals and/or populations to clarify each member's responsibility in executing components of an intervention plan; and

- Be prepared to advocate as a professional for the occupational therapy services offered and for the recipients of those services.

After completing the OTA didactic and fieldwork requirements, the OTA graduate is eligible to sit for the national certification examination for OTAs. On successful completion, the certified occupational therapy assistant (COTA) may apply for the appropriate state credential and, under specified supervision, render occupational therapy services.

Occupational Therapist Master's: Entry-Level and Postprofessional

In January 2007 the master's degree became the minimum degree level to enter the profession as an occupational therapist. Some entry-level programs require students to earn a baccalaureate degree in a related field before entering the master's degree program in occupational therapy. Other entry-level programs may require extensive prerequisite coursework but not mandate a baccalaureate degree. For example, the course of study may comprise two semesters beyond an undergraduate degree in a major such as occupational science; in other programs, the course of study may be a 5-year program leading to a master's degree. Coursework that is considered prerequisite is not generally included in the total credits required for the master's degree. On successful completion of the academic and fieldwork requirements, the graduate is eligible to take the national certification examination, then apply for state licensure and provide occupational therapy services at the professional level.

Postprofessional master's degree programs are available to individuals who have a professional degree in occupational therapy (e.g., baccalaureate, entry-level master's, entry-level doctorate degree). Such postprofessional degrees are typical of master's degree programs in other disciplines with a range of 30 to 36 credits. Many postprofessional programs are developed to enhance occupational therapy skills in a specific area (e.g., pediatrics, assistive technology, gerontology). Other master's degree programs may provide a general program with a curricular emphasis (e.g., leadership, research).

Doctorate: Clinical/Professional and Research

Currently, doctoral-level occupational therapy offerings include the clinical or professional and research doctorates. Some programs offer the PhD degree in occupational therapy. These doctoral programs focus on preparing graduates who are independent researchers and who will develop original knowledge pertinent to occupational therapy. Other doctoral degree programs related to occupational therapy exist, such as the PhD degree in rehabilitation science or occupational science or the ScD. Although many of these programs focus on the application of occupational therapy, it is beyond the scope of this document to describe the variations in doctoral programs closely aligned with occupational therapy.

The clinical or professional doctorate degree in occupational therapy confers the degree of occupational therapy doctorate (OTD) or doctor of occupational therapy (DrOT). Two pathways exist for pursuing the clinical or professional doctorate degree. The first is available to postprofessional students, that is, students who have an entry-level degree in occupational therapy and are occupational therapists. The second pathway is an entry-level doctorate. Entry-level professional doctorate degree programs are available for individuals who do not have an entry-level degree in occupational therapy but who have completed specified prerequisite coursework and, as of 2010, a baccalaureate degree.

Although clinical doctorate degree programs vary in philosophy, curriculum, and delivery method (particularly postprofessional programs, which often offer part-time and/or online options), typically the postprofessional clinical doctorate programs are shorter in duration and/or require less coursework than entry-level clinical doctorate programs. The rationale for the difference in program length is that postprofessional clinical doctorate students are occupational therapists who have previously completed an entry-level occupational therapy degree and also in consideration of the amount of clinical practice experience applicants possess. Unlike entry-level clinical doctorate programs, postprofessional clinical doctorate degrees are not currently accredited by ACOTE.

Accreditation

Institutions of higher education may choose to pursue *accreditation,* an external review to ensure that established standards are met. There are two types of accreditation: *institutional accreditation* and *program* (or *specialized*) *accreditation* (USDE, 2015). Accreditation of occupational therapy programs is the second type—program (or specialized)—and is completed by ACOTE, which is recognized by the USDE as well as by the Council for Higher Education Accreditation.

Institutional Accreditation

Regional and national accrediting bodies are recognized by the USDE and accredit institutions based upon established evaluation criteria (USDE, 2015). There are six regional agencies that accredit institutions located in distinct geographic areas. Accreditation standards from regional or national accrediting bodies influence ACOTE in that ACOTE standards must be aligned with requirements from the USDE and the Council for Higher Education Accreditation (Kramer & Graves, 2005).

Program or Specialized Accreditation

Program or specialized accreditation "applies to a particular school, department or program within the institution" and "may also apply to an entire institution if it is a free-standing, specialized institution . . . whose curriculum is all in the same program area" (Kaplin & Lee, 1995, p. 873). Currently ACOTE accredits OTA programs as well as entry-level programs in occupational therapy. The educational standards are developed through ACOTE with input from stakeholders. For postprofessional occupational therapy programs, there is no specialized accrediting body. However, institutional accrediting bodies can require a focus visit of a particular program. A focus visit does not result in the accrediting of a specific program.

Suggested Considerations When Choosing an Occupational Therapy Educational Program

When choosing an occupational therapy educational program, important factors must be considered (Box 1).

A variety of resources provide information about specific education programs. Institutional websites can be helpful in acquiring information about a program's curriculum and faculty. Brochures, catalogs, and bulletin descriptions often present the program's mission, philosophy, curriculum, or policies. These materials can be requested from the admissions office of each institution. Contacting faculty within the program is frequently useful to answer specific questions. Prospective students may request contact with a current student or with alumni to gain a consumer's perspective of the program.

In addition, it is important to answer the following questions:

• What are my future career goals?

• Does the degree offered contribute to accomplishing my short-term and long-term goals?

• If considering an online program, do I have the necessary skills to be successful (e.g., motivation, self-initiative, technical skills)?

Box 1. Considerations for Occupational Therapy Entry-Level and Postprofessional Education

- Location of program
- Tuition, return on investment, cost–salary considerations
- Length of program
- Availability of student scholarships
- Full- or part-time programs
- On-campus, distance-formatted, hybrid, or bridge-weekend programs
- Admission requirements
  - Interview
  - Entrance exams (e.g., Miller's Analogy, Graduate Record Exam)
  - Letters of recommendation, essays
  - Prerequisite classes or degree
  - Observation hours in occupational therapy
  - Undergraduate and prerequisite GPA
  - Community service and work experience
- Type of program
  - Degree awarded (e.g., AA, MS, MA, MOT, PhD, ScD, OTD)
  - Thesis requirement
  - Dissertation requirement
  - Curriculum (e.g., courses offered, course descriptions printed in catalog)
  - Program mission and philosophical grounding
  - Specialization (e.g., gerontology, pediatrics, entrepreneurialism)
  - Experiential components
    - Fieldwork, internships, rotations, etc.
    - Length of clinical preparation
    - Opportunities for post-degree experiences (e.g., residencies/fellowships)
- Institutional variables
  - Carnegie Classification
  - Library resources
  - Information technology/computer support
  - Stability of program as measured by accreditation status, retention and degree completion rates
  - Graduate or professional school
  - Ratings and rankings of programs
  - Community partnerships and international collaborations
- Graduate/alumni accomplishments
  - Graduation rate
  - Employment rates, sites
  - Employer satisfaction with graduates
  - Consumer satisfaction with graduate performance
  - NBCOT® exam pass rate
  - Graduate scholarly activity
- Faculty
  - Faculty credentials (e.g., doctorally prepared, specialty certified)
  - Faculty-to-student ratios
  - Faculty accessibility
  - Faculty projects (e.g., grants, publications)
  - Faculty clinical practice
  - Faculty community engagement, university citizenship, and professional service

References

Accreditation Council for Occupational Therapy Education. (1999, August). *ACOTE Motion and Resolution J (Minutes at the meeting of the Accreditation Council for Occupational Therapy Education)*. Bethesda, MD: Author.

Accreditation Council for Occupational Therapy Education. (2016, April). *Accreditation Council for Occupational Therapy Education standards and interpretive guide*. Retrieved May 3, 2016, from http://www.aota.org/-/media/Corporate/Files/EducationCareers/Accredit/Standards/2011-Standards-and-Interpretive-Guide.pdf

American Occupational Therapy Association. (n.d.). *Approved and candidate residency sites*. Retrieved from http://www.aota.org/Education-Careers/Advance-Career/Residency/ResidencySites.aspx

American Occupational Therapy Association. (2014). *AOTA Residency Program policy manual*. Bethesda, MD: Author. Retrieved from http://www.aota.org/-/media/corporate/files/educationcareers/advance/residency-policy-manual.pdf

Bok, D. (2013). *Higher education in America*. Princeton, NJ: Princeton University.

Di Fabio, R. P. (1999). Clinical expertise and the DPT: A need for residency training. *Journal of Orthopaedic and Sports Physical Therapy, 29,* 80–82. http://dx.doi.org/10.2519/jospt.1999.29.2.80

Edens, G. E., & Labadie, G. C. (1987). Opinions about the professional doctorate in nursing. *Nursing Outlook, 35,* 136–140.

Faut-Callahan, M. (1992). Graduate education for nurse anesthetists: Master's versus a clinical doctorate. *Journal of the American Association of Nurse Anesthetists, 60,* 98–103.

Hummer, L. A., Hunt, K. S., & Figuers, C. C. (1994). Predominant thought regarding entry-level doctor of physical therapy programs. *Journal of Physical Therapy Education, 8,* 60–66.

Indiana University Center for Postsecondary Research. (n.d.). *The Carnegie classification of institutions of higher education* (2015 ed.). Bloomington Author.

Kapel, D. E., Gifford, C. S., & Kapel, M. B. (1991). *American educators' encyclopedia* (rev. ed.). Westport, CT: Greenwood.

Kaplin, W. A., & Lee, B. A. (1995). *The law of higher education* (3rd ed.). San Francisco: Jossey-Bass.

Kidd, G. D., Jr., Cox, L. C., & Matthies, M. L. (2003). Boston University doctor of science degree program: Clinical doctorate in audiology. *American Journal of Audiology, 12,* 3–6. http://dx.doi.org/10.1044/1059-0889(2003/002)

Kramer, P., & Graves, S. (2005, March). Accreditation 101: Understanding the broad world of accreditation. *Education Special Interest Section Quarterly, 15,* 1–2.

Manathunga, C., & Pitt, R. (2009). Research students' graduate attribute development: Cooperative Research Center (CRC) graduate perceptions and employment outcomes. *Assessment and Evaluation in Higher Education, 34,* 91–103. http://dx.doi.org/10.1080/02602930801955945

Nerad, M. (2011). It takes a global village to develop the next generation of PhDs and postdoctoral fellows. *Acta Academica Supplementum, 2,* 198–216.

Pierce, D., & Peyton, C. (1999). A historical cross-disciplinary perspective on the professional doctorate in occupational therapy. *American Journal of Occupational Therapy, 53,* 64–71. http://dx.doi.org/10.5014/ajot.53.1.64

Shafritz, J. M., Koeppe, R. P., & Soper, E. W. (1988). *American educators' encyclopedia*. Westport, CT: Greenwood Press.

Sullivan, W. M. (2012). Professional education: Aligning knowledge, expertise and public purpose. In E. C. Langemann & H. Lewis (Eds.), *What is college for? The public purpose of higher education* (pp. 104–131). New York: Columbia University.

Unger, H. G. (1996). *Encyclopedia of American education*. New York: Facts on File.

U.S. Department of Education. (2008a). *Structure of the U.S. education system: Associate degrees*. Retrieved from https://www2.ed.gov/about/offices/list/ous/international/usnei/us/associate.doc

U.S. Department of Education. (2008b). *Structure of the U.S. education system: Bachelor's degrees*. Retrieved from http://www2.ed.gov/about/offices/list/ous/international/usnei/us/bachelor.doc

U.S. Department of Education. (2008c). *Structure of the U.S. education system: Master's degrees*. Retrieved from http://www2.ed.gov/about/offices/list/ous/international/usnei/us/master.doc

U.S. Department of Education. (2015). *Accreditation in the United States*. Retrieved from http://www2.ed.gov/admins/finaid/accred/accreditation.html

Watson, J. (1988). *The professional doctorate as an entry level into practice: Perspectives in nursing—1987–1989*. New York: National League for Nursing.

Resources

American Society of Health-System Pharmacists. (2001). *The residency learning system (RLS) model* (2nd ed.). Bethesda, MD: Author.

Farrell, J. P. (1996). In search of clinical excellence. *Journal of Orthopaedic and Sports Physical Therapy, 24,* 115–121. http://dx.doi.org/10.2519/jospt.1996.24.3.115

Glazer, J. S. (1988). *The master's degree* (Report No. EDO-HE-88-3). Washington, DC: Office of Educational Research and Improvement. (ERIC Document Reproduction Service No. ED301140)

LaPidus, J. B. (2000). Postbaccalaureate and graduate education: A dynamic balance. In K. Kohl & J. LaPidus (Eds.), *Postbaccalaureate futures* (pp. 3–9). Phoenix: Oryx.

Mayhew, L. B., & Ford, P. J. (1971). *Changing the curriculum*. San Francisco: Jossey-Bass.

Mayhew, L. B., & Ford, P. J. (1974). *Reform in graduate and professional education*. San Francisco: Jossey-Bass.

Medeiros, J. M. (1998). Post professional clinical residency programs. *Journal of Manual and Manipulative Therapy, 6,* 10.

Medeiros, J. M. (2000). Educational standards for residency education. *Journal of Manual and Manipulative Therapy, 8,* 50. http://dx.doi.org/10.1179/106698100790819500

Miller, S., & Clarke, A. (2002). Impact of postdoctoral specialty residencies in drug information on graduates' career paths. *American Journal of Health-System Pharmacists, 59,* 961–963.

Rogers, J. C. (1980a). Design of the master's degree in occupational therapy, part 1. A logical approach. *American Journal of Occupational Therapy, 34,* 113–118. http://dx.doi.org/10.5014/ajot.34.2.113

Rogers, J. C. (1980b). Design of the master's degree in occupational therapy, part 2. An empirical approach. *American Journal of Occupational Therapy, 34,* 176–184. http://dx.doi.org/10.5014/ajot.34.3.176

Authors

Andrea Bilics, PhD, OTR/L, FAOTA
Michael Iwama, PhD, OT(C)
Pamalyn Kearney, EdD, OTR
Judith Parker Kent, OTD, EdS, MS, OTR/L, FAOTA
Karen Romanowski, MS, OTR/L
Steven Taft, PhD, OTR, FAOTA

for

The Commission on Education
Andrea Bilics, PhD, OTR/L, FAOTA, *Chairperson*
Tina DeAngelis, EdD, OTR/L
Jamie Geraci, MS, OTR/L
Julie McLaughlin Gray, PhD, OTR/L
Michael Iwama, PhD, OT(C)
Julie Kugel, OTD, MOT, OTR/L
Kate McWilliams, MSOT, OTR/L
Maureen Nardella, MS, OTR/L
Renee Ortega, MA, COTA
Kim Qualls, MS, OTR/L
Tamra Trenary, OTD, OTR/L, BCPR
Neil Harvison, PhD, OTR/L, FAOTA, *AOTA Headquarters Liaison*

Adopted by the Representative Assembly 2015

Note. This document replaces the 2007 document *A Descriptive Review of Occupational Therapy Education,* previously published and copyrighted in 2007 by the American Occupational Therapy Association in the *American Journal of Occupational Therapy, 61,* 672–677. http://dx.doi.org/10.5014/ajot.61.6.672

Copyright © 2016 by the American Occupational Therapy Association.

Citation. American Occupational Therapy Association. (2016). A descriptive review of occupational therapy education. *American Journal of Occupational Therapy, 70,* 7012410040. http://dx.doi.org/10.5014/ajot.2016.706S03

The Role of Occupational Therapy in Disaster Preparedness, Response, and Recovery: A Concept Paper

Purpose

The focus of occupational therapy is to support people's health and participation in life through engagement in occupations (American Occupational Therapy Association [AOTA], 2008). Natural and human-created disasters are increasing in frequency throughout the world (Rodriguez, Vos, Below, & Guha-Sapir, 2009) and have a significant negative impact, both short- and long-term, on the health and occupational engagement of individuals, families, and communities. The purpose of this concept paper is to provide occupational therapy practitioners[1] with a basic understanding of disasters so those occupational therapy practitioners can support people's health and participation in life across the spectrum of disaster preparedness, response, and recovery. Beyond reading this concept paper, time for additional training and reflecting on one's own preparedness and motivation is needed prior to engaging in this important work.

Overview

When a societal crisis occurs, individuals, families, communities, institutions, and society as a whole become "disabled"—that is, limited in their ability to perform normal daily activities; restricted by environmental barriers; prohibited from participating in usual life roles; threatened by personal and financial losses; and subjected to a variety of psychological reactions, including fear, helplessness, and loss of confidence (Scaffa, 2003). Along with other people who experience a natural or technological (human-made) disaster, occupational therapists and occupational therapy assistants are victims and survivors of these experiences. However, occupational therapy practitioners also have the opportunity to be part of the solution for helping people prepare for, respond to, and recover from the disaster. They can use their understanding of occupations, occupational disruption, and activity analysis to increase individual and community readiness for and response to the disaster; to minimize or prevent maladaptation or further injury; and, ultimately, to promote health and recovery through an occupation-based approach.

Occupational therapy scholars have proposed several ways in which occupation can mediate the effects of stressful situations and promote health (McColl, 2002). Occupation can contribute to a person's sense of mastery and reinforce identity. It can restore habits and normalcy and can re-establish routines and meaningful roles. Many occupations that focus on taking care of self and others are health-promoting and are essential in responding to and recovering from trauma. Finally, occupation is a means through which people support themselves and others and through which they connect to their larger communities and social networks.

In this paper, disasters are defined, and the five stages of a disaster are presented. Next, assumptions that inform occupational therapy practitioners' participation in disaster relief are identified, followed by a discussion of occupational therapy's potential contributions before and during times of disaster. The

---

[1]When the term *occupational therapy practitioner* is used in this document, it refers to both occupational therapists and occupational therapy assistants (AOTA, 2006a). *Occupational therapists* are responsible for all aspects of occupational therapy service delivery and are accountable for the safety and effectiveness of the occupational therapy service delivery process. *Occupational therapy assistants* deliver occupational therapy services under the supervision of and in partnership with an occupational therapist (AOTA, 2009).

role occupational therapy practitioners can play in the stages of disaster work—disaster preparedness, disaster response, and disaster recovery—is outlined and provides an overview of how to initiate involvement in any of these stages. Finally, the relationship of disaster preparedness and relief to the *Occupational Therapy Code of Ethics and Ethics Standards (2010)* (AOTA, 2010a) is provided, followed by a call for involvement in disaster work and research.

Definitions and Background

In 1961, Charles E. Fritz, a pioneer in disaster research, defined *disasters* as

> Actual or threatened accidental or uncontrollable events that are concentrated in time and space, in which a society or a relatively self-sufficient subdivision of a society undergoes severe danger, and incurs such losses to its members and physical appurtenances that the social structure is disrupted and the fulfillment of all or some of the essential functions of the society, or its subdivision, is prevented. (p. 655)

This definition describes not only the physical damage and personal injuries that are typically sustained during a disaster but also the potential widespread social and economic disruption of daily-life routines.

Typically, disasters are classified into two categories: (1) natural and (2) technological (or human-made). Natural disasters include earthquakes, fires or wildfires, floods, heat waves, hurricanes, landslides and debris flow, thunderstorms, tornadoes, tsunamis, volcanoes, and winter storms/extreme cold. Technological disasters include biological threats, chemical emergencies/threats, computer attacks/viruses, dam failure, explosions, hazardous material leaks (e.g., oil spills), mass transportation accidents, mining accidents, nuclear blasts, nuclear power plant emergencies, prolonged or widespread power failures, radiological dispersion device activations, and any other terrorist activities (Federal Emergency Management Agency [FEMA], 2010; Fischer, 1998; Schneid & Collins, 2001).

Disasters progress through five stages, each requiring different behavioral and organizational responses:

- In the first stage, the *pre-impact period*, a warning of impending disaster may allow for preparation. For example, the National Weather Service may issue a hurricane warning, which prompts individuals, families, and institutions to put disaster response plans in effect while time permits. In some cases, though, there is no warning, and the pre-impact stage is short or nonexistent, such as when a mass shooting at an academic institution or a massive oil spill occurs unexpectedly.

- The second stage, the *impact period*, is generally the shortest in duration but the most dangerous in the life cycle of a disaster. In this stage the disaster is experienced in full force. Research has shown that altruism and an outpouring of concern for the victims of natural disasters is the norm, and people tend to share food, equipment, and supplies and assist one another in recovery efforts. Perceptions that antisocial behavior and widespread panic occur immediately following a disaster have not been substantiated by the literature (Drabek & McEntire, 2003; Fischer, 2002; Tierney, Bevc, & Kuligowski, 2006).

- In the third stage, the *immediate post-impact period*, search-and-rescue and evacuation efforts are initiated, the media generate increasing coverage of the event, and emergency organizations begin to respond.

- During the fourth stage, the *recovery period*, clearance of debris is completed, essential services such as electricity and water are restored, preliminary reconstruction plans are initiated, and daily life routines begin to normalize.

- The fifth and final stage, the *reconstruction period*, may last from several months to several years depending on the scope and the severity of the disaster. Reconstruction involves the rebuilding not only of structures but also of individual lifestyles and a sense of community.

According to Fischer (1998), the mental health effects of disasters often last longer than the physical manifestations.

Assumptions

This paper is based on the following nine assumptions gathered from the literature:

1. Natural disasters have been increasing in frequency throughout the world since 1998 (Rodriguez et al., 2009) and deprive persons of their right to participate in life-sustaining and meaningful occupations.

2. When disaster strikes, already-difficult circumstances are exacerbated for marginalized populations, such as persons with disabilities, elderly individuals, people with chronic illnesses, children, the poor population, and indigenous groups. These groups are especially vulnerable and disproportionately affected by disasters (Smith & Notaro, 2009).

3. Disaster situations generate significant personal loss and environmental changes that can adversely affect adaptive occupational performance of individuals and communities across all areas of occupation (Rosenfeld, 1982, 1989; Tuchner, Meiner, Parush, & Hartman-Maier, 2010).

4. Disasters can generate significant traumatic stress (Diamond & Precin, 2003; Tuchner et al., 2010; Young, Ford, Ruzek, Friedman, & Gusman, 1998), and survivors' usual coping strategies may prove inadequate for disaster situations (Rosenfeld, 1982; Tuchner et al., 2010; Young et al., 1998).

5. Engagement in occupation can moderate the effects of disaster (McColl, 2002; Tuchner et al., 2010).

6. Occupational therapy practitioners can contribute to interdisciplinary efforts of disaster preparedness through their use of activity analysis, skills at grading and adaptation of tasks, knowledge of contexts, and an understanding of the occupational needs of individuals and families.

7. In disaster situations, the focus of occupational therapy is to facilitate engagement in occupations in order to enhance adaptive responses to the disaster and to resume valued life habits, routines, roles, and rituals (AOTA, 2008).

8. Occupational therapy practitioners can assist individuals, families (Tuchner et al., 2010), and communities in coping with disaster situations and in returning to optimal occupational performance (Rosenfeld, 1982, 1989).

9. Occupational therapists and occupational therapy assistants can identify disruptions in occupational performance patterns and help clients develop new, effective patterns of performance by facilitating the process of occupational adaptation (Rosenfeld, 1982).

Occupational Therapy Contributions in Times of Disaster

Occupational therapy practitioners can and should be involved in disaster preparedness, response, and recovery. In working with individuals, families, and communities affected by disasters, occupational therapy practitioners bring a set of core practice skills grounded on the importance of occupational engagement. Working together with the client, occupational therapy practitioners can plan and implement interventions that enable people to reestablish balance and engagement in as many areas of occupation (e.g., activities of daily living [ADLs], instrumental activities of daily living, rest and sleep, education, work, play, leisure, social participation) as possible by

- Evaluating people's occupational balance, occupational performance (functional abilities), and performance patterns;

- Configuring contexts (i.e., cultural, personal, temporal, virtual,) and environments (i.e., social, physical) to maximize occupational engagement and social participation; and

- Analyzing occupations and activities to determine the underlying requisites for effective performance.

In addition, occupational therapy practitioners have mental health knowledge and skills (in common with other professionals) that are useful in disaster management and response. Possession of this knowledge and skill facilitates inclusion of occupational therapy practitioners on mental health intervention teams in times of disaster.

Occupational Therapy Contributions in Disaster Preparedness

Disaster preparedness involves actions taken before a disaster that enable a community to respond effectively. This requires planning at the community, organizational, and household levels. Planned interventions designed to address system-level concerns, as well as direct service interventions for the individual, are necessary to ensure safety and facilitate normalization. Organizations and businesses should develop emergency response plans, train employees in how to handle emergency situations, acquire needed supplies and equipment, and conduct response drills and exercises (Tierney, Lindell, & Perry, 2001). Individuals must know what these plans entail so that they can proactively remain safe or seek help, when needed, in a timely and efficient way.

When interfacing with disaster response teams, it is important to know the hierarchical structure of agencies and organizations involved in planning, responding, and facilitating recovery from disasters. The National Disaster Medical System is a section within the FEMA in the U.S. Department of Homeland Security. It is responsible for managing and coordinating the federal medical response to major emergencies and federally declared disasters. Its focus is to ensure medical response to a disaster area in the form of providing teams, supplies, and equipment; moving injured people from disaster sites to unaffected areas; and identifying the types of medical care available at participating hospitals in unaffected areas.

All states are divided into local regions with Disaster Medical Assistance Teams (DMATs). These teams develop and implement plans to meet physical and mental health needs during disasters in their areas. State, county, and local agencies, businesses, and community organizations, as well as individuals, may assist these teams in disaster planning, response, and recovery. Participating in "table-top" and other mock disaster drills at the local, state, and national levels as a member of a team provides needed training. Becoming affiliated with local and national organizations, such as the American Red Cross, community emergency response teams (CERTs), mental health crisis services, critical incident stress management (CISM) teams, and employee assistance programs prior to a disaster increases the credibility of the occupational therapy practitioner and facilitates involvement when a disaster occurs.

Occupational therapy practitioners should select the level of involvement and role that best matches community need as well as their personal availability, skills, and knowledge. Practitioners can apply their expertise in several settings, including health care facilities, schools, businesses, and shelters. Those who work in health care facilities should participate in discussions of existing policies and procedures, as well as the role of occupational therapy in the promotion of the safety of clients during a fire or severe weather conditions, including consideration of what to do when these conditions continue for an extended period. For example, when a predicted hurricane arrives, plans are already in place for securing facilities, moving those with special needs, and providing food and shelter and necessary medications for the short term. But if the storm is fierce and has caused extensive destruction, then staff need to be able to design and adapt spaces, modify expectations, create new physical and social environments, and provide support services for those under their care for an unknown period of time.

Schools often are the most likely place that children will be when a disaster occurs. School disaster planning is essential and typically consists of identifying school crisis teams, delineating the roles of staff during an emergency, and establishing processes for reuniting children with their parents. Occupational therapy practitioners who work in academic settings (e.g., K–12 schools, universities) can assist in school planning regarding the requirements of students with special needs. For example, occupational therapists can assess the medical and mental health resources that are available in the school environment and assist in the development of individualized emergency care plans for students with disabilities (Asher & Pollak, 2009; American Academy of Pediatrics, Council on School Health, 2008). According to Asher and Pollak (2009), occupational therapists are uniquely qualified to identify the elements of an emergency care plan, including "how the student is transported, moved, and positioned;

any personal equipment that may need to accompany the student; where to exit the building; or when to stay in the building" (p. CE3). In addition, occupational therapy practitioners can offer their expertise in planning for disasters by recommending the use of compact, easily stored supplies for age-appropriate activities during disasters such as a prolonged "lock down," flu or disease outbreak, or blizzard.

Occupational therapy practitioners can help DMATs and employers design plans to evacuate workers with disabilities effectively in the event of an emergency and can train staff and volunteers to work in shelters for people with special needs prior to disasters. Occupational therapy practitioners planning system-level interventions can ensure that shelters and other emergency sites are organized in ways that minimize environmental barriers. For example, they can ensure that people with mobility limitations will be located near restrooms to facilitate independence in self-care. Such planning also decreases the number of environmental modifications or kinds of adaptive equipment that will be required to address self-care needs and privacy concerns. Occupational therapists have the expertise needed to plan, organize, and direct programs in shelters and to train and supervise volunteers. In addition, practitioners can work with individuals or groups of individuals with disabilities on their own emergency preparedness plans (Diamond & Precin, 2003).

Knowledge of available resources and understanding of local plans for responding to such disasters are critical to effective rapid humanitarian responses. Sensitivity to occupational performance needs and facilitating choice in occupational engagement is a unique marker of the services provided by occupational therapy practitioners (Stone, 2006) and dissimilar to any that are likely to be provided by other members of the response team. It also is essential that practitioners have in place appropriate plans for their family's care during the extended period when they may need to remain on duty at their institution to help prevent conflicting demands on their energies and emotions.

Occupational Therapy Contributions in Disaster Response

Emergency response involves actions taken just prior to, during, and shortly after disaster impact to address the immediate needs of victims and to reduce damage, destruction, and disruption. Emergency response activities include detection of threats, dissemination of warnings, and evacuation of vulnerable populations. In addition, they include search for and rescue of victims, provision of emergency medical care, and furnishing of food and shelter for displaced persons (Tierney et al., 2001). The daily concerns of older adults after Hurricane Katrina included "securing basic resources, facing communication difficulties, and finding transportation" (Henderson, Roberto, & Kano, 2010, p. 48). All disaster-related interventions should recognize and be delivered within the hierarchy of needs framework, typically survival, safety and security, and food and shelter needs are primary, followed by health, both physical and mental (National Institute of Mental Health [NIMH], 2002).

During times of disaster or emergency, all professionals are called on to provide their expertise voluntarily in the service of others. Occupational therapy practitioners are qualified to provide disaster response services to people with special needs. FEMA defines *special-needs populations* as people in the community with physical, mental, or medical care needs who may require assistance before, during, or after a disaster or an emergency, after exhausting their usual resources and support network. During a disaster, people with special needs may be moved to regular shelters or shelters for people with special needs, or they may *shelter-in-place* (i.e., remain in their personal homes or other residences, such as assisted living facilities, foster and group homes, and long-term care facilities). People with mobility or sensory disabilities often are moved to a temporary emergency location not specifically designed to accommodate their needs. Occupational therapy practitioners can—within their skill level and arena of practice—modify and adapt these environments to promote safety and more independent function. Occupational therapy services may include supervising staff and volunteers at special-needs shelters, making home visits or telephone calls to those sheltering-in-place, and facilitating support groups designed to reduce anxiety and stress.

Occupational therapy practitioners also may provide support for displaced, confused adults and children until their caregivers can be identified and located. Occupational therapists can identify children who are having difficulty coping and address their mental health concerns, as well as provide guidance for their caregivers.

Occupational therapy practitioners can provide a variety of services to individuals and families who have evacuated their homes and workplaces and are living in emergency shelters or who are sheltering-in-place. People who are displaced from their homes and workplaces to emergency shelters face a variety of challenges. People of various cultures and ethnic backgrounds with different beliefs and habits often are forced to live in one large room with no privacy. Children are bored, a general sense of uneasiness pervades, and stress levels increase. Using a client-centered approach, occupational therapy practitioners can evaluate the needs of people in the shelter and provide appropriate services. Interventions might include providing structure in daily routines, identifying and emphasizing people's strengths, encouraging creative expression of feelings, coordinating age-appropriate play for children, and providing opportunities for stress management (Newton, 2000).

In addition, occupational therapy practitioners with appropriate knowledge and skills who are part of a disaster response team can provide short-term, supportive mental health services to victims, families, first responders, and volunteers (AOTA, 2010c). This is referred to as *psychological first aid* (NIMH, 2008; Watson & Shalev, 2005) or *mental health first aid* and is provided only to those who seek the service. Mental health first aid can be defined as "help provided to a person developing a mental health problem or in a mental health crisis. The first aid is given until appropriate professional treatment is received or until the crisis resolves" (Kitchener & Jorm, 2007, p. 2). The goals of mental health first aid are to

- Prevent injury or death when a person is a danger to themselves or others,

- Protect survivors from further harm,

- Reduce distress,

- Prevent the mental health problem from developing into a more serious condition,

- Promote the recovery of positive mental health,

- Reduce physiological arousal,

- Provide comfort to the person coping with a mental health crisis,

- Facilitate reunion with loved ones, and

- Guide the person toward appropriate professional help (Kitchener & Jorm, 2007; NIMH, 2002).

The mental health first aid process generally consists of several components:

- Assessing risk of suicide or harm,

- Listening in an active empathic manner,

- Providing reassurance and information/education,

- Facilitating self-help strategies and access to community resources,

- Reducing secondary stressors, and

- Encouraging the person to seek appropriate professional help when needed (Kitchener & Jorm, 2007; Shalev, Tuval-Mashiach, & Hadar, 2004).

First responders, including firefighters, police, and emergency medical personnel, also may benefit from occupational therapy. These individuals work long hours under difficult circumstances and often are away from home. Occupational therapists can observe first responders and volunteers for signs of distress and can provide respite, psychological first aid, or other appropriate interventions (Newton, 2000).

Occupational therapy is based on the premise that engagement in occupations facilitates adaptation. Occupation can help disaster survivors reestablish their sense of control. Focused, constructive activity, such as helping others, moves people beyond shock and denial. This strategy is especially effective for survivors who are being disruptive. Engaging survivors as active participants in their ongoing survival and adjustment to change can help them regain their sense of mastery and overcome any sense of guilt from a perceived failure to prepare for the disaster or to protect their family. By engaging in play, vigorous physical activity, or valued leisure occupations, survivors can get a brief respite from recurring thoughts, worries, and concerns about the future.

Occupational Therapy Contributions in Disaster Recovery

Post-disaster recovery involves repair and rebuilding of property, reestablishment of public utilities, and restoration of disrupted social and economic activities, and routines. For example, the restoration of the school community provides age-appropriate occupational engagement for students (Hobfoll et al., 2007). According to the Council on School Health of the American Academy of Pediatrics (2008), "Although returning to the classroom does not ensure that children are ready to address learning tasks, evidence points to the restorative power of the educational routine in guiding children through emotional crises" (p. 898). Post-disaster recovery also includes efforts to reduce acute stress, foster resilience, re-establish roles and routines, and enhance the psychosocial well-being and the quality of life of the community members affected (Tierney et al., 2001).

Following disasters, many survivors experience acute stress reactions (see Table 1). Hobfoll et al. (2007) identified five essential elements to trauma intervention including: (1) promotion of sense of safety, (2) promotion of calming, (3) promotion of sense of self-efficacy and collective efficacy, (4) promotion of

Table 1. Common Acute Stress Reactions to Disaster

Emotional Effects	Cognitive Effects
Shock	Impaired concentration
Anger	Impaired decision-making ability
Despair	Memory impairment
Emotional numbing	Disbelief
Terror	Confusion
Guilt	Distortion
Grief or sadness	Decreased self-esteem
Irritability	Decreased self-efficacy
Helplessness	Self-blame
Loss of derived pleasure from regular activities	Intrusive thoughts and memories
Dissociation (e.g., perceptual experience seems "dreamlike," "tunnel vision," "spacey," or "on automatic pilot")	Worry
Mood swings	

Physical Effects	Interpersonal Effects
Fatigue	Alienation
Insomnia	Social withdrawal
Sleep disturbance	Increased conflict within relationships
Hyperarousal	Vocational impairment
Somatic complaints	School impairment
Impaired immune response	
Headaches	
Gastrointestinal problems	
Decreased appetite	
Decreased libido	
Startle response	

Note. From *Disaster Mental Health Services: A Guidebook for Clinicians and Administrators,* by B. H. Young, J. D. Ford, J. I. Ruzek, M. J. Friedman, & F. D. Gusman, 1998, Menlo Park, CA: National Center for Post-Traumatic Stress Disorder, Department of Veterans Affairs. Available at www.ncptsd.org/publications/disaster/.

connectedness, and (5) promotion of hope. A sense of safety can be instilled by providing the facts of the current situation without the hyperbole of some media reports. Calming is required for the occupational performance of restorative sleep, which is commonly adversely affected. Occupational therapists can promote a sense of self-efficacy as they help clients to problem-solve and successfully address disaster-related issues. It is imperative to facilitate connectedness to ensure social participation necessary for well-being. Finally, hope can be instilled by providing a realistic but noncatastrophic view of the future (Hobfoll et al., 2007).

Fostering resilience as well as psychological and social recovery are major goals in this stage of disaster. Strategies to facilitate resilience and psychological and social recovery include providing education on acute stress responses and coping skills training, fostering natural social supports, encouraging social interactions, facilitating spiritual support, and offering group and family interventions (AOTA, 2010b, 2010c; NIMH, 2002).

The profession of occupational therapy has long recognized the importance of roles, habits, and routines to occupational engagement (American Occupational Therapy Foundation [AOTF], 2010). Disasters can seriously disrupt role engagement and the habits and routines that sustain them. Roles help give people an identity and a sense of self, as well as identify the responsibilities associated with that identity (Deeny & McFetridge, 2005; Kielhofner, Forsyth, & Barrett, 2003). After a disaster, roles such as student, worker, leisure participant, or others may be lost. In the case of displacement from a person's home and community, some roles, like those of family member or friend, must be maintained from a distance, or worse, relinquished. Other roles may need to be expanded, such as homeowner, as insurance issues will require significant time and attention. Often, changes in context require the adoption of new roles, such as volunteer, renter, or home remodeler. Occupational therapy practitioners are adept at helping clients successfully negotiate periods of transition and can help clients adapt to role changes dictated by the disaster.

Occupation and activity can help clients cope with traumatic stress and meet survival needs. Occupational engagement reduces the intensity of stressful events and helps reestablish a sense of mastery in a situation in which a person feels a loss of control. The military has long used occupational therapy to help soldiers overcome occupational dysfunction due to the stress of war (Ellsworth, Laedtke, & McPhee, 1993; Laedtke, 1996), to support their role identity, and to restore their confidence in their ability to function (Gerardi, 1996, 1999; Gerardi & Newton, 2004). Participation in occupation facilitates restoration of adaptive habits and routines, supports a person's sense of identity, and helps establish a spiritual connection in the disaster situation (McColl, 2002). As part of the intervention team, occupational therapy practitioners can help clients develop coping skills to deal with the aftereffects of their experience. Additionally, through engagement in occupation, disaster survivors can restructure their habits and routines to cope more effectively with stress and anxiety, to enhance their sense of mastery over their environment, and to participate in their valued life roles.

Some survivors may experience lasting psychological effects from the traumatic stress of their experience. These posttraumatic stress symptoms may be severe enough to manifest themselves as depression or an anxiety disorder such as posttraumatic stress disorder (PTSD). Characteristic of PTSD is persistent re-experiencing of the event (e.g., in nightmares and flashbacks), avoidance of reminders of the trauma and numbing of emotions (e.g., difficulty recalling aspects of the trauma and detachment from others), and heightened physiological arousal (e.g., insomnia, irritability, exaggerated startle response), all lasting more than one month (American Psychiatric Association, 1994). In addition—and of primary concern to the occupational therapy practitioner—a person with PTSD may experience significant occupational dysfunction. Providing occupational therapy in a group format offers a supportive environment and can enhance function and provide a renewed sense of self-efficacy (Ziv & Roitman, 2008).

For persons diagnosed with PTSD, occupation can be used to recover and enhance skills required in daily life roles. Such interventions may focus on ADLs to enhance independent living; on coping skills (e.g., relaxation, biofeedback) to deal with stress, anxiety, and physiological arousal; and on socialization skills to decrease emotional and social withdrawal and to increase socialization (Davis & Kutter, 1998;

Froelich, 1992; Rosenfeld, 1982, 1989; Short-Degraff & Engelman, 1992). Expressive media can be used to help clients re-experience their trauma in a safe supportive environment. This enables them to explore and discover how they have been affected by the event and to practice skills to deal more effectively with their physiological and emotional responses (Davis, 1999; Froelich, 1992; Morgan & Johnson, 1995; Short-Degraff & Engelman, 1992).

Contributions of Occupational Therapy Organizations in Times of Disaster

The AOTF, AOTA, and the World Federation of Occupational Therapists (WFOT) have been involved in disaster work. In 2002, following the terrorist attacks of 9/11, the AOTF established the Task Force on Occupation in Societal Crises. This group, made up of civilian and military personnel and occupational therapists from Canada and the United States, worked in collaboration with AOTA's Commission on Practice to write the first version of this concept paper (AOTA, 2006b).

AOTA has been responsive after hurricanes Katrina, Rita, and Ike, as well as other disasters. In large-scale disasters, where citizens of affected communities are simply struggling to survive, it is imperative that entities outside the immediate disaster zone provide assistance to ensure safe living arrangements, mental health support, job opportunities, and continued curriculum or equal educational opportunities. Local and regional, trained and networked occupational therapy practitioners are best prepared to help and to serve as conduits of information regarding needs to professional associations at the state, national, and international levels. However, before disasters occur, professional associations can provide guidance through official documents and other training materials. For example, in response to the 2004 Indian Ocean Tsunami, WFOT produced a Disaster Preparedness and Response information package and is supporting the development of a textbook on the same topic (WFOT, n.d.). AOTA also has produced disaster-related materials; links to these resources and those of the WFOT appear in Table 2. While professional associations have a role in educating members and society about the potential role of occupational therapy, ultimately it is individual occupational therapy practitioners who need to take the initiative to be trained and ready to serve if disaster occurs in their institution, community, or region (Stone, 2006).

Occupational Justice, Ethics, and Research in Disaster Preparedness, Response, and Recovery

The term *occupational justice* conveys the profession's commitment to populations and individuals in need as well as the strong belief that access to occupation is a right and a necessity for health and quality of life (AOTA, 2008; Townsend & Wilcock, 2004). Disaster survivors often are vulnerable and in need of the services of occupational therapy practitioners. Stone (2006) reports that the best method to provide recovery services is in the community (when possible) by local, pre-trained providers who are part of an established network.

To be able to assist in an ethical manner, occupational therapy practitioners must

- Be keenly aware of their motivations to engage in this type of work,

- Have an individual/family disaster plan in place,

- Seek out training and secure a position from an authorized agency,

- Be competent in the tasks and services they provide,

- Not expect special privileges, and

- Not unduly take advantage of the experience or capitalize on others' misfortune.

Communities affected by disaster can provide tremendous opportunities for research (Morris, 2008). However, special care must be taken to ensure research is done in an ethical and compassionate way. A group of social scientists met after Hurricane Katrina and established eight criteria to guide research on

Table 2. Disaster Resources

Title	Link	Description
American Academy of Pediatrics, "Children and Disasters: Disaster Preparedness to Meet Children's Needs"	www.aap.org/disasters	Web site on disaster preparedness to meet the needs of children
American Occupational Therapy Association	http://www.aota.org/Practitioners/Resources/Collections/Preparedness-Library/Emergency-Resources-.aspx	Emergency preparedness and response resources compiled for occupational therapy practitioners
American Red Cross, *Disaster Preparedness for Persons With Disabilities*	http://www.redcross.org/www-files/Documents/pdf/Preparedness/Fast%20Facts/Disaster_Preparedness_for_PwD-English.pdf	Booklet
American Red Cross, *Disaster Preparedness for Seniors by Seniors*	http://www.redcross.org/www-files/Documents/pdf/Preparedness/Fast%20Facts/Disaster_Preparedness_for_Srs-English.revised_7-09.pdf	Booklet
Center for an Accessible Society, "Disaster Mitigation for Persons With Disabilities"	www.accessiblesociety.org/topics/independentliving/disasterprep.htm	Web site of resources
Federal Emergency Management Agency	www.fema.gov	Web site
Federal Emergency Management Agency, *A Citizen Guide to Disaster Preparedness*	http://webharvest.gov/peth04/20041017185751/ http://www.pueblo.gsa.gov/cic_text/family/disaster-guide/disasterguide.htm	Booklet
Federal Emergency Management Agency, National Preparedness Directorate, Emergency Management Institute	http://training.fema.gov/	Web site of nationwide training program of resident and nonresident courses to enhance U.S. emergency management practices
Inclusive Preparedness Center, "Emergency Preparedness for People With Disabilities and Other Vulnerable Populations"	http://www.inclusivepreparedness.org/	Web site focused on ensuring that all people are included in emergency planning, response, and recovery from natural and technological disasters
International Critical Incident Stress Foundation	www.icisf.org/	Web site of nonprofit, open-membership foundation dedicated to prevention and mitigation of disabling stress through provision of education, training, and support services for all emergency medical service professions; continuing education and training in emergency mental health services; and consultation in establishment of crisis and disaster response programs for varied organizations and communities worldwide
National Voluntary Organizations Active in Disaster	http://www.nvoad.org	A coalition of nonprofit organizations sharing knowledge and resources regarding disaster preparation, response, and recovery to help disaster survivors and their communities
Substance Abuse and Mental Health Services Administration, "Disaster Kit"	http://mentalhealth.samhsa.gov/disasterrelief/default.aspx	Publications on mental health and disaster
Substance Abuse and Mental Health Services Administration, *Training Manual for Mental Health and Human Service Workers in Major Disasters*	http://mentalhealth.samhsa.gov/publications/allpubs/ADM90-538/Default.asp	Manual
U.S. Department of Education, *Practical Information on Crisis Planning: A Guide for Schools and Communities*	www.ed.gov/admins/lead/safety/emergencyplan/crisisplanning.pdf	Book

(Continued)

Table 2. Disaster Resources *(cont.)*

Title	Link	Description
U.S. Department of Health and Human Services, "National Disaster Medical System"	http://ndms.dhhs.gov	Web site
World Federation of Occupational Therapists, *Disaster Preparedness and Response Information Package*	https://www.wfot.org/wfotshop/shop exd.asp?id=71	Educational CD-ROM available for purchase or free to those working in disaster relief and to countries without the financial resources to purchase
World Federation of Occupational Therapists, *WFOT Disaster Preparedness and Response Questionnaire*	http://www.wfot.org/singleNews.asp? id=163&name=WFOT%20Disaster%20 Preparedness%20and%20Response% 20-%20Questionnaire	Survey to gather information regarding disaster preparedness and relief activities around the world

the disaster (Gill et al., 2007). While all eight criteria are relevant to occupational therapy research, the following four resonate most strongly with the *Occupational Therapy Code of Ethics and Ethics Standards* (AOTA, 2010a) and occupational justice:

- "Reducing vulnerability of populations to disaster, promoting the sustainability of human and ecological systems, and enhancing the resiliency of communities" (p. 790).

- "Facilitating recovery of individuals and communities" (p. 791).

- "Enhancing stakeholder participation, collaboration, and empowerment" (p. 792).

- "Developing new knowledge of understudied disaster-related issues" (p. 792).

Conclusion

Occupational therapy practitioners can have a significant role in disaster preparedness, response, and recovery. For example, in preparation for disasters, occupational therapy practitioners can

- Participate in facility-level and community-wide planning efforts,

- Design special-needs shelters and train staff and volunteers, and

- Assist businesses and employers in developing plans for evacuating employees with disabilities.

Occupational therapy has much to offer individuals, families, organizations, institutions, and communities affected by disaster. The profession's holistic approach and its focus on occupational engagement and adaptation constitute its unique contribution to disaster management. During the disaster response, occupational therapy practitioners can

- Provide supportive mental health services to victims and their families;

- Provide supportive mental health services to first responders, such as police, firefighters, and military personnel;

- Manage special-needs shelters;

- Provide supportive services by telephone or visits to those sheltering-in-place;

- Provide occupational interventions in shelters; and

- Facilitate psychological and educational support groups to decrease anxiety and stress.

Throughout the disaster recovery phase, occupational therapy practitioners can provide occupation-based and mental health services for persons with acute stress reactions and PTSD. Interventions must be designed to be meaningful and purposeful to those engaged in them, and they must support the individual, family, community, or agency in responding to the unique characteristics of the disaster.

Occupational therapy practitioners can use their professional expertise and the power of occupational engagement to restore control, order, and quality of life and to normalize lives in crisis when individuals, families, institutions, and communities are disrupted by natural or technological disasters. However, to be effective in this arena, occupational therapy practitioners must

- Define and establish their role in disaster preparedness, response, and recovery (McDaniel, 1960);

- Be aware of existing hospital, institutional, work site, and community disaster plans;

- Be knowledgeable about how national, state, and local governments and private agencies involved in disaster management are organized and how to gain entry into these systems;

- Monitor the literature for evidence-based work on the efficacy of various approaches such as psychological/mental health first aid and other approaches;

- Develop skills and train for their role in disaster response and recovery; and

- Be personally and professionally prepared to respond effectively to disaster situations (see Table 2 for resources).

A quote from author C. S. Lewis written for another time remains relevant today as occupational therapy practitioners think about their response to disaster, both as private individuals and as professionals. When disaster comes, let it

> find us doing sensible and human things—praying, working, teaching, reading, listening to music, bathing the children, playing tennis, chatting to our friends over a pint and a game of darts . . . . (Lewis, 1986, pp. 73–74)

References

American Academy of Pediatrics, Council on School Health. (2008). Disaster planning for schools. *Pediatrics, 122*(4), 895–901.

American Occupational Therapy Association. (2006a). Policy 1.44: Categories of occupational therapy personnel. In *Policy manual* (2009 ed.). Bethesda, MD: Author.

American Occupational Therapy Association. (2006b). The role of occupational therapy in disaster preparedness, response, and recovery. *American Journal of Occupational Therapy, 60*(6), 642–649.

American Occupational Therapy Association. (2008). Occupational therapy practice framework: Domain and process (2nd ed.). *American Journal of Occupational Therapy, 62*, 625–683.

American Occupational Therapy Association. (2009). Guidelines for supervision, roles, and responsibilities during the delivery of occupational therapy services. *American Journal of Occupational Therapy, 63*, 796–803.

American Occupational Therapy Association. (2010a). Occupational therapy code of ethics and ethics standards (2010). *American Journal of Occupational Therapy, 64*(Suppl.), S17–S26.

American Occupational Therapy Association. (2010b). Occupational therapy services in the promotion of psychological and social aspects of mental health. *American Journal of Occupational Therapy, 64*(Suppl.), S78–S91.

American Occupational Therapy Association. (2010c). Specialized knowledge and skills in mental health promotion, prevention, and intervention in occupational therapy practice. *American Journal of Occupational Therapy, 64*(Suppl.), S30–S43.

American Occupational Therapy Foundation. (2010, January). The making of New Year's resolutions and a key concept of occupational therapy. *Research Resources: A Monthly Newsletter of the AOTF Institute for the Study of Occupation and Health.* Available online at http://www.aotf.org/Portals/ 0/documents/ News/Research-Resources/January%2012%202010%20Research%20Resources.pdf

American Psychiatric Association. (1994). *Diagnostic and statistical manual of mental disorders* (4th ed., text rev.). Washington, DC: Author.

Asher, A., & Pollak, J. R. (2009). Planning emergency evacuations for students with unique needs: Role of occupational therapy. *OT Practice, 14*(21), CE1–CE7.

Davis, J. (1999). Effects of trauma on children: Occupational therapy to support recovery. *Occupational Therapy International, 6,* 126–142.

Davis, J., & Kutter, C. J. (1998). Independent living skills and posttraumatic stress disorder in women who are homeless: Implications for future practice. *American Journal of Occupational Therapy, 52,* 39–44.

Deeny, P., & McFetridge, B. (2005). The impact of disaster on culture, self, and identity: Increased awareness by health care professionals is needed. *Nursing Clinics of North America, 40*(3), 431–440.

Diamond, H., & Precin, P. (2003). Disabled and experiencing disaster: Personal and professional accounts. *Occupational Therapy in Mental Health, 19*(3/4), 27–42.

Drabek, T. E., & McEntire, D. A. (2003). Emergent phenomena and the sociology of disaster: Lessons, trends, and opportunities. *Disaster Prevention and Management, 12*(2), 97–112.

Ellsworth, P. D., Laedtke, M. E., & McPhee, S. D. (1993). Utilization of occupational therapy in combat stress control during the Persian Gulf War. *Military Medicine, 158,* 381–385.

Federal Emergency Management Agency. (2010). *Are you ready? An in-depth guide to citizen preparedness.* Retrieved March 18, 2010, from http://www.fema.gov/areyouready/

Fischer, H. W. (1998). *Response to disaster: Fact versus fiction and its perpetuation: The sociology of disaster* (2nd ed.). Lanham, MD: University Press of America.

Fischer, H. W. (2002). Terrorism and 11 September 2001: Does the "behavioral response to disaster" model fit? *Disaster Prevention and Management, 11*(2), 123–127.

Fritz, C. E. (1961). Disasters. In R. K. Merton & R. A. Nisbet (Eds.), *Contemporary social problems* (pp. 651–694). New York: Harcourt.

Froelich, J. (1992). Occupational therapy interventions with survivors of sexual abuse. *Occupational Therapy in Health Care, 8*(2/3), 1–25.

Gerardi, S. M. (1996). The management of battle-fatigued soldiers: An occupational therapy model. *Military Medicine, 161,* 483–488.

Gerardi, S. M. (1999). Part I. Work hardening for warriors: Occupational therapy for combat stress casualties. *Work, 13,* 185–195.

Gerardi, S. M., & Newton, S. M. (2004, July–September). The role of the occupational therapist in CSC (combat stress control) operations. *U.S. Army Medical Department Journal,* pp. 20–27.

Gill, D. A., Clarke, L., Cohen, M. J., Ritchie, L. A., Ladd, A. E., Meinhold, S., et al. (2007). Post-Katrina guiding principles of disaster social science research. *Sociological Spectrum, 27,* 789–792.

Henderson, T. L., Roberto, K. A., & Kamo, K. A. (2010). Older adults' responses to Hurricane Katrina: Daily hassles and coping strategies. *Journal of Applied Gerontology, 29*(1), 48–69.

Hobfoll, S. E., Watson, P., Bell, C. C., Bryant, R. A., Brymer, M. J., Friedman, M. J., et al. (2007). Five essential elements of immediate and mid-term mass trauma intervention: Empirical evidence. *Psychiatry, 70*(4), 283–315.

Kielhofner, G., Forsyth, K., & Barrett, L. (2003). The Model of Human Occupation. In E. B. Crepeau, E. S. Cohn, & B. A. Boyt Schell (Eds.), *Willard and Spackman's occupational therapy* (pp. 212–219). Philadelphia: Lippincott Williams & Wilkins.

Kitchener, B., & Jorm, A. (2007). *Mental health first aid manual*. Melbourne: University of Melbourne, ORYGEN Research Centre. Available online at http://www.burdekinmentalhealthfoundation.org/Mental%20Health%20First%20Aid%20Manual.pdf

Laedtke, M. E. (1996). Occupational therapy and the treatment of combat stress. In J. A. Martin, L. R. Sparacinco, & G. Belenky (Eds.), *The Gulf War and mental health: A comprehensive guide* (pp. 145–152). Westport, CT: Praeger.

Lewis, C. S. (1986). *Present concerns: A compelling collection of timely journalistic essays*. London: C. S. Lewis PTE.

McColl, M. A. (2002). Occupation in stressful times. *American Journal of Occupational Therapy, 56*, 350–353.

McDaniel, M. L. (1960). The role of the occupational therapist in natural disaster situations. *American Journal of Occupational Therapy, 14*, 195–198.

Morgan, C. A., & Johnson, D. R. (1995). Use of a drawing task in the treatment of nightmares in combat-related post-traumatic stress disorder. *Art Therapy, 12*, 244–247.

Morris, A. S. (2008). Making it through a traumatic life experience: Applications for teaching, research, and personal adjustment. *Training and Education in Professional Psychology, 2*(2), 89–95.

National Institute of Mental Health. (2002). *Mental health and mass violence: Evidence-based early intervention for victims/survivors of mass violence* (NIH Pub. 02-5138). Washington, DC: U.S. Government Printing Office.

National Institute of Mental Health. (2008). *Post-traumatic stress disorder (PTSD)* (NIH Pub. 08-6388). Washington, DC: U.S. Government Printing Office.

Newton, S. (2000, November). *Matching occupational therapy skills to new opportunities: Working on a natural disaster*. Poster session presented at the annual meeting of the Occupational Therapy Association of California.

Rodriguez, J., Vos, F., Below, R., & Guha-Sapir, D. (2009). *Annual disaster statistical review 2008*. Brussels, Belgium: Centre for Research on the Epidemiology of Disasters.

Rosenfeld, M. S. (1982). A model for activity intervention in disaster-stricken communities. *American Journal of Occupational Therapy, 36*, 229–235.

Rosenfeld, M. S. (1989). Occupational disruption and adaptation: A study of house fire victims. *American Journal of Occupational Therapy, 43*, 89–96.

Scaffa, M. (2003, Spring). Competence, mastery, and independence: Our cultural heritage. *American Occupational Therapy Foundation Connection, 10*(1), 6–7.

Schneid, T. D., & Collins, L. (2001). *Disaster management and preparedness*. Boca Raton, FL: Lewis.

Shalev, A. Y., Tuval-Mashiach, R., & Hadar, H. (2004). Posttraumatic stress disorder as a result of mass trauma. *Journal of Clinical Psychiatry, 65*(Suppl. 1), 4–10.

Short-Degraff, M. A., & Engelman, T. (1992). Activities in the treatment of combat-related post-traumatic stress disorder. *Occupational Therapy in Health Care, 8*(2/3), 27–47.

Smith, D. L., & Notaro, S. J. (2009). Personal emergency preparedness for people with disabilities from the 2006–2007 Behavioral Risk Factor Surveillance System. *Disability and Health Journal, 2*(2), 86–94.

Stone, G. V. M. (2006). Occupational therapy in times of disaster. *American Journal of Occupational Therapy, 60*(1), 7–8.

Tierney, K., Bevc, C., & Kuligowski, E. (2006). Metaphor matter: Disaster myths, media frames, and their consequences in Hurricane Katrina. *Annals of the American Academy of Political and Social Science, 604*(1), 57–81.

Tierney, K. J., Lindell, M. K., & Perry, R. W. (Eds.). (2001). *Facing the unexpected: Disaster preparedness and response in the United States.* Washington, DC: Joseph Henry Press & National Academy of Sciences.

Townsend, E., & Wilcock, A. (2004). Occupational justice and client-centered practice: A dialogue in progress. *Canadian Journal of Occupational Therapy, 71*(2), 75–87.

Tuchner, M., Meiner, Z., Parush, S., & Hartman-Maier, A. (2010). Relationships between sequela of injury, participation, and quality of life in survivors of terrorists' attacks. *OTJR: Occupation, Participation and Health, 20*(1), 29–38.

Watson, P. J., & Shalev, A. Y. (2005). Assessment and treatment of adult acute responses to traumatic stress following mass traumatic events. *CNS Spectrums, 10*(2), 123–131.

World Federation of Occupational Therapists. (n.d.). *WFOT disaster preparedness and response questionnaire.* Retrieved April 6, 2010, from http://www.wfot.org/singleNews.asp?id= 163&name=WFOT%20 Disaster%20Preparedness%20and%20Response%20-%20Questionnaire

Young, B. H., Ford J. D., Ruzek, J. I., Friedman, M. J., & Gusman, F. D. (1998). *Disaster mental health services: A guidebook for clinicians and administrators.* Menlo Park, CA, & White River Junction, VT: Department of Veterans Affairs, National Center for Post-Traumatic Stress Disorder. Available online at www.ncptsd.org//publications/disaster/

Ziv, N., & Roitman, D. M. (2008). Addressing the needs of elderly clients whose lives have been compounded by traumatic histories. *Occupational Therapy in Health Care, 22*(2/3), 85–93.

Authors
Marjorie E. Scaffa, PhD, OTR/L, FAOTA
S. Maggie Reitz, PhD, OTR/L, FAOTA
Theresa Marie Smith, PhD, OTR/L, CLVT

for

The Commission on Practice
Janet V. DeLany, DEd, OTR/L, FAOTA, *Chairperson*

Adopted by the Representative Assembly Coordinating Council (RACC) for the Representative Assembly

Revised by the Commission on Practice 2011

Note. This revision replaces the 2005 document *The Role of Occupational Therapy in Disaster Preparedness, Response, and Recovery: A Concept Paper* (previously published and copyrighted in 2006 by the American Occupational Therapy Association in the *American Journal of Occupational Therapy, 60,* 642–649).

Scholarship in Occupational Therapy

Background

In this document, we present the position of the American Occupational Therapy Association (AOTA) on the importance of scholarship to the growth, development, and vitality of the profession, and we describe the range of scholarly activities that will advance the profession. In addition, this document serves to inform both internal and external audiences concerning the expectations for—and the role of—scholarship in occupational therapy practice.

It is important to distinguish between scholarly practice and scholarship. *Scholarly practice* involves using the knowledge base of the profession or discipline in one's practice. As occupational therapy practitioners, we call this scholarly practice *evidence-based practice*. When engaged in scholarly teaching, educators draw on the "knowledge base on teaching and learning" (McKinney, 2007, p. 9) and their discipline or professional knowledge bases. Occupational therapy practitioners engaged in scholarly practice or scholarly teaching are reflective practitioners who assess and discuss their actions in light of the current knowledge base (McKinney, 2007, 2013; Schön, 1983). In contrast, *scholarship* or *research* is "a systematic investigation . . . designed to develop or to contribute to generalizable knowledge" (U.S. Department of Health and Human Services, 2005). Scholarship is made public, subject to review, and part of the discipline or professional knowledge base (Glassick, Huber, & Maeroff, 1997). It allows others to build on it and further advance the field.

Occupational therapy practitioners view scholarship as a vitally important contribution to the profession, the academy, and ultimately to society. Hence, practitioners see that engaging in scholarship is a professional responsibility. Every occupational therapy practitioner should contribute independently or collaboratively to building the evidence base for occupational therapy practice and occupational therapy education (Accreditation Council for Occupational Therapy Education, 2016; AOTA, 2007).

Occupational therapy practitioners are committed to engagement in scholarship that honors societal ethical standards and adheres to the standards of rigor accepted by the scientific community. Occupational therapy scholars value empiricism as the means by which knowledge must emerge, recognizing that through a variety of experimental and naturalistic means one may achieve knowledge and understanding (DePoy & Gitlin, 2011; Kielhofner, 2006). Moreover, they recognize that knowledge is established not in isolation but through interdisciplinary collaboration and intellectual discourse (Yerxa, 1987). As providers of therapeutic and educational services, occupational therapy practitioners are committed to continually developing foundational and theoretical knowledge that underlies practice; understanding the process and outcomes of service; and finally, establishing evidence of efficacious therapy and educational outcomes (Kielhofner, 2006).

The profession recognizes the necessity of a broad range of scholarly endeavors that will serve to describe and interpret the scope of the profession, establish new knowledge, interpret and appropriately apply this knowledge to practice, and engage learners in their development and understanding of the profession. Therefore, we acknowledge the relevance and legitimacy of the variety of scholarly approaches as described by Boyer (1990): the Scholarship of Discovery, the Scholarship of Integration, the Scholarship of Application, and the Scholarship of Teaching. This range of scholarship is particularly relevant considering the diversity in the field of occupational therapy represented by stakeholders with varying educational backgrounds. The four types of scholarship are discussed in the order Boyer (1990) presented them in *Scholarship Reconsidered: Priorities of the Professoriate*. He did not identify a hierarchy among the four types of scholarship, and none is intended in this document.

Scholarship of Discovery

According to Boyer (1990), the *Scholarship of Discovery* is the engagement in activity that leads to the development of "knowledge for its own sake" (p. 17). The Scholarship of Discovery encompasses original research that contributes to expanding the knowledge base of a discipline. It is the type of research that the academic community most easily recognizes and accepts and, as such, is often the expected vehicle for intellectual discourse within the academy. Traditionally, faculty members who are trained to be independent researchers in research universities conduct discovery scholarship. Such scholars are, according to Golde (2006), stewards of the discipline responsible for "*generating* new knowledge and defending knowledge claims against challenges and criticism; of *conserving* the most important ideas and findings that are a legacy of past and current work; and of *transforming* knowledge that has been generated and conserved by teaching well to a variety of audiences, including those outside formal classrooms."

Clearly, there is a need for scholarship in occupational therapy that expands overall understanding of the engagement in and meaning of human occupation and its role in attaining and maintaining health. Clark (2006) noted that the profession needed a critical mass of the Scholarship of Discovery to continue to build the theoretical and knowledge base for occupational therapy, to foster intellectual vitality, and to maintain and strengthen the central tenets of the discipline.

Scholarship of Integration

The *Scholarship of Integration* is concerned with making creative connections both within and across disciplines to integrate, synthesize, interpret, and create new perspectives and theories. This form of scholarship is the most similar to the Scholarship of Discovery, but the difference lies in the nature of the research questions. In this form of inquiry, the scholars' aim is to find the meaning of research findings and interpret the findings in ways that synthesize isolated facts from within and outside of the discipline and integrate them to provide a richer and more thorough understanding of the issues. In light of the complex nature of contemporary issues confronting the individual and society, the profession needs the Scholarship of Integration, which lies in the intersections of disciplinary boundaries, to generate new knowledge for occupational therapy to better understand and meet societal needs.

Scholarship of Application

Through the *Scholarship of Application,* practitioners apply the knowledge generated by Scholarships of Discovery or Integration to address real problems at all levels of society. In occupational therapy, an example would be the application of theoretical knowledge to practice interventions or to teaching in the classroom. Another example may be using knowledge about the value of occupations as a health determinant to address health disparities of populations. Some authors, in focusing their efforts on application, have coined the term *Scholarship of Practice* (Braveman, Helfrich, & Fisher, 2002; Kielhofner, 2005), which focuses on program development and occupational therapy intervention.

Another dimension of the Scholarship of Application is the *Scholarship of Engagement* (Boyer, 1990), which focuses on an interactive, participatory scholarship with persons and organizations (Barker, 2004; Boyer, 1996). In this form, multiple stakeholders, including community members, produce knowledge.

Regardless of differing terms, these activities fit best under Boyer's (1990) Scholarship of Application. In the broader context of the health sciences, the Scholarship of Application is often viewed as synonymous with Knowledge Translation (Straus, Tetroe, & Graham, 2011). However, *Knowledge Translation* refers to a type of scholarship application that often relates to the specific process of decision making in health care.

Scholarship of Teaching and Learning

Over time, the *Scholarship of Teaching* (Boyer, 1990) has been expanded to the *Scholarship of Teaching and Learning,* recognizing the interrelatedness of teaching and learning. The Scholarship of

Teaching and Learning implies a "research agenda" and "involves the systematic study of teaching and/ or learning and the public sharing and review of such work through presentations, publications, and performances" (McKinney, 2007, p. 10). Contributions must meet the rigorous standards of all forms of scholarship, be public, and be open to critical review.

Scholarship and Practice Roles

Scholarship must be generated, evaluated, and used to inform the many practice roles of occupational therapy. All occupational therapists and occupational therapy assistants, regardless of their individual practice roles, have the professional responsibility not only to use that evidence to inform their professional decision making but also to generate new evidence through independent or collaborative research, or both.

For example, research through the Scholarships of Discovery and Integration will contribute to the improved understanding of the constructs, processes, and theories (e.g., occupation and its therapeutic use) that provide the foundation for meeting society's complex occupational needs. At other times, through the Scholarship of Application, practitioners will establish evidence concerning the effectiveness of a specific intervention or the reliability, validity, and utility of an assessment tool and appropriately use the intervention or assessment on the basis of the strength of that evidence. They also may develop and use evidence derived from the Scholarship of Teaching and Learning in client education to support participation in meaningful occupations.

Practitioners challenge occupational therapy educators—including academic educators, academic fieldwork educators, and fieldwork educators—to find better ways to prepare diverse students to be competent professionals who advance the profession. Through the Scholarship of Teaching and Learning and the Scholarship of Application, they can empirically determine and apply better instructional methodologies to prepare students to meet the demands of a rapidly changing and increasingly complex health care environment, where consumers expect evidence-based practice and continuous professional development of all practitioners.

Finally, administrators can contribute to, and benefit from, evidence produced through the Scholarship of Application when determining how best to meet the needs of clients in a cost-effective manner or how to better mentor or supervise others. Additional examples and benchmarks of scholarship are provided in Appendix A.

References

Accreditation Council for Occupational Therapy Education. (2016, April). *Accreditation Council for Occupational Therapy Education standards and interpretive guidelines.* Retrieved May 3, 2016, from http://www. aota.org/-/media/Corporate/Files/EducationCareers/Accredit/Standards/2011-Standards-and-Interpretive-Guide.pdf

American Occupational Therapy Association. (2007). *AOTA's Centennial Vision and executive summary.* *American Journal of Occupational Therapy, 61,* 613–614. http://dx.doi.org/10.5014/ajot.61.6.613

Barker, D. (2004). The scholarship of engagement: A taxonomy of five emerging practices. *Journal of Higher Education Outreach and Engagement, 9,* 123–137.

Boyer, E. L. (1990). *Scholarship reconsidered: Priorities of the professoriate.* San Francisco: Jossey-Bass.

Boyer, E. L. (1996). The scholarship of engagement. *Journal of Higher Education Outreach and Engagement, 1,* 11–20.

Braveman, B. H., Helfrich, C. A., & Fisher, G. S. (2002). Developing and maintaining community partnerships within "a scholarship of practice." *Occupational Therapy in Health Care, 15,* 109–125. http:// dx.doi.org/10.1080/J003v15n01_12

Clark, F. (2006). One person's thoughts on the future of occupational science. *Journal of Occupational Science, 13,* 167–179. http://dx.doi.org/10.1080/14427591.2006.9726513

DePoy, E., & Gitlin, L. N. (2011). *Introduction to research: Understanding and applying multiple strategies* (4th ed.). St. Louis, MO: Elsevier/Mosby.

Glassick, C. E., Huber, M. T., & Maeroff, G. I. (1997). *Scholarship assessed: Evaluation of the professoriate.* San Francisco: Jossey-Bass.

Golde, C. (2006). *Preparing stewards of the discipline.* Stanford, CA: Carnegie Foundation for the Advancement of Teaching. Retrieved June 1, 2016, from http://archive.carnegiefoundation.org/perspectives/preparing-stewards-discipline

Kielhofner, G. (2005). A scholarship of practice: Creating discourse between theory, research and practice. *Occupational Therapy in Health Care, 19,* 7–16. http://dx.doi.org/10.1080/J003v19n01_02

Kielhofner, G. (Ed.). (2006). *Research in occupational therapy: Methods of inquiry for enhancing practice.* Philadelphia: F. A. Davis.

McKinney, K. (2007). *Enhancing learning through the scholarship of teaching and learning.* San Francisco: Jossey-Bass.

McKinney, K. (2013). *The scholarship of teaching and learning in and across the disciplines.* Bloomington: Indiana University Press.

Schön, D. A. (1983). *The reflective practitioner.* New York: Basic Books.

Straus, S. E., Tetroe, J. M., & Graham, I. D. (2011). Knowledge translation is the use of knowledge in health care decision making. *Journal of Clinical Epidemiology, 64,* 6–10. http://dx.doi.org/10.1016/j.jclinepi.2009.08.016

U.S. Department of Health and Human Services. (2005). *Part 46—Protection of human subjects. Code of Federal Regulations Title 45—Public Welfare.* Available online at http://www.hhs.gov/ohrp/documents/OHRPRegulation.pdf

Yerxa, E. J. (1987). The key to the development of occupational therapy as an academic discipline. *American Journal of Occupational Therapy, 41,* 415–419. http://dx.doi.org/10.5014/ajot.41.7.415.

Authors
The Commission on Education:
Andrea Bilics, PhD, OTR/L, FAOTA, *Chairperson*
Tina DeAngelis, EdD, OTR/L
Jamie Geraci, MS, OTR/L
Michael Iwama, PhD, OT(C)
Julie Kugel, OTD, MOT, OTR/L
Julie McLaughlin Gray, PhD, OTR/L, FAOTA
Kate McWilliams, MSOT, OTR/L
Maureen S. Nardella, MS, OTR/L
Renee Ortega, MA, COTA
Kim Qualls, MS, OTR/L
Tamra Trenary, OTD, OTR/L, BCPR
Neil Harvison, PhD, OTR/L, FAOTA, *AOTA Headquarters Liaison*

Adopted by the Representative Assembly Coordinating Council (RACC) for the Representative Assembly 2016

This document replaces the 2009 document *Scholarship in Occupational Therapy,* previously published and copyrighted in 2009 by the American Occupational Therapy Association in the *American Journal of Occupational Therapy, 63,* 790–796. http://dx.doi.org/10.5014/ajot.63.6.790

Citation. American Occupational Therapy Association. (2016). Scholarship in occupational therapy. *American Journal of Occupational Therapy, 70,* 7012410080. http://dx.doi.org/10.5014/ajot.2016.706S07

Appendix A.
Characteristics of Scholarship in Occupational Therapy

Type	Examples	Demonstration	Documentation
Scholarship of Discovery Contributes to the development or creation of new knowledge	• Primary empirical research • Historical research • Theory development • Methodological studies • Philosophical inquiry	• Peer-reviewed publications of research, theory, or philosophical essays • Peer-reviewed/invited professional presentations of research, theory, or philosophical essays • Grant awards in support of research or scholarship • Positive peer evaluations of the body of work	• Bibliographic citation of the accomplishments • Positive external evaluation of the body of work
Scholarship of Integration Contributes to the critical analysis and review of knowledge within disciplines or the creative synthesis of insights contained in different disciplines or fields of study	• Inquiry that advances knowledge across a range of theories, practice areas, techniques, or methodologies • Includes works that interface among occupational therapy and a variety of disciplines, including but not limited to occupational science	• Peer-reviewed publications of research, policy analysis, case studies, integrative reviews of the literature, and others • Copyrights, licenses, patents, or products • Published books • Positive peer evaluations of contributions to integrative scholarship • Reports of interdisciplinary programs or services • Interdisciplinary grant awards • Peer-reviewed/invited professional presentations • Policy papers designed to influence organizations or governments • Service on editorial board or as peer reviewer	• Bibliographic citation of the accomplishments • Positive external evaluation of the body of work • Documentation of role in editorial/review processes
Scholarship of Application, Practice, or Engagement Applies findings generated through the Scholarship of Integration or discovery to solve real problems in the professions, industry, government, and community	• Development of clinical knowledge • Application of technical or research skills to address problems • Participatory action research involving collaboration with community groups • Efficacy of treatment approach • Developing valid outcome measures	• Peer-reviewed publications of research, policy analysis, case studies, integrative reviews of the literature, and others • Activities related to the faculty member's area of expertise (e.g., consultation, technical assistance, policy analysis, program evaluation, development of practice patterns) • Peer-reviewed/invited professional presentations related to practice • Consultation reports • Reports compiling and analyzing patient or health services outcomes • Products, patents, license copyrights • Peer reviews of practice • Grant awards in support of practice • Reports of meta-analyses related to practice problems • Reports of clinical demonstration projects • Policy papers related to practice	• Formal documentation of a record of the activity and positive formal evaluation by users of the work • Bibliographic citation of the accomplishments • Positive external evaluation of the body of work • Documentation of role in multi-authored products

(Continued)

Appendix A.
Characteristics of Scholarship in Occupational Therapy *(cont.)*

Type	Examples	Demonstration	Documentation
Scholarship of Teaching and Learning Contributes to the development of critically reflective knowledge about teaching and learning	• Application of knowledge of the discipline or specialty applied in teaching–learning in the academic and/or fieldwork setting • Development of innovative teaching and evaluation methods • Program development and learning outcome evaluation of academic and/or fieldwork education • Professional role modeling	• Peer-reviewed publications of research related to teaching methodology or learning outcomes, case studies related to teaching–learning, learning theory development, and development or testing of educational models or theories • Educational effectiveness studies such as those found in comprehensive programs reports • Successful applications of technology to teaching and learning • Positive peer evaluations of innovations in teaching • Published textbooks or other learning aids • Grant awards in support of teaching and learning	• Peer-reviewed/invited professional presentations related to teaching and learning • Bibliographic citation of the accomplishments • Positive external evaluation of the body of work

Note. Adapted from Boyer (1990).

Ethics

Enforcement Procedures for the
Occupational Therapy Code of Ethics

1. Introduction

The principal purposes of the *Occupational Therapy Code of Ethics* (hereinafter referred to as the Code) are to help protect the public and to reinforce its confidence in the occupational therapy profession rather than to resolve private business, legal, or other disputes for which there are other more appropriate forums for resolution. The Code also is an aspirational document to guide occupational therapists, occupational therapy assistants, and occupational therapy students toward appropriate professional conduct in all aspects of their diverse professional and volunteer roles. It applies to any conduct that may affect the performance of occupational therapy as well as to behavior that an individual may do in another capacity that reflects negatively on the reputation of occupational therapy.

The *Enforcement Procedures for the Occupational Therapy Code of Ethics* have undergone a series of revisions by the Association's Ethics Commission (hereinafter referred to as the EC) since their initial adoption. This public document articulates the procedures that are followed by the EC as it carries out its duties to enforce the Code. A major goal of these *Enforcement Procedures* is to ensure objectivity and fundamental fairness to all individuals who may be parties in an ethics complaint. The *Enforcement Procedures* are used to help ensure compliance with the Code which delineates enforceable Principles and Standards of Conduct that apply to Association members.

Acceptance of Association membership commits individuals to adherence to the Code and cooperation with its *Enforcement Procedures.* These are established and maintained by the EC. The EC and Association's Ethics Office make the *Enforcement Procedures* public and available to members of the profession, state regulatory boards, consumers, and others for their use.

The EC urges particular attention to the following issues:

1.1. **Professional Responsibility**—All occupational therapy personnel have an obligation to maintain the Code of their profession and to promote and support these ethical standards among their colleagues. Each Association member must be alert to practices that undermine these standards and is obligated to take action that is appropriate in the circumstances. At the same time, members must carefully weigh their judgments as to potentially unethical practice to ensure that they are based on objective evaluation and not on personal bias or prejudice, inadequate information, or simply differences of professional viewpoint. It is recognized that individual occupational therapy personnel may not have the authority or ability to address or correct all situations of concern. Whenever feasible and appropriate, members should first pursue other corrective steps within the relevant institution or setting and discuss ethical concerns directly with the potential Respondent before resorting to the Association's ethics complaint process.

1.2. **Jurisdiction**—The Code applies to persons who are or were Association members at the time of the conduct in question. Later nonrenewal or relinquishment of membership does not affect Association jurisdiction. The *Enforcement Procedures* that shall be utilized in any complaint shall be those in effect at the time the complaint is initiated.

1.3. Disciplinary Actions/Sanctions (Pursuing a Complaint)—If the EC determines that unethical conduct has occurred, it may impose sanctions, including reprimand, censure, probation (with terms) suspension, or permanent revocation of Association membership. In all cases, except those involving only reprimand (and educative letters), the Association will report the conclusions and sanctions in its official publications and also will communicate to any appropriate persons or entities. If an individual is on either the Roster of Fellows (ROF) or the Roster of Honor (ROH), the EC Chairperson (via the EC Staff Liaison) shall notify the VLDC Chairperson and Association Executive Director (ED) of their membership suspension or revocation. That individual shall have their name removed from either the ROF or the ROH and no longer has the right to use the designated credential of FAOTA or ROH during the period of suspension or permanently, in the case of revocation.

The EC Chairperson shall also notify the Chairperson of the Board for Advanced and Specialty Certification (BASC) (via Association staff liaison, in writing) of final disciplinary actions from the EC in which an individual's membership has been suspended or revoked. These individuals are not eligible to apply for or renew certification.

The potential sanctions are defined as follows:

1.3.1. Reprimand—A formal expression of disapproval of conduct communicated privately by letter from the EC Chairperson that is nondisclosable and noncommunicative to other bodies (e.g., state regulatory boards [SRBs], National Board for Certification in Occupational Therapy® [NBCOT®]). Reprimand is not publicly reported.

1.3.2. Censure—A formal expression of disapproval that is publicly reported.

1.3.3. Probation of Membership Subject to Terms—Continued membership is conditional, depending on fulfillment of specified terms. Failure to meet terms will subject an Association member to any of the disciplinary actions or sanctions. Terms may include but are not limited to

a.   Remedial activity, applicable to the violation, with proof of satisfactory completion, by a specific date; and

b.   The corrected behavior which is expected to be maintained.

Probation is publicly reported.

1.3.4. Suspension—Removal of Association membership for a specified period of time. Suspension is publicly reported.

1.3.5. Revocation—Permanent denial of Association membership. Revocation is publicly reported.

1.4. Educative Letters—If the EC determines that the alleged conduct may or may not be a true breach of the Code but in any event does not warrant any of the sanctions set forth in Section 1.3. or is not completely in keeping with the aspirational nature of the Code or within the prevailing standards of practice or professionalism, the EC may send a private letter to educate the Respondent about relevant standards of practice and/or appropriate professional behavior. In addition, a different private educative letter, if appropriate, may be sent to the Complainant.

1.5. Advisory Opinions—The EC may issue general advisory opinions on ethical issues to inform and educate the Association membership. These opinions shall be publicized to the membership and are available in the *Reference Guide to the Occupational Therapy Code of Ethics* as well as on the Association website.

1.6. Rules of Evidence—The EC proceedings shall be conducted in accordance with fundamental fairness. However, formal rules of evidence that are used in legal proceedings do not apply to these

Enforcement Procedures. The Disciplinary Council (see Section 5) and the Appeal Panel (see Section 6) can consider any evidence that they deem appropriate and pertinent.

1.7. Confidentiality and Disclosure—The EC develops and adheres to strict rules of confidentiality in every aspect of its work. This requires that participants in the process refrain from any communication relating to the existence and subject matter of the complaint other than with those directly involved in the enforcement process. Maintaining confidentiality throughout the investigation and enforcement process of a formal ethics complaint is essential in order to ensure fairness to all parties involved. These rules of confidentiality pertain not only to the EC but also apply to others involved in the complaint process. Beginning with the EC Staff Liaison and support staff, strict rules of confidentiality are followed. These same rules of confidentiality apply to Complainants, Respondents and their attorneys, and witnesses involved with the EC's investigatory process. Due diligence must be exercised by everyone involved in the investigation to avoid compromising the confidential nature of the process. Any Association member who breaches these rules of confidentiality may become subject to an ethics complaint/investigatory process himself or herself. Non–Association members may lodge an ethics complaint against an Association member, and these individuals are still expected to adhere to the Association's confidentiality rules. The Association reserves the right to take appropriate action against non–Association members who violate confidentiality rules, including notification of their appropriate licensure boards.

> **1.7.1. Disclosure**—When the EC investigates a complaint, it may request information from a variety of sources. The process of obtaining additional information is carefully executed in order to maintain confidentiality. The EC may request information from a variety of sources, including state licensing agencies, academic councils, courts, employers, and other persons and entities. It is within the EC's purview to determine what disclosures are appropriate for particular parties in order to effectively implement its investigatory obligations. Public sanctions by the EC, Disciplinary Council, or Appeal Panel will be publicized as provided in these *Enforcement Procedures.* Normally, the EC does not disclose information or documentation reviewed in the course of an investigation unless the EC determines that disclosure is necessary to obtain additional, relevant evidence or to administer the ethics process or is legally required.

Individuals who file a complaint (i.e., *Complainant*) and those who are the subject of one (i.e., *Respondent*) must not disclose to anyone outside of those involved in the complaint process their role in an ethics complaint. Disclosing this information in and of itself may jeopardize the ethics process and violate the rules of fundamental fairness by which all parties are protected. Disclosure of information related to any case under investigation by the EC is prohibited and, if done, will lead to repercussions as outlined in these *Enforcement Procedures* (see Section 2.2.3.).

2. Complaints

2.1. Interested Party Complaints

> **2.1.1.** Complaints stating an alleged violation of the Code may originate from any individual, group, or entity within or outside the Association. All complaints must be in writing, signed by the Complainant(s), and submitted to the Ethics Office at the Association headquarters. Complainants must complete the Formal Statement of Complaint Form at the end of this document. All complaints shall identify the person against whom the complaint is directed (the Respondent), the ethical principles that the Complainant believes have been violated, and the key facts and date(s) of the alleged ethical violations. If lawfully available, supporting documentation should be attached. Hard-copy complaints must be sent to the address indicated on the complaint form.

Complaints that are emailed must be sent as a pdf attachment, marked "Confidential" with "Complaint" in the subject line to ethics@aota.org and must include the complaint form and supporting documentation.

2.1.2. Within 90 days of receipt of a complaint, the EC shall make a preliminary assessment of the complaint and decide whether it presents sufficient questions as to a potential ethics violation that an investigation is warranted in accordance with Section 3. Commencing an investigation does not imply a conclusion that an ethical violation has in fact occurred or any judgment as to the ultimate sanction, if any, that may be appropriate. In the event the EC determines at the completion of an investigation that the complaint does rise to the level of an ethical violation, the EC may issue a decision as set forth in Section 4 below. In the event the EC determines that the complaint does not rise to the level of an ethical violation, the EC may direct the parties to utilize other conflict resolution resources or authorities via an educative letter. This applies to all complaints, including those involving Association elected/volunteer leadership related to their official roles.

2.2. Complaints Initiated by the EC

2.2.1. The EC itself may initiate a complaint (a *sua sponte* complaint) when it receives information from a governmental body, certification or similar body, public media, or other source indicating that a person subject to its jurisdiction may have committed acts that violate the Code. The Association will ordinarily act promptly after learning of the basis of a *sua sponte* complaint, but there is no specified time limit.

If the EC passes a motion to initiate a *sua sponte* complaint, the Association staff liaison to the EC will complete the Formal Statement of Complaint Form (at the end of this document) and will describe the nature of the factual allegations that led to the complaint and the manner in which the EC learned of the matter. The Complaint Form will be signed by the EC Chairperson on behalf of the EC. The form will be filed with the case material in the Association's Ethics Office.

2.2.2. *De Jure* **Complaints**—Where the source of a *sua sponte* complaint is the findings and conclusions of another official body, the EC classifies such *sua sponte* complaints as *de jure*. The procedure in such cases is addressed in Section 4.2.

2.2.3. The EC shall have the jurisdiction to investigate or sanction any matter or person for violations based on information learned in the course of investigating a complaint under Section 2.2.2.

2.3. Continuation of Complaint Process—If an Association member relinquishes membership, fails to renew membership, or fails to cooperate with the ethics investigation, the EC shall nevertheless continue to process the complaint, noting in its report the circumstances of the Respondent's action. Such actions shall not deprive the EC of jurisdiction. All correspondence related to the EC complaint process is in writing and sent by mail with signature and proof of date received. In the event that any written correspondence does not have delivery confirmation, the Association Ethics Office will make an attempt to search for an alternate physical or electronic address or make a second attempt to send to the original address. If the Respondent does not claim correspondence after two attempts to deliver, delivery cannot be confirmed or correspondence is returned to the Association as undeliverable, the EC shall consider that it has made good-faith effort and shall proceed with the ethics enforcement process.

3. EC Review and Investigations

3.1. Initial Action—The purpose of the preliminary review is to decide whether or not the information submitted with the complaint warrants opening the case. If in its preliminary review of the complaint the EC determines that an investigation is not warranted, the Complainant will be so notified.

3.2. Dismissal of Complaints—The EC may at any time dismiss a complaint for any of the following reasons:

    3.2.1. Lack of Jurisdiction—The EC determines that it has no jurisdiction over the Respondent (e.g., a complaint against a person who is or was not an Association member at the time of the alleged incident or who has never been a member).

    3.2.2. Absolute Time Limit/Not Timely Filed—The EC determines that the violation of the Code is alleged to have occurred more than 7 years prior to the filing of the complaint.

    3.2.3. Subject to Jurisdiction of Another Authority—The EC determines that the complaint is based on matters that are within the authority of and are more properly dealt with by another governmental or nongovernmental body, such as an SRB, NBCOT®, an Association component other than the EC, an employer, educational institution, or a court.

    3.2.4. No Ethics Violation—The EC finds that the complaint, even if proven, does not state a basis for action under the Code (e.g., simply accusing someone of being unpleasant or rude on an occasion).

    3.2.5. Insufficient Evidence—The EC determines that there clearly would not be sufficient factual evidence to support a finding of an ethics violation.

    3.2.6. Corrected Violation—The EC determines that any violation it might find already has been or is being corrected and that this is an adequate result in the given case.

    3.2.7. Other Good Cause.

3.3. Investigator and EC (Avoidance of Conflict of Interest)—The investigator chosen shall not have a conflict of interest (i.e., shall never have had a substantial professional, personal, financial, business, or volunteer relationship with either the Complainant or the Respondent). In the event that the EC Staff Liaison has such a conflict, the EC Chairperson shall appoint an alternate investigator who has no conflict of interest. Any member of the EC with a possible conflict of interest must disclose and may be recused.

3.4. Investigation—If an investigation is deemed warranted, the EC Chairperson shall do the following within thirty (30) days: Appoint the EC Staff Liaison at the Association headquarters to investigate the complaint and notify the Respondent by mail (requiring signature and proof of date of receipt) that a complaint has been received and an investigation is being conducted. A copy of the complaint and supporting documentation shall be enclosed with this notification. The Complainant also will receive notification by mail (requiring signature and proof of date of receipt) that the complaint is being investigated.

    3.4.1. Ordinarily, the Investigator will send questions formulated by the EC to be answered by the Complainant and/or the Respondent.

    3.4.2. The Complainant shall be given thirty (30) days from receipt of the questions (if any) to respond in writing to the investigator.

    3.4.3. The Respondent shall be given thirty (30) days from receipt of the questions to respond in writing to the Investigator.

    3.4.4. The EC ordinarily will notify the Complainant of any substantive new evidence adverse to the Complainant's initial complaint that is discovered in the course of the ethics investigation and allow the Complainant to respond to such adverse evidence. In such cases, the Complainant will be given a copy of such evidence and will have fourteen (14) days in which to submit a written response. If the new evidence clearly shows that there has been no ethics violation, the

EC may terminate the proceeding. In addition, if the investigation includes questions for both the Respondent and the Complainant, the evidence submitted by each party in response to the investigatory questions shall be provided to the Respondent and available to the Complainant on request. The EC may request reasonable payment for copying expenses depending on the volume of material to be sent.

3.4.5. The Investigator, in consultation with the EC, may obtain evidence directly from third parties without permission from the Complainant or Respondent.

3.5. Investigation Timeline—The investigation will be completed within ninety (90) days after receipt of notification by the Respondent or his or her designee that an investigation is being conducted, unless the EC determines that special circumstances warrant additional time for the investigation. All timelines noted here can be extended for good cause at the discretion of the EC, including the EC's schedule and additional requests of the Respondent. The Respondent and the Complainant shall be notified in writing if a delay occurs or if the investigational process requires more time.

3.6. Case Files—The investigative files shall include the complaint and any documentation on which the EC relied in initiating the investigation.

3.7. Cooperation by Respondent—Every Association Respondent has a duty to cooperate reasonably with enforcement processes for the Code. Failure of the Respondent to participate and/or cooperate with the investigative process of the EC shall not prevent continuation of the ethics process, and this behavior itself may constitute a violation of the Code.

3.8. Referral of Complaint—The EC may at any time refer a matter to NBCOT®, the SRB, ACOTE®, or other recognized authorities for appropriate action. Despite such referral to an appropriate authority, the EC shall retain jurisdiction. EC action may be stayed for a reasonable period pending notification of a decision by that authority, at the discretion of the EC (and such delays will extend the time periods under these *Procedures*). A stay in conducting an investigation shall not constitute a waiver by the EC of jurisdiction over the matters. The EC shall provide written notice by mail (requiring signature and proof of date of receipt) to the Respondent and the Complainant of any such stay of action.

4. EC Review and Decision

4.1. Regular Complaint Process

4.1.1. Decision—If at the conclusion of the investigation the EC determines that the Respondent has engaged in conduct that constitutes a breach of the Code, the EC shall notify the Respondent and Complainant by mail with signature and proof of date received. The notice shall describe in sufficient detail the conduct that constitutes a violation of the Code and indicate the sanction that is being imposed in accordance with these *Enforcement Procedures*.

4.1.2. Respondent's Response—Within 30 days of notification of the EC's decision and sanction, if any, the Respondent shall

4.1.2.1. Accept the decision of the EC (as to both the ethics violation and the sanction) and waive any right to a Disciplinary Council hearing, or

4.1.2.2. Accept the decision that he/she committed unethical conduct but within thirty (30) days, submit to the EC a statement (with any supporting documentation) setting forth the reasons why any sanction should not be imposed or reasons why the sanction should be mitigated or reduced.

4.1.2.3. Advise the EC Chairperson in writing that he or she contests the EC's decision and sanction and requests a hearing before the Disciplinary Council.

Failure of the Respondent to take one of these actions within the time specified will be deemed to constitute acceptance of the decision and sanction. If the Respondent requests a Disciplinary Council hearing, it will be scheduled. If the Respondent does not request a Disciplinary Council hearing but accepts the decision, the EC will notify all relevant parties and implement the sanction. Correspondence with the Respondent will also indicate that public sanctions may have an impact on their ability to serve in Association positions, whether elected or appointed, for a designated period of time.

4.2. *De Jure* Complaint Process

4.2.1. The EC Staff Liaison will present to the EC any findings from external sources (as described above) that come to his or her attention and that may warrant *sua sponte* complaints pertaining to individuals who are or were Association members at the time of the alleged incident.

4.2.2. Because *de jure* complaints are based on the findings of fact or conclusions of another official body, the EC will decide whether or not to act based on such findings or conclusions and will not ordinarily initiate another investigation, absent clear and convincing evidence that such findings and conclusions were erroneous or not supported by substantial evidence. Based on the information presented by the EC Staff Liaison, the EC will determine whether the findings of the public body also are sufficient to demonstrate an egregious violation of the Code and therefore warrant taking disciplinary action.

4.2.3. If the EC decides that a breach of the Code has occurred, the EC Chairperson will notify the Respondent in writing of the violation and the disciplinary action that is being taken. Correspondence with the Respondent will also indicate that public sanctions may have an impact on their ability to serve in Association positions, whether elected or appointed, for a designated period of time. In response to the *de jure sua sponte* decision and sanction by the EC, the Respondent may

4.2.3.1. Accept the decision of the EC (as to both the ethics violation and the sanction) based solely on the findings of fact and conclusions of the EC or the public body, and waive any right to a Disciplinary Council hearing;

4.2.3.2. Accept the decision that the Respondent committed unethical conduct but within thirty (30) days submit to the EC a statement (with any supporting documentation) setting forth the reasons why any sanction should not be imposed or reasons why the sanction should be mitigated or reduced; or

4.2.3.3. Within thirty (30) days, present information showing the findings of fact of the official body relied on by the EC to impose the sanction are clearly erroneous and request reconsideration by the EC. The EC may have the option of opening an investigation or modifying the sanction in the event they find clear and convincing evidence that the findings and the conclusions of the other body are erroneous.

4.2.4. In cases of *de jure* complaints, a Disciplinary Council hearing can later be requested (pursuant to Section 5 below) only if the Respondent has first exercised Options 4.2.3.2 or 4.2.3.3.

4.2.5. Respondents in an ethics case may utilize Options 4.2.3.2 or 4.2.3.3 (reconsideration) once in responding to the EC. Following one review of the additional information submitted by the Respondent, if the EC reaffirms its original sanction, the Respondent has the option of accepting the violation and proposed sanction or requesting a Disciplinary Council hearing. Repeated requests for reconsideration will not be accepted by the EC.

5. Disciplinary Council

5.1. Purpose—The purpose of the Disciplinary Council (hereinafter to be known as the Council) hearing is to provide the Respondent an opportunity to present evidence and witnesses to answer and refute the decision and/or sanction and to permit the EC Chairperson or designee to present evidence and witnesses in support of his or her decision. The Council shall consider the matters alleged in the complaint; the matters raised in defense as well as other relevant facts, ethical principles, and federal or state law, if applicable. The Council may question the parties concerned and determine ethical issues arising from the factual matters in the case even if those specific ethical issues were not raised by the Complainant. The Council also may choose to apply Principles or other language from the Code not originally identified by the EC. The Council may affirm the decision of the EC or reverse or modify it if it finds that the decision was clearly erroneous or a material departure from its written procedure.

5.2. Parties—The parties to a Council Hearing are the Respondent and the EC Chairperson.

5.3. Criteria and Process for Selection of Council Members

5.3.1. Criteria

    5.3.1.1. Association Administrative Standard Operating Procedures (SOP) and Association Policy 2.6 shall be considered in the selection of qualified potential candidates for the Council, which shall be composed of qualified individuals and Association members drawn from a pool of candidates who meet the criteria outlined below. Members ideally will have some knowledge or experience in the areas of activity that are at issue in the case. They also will have experience in disciplinary hearings and/or general knowledge about ethics as demonstrated by education, presentations, and/or publications.

    5.3.1.2. No conflict of interest may exist with either the Complainant or the Respondent (refer to Association Policy A.13—Conflict of Interest for guidance).

    5.3.1.3. No individual may serve on the Council who is currently a member of the EC or the Board of Directors

    5.3.1.4. No individual may serve on the Council who has previously been the subject of an ethics complaint that resulted in a public EC disciplinary action within the past three (3) years.

    5.3.1.5. The public member on the Council shall have knowledge of the profession and ethical issues.

    5.3.1.6. The public member shall not be an occupational therapist or occupational therapy assistant (practitioner, educator, or researcher.)

5.4. Criteria and Process for Selection of Council Chairperson

5.4.1. Criteria

    5.4.1.1. Must have experience in analyzing/reviewing cases.

    5.4.1.2. May be selected from the pool of candidates for the Council or a former EC member who has been off the EC for at least three (3) years.

    5.4.1.3. The EC Chairperson shall not serve as the Council Chairperson.

5.4.2. Process

5.4.2.1. The Representative Assembly (RA) Speaker (in consultation with EC Staff Liaison) will select the Council Chairperson.

5.4.2.2. If the RA Speaker needs to be recused from this duty, the RA Vice Speaker will select the Council Chairperson.

5.5. Process

5.5.1. Potential candidates for the Council pool will be recruited through public postings in official publications and via the electronic forums. Association leadership will be encouraged to recruit qualified candidates. Potential members of the Council shall be interviewed to ascertain the following:

a.   Willingness to serve on the Council and availability for a period of three (3) years and

b.   Qualifications per criteria outlined in Section 5.3.1.

5.5.2. The President and EC Staff Liaison will maintain a pool of no fewer than six (6) and no more than twelve (12) qualified individuals.

5.5.3. The President, with input from the EC Staff Liaison, will select from the pool the members of each Council within thirty (30) days of notification by a Respondent that a Council is being requested.

5.5.4. Each Council shall be composed of three (3) Association members in good standing and a public member.

5.5.5. The EC Staff Liaison will remove anyone with a potential conflict of interest in a particular case from the potential Council pool.

5.6. Notification of Parties (EC Chairperson, Complainant, Respondent, Council Members)

5.6.1. The EC Staff Liaison shall schedule a hearing date in coordination with the Council Chairperson.

5.6.2. The Council (via the EC Staff Liaison) shall notify all parties at least forty-five (45) days prior to the hearing of the date, time, and place.

5.6.3. Case material will be sent to all parties and the Council members by national delivery service or mail with signature required and/or proof of date received.

5.7. Hearing Witnesses, Materials, and Evidence

5.7.1. Within thirty (30) days of notification of the hearing, the Respondent shall submit to the Council a written response to the decision and sanction, including a detailed statement as to the reasons that he or she is appealing the decision and a list of potential witnesses (if any) with a statement indicating the subject matter they will be addressing.

5.7.2. The Complainant before the Council also will submit a list of potential witnesses (if any) to the Council with a statement indicating the subject matter they will be addressing. Only under limited circumstances may the Council consider additional material evidence from the Respondent or the Complainant not presented or available prior to the issuance of their proposed sanction. Such new or additional evidence may be considered by the Council if the Council is satisfied that the Respondent or the Complainant has demonstrated the new evidence was previously unavailable and provided it is submitted to all parties in writing no later than fifteen (15) days prior to the hearing.

5.7.3. The Council Chairperson may permit testimony by conference call (at no expense to the participant), limit participation of witnesses in order to curtail repetitive testimony, or prescribe other reasonable arrangements or limitations. The Respondent may elect to appear (at Respondent's own expense) and present testimony. If alternative technology options are available for the hearing, the Respondent, Council members, and EC Chairperson shall be so informed when the hearing arrangements are sent.

5.8. **Counsel**—The Respondent may be represented by legal counsel at his or her own expense. Association Legal Counsel shall advise and represent the Association at the hearing. Association Legal Counsel also may advise the Council regarding procedural matters to ensure fairness to all parties. All parties and the Association Legal Counsel (at the request of the EC or the Council) shall have the opportunity to question witnesses.

5.9. **Hearing**

5.9.1. The Council hearing shall be recorded by a professional transcription service or telephone recording transcribed for Council members and shall be limited to two (2) hours.

5.9.2. The Council Chairperson will conduct the hearing and does not vote.

5.9.3. Each person present shall be identified for the record, and the Council Chairperson will describe the procedures for the Council hearing. An oral affirmation of truthfulness will be requested from each participant who gives factual testimony in the Council hearing.

5.9.4. The Council Chairperson shall allow for questions.

5.9.5. The EC Chairperson shall present the ethics complaint, a summary of the evidence resulting from the investigation, and the EC decision and disciplinary action imposed against the Respondent.

5.9.6. The Respondent may present a defense to the decision and sanction after the EC presents its case.

5.9.7. Each party and/or his or her legal representative shall have the opportunity to call witnesses to present testimony and to question any witnesses including the EC Chairperson or his or her designee. The Council Chairperson shall be entitled to provide reasonable limits on the extent of any witnesses' testimony or any questioning.

5.9.8. The Council Chairperson may recess the hearing at any time.

5.9.9. The Council Chairperson shall call for final statements from each party before concluding the hearing.

5.9.10. Decisions of the Council will be by majority vote.

5.10. **Disciplinary Council Decision**

5.10.1. An official copy of the transcript shall be sent to each Council member, the EC Chairperson, the Association Legal Counsel, the EC Staff Liaison, and the Respondent and his or her counsel as soon as it is available from the transcription company.

5.10.2. The Council Chairperson shall work with the EC Staff Liaison and the Association Legal Counsel in preparing the text of the final decision.

5.10.3. The Council shall issue a decision in writing to the Association ED within thirty (30) days of receiving the written transcription of the hearing (unless special circumstances warrant additional time). The Council decision shall be based on the record and evidence presented and may affirm, modify, or reverse the decision of the EC, including increasing or decreasing the level of sanction or determining that no disciplinary action is warranted.

5.11. Action, Notification, and Timeline Adjustments

5.11.1. A copy of the Council's official decision and appeal process (Section 6) is sent to the Respondent, the EC Chairperson, and other appropriate parties within fifteen (15) business days via mail (with signature and proof of date received) after notification of the Association ED.

5.11.2. The time limits specified in the *Enforcement Procedures for the Occupational Therapy Code of Ethics* may be extended by mutual consent of the Respondent, Complainant, and Council Chairperson for good cause by the Chairperson.

5.11.3. Other features of the preceding *Enforcement Procedures* may be adjusted in particular cases in light of extraordinary circumstances, consistent with fundamental fairness.

5.12. Appeal—Within thirty (30) days after notification of the Council's decision, a Respondent upon whom a sanction was imposed may appeal the decision as provided in Section 6. Within thirty (30) days after notification of the Council's decision, the EC also may appeal the decision as provided in Section 6. If no appeal is filed within that time, the Association ED or EC Staff Liaison shall publish the decision in accordance with these procedures and make any other notifications deemed necessary.

6. Appeal Process

6.1. Appeals—Either the EC or the Respondent may appeal. Appeals shall be written, signed by the appealing party, and sent by mail requiring signature and proof of date of receipt to the Association ED in care of the Association Ethics Office. The grounds for the appeal shall be fully explained in this document. When an appeal is requested, the other party will be notified.

6.2. Grounds for Appeal—Appeals shall generally address only the issues, procedures, or sanctions that are part of the record before the Council. However, in the interest of fairness, the Appeal Panel may consider newly available evidence relating to the original complaint only under extraordinary circumstances.

6.3. Composition and Leadership of Appeal Panel—The Vice-President, Secretary, and Treasurer shall constitute the Appeal Panel. In the event of vacancies in these positions or the existence of a conflict of interest, the Vice President shall appoint replacements drawn from among the other Board of Directors members. If the entire Board has a conflict of interest, the Board Appeal process (Attachment C of EC SOP) shall be followed. The President shall not serve on the Appeal Panel. No individual may serve on the Council who has previously been the subject of an ethics complaint that resulted in a specific EC disciplinary action.

The Appeal Panel Chairperson will be selected by its members from among themselves.

6.4. Appeal Process—The Association ED shall forward any letter of appeal to the Appeal Panel within fifteen (15) business days of receipt. Within thirty (30) days after the Appeal Panel receives the appeal, the Panel shall determine whether a hearing is warranted. If the Panel decides that a hearing is warranted, timely notice for such hearing shall be given to the parties. Participants at the hearing shall be limited to the Respondent and legal counsel (if so desired), the EC Chairperson, the Council Chairperson, the Association Legal Counsel, or others approved in advance by the Appeal Panel as necessary to the proceedings.

6.5. Decision

6.5.1. The Appeal Panel shall have the power to (a) affirm the decision; (b) modify the decision; or (c) reverse or remand to the EC, but only if there were procedural errors materially prejudicial to the outcome of the proceeding or if the Council decision was against the clear weight of the evidence.

6.5.2. Within thirty (30) days after receipt of the appeal if no hearing was granted, or within thirty (30) days after receipt of the transcript of an Appeal hearing if held, the Appeal Panel shall notify the Association ED of its decision. The Association ED shall promptly notify the Respondent, the original Complainant, appropriate Association bodies, and any other parties deemed appropriate (e.g., SRB, NBCOT®). For Association purposes, the decision of the Appeal Panel shall be final.

7. Notifications

All notifications referred to in these *Enforcement Procedures* shall be in writing and shall be delivered by national delivery service or mail with signature and proof of date received.

8. Records and Reports

At the completion of the enforcement process, the written records and reports that state the initial basis for the complaint, material evidence, and the disposition of the complaint shall be retained in the Association Ethics Office for a period of five (5) years.

9. Publication

Final decisions will be publicized only after any appeal process has been completed.

10. Modification

The Association reserves the right to (a) modify the time periods, procedures, or application of these *Enforcement Procedures* for good cause consistent with fundamental fairness in a given case and (b) modify its *Code* and/or these *Enforcement Procedures,* with such modifications to be applied only prospectively.

Adopted by the Representative Assembly 2015NovCO13 as Attachment A of the Standard Operating Procedures (SOP) of the Ethics Commission

Reviewed by BPPC 1/04, 1/05, 9/06, 1/07, 9/09, 9/11, 9/13, 9/15

Adopted by RA 4/96, 5/04, 5/05, 11/06, 4/07, 11/09, 12/13

Revised by SEC 4/98, 4/00, 1/02, 1/04, 12/04, 9/06

Revised by EC 12/06, 2/07, 8/09, 9/13, 9/15

This document replaces the 2014 document *Enforcement Procedures for the Occupational Therapy Code of Ethics and Ethics Standards,* previously published and copyrighted in 2014 by the American Occupational Therapy Association in the *American Journal of Occupational Therapy, 68*(Suppl. 3), S3–S15. http://dx.doi.org/10.5014/ajot.2014.686S02

Citation: American Occupational Therapy Association. (2015). Enforcement procedures for the *Occupational Therapy Code of Ethics. American Journal of Occupational Therapy, 69*(Suppl. 3), 6913410012. http://dx.doi.org/10.5014/ajot.2014.696S19

AMERICAN OCCUPATIONAL THERAPY ASSOCIATION
ETHICS COMMISSION

Formal Complaint of Alleged Violation of the Occupational Therapy Code of Ethics

If an investigation is deemed necessary, a copy of this form will be provided to the individual against whom the complaint is filed.

Date _____

Complainant: (Information regarding individual filing the complaint)

NAME	SIGNATURE
ADDRESS	TELEPHONE
	E-MAIL ADDRESS

Respondent: (Information regarding individual against whom the complaint is directed)

NAME	SIGNATURE
ADDRESS	TELEPHONE
	E-MAIL ADDRESS

1. **Summarize** in a written attachment the **facts and circumstances, including dates and events,** that support a violation of the Occupational Therapy Code of Ethics and this complaint. Include steps, if any, that have been taken to resolve this complaint before filing.

2. **Please sign and date all documents you have written and are submitting.** Do not include confidential documents such as patient or employment records.

3. **If you have filed a complaint about this same matter with any other agency (e.g., NBCOT®; SRB; academic institution; any federal, state, or local official), indicate to whom it was submitted, the approximate date(s), and resolution if known.**

I certify that the statements/information within this complaint are correct and truthful to the best of my knowledge and are submitted in good faith, not for resolution of private business, legal, or other disputes for which other appropriate forums exist.

_____
Signature

Send completed form, with accompanying documentation, **IN AN ENVELOPE MARKED CONFIDENTIAL to**

**Ethics Commission
American Occupational Therapy Association, Inc.
Attn: Ethics Program Manager/Ethics Office
4720 Montgomery Lane, Suite 200
Bethesda, MD 20814-3449**

**OR email all material in pdf format to
ethics@aota.org with "Complaint" in subject line**

Office Use Only:
Membership Verified? ❑ Yes ❑ No
By: _____

Occupational Therapy Code of Ethics (2015)

Preamble

The 2015 *Occupational Therapy Code of Ethics* (Code) of the American Occupational Therapy Association (AOTA) is designed to reflect the dynamic nature of the profession, the evolving health care environment, and emerging technologies that can present potential ethical concerns in research, education, and practice. AOTA members are committed to promoting inclusion, participation, safety, and well-being for all recipients in various stages of life, health, and illness and to empowering all beneficiaries of service to meet their occupational needs. Recipients of services may be individuals, groups, families, organizations, communities, or populations (AOTA, 2014b).

The Code is an AOTA Official Document and a public statement tailored to address the most prevalent ethical concerns of the occupational therapy profession. It outlines Standards of Conduct the public can expect from those in the profession. It should be applied to all areas of occupational therapy and shared with relevant stakeholders to promote ethical conduct.

The Code serves two purposes:

1. It provides aspirational Core Values that guide members toward ethical courses of action in professional and volunteer roles.

2. It delineates enforceable Principles and Standards of Conduct that apply to AOTA members.

Whereas the Code helps guide and define decision-making parameters, ethical action goes beyond rote compliance with these Principles and is a manifestation of moral character and mindful reflection. It is a commitment to benefit others, to virtuous practice of artistry and science, to genuinely good behaviors, and to noble acts of courage. Recognizing and resolving ethical issues is a systematic process that includes analyzing the complex dynamics of situations, weighing consequences, making reasoned decisions, taking action, and reflecting on outcomes. Occupational therapy personnel, including students in occupational therapy programs, are expected to abide by the Principles and Standards of Conduct within this Code. Personnel roles include clinicians (e.g., direct service, consultation, administration); educators; researchers; entrepreneurs; business owners; and those in elected, appointed, or other professional volunteer service.

The process for addressing ethics violations by AOTA members (and associate members, where applicable) is outlined in the Code's Enforcement Procedures (AOTA, 2014a).

Although the Code can be used in conjunction with licensure board regulations and laws that guide standards of practice, the Code is meant to be a free-standing document, guiding ethical dimensions of professional behavior, responsibility, practice, and decision making. This Code is not exhaustive; that is, the Principles and Standards of Conduct cannot address every possible situation. Therefore, before making complex ethical decisions that require further expertise, occupational therapy personnel should seek out resources to assist in resolving ethical issues not addressed in this document. Resources can include, but are not limited to, ethics committees, ethics officers, the AOTA Ethics Commission or Ethics Program Manager, or an ethics consultant.

Core Values

The profession is grounded in seven long-standing Core Values: (1) Altruism, (2) Equality, (3) Freedom, (4) Justice, (5) Dignity, (6) Truth, and (7) Prudence. *Altruism* involves demonstrating concern for the welfare of others. *Equality* refers to treating all people impartially and free of bias. *Freedom* and personal choice are paramount in a profession in which the values and desires of the client guide our interventions. *Justice* expresses a state in which diverse communities are inclusive; diverse communities are organized and structured such that all members can function, flourish, and live a satisfactory life. Occupational therapy personnel, by virtue of the specific nature of the practice of occupational therapy, have a vested interest in addressing unjust inequities that limit opportunities for participation in society (Braveman & Bass-Haugen, 2009).

Inherent in the practice of occupational therapy is the promotion and preservation of the individuality and *Dignity* of the client by treating him or her with respect in all interactions. In all situations, occupational therapy personnel must provide accurate information in oral, written, and electronic forms (*Truth*). Occupational therapy personnel use their clinical and ethical reasoning skills, sound judgment, and reflection to make decisions in professional and volunteer roles (*Prudence*).

The seven Core Values provide a foundation to guide occupational therapy personnel in their interactions with others. Although the Core Values are not themselves enforceable standards, they should be considered when determining the most ethical course of action.

Principles and Standards of Conduct

The Principles and Standards of Conduct that are enforceable for professional behavior include (1) Beneficence, (2) Nonmaleficence, (3) Autonomy, (4) Justice, (5) Veracity, and (6) Fidelity. Reflection on the historical foundations of occupational therapy and related professions resulted in the inclusion of Principles that are consistently referenced as a guideline for ethical decision making.

BENEFICENCE

Principle 1. Occupational therapy personnel shall demonstrate a concern for the well-being and safety of the recipients of their services.

Beneficence includes all forms of action intended to benefit other persons. The term *beneficence* connotes acts of mercy, kindness, and charity (Beauchamp & Childress, 2013). Beneficence requires taking action by helping others, in other words, by promoting good, by preventing harm, and by removing harm. Examples of beneficence include protecting and defending the rights of others, preventing harm from occurring to others, removing conditions that will cause harm to others, helping persons with disabilities, and rescuing persons in danger (Beauchamp & Childress, 2013).

RELATED STANDARDS OF CONDUCT

Occupational therapy personnel shall

A. Provide appropriate evaluation and a plan of intervention for recipients of occupational therapy services specific to their needs.

B. Reevaluate and reassess recipients of service in a timely manner to determine whether goals are being achieved and whether intervention plans should be revised.

C. Use, to the extent possible, evaluation, planning, intervention techniques, assessments, and therapeutic equipment that are evidence based, current, and within the recognized scope of occupational therapy practice.

D. Ensure that all duties delegated to other occupational therapy personnel are congruent with credentials, qualifications, experience, competency, and scope of practice with respect to service delivery, supervision, fieldwork education, and research.

E. Provide occupational therapy services, including education and training, that are within each practitioner's level of competence and scope of practice.

F. Take steps (e.g., continuing education, research, supervision, training) to ensure proficiency, use careful judgment, and weigh potential for harm when generally recognized standards do not exist in emerging technology or areas of practice.

G. Maintain competency by ongoing participation in education relevant to one's practice area.

H. Terminate occupational therapy services in collaboration with the service recipient or responsible party when the services are no longer beneficial.

I. Refer to other providers when indicated by the needs of the client.

J. Conduct and disseminate research in accordance with currently accepted ethical guidelines and standards for the protection of research participants, including determination of potential risks and benefits.

NONMALEFICENCE

Principle 2. Occupational therapy personnel shall refrain from actions that cause harm.

Nonmaleficence "obligates us to abstain from causing harm to others" (Beauchamp & Childress, 2013, p. 150). The Principle of *Nonmaleficence* also includes an obligation to not impose risks of harm even if the potential risk is without malicious or harmful intent. This Principle often is examined under the context of due care. The standard of *due care* "requires that the goals pursued justify the risks that must be imposed to achieve those goals" (Beauchamp & Childress, 2013, p. 154). For example, in occupational therapy practice, this standard applies to situations in which the client might feel pain from a treatment intervention; however, the acute pain is justified by potential longitudinal, evidence-based benefits of the treatment.

RELATED STANDARDS OF CONDUCT

Occupational therapy personnel shall

A. Avoid inflicting harm or injury to recipients of occupational therapy services, students, research participants, or employees.

B. Avoid abandoning the service recipient by facilitating appropriate transitions when unable to provide services for any reason.

C. Recognize and take appropriate action to remedy personal problems and limitations that might cause harm to recipients of service, colleagues, students, research participants, or others.

D. Avoid any undue influences that may impair practice and compromise the ability to safely and competently provide occupational therapy services, education, or research.

E. Address impaired practice and, when necessary, report it to the appropriate authorities.

F. Avoid dual relationships, conflicts of interest, and situations in which a practitioner, educator, student, researcher, or employer is unable to maintain clear professional boundaries or objectivity.

G. Avoid engaging in sexual activity with a recipient of service, including the client's family or significant other, student, research participant, or employee, while a professional relationship exists.

H. Avoid compromising the rights or well-being of others based on arbitrary directives (e.g., unrealistic productivity expectations, falsification of documentation, inaccurate coding) by exercising professional judgment and critical analysis.

I. Avoid exploiting any relationship established as an occupational therapy clinician, educator, or researcher to further one's own physical, emotional, financial, political, or business interests at the expense of recipients of services, students, research participants, employees, or colleagues.

J. Avoid bartering for services when there is the potential for exploitation and conflict of interest.

AUTONOMY

Principle 3. Occupational therapy personnel shall respect the right of the individual to self-determination, privacy, confidentiality, and consent.

The Principle of *Autonomy* expresses the concept that practitioners have a duty to treat the client according to the client's desires, within the bounds of accepted standards of care, and to protect the client's confidential information. Often, respect for Autonomy is referred to as the *self-determination principle*. However, respecting a person's autonomy goes beyond acknowledging an individual as a mere agent and also acknowledges a person's right "to hold views, to make choices, and to take actions based on [his or her] values and beliefs" (Beauchamp & Childress, 2013, p. 106). Individuals have the right to make a determination regarding care decisions that directly affect their lives. In the event that a person lacks decision-making capacity, his or her autonomy should be respected through involvement of an authorized agent or surrogate decision maker.

RELATED STANDARDS OF CONDUCT

Occupational therapy personnel shall

A. Respect and honor the expressed wishes of recipients of service.

B. Fully disclose the benefits, risks, and potential outcomes of any intervention; the personnel who will be providing the intervention; and any reasonable alternatives to the proposed intervention.

C. Obtain consent after disclosing appropriate information and answering any questions posed by the recipient of service or research participant to ensure voluntariness.

D. Establish a collaborative relationship with recipients of service and relevant stakeholders to promote shared decision making.

E. Respect the client's right to refuse occupational therapy services temporarily or permanently, even when that refusal has potential to result in poor outcomes.

F. Refrain from threatening, coercing, or deceiving clients to promote compliance with occupational therapy recommendations.

G. Respect a research participant's right to withdraw from a research study without penalty.

H. Maintain the confidentiality of all verbal, written, electronic, augmentative, and nonverbal communications, in compliance with applicable laws, including all aspects of privacy laws and exceptions thereto (e.g., Health Insurance Portability and Accountability Act [Pub. L. 104–191], Family Educational Rights and Privacy Act [Pub. L. 93–380]).

I. Display responsible conduct and discretion when engaging in social networking, including but not limited to refraining from posting protected health information.

J. Facilitate comprehension and address barriers to communication (e.g., aphasia; differences in language, literacy, culture) with the recipient of service (or responsible party), student, or research participant.

JUSTICE

Principle 4. Occupational therapy personnel shall promote fairness and objectivity in the provision of occupational therapy services.

The Principle of *Justice* relates to the fair, equitable, and appropriate treatment of persons (Beauchamp & Childress, 2013). Occupational therapy personnel should relate in a respectful, fair, and impartial manner to individuals and groups with whom they interact. They should also respect the applicable laws and standards related to their area of practice. Justice requires the impartial consideration and consistent following of rules to generate unbiased decisions and promote fairness. As occupational therapy personnel, we work to uphold a society in which all individuals have an equitable opportunity to achieve occupational engagement as an essential component of their life.

RELATED STANDARDS OF CONDUCT

Occupational therapy personnel shall

A. Respond to requests for occupational therapy services (e.g., a referral) in a timely manner as determined by law, regulation, or policy.

B. Assist those in need of occupational therapy services in securing access through available means.

C. Address barriers in access to occupational therapy services by offering or referring clients to financial aid, charity care, or pro bono services within the parameters of organizational policies.

D. Advocate for changes to systems and policies that are discriminatory or unfairly limit or prevent access to occupational therapy services.

E. Maintain awareness of current laws and AOTA policies and Official Documents that apply to the profession of occupational therapy.

F. Inform employers, employees, colleagues, students, and researchers of applicable policies, laws, and Official Documents.

G. Hold requisite credentials for the occupational therapy services they provide in academic, research, physical, or virtual work settings.

H. Provide appropriate supervision in accordance with AOTA Official Documents and relevant laws, regulations, policies, procedures, standards, and guidelines.

I. Obtain all necessary approvals prior to initiating research activities.

J. Refrain from accepting gifts that would unduly influence the therapeutic relationship or have the potential to blur professional boundaries, and adhere to employer policies when offered gifts.

K. Report to appropriate authorities any acts in practice, education, and research that are unethical or illegal.

L. Collaborate with employers to formulate policies and procedures in compliance with legal, regulatory, and ethical standards and work to resolve any conflicts or inconsistencies.

M. Bill and collect fees legally and justly in a manner that is fair, reasonable, and commensurate with services delivered.

N. Ensure compliance with relevant laws, and promote transparency when participating in a business arrangement as owner, stockholder, partner, or employee.

O. Ensure that documentation for reimbursement purposes is done in accordance with applicable laws, guidelines, and regulations.

P. Refrain from participating in any action resulting in unauthorized access to educational content or exams (including but not limited to sharing test questions, unauthorized use of or access to content or codes, or selling access or authorization codes).

VERACITY

Principle 5. Occupational therapy personnel shall provide comprehensive, accurate, and objective information when representing the profession.

Veracity is based on the virtues of truthfulness, candor, and honesty. The Principle of *Veracity* refers to comprehensive, accurate, and objective transmission of information and includes fostering understanding of such information (Beauchamp & Childress, 2013). Veracity is based on respect owed to others, including but not limited to recipients of service, colleagues, students, researchers, and research participants.

In communicating with others, occupational therapy personnel implicitly promise to be truthful and not deceptive. When entering into a therapeutic or research relationship, the recipient of service or research participant has a right to accurate information. In addition, transmission of information is incomplete without also ensuring that the recipient or participant understands the information provided.

Concepts of veracity must be carefully balanced with other potentially competing ethical principles, cultural beliefs, and organizational policies. Veracity ultimately is valued as a means to establish trust and strengthen professional relationships. Therefore, adherence to the Principle of Veracity also requires thoughtful analysis of how full disclosure of information may affect outcomes.

RELATED STANDARDS OF CONDUCT

Occupational therapy personnel shall

A. Represent credentials, qualifications, education, experience, training, roles, duties, competence, contributions, and findings accurately in all forms of communication.

B. Refrain from using or participating in the use of any form of communication that contains false, fraudulent, deceptive, misleading, or unfair statements or claims.

C. Record and report in an accurate and timely manner and in accordance with applicable regulations all information related to professional or academic documentation and activities.

D. Identify and fully disclose to all appropriate persons errors or adverse events that compromise the safety of service recipients.

E. Ensure that all marketing and advertising are truthful, accurate, and carefully presented to avoid misleading recipients of service, research participants, or the public.

F. Describe the type and duration of occupational therapy services accurately in professional contracts, including the duties and responsibilities of all involved parties.

G. Be honest, fair, accurate, respectful, and timely in gathering and reporting fact-based information regarding employee job performance and student performance.

H. Give credit and recognition when using the ideas and work of others in written, oral, or electronic media (i.e., do not plagiarize).

I. Provide students with access to accurate information regarding educational requirements and academic policies and procedures relative to the occupational therapy program or educational institution.

J. Maintain privacy and truthfulness when using telecommunication in the delivery of occupational therapy services.

FIDELITY

Principle 6. Occupational therapy personnel shall treat clients, colleagues, and other professionals with respect, fairness, discretion, and integrity.

The Principle of Fidelity comes from the Latin root *fidelis,* meaning loyal. *Fidelity* refers to the duty one has to keep a commitment once it is made (Veatch, Haddad, & English, 2010). In the health professions, this commitment refers to promises made between a provider and a client or patient based on an expectation of loyalty, staying with the client or patient in a time of need, and compliance with a code of ethics. These promises can be implied or explicit. The duty to disclose information that is potentially meaningful in making decisions is one obligation of the moral contract between provider and client or patient (Veatch et al., 2010).

Whereas respecting Fidelity requires occupational therapy personnel to meet the client's reasonable expectations, the Principle also addresses maintaining respectful collegial and organizational relationships (Purtilo & Doherty, 2011). Professional relationships are greatly influenced by the complexity of the environment in which occupational therapy personnel work. Practitioners, educators, and researchers alike must consistently balance their duties to service recipients, students, research participants, and other professionals as well as to organizations that may influence decision making and professional practice.

RELATED STANDARDS OF CONDUCT

Occupational therapy personnel shall

A. Preserve, respect, and safeguard private information about employees, colleagues, and students unless otherwise mandated or permitted by relevant laws.

B. Address incompetent, disruptive, unethical, illegal, or impaired practice that jeopardizes the safety or well-being of others and team effectiveness.

C. Avoid conflicts of interest or conflicts of commitment in employment, volunteer roles, or research.

D. Avoid using one's position (employee or volunteer) or knowledge gained from that position in such a manner as to give rise to real or perceived conflict of interest among the person, the employer, other AOTA members, or other organizations.

E. Be diligent stewards of human, financial, and material resources of their employers, and refrain from exploiting these resources for personal gain.

F. Refrain from verbal, physical, emotional, or sexual harassment of peers or colleagues.

G. Refrain from communication that is derogatory, intimidating, or disrespectful and that unduly discourages others from participating in professional dialogue.

H. Promote collaborative actions and communication as a member of interprofessional teams to facilitate quality care and safety for clients.

I. Respect the practices, competencies, roles, and responsibilities of their own and other professions to promote a collaborative environment reflective of interprofessional teams.

J. Use conflict resolution and internal and alternative dispute resolution resources as needed to resolve organizational and interpersonal conflicts, as well as perceived institutional ethics violations.

K.   Abide by policies, procedures, and protocols when serving or acting on behalf of a professional organization or employer to fully and accurately represent the organization's official and authorized positions.

L.   Refrain from actions that reduce the public's trust in occupational therapy.

M.   Self-identify when personal, cultural, or religious values preclude, or are anticipated to negatively affect, the professional relationship or provision of services, while adhering to organizational policies when requesting an exemption from service to an individual or group on the basis of conflict of conscience.

References

American Occupational Therapy Association. (2014a). Enforcement procedures for the *Occupational therapy code of ethics and ethics standards. American Journal of Occupational Therapy, 68*(Suppl. 3), S3–S15. http://dx.doi.org/10.5014/ajot.2014.686S02

American Occupational Therapy Association. (2014b). Occupational therapy practice framework: Domain and process (3rd ed.). *American Journal of Occupational Therapy, 68* (Suppl. 1), S1–S48. http://dx.doi.org/10.5014/ajot.2014.682006

Beauchamp, T. L., & Childress, J. F. (2013). *Principles of biomedical ethics* (7th ed.). New York: Oxford University Press.

Braveman, B., & Bass-Haugen, J. D. (2009). Social justice and health disparities: An evolving discourse in occupational therapy research and intervention. *American Journal of Occupational Therapy, 63,* 7–12. http://dx.doi.org/10.5014/ajot.63.1.7

Purtilo, R., & Doherty, R. (2011). *Ethical dimensions in the health professions* (5th ed.). Philadelphia: Saunders/Elsevier.

Veatch, R. M., Haddad, A. M., & English, D. C. (2010). *Case studies in biomedical ethics.* New York: Oxford University Press.

Ethics Commission

Yvette Hachtel, JD, OTR/L, *Chair (2013–2014)*
Lea Cheyney Brandt, OTD, MA, OTR/L, *Chair (2014–2015)*
Ann Moodey Ashe, MHS, OTR/L *(2011–2014)*
Joanne Estes, PhD, OTR/L *(2012–2015)*
Loretta Jean Foster, MS, COTA/L *(2011–2014)*
Wayne L. Winistorfer, MPA, OTR *(2014–2017)*
Linda Scheirton, PhD, RDH *(2012–2015)*
Kate Payne, JD, RN *(2013–2014)*
Margaret R. Moon, MD, MPH, FAAP *(2014–2016)*
Kimberly S. Erler, MS, OTR/L *(2014–2017)*
Kathleen McCracken, MHA, COTA/L *(2014–2017)*
Deborah Yarett Slater, MS, OT/L, FAOTA, *AOTA Ethics Program Manager*

Adopted by the Representative Assembly 2015AprilC3

Guidelines

Guidelines for Documentation of Occupational Therapy

Documentation of occupational therapy services is necessary whenever professional services are provided to a client. Occupational therapists and occupational therapy assistants[1] determine the appropriate type of documentation structure and then record the services provided within their scope of practice. This document, based on the *Occupational Therapy Practice Framework: Domain and Process* (2nd ed.; American Occupational Therapy Association [AOTA], 2008), describes the components and purpose of professional documentation used in occupational therapy.

AOTA's (2010) *Standards of Practice for Occupational Therapy* states that an occupational therapy practitioner[2] documents the occupational therapy services and "abides by the time frames, format, and standards established by the practice settings, government agencies, external accreditation programs, payers, and AOTA documents" (p. S108). These requirements apply to both electronic and written forms of documentation. Documentation should reflect the nature of services provided and the clinical reasoning of the occupational therapy practitioner, and it should provide enough information to ensure that services are delivered in a safe and effective manner. Documentation should describe the depth and breadth of services provided to meet the complexity of individual client[3] needs. The client's diagnosis or prognosis should not be used as the sole rationale for occupational therapy services.

The purpose of documentation is to

- Communicate information about the client from the occupational therapy perspective;

- Articulate the rationale for provision of occupational therapy services and the relationship of those services to client outcomes, reflecting the occupational therapy practitioner's clinical reasoning and professional judgment; and

- Create a chronological record of client status, occupational therapy services provided to the client, client response to occupational therapy intervention, and client outcomes.

Types of Documentation

Table 1 outlines common types of documentation reports. Reports may be named differently or combined and reorganized to meet the specific needs of the setting. Occupational therapy documentation should always record the practitioner's activity in the areas of screening, evaluation, intervention, and outcomes (AOTA, 2008) in accordance with payer, facility, and state and federal guidelines.

---

[1]*Occupational therapists* are responsible for all aspects of occupational therapy service delivery and are accountable for the safety and effectiveness of the occupational therapy service delivery process. *Occupational therapy assistants* deliver occupational therapy services under the supervision of and in partnership with an occupational therapist (AOTA, 2009).
[2]When the term *occupational therapy practitioner* is used in this document, it refers to both occupational therapists and occupational therapy assistants (AOTA, 2006).
[3]In this document, *client* may refer to an individual, organization, or population.

Table 1. Common Types of Occupational Therapy Documentation Reports

Process Areas	Type of Report
I. Screening	A. Screening Report
II. Evaluation	A. Evaluation Report
	B. Reevaluation Report
III. Intervention	A. Intervention Plan
	B. Contact Report Note or Communiqué
	C. Progress Report/Note
	D. Transition Plan
IV. Outcomes	A. Discharge/Discontinuation Report

Content of Reports

I. Screening

A. Documents referral source, reason for occupational therapy screening, and need for occupational therapy evaluation and service.

1. Phone referrals should be documented in accordance with payer, facility, and state and federal guidelines and include

a. Names of individuals spoken with,

b. Purpose of screening,

c. Date of request,

d. Number of contact for referral source, and

e. Description of client's prior level of occupational performance.

B. Consists of an initial brief assessment to determine client's need for an occupational therapy evaluation or for referral to another service if not appropriate for occupational therapy services.

C. Suggested content:

1. *Client information*—Name/agency; date of birth; gender; health status; and applicable medical/ educational/developmental diagnoses, precautions, and contraindications

2. *Referral information*—Date and source of referral, services requested, reason for referral, funding source, and anticipated length of service

3. *Brief occupational profile*—Client's reason for seeking occupational therapy services, current areas of occupation that are successful and problematic, contexts and environments that support and hinder occupations, medical/educational/work history, occupational history (e.g., patterns of living, interest, values), client's priorities, and targeted goals

4. *Assessments used and results*—Types of assessments used and results (e.g., interviews, record reviews, observations)

5. *Recommendation*—Professional judgments regarding appropriateness of need for complete occupational therapy evaluation.

II. Evaluation

A. Evaluation Report

1. Documents referral source and data gathered through the evaluation process in accordance with payer, facility, state, and/or federal guidelines. Includes

    a. Analysis of occupational performance and identification of factors that support and hinder performance and participation and

    b. Identification of specific areas of occupation and occupational performance to be addressed, interventions, and expected outcomes.

2. Suggested content:

    a. *Client information*—Name; date of birth; gender; health status; medical history; and applicable medical/educational/developmental diagnoses, precautions, and contraindications

    b. *Referral information*—Date and source of referral, services requested, reason for referral, funding source, and anticipated length of service

    c. *Occupational profile*—Client's reason for seeking occupational therapy services, current areas of occupation that are successful and problematic, contexts and environments that support or hinder occupations, medical/educational/work history, occupational history (e.g., patterns of living, interest, values), client's priorities, and targeted outcomes

    d. *Assessments used and results*—Types of assessments used and results (e.g., interviews, record reviews, observations, standardized and/or nonstandardized assessments)

    e. *Analysis of occupational performance*—Description of and judgment about performance skills, performance patterns, contexts and environments, activity demands, outcomes from standardized measures and/or nonstandardized assessments,[4] and client factors that will be targeted for intervention and outcomes expected

    f. *Summary and analysis*—Interpretation and summary of data as related to occupational profile and referring concern

    g. *Recommendation*—Judgment regarding appropriateness of occupational therapy services or other services.

    Note. The intervention plan, including intervention goals addressing anticipated outcomes, objectives, and frequency of therapy, is described in the "Intervention Plan" section that follows.

B. Reevaluation Report

1. Documents the results of the reevaluation process. Frequency of reevaluation depends on the needs of the setting, the progress of the client, and client changes.

2. Suggested content:

    a. *Client information*—Name; date of birth; gender; and applicable medical/educational/developmental diagnoses, precautions, and contraindications

    b. *Occupational profile*—Updates on current areas of occupation that are successful and problematic, contexts and environments that support or hinder occupations, summary of any new

---

[4]*Nonstandardized assessment tools* are considered a valid form of information gathering that allows for flexibility and individualization when measuring outcomes related to the status of an individual or group through an intrapersonal comparison. Although not uniform in administration or scoring or possessing full and complete psychometric data, nonstandardized assessment tools possess strong internal validity and represent an evidence- based approach to occupational therapy practice (Hinojosa, Kramer, & Christ, 2010). Nonstandardized tools should be selected on the basis of the best available evidence and the clinical reasoning of the practitioner.

medical/educational/work information, and updates or changes to client's priorities and targeted outcomes

c. *Reevaluation results*—Focus of reevaluation, specific types of outcome measures from standardized and/or nonstandardized assessments used, and client's performance and subjective responses

d. *Analysis of occupational performance*—Description of and judgment about performance skills, performance patterns, contexts and environments, activity demands, outcomes from standardized measures and/or nonstandardized assessments, and client factors that will be targeted for intervention and outcomes expected

e. *Summary and analysis*—Interpretation and summary of data as related to referring concern and comparison of results with previous evaluation results

f. *Recommendations*—Changes to occupational therapy services, revision or continuation of interventions, goals and objectives, frequency of occupational therapy services, and recommendation for referral to other professionals or agencies as applicable.

III. Intervention

A. Intervention Plan

1. Documents the goals, intervention approaches, and types of interventions to be used to achieve the client's identified targeted outcomes and is based on results of evaluation or reevaluation processes. Includes recommendations or referrals to other professionals and agencies in adherence with each payer source documentation requirements (e.g., pain levels, time spent on each modality).

2. Suggested content:

   a. *Client information*—Name, date of birth, gender, precautions, and contraindications

   b. *Intervention goals*—Measurable and meaningful occupation-based long-term and short-term objective goals directly related to the client's ability and need to engage in desired occupations

   c. *Intervention approaches and types of interventions to be used*—Intervention approaches that include create/promote, establish/restore, maintain, modify, and/or prevent; types of interventions that include consultation, education process, advocacy, and/or the therapeutic use of occupations or activities

   d. *Service delivery mechanisms*—Service provider, service location, and frequency and duration of services

   e. *Plan for discharge*—Discontinuation criteria, discharge setting (e.g., skilled nursing facility, home, community, classroom) and follow-up care

   f. *Outcome measures*—Tools that assess occupational performance, adaptation, role competence, improved health and wellness, improved quality of life, self-advocacy, and occupational justice. Standardized and/or nonstandardized assessments used at evaluation should be readministered periodically to monitor measurable progress and report functional outcomes as required by client's payer source and/or facility requirements.

   g. *Professionals responsible and date of plan*—Names and positions of persons overseeing plan, date plan was developed, and date when plan was modified or reviewed.

B. Service Contacts

1. Documents contacts between the client and the occupational therapy practitioner. Records the types of interventions used and client's response, which can include telephone contacts, interventions, and meetings with others.

2. Suggested content:

    a. *Client information*—Name; date of birth; gender; and diagnosis, precautions, and contraindications

    b. *Therapy log*—Date, type of contact, names/positions of persons involved, summary or significant information communicated during contacts, client attendance and participation in intervention, reason service is missed, types of interventions used, client's response, environmental or task modification, assistive or adaptive devices used or fabricated, statement of any training education or consultation provided, and the client's present level of performance. Documentation of services provided should reflect the complexity of the client and the professional clinical reasoning and expertise of an occupational therapy practitioner required to provide an effective outcome in occupational performance. The client's diagnosis or prognosis should not be the sole rationale for the skilled interventions provided. Measures used to assess outcomes should be repeated in accordance with payer and facility requirements and documented to demonstrate measurable functional progress of the client.

    c. *Intervention/procedure coding* (i.e., *CPT*™),[5] if applicable.

C. Progress Report/Note

1. Summarizes intervention process and documents client's progress toward achievement of goals. Includes new data collected; modifications of treatment plan; and statement of need for continuation, discontinuation, or referral.

2. Suggested content:

    a. *Client information*—Name; date of birth; gender; and diagnosis, precautions, and contraindications

    b. *Summary of services provided*—Brief statement of frequency of services and length of time services have been provided; techniques and strategies used; measurable progress or lack thereof using age-appropriate current functional standardized and/or nonstandardized outcome measures; environmental or task modifications provided; adaptive equipment or orthotics provided; medical, educational, or other pertinent client updates; client's response to occupational therapy services; and programs or training provided to the client or caregivers

    c. *Current client performance*—Client's progress toward the goals and client's performance in areas of occupations

    d. *Plan or recommendations*—Recommendations and rationale as well as client's input to changes or continuation of plan.

D. Transition Plan

1. Documents the formal transition plan and is written when client is transitioning from one service setting to another within a service delivery system.

2. Suggested content:

    a. *Client information*—Name; date of birth; gender; and diagnosis, precautions, and contraindications

    b. *Client's current status*—Client's current performance in occupations

    c. *Transition plan*—Name of current service setting and name of setting to which client will transition, reason for transition, time frame in which transition will occur, and outline of activities to be carried out during the transition plan

---

[5]*CPT* is a trademark of the American Medical Association (AMA). *CPT* five-digit codes, nomenclature, and other data are copyright © 2011 by the AMA. All rights reserved.

    d. *Recommendations*—Recommendations and rationale for occupational therapy services, modifications or accommodations needed, and assistive technology and environmental modifications needed.

IV. Outcomes

  A. Discharge Report—Summary of Occupational Therapy Services and Outcomes

    1. Summarizes the changes in client's ability to engage in occupations between the initial evaluation and discontinuation of services and makes recommendations as applicable.

    2. Suggested content with examples include

      a. *Client information*—name/agency, date of birth, gender, diagnosis, precautions, and contraindications

      b. *Summary of intervention process*—date of initial and final service; frequency, number of sessions, summary of interventions used; summary of progress toward goals; and occupational therapy outcomes—initial client status and ending status regarding engagement in occupations, client's assessment of efficacy of occupational therapy services

      c. *Recommendations*—recommendations pertaining to the client's future needs; specific follow-up plans, if applicable; and referrals to other professionals and agencies, if applicable.

Each occupational therapy client has a client record maintained as a permanent file. The record is maintained in a professional and legal fashion (i.e., organized, legible, concise, clear, accurate, complete, current, grammatically correct, and objective; see Box 1 for more information).

Box 1. Fundamentals of Documentation

- Client's full name and case number (if applicable) on each page of documentation
- Date
- Identification of type of documentation (e.g., evaluation report, progress report/note)
- Occupational therapy practitioner's signature with a minimum of first name or initial, last name, and professional designation
- When applicable, signature of the recorder directly after the documentation entry. If additional information is needed, a signed addendum must be added to the record.
- Cosignature of an occupational therapist or occupational therapy assistant on student documentation, as required by payer policy, governing laws and regulations, and/or employer
- Compliance with all laws, regulations, payer, and employer requirements
- Acceptable terminology defined within the boundaries of setting
- Abbreviations usage as acceptable within the boundaries of setting
- All errors noted and signed
- Adherence to professional standards of technology, when used to document occupational therapy services with electronic claims or records.
- Disposal of records (electronic and traditionally written) within law or agency requirements
- Compliance with confidentiality standards
- Compliance with agency or legal requirements of storage of records
- Documentation should reflect professional clinical reasoning and expertise of an occupational therapy practitioner and the nature of occupational therapy services delivered in a safe and effective manner. The client's diagnosis or prognosis should not be the sole rationale for occupational therapy services.

References

American Medical Association. (2010). *Current procedural terminology.* Chicago: Author.

American Occupational Therapy Association. (2006). Policy 1.41. Categories of occupational therapy personnel. In *Policy manual* (2011 ed.). Bethesda, MD: Author.

American Occupational Therapy Association. (2008). Occupational therapy practice framework: Domain and process (2nd ed.). *American Journal of Occupational Therapy, 62,* 625–683. http://dx.doi.org/10.5014/ajot.62.6.625

American Occupational Therapy Association. (2009). Guidelines for supervision, roles, and responsibilities during the delivery of occupational therapy services. *American Journal of Occupational Therapy, 63,* 797–803. http://dx.doi.org/10.5014/ajot.63.6.797

American Occupational Therapy Association. (2010). Standards of practice for occupational therapy. *American Journal of Occupational Therapy, 64*(Suppl.), S106–S111. http://dx.doi.org/10.5014/ajot.2010.64S106

Hinojosa, J., Kramer, P., & Crist, P. (2010). *Evaluation: Obtaining and interpreting data* (3rd ed.). Bethesda, MD: AOTA Press.

Authors
Gloria Frolek Clark, MS, OTR/L, FAOTA
Mary Jane Youngstrom, MS, OTR/L, FAOTA

for

The Commission on Practice
Sara Jane Brayman, PhD, OTR/L, FAOTA, *Chairperson*

Adopted by the Representative Assembly 2003M16

Edited by the Commission on Practice 2007

Edited by the Commission on Practice 2012
Debbie Amini, EdD, OTR/L, CHT, *Chairperson*

Adopted by the Representative Assembly Coordinating Council (RACC) for the Representative Assembly, 2012

Note. This revision replaces the 2007 document previously published and copyrighted in 2008 by the American Occupational Therapy Association in the *American Journal of Occupational Therapy, 62,* 684–690.

Guidelines for Supervision, Roles, and Responsibilities During the Delivery of Occupational Therapy Services

This document is a set of guidelines describing the supervision, roles, and responsibilities of occupational therapy practitioners. Intended for both internal and external audiences, it also provides an outline of the roles and responsibilities of occupational therapists, occupational therapy assistants, and occupational therapy aides during the delivery of occupational therapy services.

General Supervision

These guidelines provide a definition of supervision and outline parameters regarding effective supervision as it relates to the delivery of occupational therapy services. The guidelines themselves cannot be interpreted to constitute a standard of supervision in any particular locality. Occupational therapists, occupational therapy assistants, and occupational therapy aides are expected to meet applicable state and federal regulations, adhere to relevant workplace and payer policies and to the *Occupational Therapy Code of Ethics and Ethics Standards* (American Occupational Therapy Association [AOTA], 2010), and participate in ongoing professional development activities to maintain continuing competency.

Within the scope of occupational therapy practice, *supervision* is a process aimed at ensuring the safe and effective delivery of occupational therapy services and fostering professional competence and development. In addition, in these guidelines, supervision is viewed as a cooperative process in which two or more people participate in a joint effort to establish, maintain, and/or elevate a level of competence and performance. Supervision is based on mutual understanding between the supervisor and the supervisee about each other's competence, experience, education, and credentials. It fosters growth and development, promotes effective utilization of resources, encourages creativity and innovation, and provides education and support to achieve a goal.

Supervision of Occupational Therapists and Occupational Therapy Assistants

Occupational Therapists

Based on education and training, occupational therapists, after initial certification and relevant state licensure or other governmental requirements, are autonomous practitioners who are able to deliver occupational therapy services independently. Occupational therapists are responsible for all aspects of occupational therapy service delivery and are accountable for the safety and effectiveness of occupational therapy services and the service delivery process. Occupational therapists are encouraged to seek peer supervision and mentoring for ongoing development of best practice approaches and promotion of professional growth.

Occupational Therapy Assistants

Based on education and training, occupational therapy assistants, after initial certification and meeting of state regulatory requirements, must receive supervision from an occupational therapist to deliver occupational therapy services. Occupational therapy assistants deliver occupational therapy services under the supervision of and in partnership with occupational therapists. Occupational therapists and occupational therapy assistants are equally responsible for developing a collaborative plan for supervision. The occupational therapist is ultimately responsible for the implementation of appropriate supervision, but the occupational therapy assistant also has a responsibility to seek and obtain appropriate supervision to ensure proper occupational therapy is being provided.

General Principles

1. Supervision involves guidance and oversight related to the delivery of occupational therapy services and the facilitation of professional growth and competence. It is the responsibility of the occupational therapy assistant to seek the appropriate quality and frequency of supervision to ensure safe and effective occupational therapy service delivery. It is the responsibility of the occupational therapist to provide adequate and appropriate supervision.

2. To ensure safe and effective occupational therapy services, it is the responsibility of occupational therapists to recognize when they require peer supervision or mentoring that supports current and advancing levels of competence and professional growth.

3. The specific frequency, methods, and content of supervision may vary and are dependent on the

    a. Complexity of client needs,

    b. Number and diversity of clients,

    c. Knowledge and skill level of the occupational therapist and the occupational therapy assistant,

    d. Type of practice setting,

    e. Requirements of the practice setting, and

    f. Other regulatory requirements.

4. Supervision of the occupational therapy assistant that is more frequent than the minimum level required by the practice setting or regulatory requirements may be necessary when

    a. The needs of the client and the occupational therapy process are complex and changing,

    b. The practice setting provides occupational therapy services to a large number of clients with diverse needs, or

    c. The occupational therapist and occupational therapy assistant determine that additional supervision is necessary to ensure safe and effective delivery of occupational therapy services.

5. There are a variety of types and methods of supervision. Methods can include but are not limited to direct, face-to-face contact and indirect contact. Examples of methods or types of supervision that involve direct face-to-face contact include observation, modeling, client demonstration, discussions, teaching, and instruction. Examples of methods or types of supervision that involve indirect contact include phone conversations, written correspondence, and electronic exchanges.

6. Occupational therapists and occupational therapy assistants must abide by facility and state requirements regarding the documentation of a supervision plan and supervision contacts. Documentation may include the

    a. Frequency of supervisory contact,

    b. Methods or types of supervision,

    c. Content areas addressed,

d. Evidence to support areas and levels of competency, and

e. Names and credentials of the persons participating in the supervisory process.

7. Peer supervision and mentoring related to professional growth, such as leadership and advocacy skills development, may differ from the peer supervision mentoring needed to provide occupational therapy services. The person providing this supervision, as well as the frequency, method, and content of supervision, should be responsive to the supervisee's advancing levels of professional growth.

Supervision Outside the Delivery of Occupational Therapy Services

The education and expertise of occupational therapists and occupational therapy assistants prepare them for employment in arenas other than those related to the delivery of occupational therapy. In these other arenas, supervision may be provided by non–occupational therapy professionals.

1. The guidelines of the setting, regulatory agencies, and funding agencies direct the supervision requirements.

2. The occupational therapist and occupational therapy assistant should obtain and use credentials or job titles commensurate with their roles in these other employment arenas.

3. The following can be used to determine whether the services provided are related to the delivery of occupational therapy:

a. State practice acts;

b. Regulatory agency standards and rules;

c. *Occupational Therapy Practice Framework: Domain and Process* (AOTA, 2014) and other AOTA official documents; and

d. Written and verbal agreement among the occupational therapist, the occupational therapy assistant, the client, and the agency or payer about the services provided.

Roles and Responsibilities of Occupational Therapists and Occupational Therapy Assistants During the Delivery of Occupational Therapy Services

Overview

The focus of occupational therapy is to assist the client in "achieving health, well-being, and participation in life through engagement in occupation" (AOTA, 2014, p. S2). Occupational therapy addresses the needs and goals of the client related to engaging in areas of occupation and considers the performance skills, performance patterns, context and environment, and client factors that may influence performance in various areas of occupation.

1. The occupational therapist is responsible for all aspects of occupational therapy service delivery and is accountable for the safety and effectiveness of the occupational therapy service delivery process. The occupational therapy service delivery process involves evaluation, intervention planning, intervention implementation, intervention review, and targeting of outcomes and outcomes evaluation.

2. The occupational therapist must be directly involved in the delivery of services during the initial evaluation and regularly throughout the course of intervention, intervention review, and outcomes evaluation.

3. The occupational therapy assistant delivers safe and effective occupational therapy services under the supervision of and in partnership with the occupational therapist.

4. It is the responsibility of the occupational therapist to determine when to delegate responsibilities to an occupational therapy assistant. It is the responsibility of the occupational therapy assistant who performs the delegated responsibilities to demonstrate service competency and also to not accept delegated responsibilities that go beyond the scope of an occupational therapy assistant.

5. The occupational therapist and the occupational therapy assistant demonstrate and document service competency for clinical reasoning and judgment during the service delivery process as well as for the performance of specific techniques, assessments, and intervention methods used.

6. When delegating aspects of occupational therapy services, the occupational therapist considers the following factors:

   a. Complexity of the client's condition and needs,

   b. Knowledge, skill, and competence of the occupational therapy assistant,

   c. Nature and complexity of the intervention,

   d. Needs and requirements of the practice setting, and

   e. Appropriate scope of practice of an occupational therapy assistant under state law and other requirements.

Roles and Responsibilities

Regardless of the setting in which occupational therapy services are delivered, occupational therapists and occupational therapy assistants assume the following general responsibilities during evaluation; intervention planning, implementation, and review; and targeting and evaluating outcomes.

Evaluation

1. The occupational therapist directs the evaluation process.

2. The occupational therapist is responsible for directing all aspects of the initial contact during the occupational therapy evaluation, including

   a. Determining the need for service,

   b. Defining the problems within the domain of occupational therapy to be addressed,

   c. Determining the client's goals and priorities,

   d. Establishing intervention priorities,

   e. Determining specific further assessment needs, and

   f. Determining specific assessment tasks that can be delegated to the occupational therapy assistant.

3. The occupational therapist initiates and directs the evaluation, interprets the data, and develops the intervention plan.

4. The occupational therapy assistant contributes to the evaluation process by implementing delegated assessments and by providing verbal and written reports of observations, assessments, and client capacities to the occupational therapist.

5. The occupational therapist interprets the information provided by the occupational therapy assistant and integrates that information into the evaluation and decision-making process.

Intervention Planning

1. The occupational therapist has overall responsibility for the development of the occupational therapy intervention plan.

2. The occupational therapist and the occupational therapy assistant collaborate with the client to develop the plan.

3. The occupational therapy assistant is responsible for being knowledgeable about evaluation results and for providing input into the intervention plan, based on client needs and priorities.

Intervention Implementation

1. The occupational therapist has overall responsibility for intervention implementation.

2. When delegating aspects of the occupational therapy intervention to the occupational therapy assistant, the occupational therapist is responsible for providing appropriate supervision.

3. The occupational therapy assistant is responsible for being knowledgeable about the client's occupational therapy goals.

4. The occupational therapy assistant in collaboration with the occupational therapist selects, implements, and makes modifications to occupational therapy interventions, including, but not limited to, occupations and activities, preparatory methods and tasks, client education and training, and group interventions consistent with demonstrated competency levels, client goals, and the requirements of the practice setting.

Intervention Review

1. The occupational therapist is responsible for determining the need for continuing, modifying, or discontinuing occupational therapy services.

2. The occupational therapy assistant contributes to this process by exchanging information with and providing documentation to the occupational therapist about the client's responses to and communications during intervention.

Targeting and Evaluating Outcomes

1. The occupational therapist is responsible for selecting, measuring, and interpreting outcomes that are related to the client's ability to engage in occupations.

2. The occupational therapy assistant is responsible for being knowledgeable about the client's targeted occupational therapy outcomes and for providing information and documentation related to outcome achievement.

3. The occupational therapy assistant may implement outcome measurements and provide needed client discharge resources.

Supervision of Occupational Therapy Aides[1]

An *aide,* as used in occupational therapy practice, is an individual who provides supportive services to the occupational therapist and the occupational therapy assistant. Aides do not provide skilled occupational therapy services. An aide is trained by an occupational therapist or an occupational therapy assistant

---

[1]Depending on the setting in which service is provided, aides may be referred to by various names. Examples include, but are not limited to, *rehabilitation aides, restorative aides, extenders, paraprofessionals,* and *rehab techs* (AOTA, 2009).

to perform specifically delegated tasks. The occupational therapist is responsible for the overall use and actions of the aide. An aide first must demonstrate competency to be able to perform the assigned, delegated client and non-client tasks.

1. The occupational therapist must oversee the development, documentation, and implementation of a plan to supervise and routinely assess the ability of the occupational therapy aide to carry out non–client- and client-related tasks. The occupational therapy assistant may contribute to the development and documentation of this plan.

2. The occupational therapy assistant can supervise the aide.

3. *Non–client-related tasks* include clerical and maintenance activities and preparation of the work area or equipment.

4. *Client-related tasks* are routine tasks during which the aide may interact with the client. The following factors must be present when an occupational therapist or occupational therapy assistant delegates a selected client-related task to the aide:

   a. The outcome anticipated for the delegated task is predictable.

   b. The situation of the client and the environment is stable and will not require that judgment, interpretations, or adaptations be made by the aide.

   c. The client has demonstrated some previous performance ability in executing the task.

   d. The task routine and process have been clearly established.

5. When performing delegated client-related tasks, the supervisor must ensure that the aide

   a. Is trained and able to demonstrate competency in carrying out the selected task and using equipment, if appropriate;

   b. Has been instructed on how to specifically carry out the delegated task with the specific client; and

   c. Knows the precautions, signs, and symptoms for the particular client that would indicate the need to seek assistance from the occupational therapist or occupational therapy assistant.

6. The supervision of the aide needs to be documented. Documentation includes information about frequency and methods of supervision used, the content of supervision, and the names and credentials of all persons participating in the supervisory process.

Summary

These guidelines about supervision, roles, and responsibilities are to assist in the appropriate utilization of occupational therapists, occupational therapy assistants, and occupational therapy aides and in the appropriate and effective provision of occupational therapy services. It is expected that occupational therapy services are delivered in accordance with applicable state and federal regulations, relevant workplace policies, the *Occupational Therapy Code of Ethics and Ethics Standards* (AOTA, 2010), and continuing competency and professional development guidelines. For information regarding the supervision of occupational therapy students, please refer to *Fieldwork Level II and Occupational Therapy Students: A Position Paper* (AOTA, 2012).

References

American Occupational Therapy Association. (2009). Guidelines for supervision, roles, and responsibilities during the delivery of occupational therapy services. *American Journal of Occupational Therapy, 63,* 797–803. http://dx.doi.org/10/5014/ajot.63.6.797

American Occupational Therapy Association. (2010). Occupational therapy code of ethics and ethics standards (2010). *American Journal of Occupational Therapy, 64*(6, Suppl.), S17–S26. http://dx.doi.org/10.5014/ajot.2010.64S17

American Occupational Therapy Association. (2012). Fieldwork Level II and occupational therapy students: A position paper. *American Journal of Occupational Therapy, 66*(6, Suppl.), S75–S77. http://dx.doi.org/10.5014/ajot.2012.66S75

American Occupational Therapy Association. (2014). Occupational therapy practice framework: Domain and process (3rd ed.). *American Journal of Occupational Therapy, 68*(Suppl. 1), S1–S48. http://dx.doi.org/10.5014/ajot.2014.682005

Additional Reading

American Occupational Therapy Association. (2010). Standards of practice for occupational therapy. *American Journal of Occupational Therapy, 64*(Suppl.), S106–S111. http://dx.doi.org/10.5014/ajot.2010.64S106

Authors

Sara Jane Brayman, PhD, OTR/L, FAOTA
Gloria Frolek Clark, MS, OTR/L, FAOTA
Janet V. DeLany, DEd, OTR/L
Eileen R. Garza, PhD, OTR, ATP
Mary V. Radomski, MA, OTR/L, FAOTA
Ruth Ramsey, MS, OTR/L
Carol Siebert, MS, OTR/L
Kristi Voelkerding, BS, COTA/L
Patricia D. LaVesser, PhD, OTR/L, *SIS Liaison*
Lenna Aird, *ASD Liaison*
Deborah Lieberman, MHSA, OTR/L, FAOTA, *AOTA Headquarters Liaison*

for

The Commission on Practice
Sara Jane Brayman, PhD, OTR/L, FAOTA, *Chairperson*

Adopted by the Representative Assembly 2004C24

Edited by the Commission on Practice 2014
Debbie Amini, EdD, OTR/L, CHT, FAOTA, *Chairperson*

Adopted by the Representative Assembly Coordinating Council (RACC) for the Representative Assembly, 2014

Guidelines for Reentry Into the Field of Occupational Therapy

Purpose of the Guidelines

These guidelines are designed to assist occupational therapists and occupational therapy assistants who have left the field of occupational therapy for 24 months or more and have chosen to return to the profession and deliver occupational therapy services. The guidelines represent minimum recommendations only and are designed to support practitioners in meeting their ethical obligation to maintain high standards of competence.

It is expected that practitioners will identify and meet requirements outlined in applicable state and federal regulations, relevant workplace policies, the *Occupational Therapy Code of Ethics (2015)* (American Occupational Therapy Association [AOTA], 2015a), and continuing competence and professional development guidelines prior to reentering the field.

Clarification of Terms

Reentry—For the purpose of this document, reentering occupational therapists and occupational therapy assistants are individuals who

- Have practiced in the field of occupational therapy; and

- Have not engaged in the practice of occupational therapy (may include direct intervention, supervision, teaching, consultation, administration, case or care management, community programming, or research) for a minimum of 24 months; and

- Wish to return to the profession in the capacity of delivering occupational therapy services to clients.

Formal Learning—This term refers to any learning that has established goals and objectives that are measureable. It may include activities such as

- Attending workshops, seminars, lectures, and professional conferences;

- Auditing or participating in formal academic coursework;

- Participating in external self-study series (e.g., AOTA Self-Paced Clinical Courses); or

- Participating in independent distance learning, either synchronous or asynchronous (e.g., continuing education articles, video, audio, or online courses) with established goals and objectives that are measurable.

Supervised Service Delivery—For this document, *supervised service delivery* refers to provision of occupational therapy services under the supervision of a qualified occupational therapist. The *Guidelines for Supervision, Roles, and Responsibilities During the Delivery of Occupational Therapy Services* (AOTA, 2014a) state that within the scope of occupational therapy practice, *supervision* is a process aimed at ensuring the safe and effective delivery of occupational therapy services and fostering professional competence and development. [It is] a cooperative process in which two or more people participate in a joint effort to establish, maintain, and/or elevate a level of competence and performance. (p. S16)

Specific Guidelines for Reentry

Practitioners who are seeking reentry must abide by state licensure and practice regulations and any requirements established by the workplace. In addition, the following suggested guidelines are recommended:

1. Engage in a formalized process of self-assessment (e.g., self-assessment tools, such as AOTA's [2003] *Professional Development Tool*), and complete a professional development plan that addresses the *Standards for Continuing Competence* (AOTA, 2015b).

2. Attend a minimum of 10 hours of formal learning related to occupational therapy service delivery for each 12 consecutive months out of practice. At least 20 hours of the formal learning must have occurred within the past 24 months of re-entry.

3. Attain relevant updates to core knowledge of the profession of occupational therapy and the responsibilities of occupational therapy practitioners that are consistent with material found in AOTA official documents such as the *Occupational Therapy Practice Framework: Domain and Process* (3rd ed.; AOTA, 2014b), the *Occupational Therapy Code of Ethics (2015)* (AOTA, 2015a), *Standards for Continuing Competence* (AOTA, 2015b), *Standards of Practice for Occupational Therapy* (AOTA, 2010), and *Guidelines for Supervision, Roles, and Responsibilities During the Delivery of Occupational Therapy Services* (AOTA, 2014a).

4. Complete of a minimum of 30 hours of documented supervised service delivery in occupational therapy, which is recommended for practitioners who have been out of practice for 3 or more years.

   a. The supervised service delivery should be completed between the 12 months prior to anticipated reentry and the first 30 days of employment.

   b. The reentering practitioner, in conjunction with the supervising occupational therapy practitioner(s), should establish specific goals and objectives for the 30 hours. Goals, objectives, and related assessment of performance may be developed or adapted from a variety of sources, including competency and performance review resources existing within the setting as well as AOTA resources such as the *Fieldwork Performance Evaluation for the Occupational Therapy Student*© forms (AOTA, 2002a, 2002b).

   c. The supervised service delivery experience should focus on the area of practice to which the practitioner intends to return.

   d. Supervised service delivery should occur with a practitioner at the same or greater professional level (i.e., an occupational therapist, not an occupational therapy assistant, supervises a returning therapist).

   e. Supervision should be direct face-to-face contact, which may include observation, modeling, cotreatment, discussions, teaching, and instruction (AOTA, 2014a) and may be augmented by indirect methods such as electronic communications.

Ongoing Continuing Competence

Once practitioners have successfully returned to the delivery of occupational therapy services, they are encouraged to engage in activities that support them in their ongoing continuing competence, such as

- Seeking mentoring, consultation, or supervision—especially during the first year of return to practice;

- Engaging in relevant AOTA Special Interest Section forums to build a professional network and facilitate opportunities for practice guidance;

- Exploring relevant AOTA Board and Specialty Certifications and using the identified criteria as a blueprint for ongoing professional development; and

- Joining and becoming active in both AOTA and the state occupational therapy association to stay abreast of practice trends and increase opportunities for networking.

References and Resources

American Occupational Therapy Association. (2002a). *Fieldwork performance evaluation for the occupational therapy assistant student.* Bethesda, MD: AOTA Press.

American Occupational Therapy Association. (2002b). *Fieldwork performance evaluation for the occupational therapy student.* Bethesda, MD: AOTA Press.

American Occupational Therapy Association. (2003, May). *Professional development tool.* Retrieved October 12, 2014, from http://www1.aota.org/pdt/index.asp

American Occupational Therapy Association. (2010). Standards of practice for occupational therapy. *American Journal of Occupational Therapy, 64*(6, Suppl.), S106–S111. http://dx.doi.org/10.5014/ajot.2010.64S106

American Occupational Therapy Association. (2014a). Guidelines for supervision, roles, and responsibilities during the delivery of occupational therapy services. *American Journal of Occupational Therapy, 68*(Suppl. 3), S16–S22. http://dx.doi.org/10.5014/ajot.2014.686S03

American Occupational Therapy Association. (2014b). Occupational therapy practice framework: Domain and process (3rd ed.). *American Journal of Occupational Therapy, 68*(Suppl. 1), S1–S48. http://dx.doi.org/10.5014/ajot.2014.682006

American Occupational Therapy Association. (2015a). Occupational therapy code of ethics (2015). *American Journal of Occupational Therapy, 69*(Suppl. 3), 6913410030. http://dx.doi.org/10.5014/ajot.2015.696S03

American Occupational Therapy Association. (2015b). Standards for continuing competence. *American Journal of Occupational Therapy, 69*(Suppl. 3), 6913410055. http://dx.doi.org/10.5014/ajot.2015.696S16

Authors

Melisa Tilton, BS, COTA/L ROH, *Chair*
Clare Giuffrida, PhD, MS, OTR/L, FAOTA
Christy L. A. Nelson, PhD, OTR/L, FAOTA
Winifred Schultz-Krohn, PhD, OTR/L, BCP, FAOTA, *Chairperson*
Maria Elena E. Louch, *AOTA Staff Liaison for the Commission on Continuing Competence and Professional Development*

Adopted by the Representative Assembly 2010CApr11

Revisions adopted 2015Apr16

Note. This revision replaces the 2010 document *Guidelines for Re-Entry Into the Field of Occupational Therapy,* previously published and copyrighted in 2010 by the American Occupational Therapy Association in the *American Journal of Occupational Therapy,* 64(6, Suppl.), S27–S29. http://dx.doi.org/10.5014/ajot.2010.64S27

Citation. American Occupational Therapy Association. (2015). Guidelines for reentry into the field of occupational therapy. *American Journal of Occupational Therapy, 69*(Suppl. 3), 6913410015. http://dx.doi.org/10.5014/ajot.2015.696S15

OCCUPATIONAL THERAPY PRACTICE
FRAMEWORK:
Domain & Process
3rd Edition

Contents

When citing this document the preferred reference is: American Occupational Therapy Association. (2014). Occupational therapy practice framework: Domain and process (3rd ed.). *American Journal of Occupational Therapy, 68*(Suppl. 1), S1–S48. http://dx.doi.org/10.5014/ajot.2014.682006

PREFACE

The *Occupational Therapy Practice Framework: Domain and Process,* 3rd edition (hereinafter referred to as "the *Framework*"), is an official document of the American Occupational Therapy Association (AOTA). Intended for occupational therapy practitioners and students, other health care professionals, educators, researchers, payers, and consumers, the *Framework* presents a summary of interrelated constructs that describe occupational therapy practice.

Definitions

Within the *Framework, occupational therapy* is defined as
the therapeutic use of everyday life activities (occupations) with individuals or groups for the purpose of enhancing or enabling participation in roles, habits, and routines in home, school, workplace, community, and other settings. Occupational therapy practitioners use their knowledge of the transactional relationship among the person, his or her engagement in valuable occupations, and the context to design occupation-based intervention plans that facilitate change or growth in client factors (body functions, body structures, values, beliefs, and spirituality) and skills (motor, process, and social interaction) needed for successful participation. Occupational therapy practitioners are concerned with the end result of participation and thus enable engagement through adaptations and modifications to the environment or objects within the environment when needed. Occupational therapy services are provided for habilitation, rehabilitation, and promotion of health and wellness for clients with disability- and non–disability-related needs. These services include acquisition and preservation of occupational identity for those who have or are at risk for developing an illness, injury, disease, disorder, condition, impairment, disability, activity limitation, or participation restriction. (adapted from AOTA, 2011; see Appendix A for additional definitions in a glossary)

When the term *occupational therapy practitioner* is used in this document, it refers to both occupational therapists and occupational therapy assistants (AOTA, 2006). Occupational therapists are responsible for all aspects of occupational therapy service delivery and are accountable for the safety and effectiveness of the occupational therapy service delivery process. Occupational therapy assistants deliver occupational therapy services under the supervision of and in partnership with an occupational therapist (AOTA, 2009). Additional information about the preparation and qualifications of occupational therapists and occupational therapy assistants can be found in Appendix B.

Evolution of This Document

The *Framework* was originally developed to articulate occupational therapy's distinct perspective and contribution to promoting the health and participation of persons, groups, and populations through engagement in occupation. The first edition of the *Framework* emerged from an examination of documents related to the *Occupational Therapy Product Output Reporting System and Uniform Terminology for Reporting Occupational Therapy Services* (AOTA, 1979). Originally a document that responded to a federal requirement to develop a uniform reporting system, the text gradually shifted to describing and outlining the domains of concern of occupational therapy.

The second edition of *Uniform Terminology for Occupational Therapy* (AOTA, 1989) was adopted by the AOTA Representative Assembly (RA) and published in 1989. The document focused on delineating and defining only the occupational performance areas and occupational performance components that are addressed in occupational therapy direct services. The third and final revision of *Uniform Terminology for Occupational Therapy* (AOTA, 1994) was adopted by the RA in 1994 and was "expanded to reflect current practice and to incorporate contextual aspects of performance" (p. 1047). Each revision reflected changes in practice and provided consistent terminology for use by the profession.

In Fall 1998, the AOTA Commission on Practice (COP) embarked on the journey that culminated in the *Occupational Therapy Practice Framework: Domain and Process* (AOTA, 2002b). At that time, AOTA also published *The Guide to Occupational Therapy Practice* (Moyers, 1999), which outlined contemporary practice for the profession. Using this document and the feedback received during the review process for the third edition of *Uniform Terminology for Occupational Therapy,* the COP proceeded to develop a document that more fully articulated occupational therapy.

The *Framework* is an ever-evolving document. As an official AOTA document, it is reviewed on a 5-year cycle for usefulness and the potential need for further refinements or changes. During the review period, the COP collects feedback from members, scholars, authors, practitioners, and other stakeholders. The revision process ensures that the *Framework* maintains its integrity while responding to internal and external influences that should be reflected in emerging concepts and advances in occupational therapy.

The *Framework* was first revised and approved by the RA in 2008. Changes to the document included refinement of the writing and the addition of emerging concepts and changes in occupational therapy. The rationale for specific changes can be found in Table 11 of the second edition of the *Framework* (AOTA, 2008, pp. 665–667).

In 2012, the process of review and revision of the *Framework* was initiated again. Following member review and feedback, several modifications were made to improve flow, usability, and parallelism of concepts within the document. The following major revisions were made and approved by the RA in the Fall 2013 meeting:

- The overarching statement describing occupational therapy's domain is now stated as "achieving health, well-being, and participation in life through engagement in occupation" to encompass both domain and process.
- *Clients* are now defined as persons, groups, and populations.
- The relationship of occupational therapy to organizations has been further defined.
- *Activity demands* has been removed from the domain and placed in the overview of the process to augment the discussion of the occupational therapy practitioner's basic skill of activity analysis.
- *Areas of occupation* are now called *occupations.*
- *Performance skills* have been redefined, and Table 3 has been revised accordingly.
- The following changes have been made to the interventions table (Table 6):
  - *Consultation* has been removed and has been infused throughout the document as a method of service delivery.
  - Additional intervention methods used in practice have been added, and a clearer distinction is made among the interventions of *occupations, activities,* and *preparatory methods and tasks.*
  - *Self-advocacy* and *group interventions* have been added.
  - *Therapeutic use of self* has been moved to the process overview to ensure the understanding that use of the self as a therapeutic agent is integral to the practice of occupational therapy and is used in all interactions with all clients.
- Several additional, yet minor, changes have been made, including the creation of a preface, reorganization for flow of content, and modifications to several definitions. These changes reflect feedback received from AOTA members, educators, and other stakeholders.

Vision for This Work

Although this revision of the *Framework* represents the latest in the profession's efforts to clearly articulate the occupational therapy domain and process, it builds on a set of values that the profession has held since its founding in 1917. This founding vision had at its center a profound belief in the value of therapeutic occupations as a way to remediate illness and maintain health (Slagle, 1924). The founders emphasized the importance of establishing a therapeutic relationship with each client and designing a treatment plan based on knowledge about the client's environment, values, goals, and desires (Meyer, 1922). They advocated for scientific practice based on systematic observation and treatment (Dunton, 1934). Paraphrased using today's lexicon, the founders proposed a vision that was occupation based, client centered, contextual, and evidence based—the vision articulated in the *Framework.*

INTRODUCTION

The purpose of a *framework* is to provide a structure or base on which to build a system or a concept (*American Heritage Dictionary of the English Language,* 2003). The *Occupational Therapy Practice Framework: Domain and Process* describes the central concepts that ground occupational therapy practice and builds a common understanding of the basic tenets and vision of the profession. The *Framework* does not serve as a taxonomy, theory, or model of occupational therapy.

By design, the *Framework* must be used to guide occupational therapy practice in conjunction with the knowledge and evidence relevant to occupation and occupational therapy within the identified areas of practice and with the appropriate clients. Embedded in this document is the profession's core belief in the positive relationship between occupation and health and its view of people as occupational beings. Occupational therapy practice emphasizes the occupational nature of humans and the importance of occupational identity (Unruh, 2004) to healthful, productive, and satisfying living. As Hooper and Wood (2014) stated,

> A core philosophical assumption of the profession, therefore, is that by virtue of our biological endowment, people of all ages and abilities require occupation to grow and thrive; in pursuing occupation, humans express the totality of their being, a mind–body–spirit union. Because human existence could not otherwise be, humankind is, in essence, occupational by nature. (p. 38)

The clients of occupational therapy are typically classified as *persons* (including those involved in care of a client), *groups* (collectives of individuals, e.g., families, workers, students, communities), and *populations* (collectives of groups of individuals living in a similar locale—e.g., city, state, or country—or sharing the same or like characteristics or concerns). Services are provided directly to clients using a collaborative approach or indirectly on behalf of clients through advocacy or consultation processes.

Organization- or systems-level practice is a valid and important part of occupational therapy for several reasons. First, organizations serve as a mechanism through which occupational therapy practitioners provide interventions to support participation of those who are members of or served by the organization (e.g., falls prevention programming in a skilled nursing facility, ergonomic changes to an assembly line to reduce cumulative trauma disorders). Second, organizations support occupational therapy practice and occupational therapy practitioners as stakeholders in carrying out the mission of the organization. It is the fiduciary responsibility of practitioners to ensure that services provided to organizational stakeholders (e.g., third-party payers, employers) are of high quality and delivered in an efficient and efficacious manner. Finally, organizations employ occupational therapy practitioners in roles in which they use their knowledge of occupation and the profession of occupational therapy indirectly. For example, practitioners can serve in positions such as dean, administrator, and corporate leader; in these positions, practitioners support and enhance the organization but do not provide client care in the traditional sense.

The *Framework* is divided into two major sections: (1) the *domain,* which outlines the profession's purview and the areas in which its members have an established body of knowledge and expertise, and (2) the *process,* which describes the actions practitioners take when providing services that are client centered and focused on engagement in occupations. The profession's understanding of the domain and process of occupational therapy guides practitioners as they seek to support clients' participation in daily living that results from the dynamic intersection of clients, their desired engagements, and the context and environment (Christiansen

& Baum, 1997; Christiansen, Baum, & Bass-Haugen, 2005; Law, Baum, & Dunn, 2005).

Although the domain and process are described separately, in actuality they are linked inextricably in a transactional relationship. The aspects that constitute the domain and those that constitute the process exist in constant interaction with one another during the delivery of occupational therapy services. In other words, it is through simultaneous attention to the client's body functions and structures, skills, roles, habits, routines, and context—combined with a focus on the client as an occupational being and the practitioner's knowledge of the health- and performance-enhancing effects of occupational engagements—that outcomes such as occupational performance, role competence, and participation in daily life are produced.

Achieving health, well-being, and participation in life through engagement in occupation is the overarching statement that describes the domain and process of occupational therapy in its fullest sense. This statement acknowledges the profession's belief that active engagement in occupation promotes, facilitates, supports, and maintains health and participation. These interrelated concepts include

- *Health*—"a state of complete physical, mental, and social well-being, and not merely the absence of disease or infirmity" (World Health Organization [WHO], 2006, p. 1).
- *Well-being*—"a general term encompassing the total universe of human life domains, including physical, mental, and social aspects" (WHO, 2006, p. 211).
- *Participation*—"involvement in a life situation" (WHO, 2001, p. 10). Participation naturally occurs when clients are actively involved in carrying out occupations or daily life activities they find purposeful and meaningful. More specific outcomes of

occupational therapy intervention are multidimensional and support the end result of participation.

- *Engagement in occupation*—performance of occupations as the result of choice, motivation, and meaning within a supportive context and environment. Engagement includes objective and subjective aspects of clients' experiences and involves the transactional interaction of the mind, body, and spirit. Occupational therapy intervention focuses on creating or facilitating opportunities to engage in occupations that lead to participation in desired life situations (AOTA, 2008).

Domain

Exhibit 1 identifies the aspects of the domain, and Figure 1 illustrates the dynamic interrelatedness among them. All aspects of the domain, including occupations, client factors, performance skills, performance patterns, and context and environment, are of equal value, and together they interact to affect the client's occupational identity, health, well-being, and participation in life.

Occupational therapists are skilled in evaluating all aspects of the domain, their interrelationships, and the client within his or her contexts and environments. In addition, occupational therapy practitioners recognize the importance and impact of the mind–body–spirit connection as the client participates in daily life. Knowledge of the transactional relationship and the significance of meaningful and productive occupations form the basis for the use of occupations as both the means and the ends of interventions (Trombly, 1995). This knowledge sets occupational therapy apart as a distinct and valuable service (Hildenbrand & Lamb, 2013) for which a focus on the whole is considered stronger than a focus on isolated aspects of human function.

OCCUPATIONS	CLIENT FACTORS	PERFORMANCE SKILLS	PERFORMANCE PATTERNS	CONTEXTS AND ENVIRONMENTS
Activities of daily living (ADLs)*	Values, beliefs, and spirituality	Motor skills	Habits	Cultural
Instrumental activities of daily living (IADLs)	Body functions	Process skills	Routines	Personal
Rest and sleep	Body structures	Social interaction skills	Rituals	Physical
Education			Roles	Social
Work				Temporal
Play				Virtual
Leisure				
Social participation				

*Also referred to as *basic activities of daily living (BADLs)* or *personal activities of daily living (PADLs)*.

Exhibit 1. Aspects of the domain of occupational therapy. All aspects of the domain transact to support engagement, participation, and health. This exhibit does not imply a hierarchy.

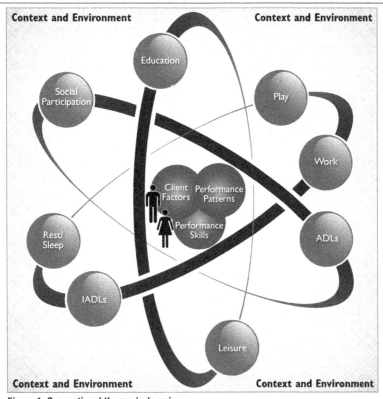

Figure 1. Occupational therapy's domain.
Note. ADLs = activities of daily living; IADLs = instrumental activities of daily living.

Occupations

The discussion that follows provides a brief explanation of each aspect of the domain. Tables included at the end of the document provide full descriptions and definitions of terms.

Occupations

Occupations are central to a client's (person's, group's, or population's) identity and sense of competence and have particular meaning and value to that client. Several definitions of *occupation* are described in the literature and can add to an understanding of this core concept:

- "Goal-directed pursuits that typically extend over time, have meaning to the performance, and involve multiple tasks" (Christiansen et al., 2005, p. 548).
- "The things that people do that occupy their time and attention; meaningful, purposeful activity; the personal activities that individuals choose or need to engage in and the ways in which each individual actually experiences them" (Boyt Schell, Gillen, & Scaffa, 2014a, p. 1237).
- "When a person engages in purposeful activities out of personal choice and they are valued, these clusters of purposeful activities form occupations

(Hinojosa, Kramer, Royeen, & Luebben, 2003). Thus, occupations are unique to each individual and provide personal satisfaction and fulfillment as a result of engaging in them (AOTA, 2002b; Pierce, 2001)" (Hinojosa & Blount, 2009, pp. 1–2).

- "In occupational therapy, occupations refer to the everyday activities that people do as individuals, in families and with communities to occupy time and bring meaning and purpose to life. Occupations include things people need to, want to and are expected to do" (World Federation of Occupational Therapists, 2012).
- "Activities . . . of everyday life, named, organized, and given value and meaning by individuals and a culture. Occupation is everything people do to occupy themselves, including looking after themselves . . . enjoying life . . . and contributing to the social and economic fabric of their communities" (Law, Polatajko, Baptiste, & Townsend, 1997, p. 32).
- "A dynamic relationship among an occupational form, a person with a unique developmental structure, subjective meanings and purpose, and the

resulting occupational performance" (Nelson & Jepson-Thomas, 2003, p. 90).

- "Occupation is used to mean all the things people want, need, or have to do, whether of physical, mental, social, sexual, political, or spiritual nature and is inclusive of sleep and rest. It refers to all aspects of actual human doing, being, becoming, and belonging. The practical, everyday medium of self-expression or of making or experiencing meaning, occupation is the activist element of human existence whether occupations are contemplative, reflective, and meditative or action based" (Wilcock & Townsend, 2014, p. 542).

The term *occupation*, as it is used in the *Framework*, refers to the daily life activities in which people engage. Occupations occur in context and are influenced by the interplay among client factors, performance skills, and performance patterns. Occupations occur over time; have purpose, meaning, and perceived utility to the client; and can be observed by others (e.g., preparing a meal) or be known only to the person involved (e.g., learning through reading a textbook). Occupations can involve the execution of multiple activities for completion and can result in various outcomes. The *Framework* identifies a broad range of occupations categorized as activities of daily living (ADLs), instrumental activities of daily living (IADLs), rest and sleep, education, work, play, leisure, and social participation (Table 1).

When occupational therapy practitioners work with clients, they identify the many types of occupations clients engage in while alone or with others. Differences among persons and the occupations they engage in are complex and multidimensional. The client's perspective on how an occupation is categorized varies depending on that client's needs and interests as well as the context. For example, one person may perceive doing laundry as work, whereas another may consider it an IADL. One group may engage in a quiz game and view their participation as play, but another group may engage in the same quiz game and view it as education.

The ways in which clients prioritize engagement in selected occupations may vary at different times. For example, clients in a community psychiatric rehabilitation setting may prioritize registering to vote during an election season and food preparation during holidays. The unique features of occupations are noted and analyzed by occupational therapy practitioners, who consider all components of the engagement and use them effectively as both a therapeutic tool and a way to achieve the targeted outcomes of intervention.

The extent to which a person is involved in a particular occupational engagement is also important. Occupations can contribute to a well-balanced and fully functional lifestyle or to a lifestyle that is out of balance and characterized by occupational dysfunction. For example, excessive work without sufficient regard for other aspects of life, such as sleep or relationships, places clients at risk for health problems (Hakansson, Dahlin-Ivanoff, & Sonn, 2006).

Sometimes occupational therapy practitioners use the terms *occupation* and *activity* interchangeably to describe participation in daily life pursuits. Some scholars have proposed that the two terms are different (Christiansen & Townsend, 2010; Pierce, 2001; Reed, 2005). In the *Framework*, the term *occupation* denotes life engagements that are constructed of multiple activities. Both occupations and activities are used as interventions by practitioners. Participation in occupations is considered the end result of interventions, and practitioners use occupations during the intervention process as the means to the end.

Occupations often are shared and done with others. Those that implicitly involve two or more individuals may be termed *co-occupations* (Zemke & Clark, 1996). Caregiving is a co-occupation that involves active participation on the part of both the caregiver and the recipient of care. For example, the co-occupations required during parenting, such as the socially interactive routines of eating, feeding, and comforting, may involve the parent, a partner, the child, and significant others (Olson, 2004); the activities inherent in this social interaction are reciprocal, interactive, and nested co-occupations (Dunlea, 1996; Esdaile & Olson, 2004). Consideration of co-occupations supports an integrated view of the client's engagement in context in relationship to significant others.

Occupational participation occurs individually or with others. It is important to acknowledge that clients can be independent in living regardless of the amount of assistance they receive while completing activities. Clients may be considered independent when they perform or direct the actions necessary to participate, regardless of the amount or kind of assistance required, if they are satisfied with their performance. In contrast with definitions of independence that imply a level of physical interaction with the environment or objects within the environment, occupational therapy practitioners consider clients to be independent whether they perform the component activities by themselves, perform the occupation in an adapted or modified environment, use various devices or alternative strategies, or oversee activity completion by others (AOTA, 2002a). For example, people with a spinal cord injury who direct a personal care assistant to assist them with their ADLs are demonstrating independence in this essential aspect of their lives.

Occupational therapy practitioners recognize that health is supported and maintained when clients are able to engage in home, school, workplace, and community life. Thus, practitioners are concerned not only with occupations but also with the variety of factors that empower and make possible clients' engagement and participation in positive health-promoting occupations (Wilcock & Townsend, 2014).

Client Factors

Client factors are specific capacities, characteristics, or beliefs that reside within the person and that influence performance in occupations (Table 2). Client factors are affected by the presence or absence of illness, disease, deprivation, disability, and life experiences. Although client factors are not to be confused with performance skills, client factors can affect performance skills. Thus, client factors may need to be present in whole or in part for a person to complete an action (skill) used in the execution of an occupation. In addition, client factors are affected by performance skills, performance patterns, contexts and environments, and performance and participation in activities and occupations. It is through this cyclical relationship that preparatory methods, activities, and occupations can be used to affect client factors and vice versa.

Values, beliefs, and spirituality influence a person's motivation to engage in occupations and give his or her life meaning. *Values* are principles, standards, or qualities considered worthwhile by the client who holds them. *Beliefs* are cognitive content held as true (Moyers & Dale, 2007). *Spirituality* is "the aspect of humanity that refers to the way individuals seek and express meaning and purpose and the way they experience their connectedness to the moment, to self, to others, to nature, and to the significant or sacred" (Puchalski et al., 2009, p. 887).

Body functions and *body structures* refer to the "physiological function of body systems (including psychological functions) and anatomical parts of the body such as organs, limbs, and their components," respectively (WHO, 2001, p. 10). Examples of body functions include sensory, musculoskeletal, mental (affective, cognitive, perceptual), cardiovascular, respiratory, and endocrine functions. Examples of body structures include the heart and blood vessels that support cardiovascular function (for additional examples, see Table 2). Body structures and body functions are interrelated, and occupational therapy practitioners must consider them when seeking to promote clients' ability to engage in desired occupations.

Moreover, occupational therapy practitioners understand that, despite their importance, the presence, absence, or limitation of specific body functions and body structures does not necessarily ensure a client's success or difficulty with daily life occupations. Occupational performance and various types of client factors may benefit from supports in the physical or social environment that enhance or allow participation. It is through the process of observing clients engaging in occupations and activities that occupational therapy practitioners are able to determine the transaction between client factors and performance and to then create adaptations and modifications and select activities that best promote enhanced participation.

Client factors can also be understood as pertaining to individuals at the group and population level. Although client factors may be described differently when applied to a group or population, the underlying tenets do not change substantively.

Performance Skills

Various approaches have been used to describe and categorize performance skills. The occupational therapy literature from research and practice offers multiple perspectives on the complexity and types of skills used during performance.

Performance skills are goal-directed actions that are observable as small units of engagement in daily life occupations. They are learned and developed over time and are situated in specific contexts and environments (Fisher & Griswold, 2014). Fisher and Griswold (2014) categorized performance skills as motor skills, process skills, and social interaction skills (Table 3). Various body structures, as well as personal and environmental contexts, converge and emerge as occupational performance skills. In addition, body functions, such as mental, sensory, neuromuscular, and movement-related functions, are identified as the capacities that reside within the person and also converge with structures and environmental contexts to emerge as performance skills. This description is consistent with WHO's (2001) *International Classification of Functioning, Disability and Health.*

Performance skills are the client's demonstrated abilities. For example, praxis capacities, such as imitating, sequencing, and constructing, affect a client's motor performance skills. Cognitive capacities, such as perception, affect a client's process performance skills and ability to organize actions in a timely and safe manner. Emotional regulation capacities can affect a client's ability to effectively respond to the demands of occupation with a range of emotions. It is important to remember that many body functions underlie each performance skill.

Performance skills are also closely linked and are used in combination with one another as a client engages in an occupation. A change in one performance skill can affect other performance skills. Occupational therapy practitioners observe and analyze performance skills to understand the transactions among client factors, context and environment, and activity or occupational demands, which support or hinder performance skills and occupational performance (Chisholm & Boyt Schell, 2014; Hagedorn, 2000).

In practice and in some literature, underlying body functions are labeled as *performance skills* and are seen in various combinations such as perceptual–motor skills and social–emotional skills. Although practitioners may focus on underlying capacities such as cognition, body structures, and emotional regulation, the *Framework* defines performance skills as those that are observable and that are key aspects of successful occupational participation. Table 3 provides definitions of the various skills in each category.

Resources informing occupational therapy practice related to performance skills include Fisher (2006); Polatajko, Mandich, and Martini (2000); and Fisher and Griswold (2014). Detailed information about the ways performance skills are used in occupational therapy practice may be found in the literature on specific theories and models such as the Model of Human Occupation (Kielhofner, 2008), the Cognitive Orientation to Daily Occupational Performance (Polatajko & Mandich, 2004), the Occupational Therapy Intervention Process Model (Fisher, 2009), sensory integration theory (Ayres, 1972, 2005), and motor learning and motor control theory (Shumway-Cook & Woollacott, 2007).

Performance Patterns

Performance patterns are the habits, routines, roles, and rituals used in the process of engaging in occupations or activities that can support or hinder occupational performance. *Habits* refers to specific, automatic behaviors; they may be useful, dominating, or impoverished (Boyt Schell, Gillen, & Scaffa, 2014b; Clark, 2000; Dunn, 2000). *Routines* are established sequences of occupations or activities that provide a structure for daily life; routines also can promote or damage health (Fiese, 2007; Koome, Hocking, & Sutton, 2012; Segal, 2004).

Roles are sets of behaviors expected by society and shaped by culture and context; they may be further conceptualized and defined by a client (person, group, or population). Roles can provide guidance in selecting occupations or can be used to identify activities connected with certain occupations in which a client engages.

When considering roles, occupational therapy practitioners are concerned with how clients construct their occupations to fulfill their perceived roles and identity and whether their roles reinforce their values and beliefs. Some roles lead to stereotyping and restricted engagement patterns. Jackson (1998a, 1998b) cautioned that describing people by their roles can be limiting and can promote segmented rather than enfolded occupations.

Rituals are symbolic actions with spiritual, cultural, or social meaning. Rituals contribute to a client's identity and reinforce the client's values and beliefs (Fiese, 2007; Segal, 2004).

Performance patterns develop over time and are influenced by all other aspects of the occupational therapy domain. Practitioners who consider clients' performance patterns are better able to understand the frequency and manner in which performance skills and occupations are integrated into clients' lives. Although clients may have the ability to engage in skilled performance, if they do not embed essential skills in a productive set of engagement patterns, their health, well-being, and participation may be negatively affected. For example, a client who has the skills and resources to engage in appropriate grooming, bathing, and meal preparation but does not embed them into a consistent routine may struggle with poor nutrition and social isolation. Table 4 provides examples of performance patterns for persons and groups or populations.

Context and Environment

Engagement and participation in occupation take place within the social and physical environment situated within context. In the literature, the terms *environment* and *context* often are used interchangeably. In the *Framework,* both terms are used to reflect the importance of considering the wide array of interrelated variables that influence performance. Understanding the environments and contexts in which occupations can and do occur provides practitioners with insights into their overarching, underlying, and embedded influences on engagement.

The *physical environment* refers to the natural (e.g., geographic terrain, plants) and built (e.g., buildings, furniture) surroundings in which daily life occupations occur. Physical environments can either support or present barriers to participation in meaningful occupations. Examples of barriers include doorway widths that do not allow for wheelchair passage or absence of healthy social opportunities for people abstaining from alcohol use. Conversely, environments can provide supports and resources for service delivery (e.g., community, health care facility, home). The *social environment* consists of the presence of, relationships with, and expectations of persons, groups, and populations with whom clients have contact (e.g., availability and expectations of significant individuals, such as spouse, friends, and caregivers).

The term *context* refers to elements within and surrounding a client that are often less tangible than physical and social environments but nonetheless exert a strong influence on performance. Contexts, as described in the *Framework,* are cultural, personal, temporal, and virtual.

The *cultural context* includes customs, beliefs, activity patterns, behavioral standards, and expectations accepted by the society of which a client is a member. The cultural context influences the client's identity and activity choices, and practitioners must be aware, for example, of norms related to eating or deference to medical professionals when working with someone from another culture and of socioeconomic status when providing a discharge plan for a young child and family. *Personal context* refers to demographic features of the individual, such as age, gender, socioeconomic status, and educational level, that are not part of a health condition (WHO, 2001). *Temporal context* includes stage of life, time of day or year, duration or rhythm of activity, and history.

Finally, *virtual context* refers to interactions that occur in simulated, real-time, or near-time situations absent of physical contact. The virtual context is becoming increasingly important for clients as well as occupational therapy practitioners and other health care providers. Clients may require access to and the ability to use technology such as cell or smartphones, computers or tablets, and videogame consoles to carry out their daily routines and occupations.

Contexts and environments affect a client's access to occupations and influence the quality of and satisfaction with performance. A client who has difficulty performing effectively in one environment or context may be successful when the environment or context is changed. The context within which the engagement in occupations occurs is specific for each client. Some contexts are external to clients (e.g., virtual), some are internal to clients (e.g., personal), and some have both external features and internalized beliefs and values (e.g., cultural).

Occupational therapy practitioners recognize that for clients to truly achieve an existence of full participation, meaning, and purpose, clients must not only function but also engage comfortably with their world, which consists of a unique combination of contexts and environments (Table 5).

Interwoven throughout all contexts and environments is the concept of *occupational justice,* defined as "a justice that recognizes occupational rights to inclusive participation in everyday occupations for all persons in society, regardless of age, ability, gender, social class, or other differences" (Nilsson & Townsend, 2010, p. 58). Occupational justice describes the concern that occupational therapy practitioners have with the ethical, moral, and civic aspects of clients' environments and contexts. As part of the occupational therapy domain, practitioners consider how these aspects can affect the implementation of occupational therapy and the target outcome of participation.

Several environments and contexts can present occupational justice issues. For example, an alternative school placement for children with psychiatric disabilities could provide academic support and counseling but limit opportunity for participation in sports, music programs, and organized social activities. A residential facility could offer safety and medical support but provide little opportunity for engagement in the role-related activities that were once a source of meaning for residents. Poor communities that lack accessibility and resources make participation especially difficult and dangerous for people with disabilities. Occupational therapy practitioners may recognize areas of occupational injustice and work to support policies, actions, and laws that allow people to engage in occupations that provide purpose and meaning in their lives.

By understanding and addressing the specific justice issues within a client's discharge environment, occupational therapy practitioners promote therapy outcomes that address empowerment and self-advocacy. Occupational therapy's focus on engagement in occupations and occupational justice complements WHO's (2001) perspective on health. In an effort to broaden the understanding of the effects of disease and disability on health, WHO recognized that health can be affected by the inability to carry out activities and participate in life situations caused both by environmental barriers and by problems that exist in body structures and body functions. The *Framework* identifies occupational justice as both an aspect of contexts and environments and an outcome of intervention.

Process

This section operationalizes the process undertaken by occupational therapy practitioners when providing services to clients. Exhibit 2 identifies the aspects of the process, and Figure 2 illustrates the dynamic interrelatedness among them. The *occupational therapy process* is

Evaluation
Occupational profile—The initial step in the evaluation process, which provides an understanding of the client's occupational history and experiences, patterns of daily living, interests, values, and needs. The client's reasons for seeking services, strengths and concerns in relation to performing occupations and daily life activities, areas of potential occupational disruption, supports and barriers, and priorities are also identified.   *Analysis of occupational performance*—The step in the evaluation process during which the client's assets and problems or potential problems are more specifically identified. Actual performance is often observed in context to identify supports for and barriers to the client's performance. Performance skills, performance patterns, context or environment, client factors, and activity demands are all considered, but only selected aspects may be specifically assessed. Targeted outcomes are identified.
Intervention
Intervention plan—The plan that will guide actions taken and that is developed in collaboration with the client. It is based on selected theories, frames of reference, and evidence. Outcomes to be targeted are confirmed.   *Intervention implementation*—Ongoing actions taken to influence and support improved client performance and participation. Interventions are directed at identified outcomes. The client's response is monitored and documented.   *Intervention review*—Review of the intervention plan and progress toward targeted outcomes.
Targeting of Outcomes
Outcomes—Determinants of success in reaching the desired end result of the occupational therapy process. Outcome assessment information is used to plan future actions with the client and to evaluate the service program (i.e., program evaluation).

Exhibit 2. Process of occupational therapy service delivery.
The process of service delivery is applied within the profession's domain to support the client's health and participation.

the client-centered delivery of occupational therapy services. The process includes evaluation and intervention to achieve targeted outcomes, occurs within the purview of the occupational therapy domain, and is facilitated by the distinct perspective of occupational therapy practitioners when engaging in clinical reasoning, analyzing activities and occupations, and collaborating with clients. This section is organized into four broad areas: (1) an overview of the process as it is applied within the profession's domain, (2) the evaluation process, (3) the intervention process, and (4) the process of targeting outcomes.

Overview of the Occupational Therapy Process

Many professions use a similar process of evaluating, intervening, and targeting intervention outcomes. However,

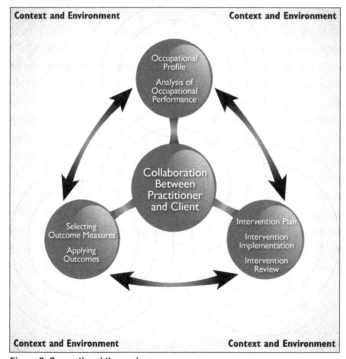

Figure 2. Occupational therapy's process.

only occupational therapy practitioners focus on the use of occupations to promote health, well-being, and participation in life. Occupational therapy practitioners use therapeutically selected occupations and activities as primary methods of intervention throughout the process (Table 6).

To help clients achieve desired outcomes, occupational therapy practitioners facilitate interactions among the client, his or her environments and contexts, and the occupations in which he or she engages. This perspective is based on the theories, knowledge, and skills generated and used by the profession and informed by available evidence (Clark et al., 2012; Davidson, Shahar, Lawless, Sells, & Tondora, 2006; Glass, de Leon, Marottoli, & Berkman, 1999; Jackson, Carlson, Mandel, Zemke, & Clark, 1998; Sandqvist, Akesson, & Eklund, 2005).

Analyzing occupational performance requires an understanding of the complex and dynamic interaction among client factors, performance skills, performance patterns, and contexts and environments, along with the activity demands of the occupation being performed. Occupational therapy practitioners attend to each aspect and gauge the influence of each on the others, individually and collectively. By understanding how these aspects influence each other, practitioners can better evaluate how each aspect contributes to clients' performance-related concerns and potentially contributes to interventions that support occupational performance.

For ease of explanation, the *Framework* describes the occupational therapy process as being linear. In reality, the process does not occur in a sequenced, step-by-step fashion. Rather, it is fluid and dynamic, allowing occupational therapy practitioners and clients to maintain their focus on the identified outcomes while continually reflecting on and changing the overall plan to accommodate new developments and insights along the way.

The broader definition of *client* included in this document is indicative of the profession's increasing involvement in providing services not only to a person but also to groups and populations. When working with a group or population, occupational therapy practitioners consider the collective occupational performance abilities of the members. Whether the client is a person, group, or population, information about the client's wants, needs, strengths, limitations, and occupational risks is gathered, synthesized, and framed from an occupational perspective.

Service Delivery Models

Occupational therapy practitioners provide services to clients directly, in settings such as hospitals, clinics, industry, schools, homes, and communities, and indirectly on behalf of clients through consultation. Direct services include interventions completed when in direct contact with the individual or group of clients. These interventions are completed through various mechanisms such as meeting in person with a client, leading a group session, or interacting with clients and families through telehealth systems (AOTA, 2013c).

When providing services to clients indirectly on their behalf, practitioners provide consultation to entities such as teachers, multidisciplinary teams, and community planning agencies. Occupational therapy practitioners also provide consultation to community organizations such as park districts and civic organizations that may or may not include people with disabilities. In addition, practitioners consult with businesses regarding the work environment, ergonomic modifications, and compliance with the Americans With Disabilities Act of 1990 (Pub. L. 101–336).

Occupational therapy practitioners can indirectly affect the lives of clients through advocacy. Common examples of advocacy include talking to legislators about improving transportation for older adults or improving services for people with mental or physical disabilities to support their living and working in the community of their choice.

Regardless of the service delivery model, the individual client may not be the exclusive focus of the intervention. For example, the needs of an at-risk infant may be the initial impetus for intervention, but the concerns and priorities of the parents, extended family, and funding agencies are also considered. Occupational therapy practitioners understand and focus intervention to include the issues and concerns surrounding the complex dynamics among the client, caregiver, and family. Similarly, services addressing independent living skills for adults coping with serious and persistent mental illness may also address the needs and expectations of state and local services agencies and of potential employers.

Clinical Reasoning

Throughout the process, occupational therapy practitioners are continually engaged in clinical reasoning about a client's occupational performance. Clinical reasoning enables practitioners to

* Identify the multiple demands, required skills, and potential meanings of the activities and occupations and
* Gain a deeper understanding of the interrelationships between aspects of the domain that affect performance and that support client-centered interventions and outcomes.

Occupational therapy practitioners use theoretical principles and models, knowledge about the effects of conditions on participation, and available evidence of the effectiveness of intervention to guide their reasoning. Clinical reasoning ensures the accurate selection and application of evaluations, interventions, and client-centered outcome measures. Practitioners also apply their knowledge and skills to enhance clients' participation in occupations and promote their health and well-being regardless of the effects of disease, disability, and occupational disruption or deprivation.

Therapeutic Use of Self

An integral part of the occupational therapy process is *therapeutic use of self*, which allows occupational therapy practitioners to develop and manage their therapeutic relationship with clients by using narrative and clinical reasoning; empathy; and a client-centered, collaborative approach to service delivery (Taylor & Van Puymbroeck, 2013). *Empathy* is the emotional exchange between occupational therapy practitioners and clients that allows more open communication, ensuring that practitioners connect with clients at an emotional level to assist them with their current life situation.

Occupational therapy practitioners use narrative and clinical reasoning to help clients make sense of the information they are receiving in the intervention process, to discover meaning, and to build hope (Peloquin, 2003; Taylor & Van Puymbroeck, 2013). Clients have identified the therapeutic relationship as critical to the outcome of occupational therapy intervention (Cole & McLean, 2003).

Occupational therapy practitioners develop a collaborative relationship with clients to understand their experiences and desires for intervention. The collaborative approach used throughout the process honors the contributions of clients along with practitioners. Through the use of interpersonal communication skills, occupational therapy practitioners shift the power of the relationship to allow clients more control in decision making and problem solving, which is essential to effective intervention.

Clients bring to the occupational therapy process their knowledge about their life experiences and their hopes and dreams for the future. They identify and share their needs and priorities. Occupational therapy practitioners bring their knowledge about how engagement in occupation affects health, well-being, and participation; they use this information, coupled with theoretical perspectives and clinical reasoning, to critically observe, analyze, describe, and interpret human performance. Practitioners and clients, together with caregivers, family members, community members, and other

stakeholders (as appropriate), identify and prioritize the focus of the intervention plan.

Activity Analysis

Activity analysis is an important process occupational therapy practitioners use to understand the demands a specific activity places on a client:

> *Activity analysis* addresses the typical demands of an activity, the range of skills involved in its performance, and the various cultural meanings that might be ascribed to it. . . . Occupation-based activity analysis places the person in the foreground. It takes into account the particular person's interests, goals, abilities, and contexts, as well as the demands of the activity itself. These considerations shape the practitioner's efforts to help the . . . person reach his/her goals through carefully designed evaluation and intervention. (Crepeau, 2003, pp. 192–193)

Occupational therapy practitioners analyze the demands of an activity or occupation to understand the specific body structures, body functions, performance skills, and performance patterns that are required and to determine the generic demands the activity or occupation makes on the client.

Activity and occupational demands are the specific features of an activity and occupation that influence its meaning for the client and the type and amount of effort required to engage in it. Activity and occupational demands include the following (see Table 7 for definitions and examples):

* *The tools and resources needed to engage in the activity*—What specific objects are used in the activity? What are their properties, and what transportation, money, or other resources are needed to participate in the activity?
* *Where and with whom the activity takes place*—What are the physical space requirements of the activity, and what are the social interaction demands?
* *How the activity is accomplished*—What process is used in carrying out the activity, including the sequence and timing of the steps and necessary procedures and rules?
* *How the activity challenges the client's capacities*—What actions, performance skills, body functions, and body structures are the individual, group, or population required to use during the performance of the activity?
* *The meaning the client derives from the activity*—What potential symbolic, unconscious, and metaphorical meanings does the individual attach to the activity (e.g., driving a car equates with independence, preparing a holiday meal connects with family tradition, voting is a rite of passage to adulthood)?

Activity and occupational demands are specific to each activity. A change in one feature of an activity may change the extent of the demand in another feature. For example, an increase in the number or sequence of steps in an activity increases the demand on attention skills.

Evaluation Process

The evaluation process is focused on finding out what a client wants and needs to do; determining what a client can do and has done; and identifying supports and barriers to health, well-being, and participation. Evaluation occurs during the initial and all subsequent interactions with a client. The type and focus of the evaluation differ depending on the practice setting.

The evaluation consists of the occupational profile and an analysis of occupational performance. The occupational profile includes information about the client's needs, problems, and concerns about performance in occupations. The analysis of occupational performance focuses on collecting and interpreting information to more specifically identify supports and barriers related to occupational performance and identify targeted outcomes.

Although the *Framework* describes the components of the evaluation process separately and sequentially, the exact manner in which occupational therapists collect client information is influenced by client needs, practice settings, and therapists' frames of reference or practice models. Information related to the occupational profile is gathered throughout the occupational therapy process.

Occupational Profile

The *occupational profile* is a summary of a client's occupational history and experiences, patterns of daily living, interests, values, and needs. Developing the occupational profile provides the occupational therapy practitioner with an understanding of a client's perspective and background.

Using a client-centered approach, the practitioner gathers information to understand what is currently important and meaningful to the client (i.e., what he or she wants and needs to do) and to identify past experiences and interests that may assist in the understanding of current issues and problems. During the process of collecting this information, the client, with the assistance of the occupational therapy practitioner, identifies priorities and desired targeted outcomes that will lead to the client's engagement in occupations that support participation in life. Only clients can identify the occupations that give meaning to their lives and select the goals and priorities that are important to them. By valuing and respecting clients' input, practitioners help foster their involvement and can more efficiently guide interventions.

Occupational therapy practitioners collect information for the occupational profile at the beginning of contact with clients to establish client-centered outcomes. Over time, practitioners collect additional information, refine the profile, and ensure that the additional information is reflected in changes subsequently made to targeted outcomes. The process of completing and refining the occupational profile varies by setting and client. The information gathered in the profile may be completed in one session or over a longer period while working with a client. For clients who are unable to participate in this process, their profiles may be compiled through interaction with family members or other significant people in their lives.

Obtaining information for the occupational profile through both formal interview techniques and casual conversation is a way to establish a therapeutic relationship with clients and their support network. The information obtained through the occupational profile leads to an individualized approach in the evaluation, intervention planning, and intervention implementation stages. Information is collected in the following areas:

- Why is the client seeking service, and what are the client's current concerns relative to engaging in occupations and in daily life activities?
- In what occupations does the client feel successful, and what barriers are affecting his or her success?
- What aspects of his or her environments or contexts does the client see as supporting engagement in desired occupations, and what aspects are inhibiting engagement?
- What is the client's occupational history (i.e., life experiences)?
- What are the client's values and interests?
- What are the client's daily life roles?
- What are the client's patterns of engagement in occupations, and how have they changed over time?
- What are the client's priorities and desired targeted outcomes related to occupational performance, prevention, participation, role competence, health and wellness, quality of life, well-being, and occupational justice?

After collecting profile data, occupational therapists view the information and develop a working hypothesis regarding possible reasons for the identified problems and concerns. Reasons could include impairments in client factors, performance skills, and performance patterns or barriers within the context and environment. Therapists then work with clients to establish preliminary goals and outcome measures. In addition, therapists note strengths and supports within all areas because these can inform the intervention plan and affect future outcomes.

Analysis of Occupational Performance

Occupational performance is the accomplishment of the selected occupation resulting from the dynamic transaction among the client, the context and environment, and the activity or occupation. In the *analysis of occupational performance,* the client's assets and problems or potential problems are more specifically identified through assessment tools designed to observe, measure, and inquire about factors that support or hinder occupational performance. Targeted outcomes also are identified. The analysis of occupational performance involves one or more of the following activities:

- Synthesizing information from the occupational profile to focus on specific occupations and contexts that need to be addressed
- Observing a client's performance during activities relevant to desired occupations, noting effectiveness of performance skills and performance patterns
- Selecting and using specific assessments to measure performance skills and performance patterns, as appropriate
- Selecting and administering assessments, as needed, to identify and measure more specifically the contexts or environments, activity demands, and client factors that influence performance skills and performance patterns
- Selecting outcome measures
- Interpreting the assessment data to identify supports and hindrances to performance
- Developing and refining hypotheses about the client's occupational performance strengths and limitations
- Creating goals in collaboration with the client that address the desired outcomes
- Determining procedures to measure the outcomes of intervention
- Delineating a potential intervention approach or approaches based on best practices and available evidence.

Multiple methods often are used during the evaluation process to assess client, environment or context, occupation or activity, and occupational performance. Methods may include an interview with the client and significant others, observation of performance and context, record review, and direct assessment of specific aspects of performance. Formal and informal, structured and unstructured, and standardized criterion- or norm-referenced assessment tools can be used. Standardized assessments are preferred, when available, to provide objective data about various aspects of the domain influencing engagement and performance. The use of valid and reliable assessments for obtaining trustworthy information can also help support and justify the need for occupational therapy services (Doucet & Gutman, 2013; Gutman, Mortera, Hinojosa, & Kramer, 2007).

Implicit in any outcome assessment used by occupational therapy practitioners are clients' belief systems and underlying assumptions regarding their desired occupational performance. Occupational therapists select outcome assessments pertinent to clients' needs and goals, congruent with the practitioner's theoretical model of practice and based on knowledge of the psychometric properties of standardized measures or the rationale and protocols of nonstandardized yet structured measures and the available evidence. In addition, clients' perception of success in engaging in desired occupations is vital to any outcomes assessment (Bandura, 1986).

Intervention Process

The intervention process consists of the skilled services provided by occupational therapy practitioners in collaboration with clients to facilitate engagement in occupation related to health, well-being, and participation. Practitioners use the information about clients gathered during the evaluation and theoretical principles to direct occupation-centered interventions. Intervention is then provided to assist clients in reaching a state of physical, mental, and social well-being; identifying and realizing aspirations; satisfying needs; and changing or coping with the environment. Types of occupational therapy interventions are discussed in Table 6.

Intervention is intended to promote health, well-being, and participation. *Health promotion* is "the process of enabling people to increase control over, and to improve, their health" (WHO, 1986). Wilcock (2006) stated,

> Following an occupation-focused health promotion approach to well-being embraces a belief that the potential range of what people can do, be, and strive to become is the primary concern, and that health is a by-product. A varied and full occupational lifestyle will coincidentally maintain and improve health and well-being if it enables people to be creative and adventurous physically, mentally, and socially. (p. 315)

Interventions vary depending on the client—person, group, or population—and the context of service delivery (Moyers & Dale, 2007). The actual term used for clients or groups of clients receiving occupational therapy varies among practice settings and delivery models. For example, when working in a hospital, the person or group might be referred to as a *patient* or *patients,* and in a school, the clients might be *students.* When providing consultation to an organization, clients may be called *consumers* or *members.* The term *person* includes others who may help or be served indirectly, such as caregiver, teacher, parent, employer, or spouse.

Interventions provided to groups and populations are directed to all the members collectively rather than individualized to specific people within the group. Practitioners direct their interventions toward current or potential disabling conditions with the goal of enhancing the health, well-being, and participation of all group members collectively. The intervention focus often is on health promotion activities, self-management, educational services, and environmental modification. For instance, occupational therapy practitioners may provide education on falls prevention and the impact of fear of falling to a group of residents in an assisted living center or provide support to people with psychiatric disability as they learn to use the Internet to identify and coordinate community resources that meet their needs. Practitioners may work with a wide variety of populations experiencing difficulty in accessing and engaging in healthy occupations because of conditions such as poverty, homelessness, and discrimination.

The intervention process is divided into three steps: (1) intervention plan, (2) intervention implementation, and (3) intervention review. During the intervention process, information from the evaluation is integrated with theory, practice models, frames of reference, and evidence. This information guides occupational therapy practitioners' clinical reasoning in the development, implementation, and review of the intervention plan.

Intervention Plan

The *intervention plan,* which directs the actions of occupational therapy practitioners, describes selected occupational therapy approaches and types of interventions to be used in reaching clients' identified outcomes. The intervention plan is developed collaboratively with clients or their proxies and is directed by

- Client goals, values, beliefs, and occupational needs;
- Client health and well-being;
- Client performance skills and performance patterns;
- Collective influence of the context and environment, activity demands, and client factors on the client;

- Context of service delivery in which the intervention is provided; and
- Best available evidence.

The selection and design of the intervention plan and goals are directed toward addressing clients' current and potential situation related to engagement in occupations or activities. Intervention planning includes the following steps:

1. Developing the plan, which involves selecting
   - Objective and measurable occupation-focused goals and related time frames;
   - The occupational therapy intervention approach or approaches, such as create or promote, establish or restore, maintain, modify, and prevent (Table 8); and
   - Methods for service delivery, including who will provide the intervention, types of interventions, and service delivery models to be used.
2. Considering potential discharge needs and plans.
3. Making recommendations or referrals to other professionals as needed.

Intervention Implementation

Intervention implementation is the process of putting the intervention plan into action. Interventions may focus on a single aspect of the domain, such as a specific occupation, or on several aspects of the domain, such as context and environment, performance patterns, and performance skills.

Given that aspects of the domain are interrelated and influence one another in a continuous, dynamic process, occupational therapy practitioners expect that a client's ability to adapt, change, and develop in one area will affect other areas. Because of this dynamic interrelationship, evaluation and intervention planning continue throughout the implementation process.

Intervention implementation includes the following steps:

1. Determining and carrying out the occupational therapy intervention or interventions to be used (see Table 6), which may include the following:
   - Therapeutic use of occupations and activities
   - Preparatory methods (e.g., splinting, assistive technology, wheeled mobility) and preparatory tasks
   - Education and training
   - Advocacy (e.g., advocacy, self-advocacy)
   - Group interventions.
2. Monitoring a client's response to specific interventions on the basis of ongoing evaluation and reevaluation of his or her progress toward goals.

Intervention Review

Intervention review is the continuous process of reevaluating and reviewing the intervention plan, the effectiveness of its delivery, and progress toward outcomes. As during intervention planning, this process includes collaboration with the client on the basis of identified goals and progress toward the associated outcomes. Reevaluation and review may lead to change in the intervention plan.

The intervention review includes the following steps:
1. Reevaluating the plan and how it is implemented relative to achieving outcomes
2. Modifying the plan as needed
3. Determining the need for continuation or discontinuation of occupational therapy services and for referral to other services.

Targeting of Outcomes

Outcomes are the end result of the occupational therapy process; they describe what clients can achieve through occupational therapy intervention. The benefits of occupational therapy are multifaceted and may occur in all aspects of the domain of concern. Outcomes are directly related to the interventions provided and to the occupations, client factors, performance skills, performance patterns, and contexts and environments targeted. Outcomes may also be traced to the improved transactional relationship among the areas of the domain that result in clients' ability to engage in desired occupations secondary to improved abilities at the client factor and performance skill level (Table 9).

In addition, outcomes may relate to clients' subjective impressions regarding goal attainment, such as improved outlook, confidence, hope, playfulness, self-efficacy, sustainability of valued occupations, resilience, and perceived well-being. An example of a subjective outcome of intervention is parents' greater perceived efficacy about their parenting through a new understanding of their child's behavior after receiving occupational therapy services (Cohn, 2001; Cohn, Miller, & Tickle-Degnen, 2000; Graham, Rodger, & Ziviani, 2013).

Interventions can also be designed for caregivers of people with dementia to improve quality of life for both care recipient and caregiver. Caregivers who received intervention reported fewer declines in occupational performance, enhanced mastery and skill, improved sense of self-efficacy and well-being, and less need for help with care recipients (Gitlin & Corcoran, 2005; Gitlin, Corcoran, Winter, Boyce, & Hauck, 2001; Gitlin et al., 2003, 2008; Graff et al., 2007).

Outcomes for groups may include improved social interaction, increased self-awareness through peer support, a larger social network, or increased workplace productivity with fewer injuries. Outcomes for populations may include health promotion, occupational justice and self-advocacy, and access to services. The impact of outcomes and the way they are defined are specific to clients and to other stakeholders such as payers and regulators. Specific outcomes and documentation of those outcomes vary by practice setting and are influenced by the stakeholders in each setting.

The focus on outcomes is woven throughout the process of occupational therapy. Occupational therapists and clients collaborate during evaluation to identify initial client outcomes related to engagement in valued occupations or daily life activities. During intervention implementation and reevaluation, clients, occupational therapists, and, when appropriate, occupational therapy assistants may modify outcomes to accommodate changing needs, contexts, and performance abilities. As further analysis of occupational performance and the development of the intervention plan occur, therapists and clients may redefine the desired outcomes.

Implementation of the outcomes process includes the following steps:
1. Selecting types of outcomes and measures, including but not limited to occupational performance, prevention, health and wellness, quality of life, participation, role competence, well-being, and occupational justice (see Table 9). Outcome measures are
   * Selected early in the intervention process (see "Evaluation Process" section);
   * Valid, reliable, and appropriately sensitive to change in clients' occupational performance;
   * Consistent with targeted outcomes;
   * Congruent with clients' goals; and
   * Selected on the basis of their actual or purported ability to predict future outcomes.
2. Using outcomes to measure progress and adjust goals and interventions by
   * Comparing progress toward goal achievement to outcomes throughout the intervention process and
   * Assessing outcome use and results to make decisions about the future direction of intervention (e.g., continue intervention, modify intervention, discontinue intervention, provide follow-up, refer for other services).

Outcomes and the other aspects of the occupational therapy process are summarized in Exhibit 3.

Evaluation		Intervention			Targeting of Outcomes
Occupational Profile ←→	**Analysis of Occupational Performance**	**Intervention Plan**	**Intervention Implementation**	**Intervention Review**	**Outcomes**

Identify the following:
• Why is the client seeking service, and what are the client's current concerns relative to engaging in activities and occupations?
• In what occupations does the client feel successful, and what barriers are affecting his or her success?
• What aspects of the contexts or environments does the client see as supporting and as inhibiting engagement in desired occupations?
• What is the client's occupational history?
• What are the client's values and interests?
• What are the client's daily life roles?
• What are the client's patterns of engagement in occupations, and how have they changed over time?
• What are the client's priorities and desired targeted outcomes related to occupational performance, prevention, participation, role competence, health and wellness, quality of life, well-being, and occupational justice?
	• Synthesize information from the occupational profile to focus on specific occupations and contexts.
	• Observe the client's performance during activities relevant to desired occupations.
	• Select and use specific assessments to identify and measure contexts or environments, activity and occupational demands, client factors, and performance skills and patterns.
	• Select outcome measures.
	• Interpret assessment data to identify supports for and hindrances to performance.
	• Develop and refine hypotheses about the client's occupational performance strengths and limitations.
	• Create goals in collaboration with the client that address desired outcomes.
	• Determine procedures to measure the outcomes of intervention.
	• Delineate a potential intervention based on best practices and available evidence.
		1. Develop the plan, which involves selecting
		  • Objective and measurable occupation-focused goals and related time frames;
		  • Occupational therapy intervention approach or approaches, such as create or promote, establish or restore, maintain, modify, or prevent; and
		  • Methods for service delivery, including who will provide the intervention, types of intervention, and service delivery models.
		2. Consider potential discharge needs and plans.
		3. Recommend or refer to other professionals as needed.
			1. Determine and carry out occupational therapy intervention or interventions, which may include the following:
			  • Therapeutic use of occupations and activities
			  • Preparatory methods and tasks
			  • Education and training
			  • Advocacy
			  • Group interventions
			2. Monitor the client's response through ongoing evaluation and reevaluation.
				1. Reevaluate the plan and implementation relative to achieving outcomes.
				2. Modify the plan as needed.
				3. Determine the need for continuation or discontinuation of occupational therapy services and for referral.
					1. Early in the intervention process, select outcomes and measures that are
					  • Valid, reliable, sensitive to change, and consistent with outcomes
					  • Congruent with client goals
					  • Based on their actual or purported ability to predict future outcomes
					2. Apply outcomes to measure progress and adjust goals and interventions.
					  • Compare progress toward goal achievement to outcomes throughout the intervention process.
					  • Assess outcome use and results to make decisions about the future direction of intervention.

←————————————Continue to renegotiate intervention plans and targeted outcomes.————————————→

←————————Ongoing interaction among evaluation, intervention, and outcomes occurs throughout the process.————————→

Exhibit 3. Operationalizing the occupational therapy process.

Conclusion

The *Framework* describes the central concepts that ground occupational therapy practice and builds a common understanding of the basic tenets and distinct contribution of the profession. The occupational therapy domain and process are linked inextricably in a transactional relationship, as illustrated in Figure 3. An understanding of this relationship supports and guides the complex decision making required in the daily practice of occupational therapy and enhances practitioners' ability to define the reasons for and direct interventions to clients (persons, groups, and populations), family members, team members, payers, and policymakers. The *Framework* highlights the distinct value of occupation and occupational therapy in contributing to client health, well-being, and participation in life.

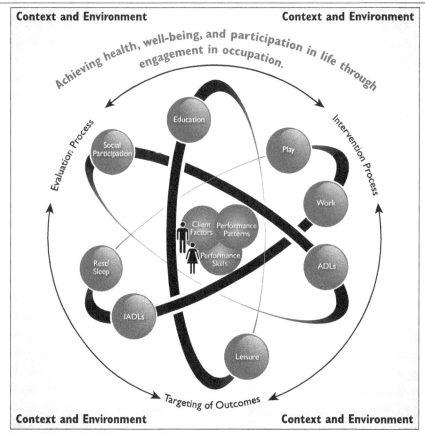

Figure 3. Occupational therapy domain and process.

March/April 2014, Volume 68(Supplement 1)

TABLE 1. OCCUPATIONS

Occupations *are various kinds of life activities in which individuals, groups, or populations engage, including activities of daily living, instrumental activities of daily living, rest and sleep, education, work, play, leisure, and social participation.*

Category	Description
▨ **ACTIVITIES OF DAILY LIVING (ADLs)**—Activities oriented toward taking care of one's own body (adapted from Rogers & Holm, 1994). ADLs also are referred to as *basic activities of daily living (BADLs)* and *personal activities of daily living (PADLs)*. These activities are "fundamental to living in a social world; they enable basic survival and well-being" (Christiansen & Hammecker, 2001, p. 156).	
Bathing, showering	Obtaining and using supplies; soaping, rinsing, and drying body parts; maintaining bathing position; and transferring to and from bathing positions
Toileting and toilet hygiene	Obtaining and using toileting supplies, managing clothing, maintaining toileting position, transferring to and from toileting position, cleaning body, and caring for menstrual and continence needs (including catheter, colostomy, and suppository management), as well as completing intentional control of bowel movements and urination and, if necessary, using equipment or agents for bladder control (Uniform Data System for Medical Rehabilitation, 1996, pp. III-20, III-24)
Dressing	Selecting clothing and accessories appropriate to time of day, weather, and occasion; obtaining clothing from storage area; dressing and undressing in a sequential fashion; fastening and adjusting clothing and shoes; and applying and removing personal devices, prosthetic devices, or splints
Swallowing/eating	Keeping and manipulating food or fluid in the mouth and swallowing it; *swallowing* is moving food from the mouth to the stomach
Feeding	Setting up, arranging, and bringing food [or fluid] from the plate or cup to the mouth; sometimes called *self-feeding*
Functional mobility	Moving from one position or place to another (during performance of everyday activities), such as in-bed mobility, wheelchair mobility, and transfers (e.g., wheelchair, bed, car, shower, tub, toilet, chair, floor). Includes functional ambulation and transportation of objects.
Personal device care	Using, cleaning, and maintaining personal care items, such as hearing aids, contact lenses, glasses, orthotics, prosthetics, adaptive equipment, glucometers, and contraceptive and sexual devices
Personal hygiene and grooming	Obtaining and using supplies; removing body hair (e.g., using razor, tweezers, lotion); applying and removing cosmetics; washing, drying, combing, styling, brushing, and trimming hair; caring for nails (hands and feet); caring for skin, ears, eyes, and nose; applying deodorant; cleaning mouth; brushing and flossing teeth; and removing, cleaning, and reinserting dental orthotics and prosthetics
Sexual activity	Engaging in activities that result in sexual satisfaction and/or meet relational or reproductive needs
▨ **INSTRUMENTAL ACTIVITIES OF DAILY LIVING (IADLs)**—Activities to support daily life within the home and community that often require more complex interactions than those used in ADLs.	
Care of others (including selecting and supervising caregivers)	Arranging, supervising, or providing care for others
Care of pets	Arranging, supervising, or providing care for pets and service animals
Child rearing	Providing care and supervision to support the developmental needs of a child
Communication management	Sending, receiving, and interpreting information using a variety of systems and equipment, including writing tools, telephones (cell phones or smartphones), keyboards, audiovisual recorders, computers or tablets, communication boards, call lights, emergency systems, Braille writers, telecommunication devices for deaf people, augmentative communication systems, and personal digital assistants
Driving and community mobility	Planning and moving around in the community and using public or private transportation, such as driving, walking, bicycling, or accessing and riding in buses, taxi cabs, or other transportation systems
Financial management	Using fiscal resources, including alternate methods of financial transaction, and planning and using finances with long-term and short-term goals
Health management and maintenance	Developing, managing, and maintaining routines for health and wellness promotion, such as physical fitness, nutrition, decreased health risk behaviors, and medication routines
Home establishment and management	Obtaining and maintaining personal and household possessions and environment (e.g., home, yard, garden, appliances, vehicles), including maintaining and repairing personal possessions (e.g., clothing, household items) and knowing how to seek help or whom to contact

(Continued)

TABLE 1. OCCUPATIONS
(Continued)

Category	Description
Meal preparation and cleanup	Planning, preparing, and serving well-balanced, nutritious meals and cleaning up food and utensils after meals
Religious and spiritual activities and expression	Participating in *religion,* "an organized system of beliefs, practices, rituals, and symbols designed to facilitate closeness to the sacred or transcendent" (Moreira-Almeida & Koenig, 2006, p. 844), and engaging in activities that allow a sense of connectedness to something larger than oneself or that are especially meaningful, such as taking time out to play with a child, engaging in activities in nature, and helping others in need (Spencer, Davidson, & White, 1997)
Safety and emergency maintenance	Knowing and performing preventive procedures to maintain a safe environment; recognizing sudden, unexpected hazardous situations; and initiating emergency action to reduce the threat to health and safety; examples include ensuring safety when entering and exiting the home, identifying emergency contact numbers, and replacing items such as batteries in smoke alarms and light bulbs
Shopping	Preparing shopping lists (grocery and other); selecting, purchasing, and transporting items; selecting method of payment; and completing money transactions; included are Internet shopping and related use of electronic devices such as computers, cell phones, and tablets
▨ **REST AND SLEEP**—Activities related to obtaining restorative rest and sleep to support healthy, active engagement in other occupations.	
Rest	Engaging in quiet and effortless actions that interrupt physical and mental activity, resulting in a relaxed state (Nurit & Michal, 2003, p. 227); included are identifying the need to relax; reducing involvement in taxing physical, mental, or social activities; and engaging in relaxation or other endeavors that restore energy and calm and renew interest in engagement
Sleep preparation	(1) Engaging in routines that prepare the self for a comfortable rest, such as grooming and undressing, reading or listening to music to fall asleep, saying goodnight to others, and engaging in meditation or prayers; determining the time of day and length of time desired for sleeping and the time needed to wake; and establishing sleep patterns that support growth and health (patterns are often personally and culturally determined). (2) Preparing the physical environment for periods of unconsciousness, such as making the bed or space on which to sleep; ensuring warmth or coolness and protection; setting an alarm clock; securing the home, such as locking doors or closing windows or curtains; and turning off electronics or lights.
Sleep participation	Taking care of personal needs for sleep, such as ceasing activities to ensure onset of sleep, napping, and dreaming; sustaining a sleep state without disruption; and performing nighttime care of toileting needs and hydration; also includes negotiating the needs and requirements of and interacting with others within the social environment such as children or partners, including providing nighttime caregiving such as breastfeeding and monitoring the comfort and safety of others who are sleeping
▨ **EDUCATION**—Activities needed for learning and participating in the educational environment.	
Formal educational participation	Participating in academic (e.g., math, reading, degree coursework), nonacademic (e.g., recess, lunchroom, hallway), extracurricular (e.g., sports, band, cheerleading, dances), and vocational (prevocational and vocational) educational activities
Informal personal educational needs or interests exploration (beyond formal education)	Identifying topics and methods for obtaining topic-related information or skills
Informal personal education participation	Participating in informal classes, programs, and activities that provide instruction or training in identified areas of interest
▨ **WORK**—"Labor or exertion; to make, construct, manufacture, form, fashion, or shape objects; to organize, plan, or evaluate services or processes of living or governing; committed occupations that are performed with or without financial reward" (Christiansen & Townsend, 2010, p. 423).	
Employment interests and pursuits	Identifying and selecting work opportunities based on assets, limitations, likes, and dislikes relative to work (adapted from Mosey, 1996, p. 342)
Employment seeking and acquisition	Advocating for oneself; completing, submitting, and reviewing appropriate application materials; preparing for interviews; participating in interviews and following up afterward; discussing job benefits; and finalizing negotiations
Job performance	Performing the requirements of a job, including work skills and patterns; time management; relationships with coworkers, managers, and customers; leadership and supervision; creation, production, and distribution of products and services; initiation, sustainment, and completion of work; and compliance with work norms and procedures
Retirement preparation and adjustment	Determining aptitudes, developing interests and skills, selecting appropriate avocational pursuits, and adjusting lifestyle in the absence of the worker role

(Continued)

TABLE 1. OCCUPATIONS
(Continued)

Category	Description
Volunteer exploration	Determining community causes, organizations, or opportunities for unpaid work in relationship to personal skills, interests, location, and time available
Volunteer participation	Performing unpaid work activities for the benefit of selected causes, organizations, or facilities
PLAY—"Any spontaneous or organized activity that provides enjoyment, entertainment, amusement, or diversion" (Parham & Fazio, 1997, p. 252).	
Play exploration	Identifying appropriate play activities, including exploration play, practice play, pretend play, games with rules, constructive play, and symbolic play (adapted from Bergen, 1988, pp. 64–65)
Play participation	Participating in play; maintaining a balance of play with other occupations; and obtaining, using, and maintaining toys, equipment, and supplies appropriately
LEISURE—"Nonobligatory activity that is intrinsically motivated and engaged in during discretionary time, that is, time not committed to obligatory occupations such as work, self-care, or sleep" (Parham & Fazio, 1997, p. 250).	
Leisure exploration	Identifying interests, skills, opportunities, and appropriate leisure activities
Leisure participation	Planning and participating in appropriate leisure activities; maintaining a balance of leisure activities with other occupations; and obtaining, using, and maintaining equipment and supplies as appropriate
SOCIAL PARTICIPATION—"The interweaving of occupations to support desired engagement in community and family activities as well as those involving peers and friends" (Gillen & Boyt Schell, 2014, p. 607); involvement in a subset of activities that involve social situations with others (Bedell, 2012) and that support social interdependence (Magasi & Hammel, 2004). Social participation can occur in person or through remote technologies such as telephone calls, computer interaction, and video conferencing.	
Community	Engaging in activities that result in successful interaction at the community level (e.g., neighborhood, organization, workplace, school, religious or spiritual group)
Family	Engaging in activities that result in "successful interaction in specific required and/or desired familial roles" (Mosey, 1996, p. 340)
Peer, friend	Engaging in activities at different levels of interaction and intimacy, including engaging in desired sexual activity

TABLE 2. CLIENT FACTORS

Client factors *include (1) values, beliefs, and spirituality; (2) body functions; and (3) body structures that reside within the client that influence the client's performance in occupations.*

VALUES, BELIEFS, AND SPIRITUALITY— Clients' perceptions, motivations, and related meaning that influence or are influenced by engagement in occupations.

Category and Definition	Examples
Values—Acquired beliefs and commitments, derived from culture, about what is good, right, and important to do (Kielhofner, 2008)	*Person:* • Honesty with self and others • Commitment to family *Group:* • Obligation to provide a service • Fairness *Population:* • Freedom of speech • Equal opportunities for all • Tolerance toward others
Beliefs—Cognitive content held as true by or about the client	*Person:* • One is powerless to influence others. • Hard work pays off. *Group and population:* • Some personal rights are worth fighting for. • A new health care policy, as yet untried, will positively affect society.
Spirituality—"The aspect of humanity that refers to the way individuals seek and express meaning and purpose and the way they experience their connectedness to the moment, to self, to others, to nature, and to the significant or sacred" (Puchalski et al., 2009, p. 887)	*Person:* • Daily search for purpose and meaning in one's life • Guidance of actions by a sense of value beyond the personal acquisition of wealth or fame *Group and population:* • Common search for purpose and meaning in life • Guidance of actions by values agreed on by the collective

BODY FUNCTIONS—"The physiological functions of body systems (including psychological functions)" (WHO, 2001, p. 10). This section of the table is organized according to the classifications of the *International Classification of Functioning, Disability and Health (ICF)*; for fuller descriptions and definitions, refer to WHO (2001).

Category	Description (not an all-inclusive list)
Mental functions (affective, cognitive, perceptual)	
Specific mental functions	
Higher-level cognitive	Judgment, concept formation, metacognition, executive functions, praxis, cognitive flexibility, insight
Attention	Sustained shifting and divided attention, concentration, distractibility
Memory	Short-term, long-term, and working memory
Perception	Discrimination of sensations (e.g., auditory, tactile, visual, olfactory, gustatory, vestibular, proprioceptive)
Thought	Control and content of thought, awareness of reality vs. delusions, logical and coherent thought
Mental functions of sequencing complex movement	Mental functions that regulate the speed, response, quality, and time of motor production, such as restlessness, toe tapping, or hand wringing, in response to inner tension
Emotional	Regulation and range of emotions; appropriateness of emotions, including anger, love, tension, and anxiety; lability of emotions
Experience of self and time	Awareness of one's identity, body, and position in the reality of one's environment and of time
Global mental functions	
Consciousness	State of awareness and alertness, including the clarity and continuity of the wakeful state
Orientation	Orientation to person, place, time, self, and others
Temperament and personality	Extroversion, introversion, agreeableness, conscientiousness, emotional stability, openness to experience, self-control, self-expression, confidence, motivation, impulse control, appetite

(Continued)

TABLE 2. CLIENT FACTORS
(Continued)

Category	Description (not an all-inclusive list)
Energy and drive	Energy level, motivation, appetite, craving, impulse control
Sleep	Physiological process, quality of sleep
Sensory functions	
Visual functions	Quality of vision, visual acuity, visual stability, and visual field functions to promote visual awareness of environment at various distances for functioning
Hearing functions	Sound detection and discrimination; awareness of location and distance of sounds
Vestibular functions	Sensation related to position, balance, and secure movement against gravity
Taste functions	Association of taste qualities of bitterness, sweetness, sourness, and saltiness
Smell functions	Sensing odors and smells
Proprioceptive functions	Awareness of body position and space
Touch functions	Feeling of being touched by others or touching various textures, such as those of food; presence of numbness, paresthesia, hyperesthesia
Pain (e.g., diffuse, dull, sharp, phantom)	Unpleasant feeling indicating potential or actual damage to some body structure; sensations of generalized or localized pain (e.g., diffuse, dull, sharp, phantom)
Sensitivity to temperature and pressure	Thermal awareness (hot and cold), sense of force applied to skin
Neuromusculoskeletal and movement-related functions	
Functions of joints and bones	
Joint mobility	Joint range of motion
Joint stability	Maintenance of structural integrity of joints throughout the body; physiological stability of joints related to structural integrity
Muscle functions	
Muscle power	Strength
Muscle tone	Degree of muscle tension (e.g., flaccidity, spasticity, fluctuation)
Muscle endurance	Sustaining muscle contraction
Movement functions	
Motor reflexes	Involuntary contraction of muscles automatically induced by specific stimuli (e.g., stretch, asymmetrical tonic neck, symmetrical tonic neck)
Involuntary movement reactions	Postural reactions, body adjustment reactions, supporting reactions
Control of voluntary movement	Eye–hand and eye–foot coordination, bilateral integration, crossing of the midline, fine and gross motor control, and oculomotor function (e.g., saccades, pursuits, accommodation, binocularity)
Gait patterns	Gait and mobility considered in relation to how they affect ability to engage in occupations in daily life activities; for example, walking patterns and impairments, asymmetric gait, stiff gait
Cardiovascular, hematological, immunological, and respiratory system functions (*Note.* Occupational therapy practitioners have knowledge of these body functions and understand broadly the interaction that occurs among these functions to support health, well-being, and participation in life through engagement in occupation.)	
Cardiovascular system functions Hematological and immunological system functions	Maintenance of blood pressure functions (hypertension, hypotension, postural hypotension), heart rate and rhythm
Respiratory system functions	Rate, rhythm, and depth of respiration
Additional functions and sensations of the cardiovascular and respiratory systems	Physical endurance, aerobic capacity, stamina, fatigability
Voice and speech functions; digestive, metabolic, and endocrine system functions; genitourinary and reproductive functions (*Note.* Occupational therapy practitioners have knowledge of these body functions and understand broadly the interaction that occurs among these functions to support health, well-being, and participation in life through engagement in occupation.)	
Voice and speech functions	Fluency and rhythm, alternative vocalization functions

(Continued)

TABLE 2. CLIENT FACTORS
(Continued)

Category	Description (not an all-inclusive list)
Digestive, metabolic, and endocrine system functions	Digestive system functions, metabolic system and endocrine system functions
Genitourinary and reproductive functions	Urinary functions, genital and reproductive functions

Skin and related structure functions
(*Note.* Occupational therapy practitioners have knowledge of these body functions and understand broadly the interaction that occurs among these functions to support health, well-being, and participation in life through engagement in occupation.)

Skin functions Hair and nail functions	Protection (presence or absence of wounds, cuts, or abrasions), repair (wound healing)

▧ **BODY STRUCTURES:** "Anatomical parts of the body, such as organs, limbs, and their components" that support body function (WHO, 2001, p. 10). The "Body Structures" section of the table is organized according to the *ICF* classifications; for fuller descriptions and definitions, refer to WHO (2001).

Category	Examples not delineated in the "Body Structure" section of this table
Structure of the nervous system **Eyes, ear, and related structures** **Structures involved in voice and speech** **Structures of the cardiovascular, immunological, and respiratory systems** **Structures related to the digestive, metabolic, and endocrine systems** **Structures related to the genitourinary and reproductive systems** **Structures related to movement** **Skin and related structures**	(*Note.* Occupational therapy practitioners have knowledge of body structures and understand broadly the interaction that occurs between these structures to support health, well-being, and participation in life through engagement in occupation.)

Note. The categorization of body function and body structure client factors outlined in Table 2 is based on the *ICF* proposed by WHO (2001). The classification was selected because it has received wide exposure and presents a language that is understood by external audiences. WHO = World Health Organization.

TABLE 3. PERFORMANCE SKILLS

Performance skills *are observable elements of action that have an implicit functional purpose; skills are considered a classification of actions, encompassing multiple capacities (body functions and body structures) and, when combined, underlie the ability to participate in desired occupations and activities. This list is not all inclusive and may not include all possible skills addressed during occupational therapy interventions.*

Skill	Definition
MOTOR SKILLS—"Occupational performance skills observed as the person interacts with and moves task objects and self around the task environment" (e.g., activity of daily living [ADL] motor skills, school motor skills; Boyt Schell, Gillen, & Scaffa, 2014a, p. 1237).	
Aligns	Interacts with task objects without evidence of persistent propping or persistent leaning
Stabilizes	Moves through task environment and interacts with task objects without momentary propping or loss of balance
Positions	Positions self an effective distance from task objects and without evidence of awkward body positioning
Reaches	Effectively extends the arm and, when appropriate, bends the trunk to effectively grasp or place task objects that are out of reach
Bends	Flexes or rotates the trunk as appropriate to the task to grasp or place task objects out of reach or when sitting down
Grips	Effectively pinches or grasps task objects such that the objects do not slip (e.g., from the person's fingers, between teeth)
Manipulates	Uses dexterous finger movements, without evidence of fumbling, when manipulating task objects (e.g., manipulating buttons when buttoning)
Coordinates	Uses two or more body parts together to manipulate, hold, and/or stabilize task objects without evidence of fumbling task objects or slipping from one's grasp
Moves	Effectively pushes or pulls task objects along a supporting surface, pulls to open or pushes to close doors and drawers, or pushes on wheels to propel a wheelchair
Lifts	Effectively raises or lifts task objects without evidence of increased effort
Walks	During task performance, ambulates on level surfaces without shuffling the feet, becoming unstable, propping, or using assistive devices
Transports	Carries task objects from one place to another while walking or moving in a wheelchair
Calibrates	Uses movements of appropriate force, speed, or extent when interacting with task objects (e.g., not crushing objects, pushing a door with enough force that it closes)
Flows	Uses smooth and fluid arm and wrist movements when interacting with task objects
Endures	Persists and completes the task without showing obvious evidence of physical fatigue, pausing to rest, or stopping to catch one's breath
Paces	Maintains a consistent and effective rate or tempo of performance throughout the entire task
PROCESS SKILLS—"Occupational performance skills [e.g., ADL process skills, school process skills] observed as a person (1) selects, interacts with, and uses task tools and materials; (2) carries out individual actions and steps; and (3) modifies performance when problems are encountered" (Boyt Schell et al., 2014a, p. 1239).	
Paces	Maintains a consistent and effective rate or tempo of performance throughout the entire task
Attends	Does not look away from what he or she is doing, interrupting the ongoing task progression
Heeds	Carries out and completes the task originally agreed on or specified by another
Chooses	Selects necessary and appropriate type and number of tools and materials for the task, including the tools and materials that the person was directed to use or specified he or she would use
Uses	Applies tools and materials as they are intended (e.g., uses a pencil sharpener to sharpen a pencil but not to sharpen a crayon) and in a hygienic fashion
Handles	Supports or stabilizes tools and materials in an appropriate manner, protecting them from being damaged, slipping, moving, and falling
Inquires	(1) Seeks needed verbal or written information by asking questions or reading directions or labels and (2) does not ask for information when he or she was fully oriented to the task and environment and had immediate prior awareness of the answer
Initiates	Starts or begins the next action or step without hesitation
Continues	Performs single actions or steps without interruptions such that once an action or task is initiated, the person continues without pauses or delays until the action or step is completed
Sequences	Performs steps in an effective or logical order and with an absence of (1) randomness or lack of logic in the ordering and (2) inappropriate repetition of steps
Terminates	Brings to completion single actions or single steps without inappropriate persistence or premature cessation
Searches/locates	Looks for and locates tools and materials in a logical manner, both within and beyond the immediate environment
Gathers	Collects related tools and materials into the same work space and regathers tools or materials that have spilled, fallen, or been misplaced

(Continued)

TABLE 3. PERFORMANCE SKILLS
(Continued)

Skill	Definition
Organizes	Logically positions or spatially arranges tools and materials in an orderly fashion within a single work space and between multiple appropriate work spaces such that the work space is not too spread out or too crowded
Restores	Puts away tools and materials in appropriate places and ensures that the immediate work space is restored to its original condition
Navigates	Moves the arm, body, or wheelchair without bumping into obstacles when moving in the task environment or interacting with task objects
Notices/responds	Responds appropriately to (1) nonverbal task-related cues (e.g., heat, movement), (2) the spatial arrangement and alignment of task objects to one another, and (3) cupboard doors and drawers that have been left open during task performance
Adjusts	Effectively (1) goes to new work spaces; (2) moves tools and materials out of the current work space; and (3) adjusts knobs, dials, or water taps to overcome problems with ongoing task performance
Accommodates	Prevents ineffective task performance
Benefits	Prevents problems with task performance from recurring or persisting
▧ **SOCIAL INTERACTION SKILLS**—"Occupational performance skills observed during the ongoing stream of a social exchange" (Boyt Schell et al., 2014a, p. 1241).	
Approaches/starts	Approaches or initiates interaction with the social partner in a manner that is socially appropriate
Concludes/disengages	Effectively terminates the conversation or social interaction, brings to closure the topic under discussion, and disengages or says good-bye
Produces speech	Produces spoken, signed, or augmentative (i.e., computer-generated) messages that are audible and clearly articulated
Gesticulates	Uses socially appropriate gestures to communicate or support a message
Speaks fluently	Speaks in a fluent and continuous manner, with an even pace (not too fast, not too slow) and without pauses or delays during the message being sent
Turns toward	Actively positions or turns the body and face toward the social partner or person who is speaking
Looks	Makes eye contact with the social partner
Places self	Positions self at an appropriate distance from the social partner during the social interaction
Touches	Responds to and uses touch or bodily contact with the social partner in a manner that is socially appropriate
Regulates	Does not demonstrate irrelevant, repetitive, or impulsive behaviors that are not part of social interaction
Questions	Requests relevant facts and information and asks questions that support the intended purpose of the social interaction
Replies	Keeps conversation going by replying appropriately to question and comments
Discloses	Reveals opinions, feelings, and private information about self or others in a manner that is socially appropriate
Expresses emotion	Displays affect and emotions in a way that is socially appropriate
Disagrees	Expresses differences of opinion in a socially appropriate manner
Thanks	Uses appropriate words and gestures to acknowledge receipt of services, gifts, or compliments
Transitions	Handles transitions in the conversation smoothly or changes the topic without disrupting the ongoing conversation
Times response	Replies to social messages without delay or hesitation and without interrupting the social partner
Times duration	Speaks for reasonable periods given the complexity of the message sent
Takes turns	Takes his or her turn and gives the social partner the freedom to take his or her turn
Matches language	Uses a tone of voice, dialect, and level of language that are socially appropriate and matched to the social partner's abilities and level of understanding
Clarifies	Responds to gestures or verbal messages signaling that the social partner does not comprehend or understand a message and ensures that the social partner is following the conversation
Acknowledges and encourages	Acknowledges receipt of messages, encourages the social partner to continue interaction, and encourages all social partners to participate in social interaction
Empathizes	Expresses a supportive attitude toward the social partner by agreeing with, empathizing with, or expressing understanding of the social partner's feelings and experiences
Heeds	Uses goal-directed social interactions focused on carrying out and completing the intended purpose of the social interaction
Accommodates	Prevents ineffective or socially inappropriate social interaction
Benefits	Prevents problems with ineffective or socially inappropriate social interaction from recurring or persisting

Source. From "Performance Skills: Implementing Performance Analyses to Evaluate Quality of Occupational Performance," by A. G. Fisher and L. A. Griswold, in *Willard and Spackman's Occupational Therapy* (12th ed., pp. 252–254), by B. A. B. Schell, G. Gillen, M. E. Scaffa, and E. S. Cohn (Eds.), 2014, Philadelphia: Wolters Kluwer/Lippincott Williams & Wilkins; http://lww.com. Copyright © 2014 by Wolters Kluwer/Lippincott Williams & Wilkins. Adapted with permission.

TABLE 4. PERFORMANCE PATTERNS

Performance patterns *are the habits, routines, roles, and rituals used in the process of engaging in occupations or activities; these patterns can support or hinder occupational performance.*

Category	Description	Examples
▨ PERSON		
Habits	"Acquired tendencies to respond and perform in certain consistent ways in familiar environments or situations; specific, automatic behaviors performed repeatedly, relatively automatically, and with little variation" (Boyt Schell, Gillen, & Scaffa, 2014a, p. 1234). Habits can be useful, dominating, or impoverished and can either support or interfere with performance in occupations (Dunn, 2000).	• Automatically puts car keys in the same place • Spontaneously looks both ways before crossing the street • Always turns off the stove burner before removing a cooking pot • Activates the alarm system before leaving the home
Routines	Patterns of behavior that are observable, regular, and repetitive and that provide structure for daily life. They can be satisfying, promoting, or damaging. Routines require momentary time commitment and are embedded in cultural and ecological contexts (Fiese, 2007; Segal, 2004).	• Follows a morning sequence to complete toileting, bathing, hygiene, and dressing • Follows the sequence of steps involved in meal preparation • Follows a daily routine of dropping children off at school, going to work, picking children up from school, doing homework, and making dinner
Rituals	Symbolic actions with spiritual, cultural, or social meaning contributing to the client's identity and reinforcing values and beliefs. Rituals have a strong affective component and consist of a collection of events (Fiese, 2007; Fiese et al., 2002; Segal, 2004).	• Uses an inherited antique hairbrush to brush hair 100 strokes nightly as her mother had done • Prepares holiday meals with favorite or traditional accoutrements using designated dishware • Kisses a sacred book before opening the pages to read • Attends a spiritual gathering on a particular day
Roles	Sets of behaviors expected by society and shaped by culture and context that may be further conceptualized and defined by the client.	• Mother of an adolescent with developmental disabilities • Student with a learning disability studying computer technology • Corporate executive returning to work after a stroke
▨ GROUP OR POPULATION		
Routines	Patterns of behavior that are observable, regular, and repetitive and that provide structure for daily life. They can be satisfying, promoting, or damaging. Routines require momentary time commitment and are embedded in cultural and ecological contexts (Segal, 2004).	• Follows health practices, such as scheduled immunizations for children and yearly health screenings for adults • Follows business practices, such as provision of services for disadvantaged populations (e.g., loans to underrepresented groups) • Follows legislative procedures, such as those associated with the Individuals With Disabilities Education Improvement Act of 2004 (Pub. L. 108–446) or Medicare • Follows social customs for greeting
Rituals	Shared social actions with traditional, emotional, purposive, and technological meaning contributing to values and beliefs within the group or population.	• Holds cultural celebrations • Has parades or demonstrations • Shows national affiliations or allegiances • Follows religious, spiritual, and cultural practices, such as touching the mezuzah or using holy water when leaving and entering or praying while facing Mecca
Roles	Sets of behaviors by the group or population expected by society and shaped by culture and context that may be further conceptualized and defined by the group or population.	• Nonprofit civic group providing housing for people with mental illness • Humanitarian group distributing food and clothing donations to refugees • Student organization in a university educating elementary school children about preventing bullying

TABLE 5. CONTEXT AND ENVIRONMENT

Context *refers to a variety of interrelated conditions that are within and surrounding the client. Contexts include cultural, personal, temporal, and virtual. The term* environment *refers to the external physical and social conditions that surround the client and in which the client's daily life occupations occur.*

Category	Definition	Examples
CONTEXTS		
Cultural	Customs, beliefs, activity patterns, behavioral standards, and expectations accepted by the society of which a client is a member. The cultural context influences the client's identity and activity choices.	• *Person:* A person delivering Thanksgiving meals to home-bound individuals • *Group:* Employees marking the end of the work week with casual dress on Friday • *Population:* People engaging in an afternoon siesta or high tea
Personal	"Features of the individual that are not part of a health condition or health status" (WHO, 2001, p. 17). The personal context includes age, gender, socioeconomic status, and educational status and can also include group membership (e.g., volunteers, employees) and population membership (e.g., members of society).	• *Person:* A 25-year-old unemployed man with a high school diploma • *Group:* Volunteers working in a homeless shelter • *Population:* Older drivers learning about community mobility options
Temporal	The experience of time as shaped by engagement in occupations; the temporal aspects of occupation that "contribute to the patterns of daily occupations" include "rhythm . . . tempo . . . synchronization . . . duration . . . and sequence" (Larson & Zemke, 2003, p. 82; Zemke, 2004, p. 610). The temporal context includes stage of life, time of day or year, duration and rhythm of activity, and history.	• *Person:* A person retired from work for 10 years • *Group:* A community organization's annual fundraising campaign • *Population:* People celebrating Independence Day on July 4
Virtual	Environment in which communication occurs by means of airwaves or computers and in the absence of physical contact. The virtual context includes simulated, real-time, or near-time environments such as chat rooms, email, video conferencing, or radio transmissions; remote monitoring via wireless sensors; or computer-based data collection.	• *Person:* Friends who text message each other • *Group:* Members who participate in a video conference, telephone conference call, instant message, or interactive white board use • *Population:* Virtual community of gamers
ENVIRONMENTS		
Physical	Natural and built nonhuman surroundings and the objects in them. The natural environment includes geographic terrain, plants, and animals, as well as the sensory qualities of the surroundings. The built environment includes buildings, furniture, tools, and devices.	• *Person:* Individual's house or apartment • *Group:* Office building or factory • *Population:* Transportation system
Social	Presence of, relationships with, and expectations of persons, groups, or populations with whom clients have contact. The social environment includes availability and expectations of significant individuals, such as spouse, friends, and caregivers; relationships with individuals, groups, or populations; and relationships with systems (e.g., political, legal, economic, institutional) that influence norms, role expectations, and social routines.	• *Person:* Friends, colleagues • *Group:* Occupational therapy students conducting a class get-together • *Population:* People influenced by a city government

Note. WHO = World Health Organization.

TABLE 6. TYPES OF OCCUPATIONAL THERAPY INTERVENTIONS

Occupational therapy interventions *include the use of occupations and activities, preparatory methods and tasks, education and training, advocacy, and group interventions to facilitate engagement in occupations to promote health and participation. The examples provided illustrate the types of interventions occupational therapy practitioners provide and are not intended to be all inclusive.*

Category	Description	Examples
OCCUPATIONS AND ACTIVITIES—Occupations and activities selected as interventions for specific clients and designed to meet therapeutic goals and address the underlying needs of the mind, body, and spirit of the client. To use occupations and activities therapeutically, the practitioner considers activity demands and client factors in relation to the client's therapeutic goals, contexts, and environments.		
Occupations	Client-directed daily life activities that match and support or address identified participation goals.	The client • Completes morning dressing and hygiene using adaptive devices • Purchases groceries and prepares a meal • Visits a friend using public transportation independently • Applies for a job in the retail industry • Plays on a playground with children and adults • Participates in a community festival by setting up a booth to sell baked goods • Engages in a pattern of self-care and relaxation activities in preparation for sleep • Engages in a statewide advocacy program to improve services to people with mental illness
Activities	Actions designed and selected to support the development of performance skills and performance patterns to enhance occupational engagement. Activities often are components of occupations and always hold meaning, relevance, and perceived utility for clients at their level of interest and motivation.	The client • Selects clothing and manipulates clothing fasteners in advance of dressing • Practices safe ways to get into and out of the bathtub • Prepares a food list and practices using cooking appliances • Reviews how to use a map and transportation schedule • Writes answers on an application form • Climbs on and off playground and recreation equipment • Greets people and initiates conversation in a role-play situation • Develops a weekly schedule to manage time and organize daily and weekly responsibilities required to live independently • Uses adaptive switches to operate the home environmental control system • Completes a desired expressive activity (e.g., art, craft, dance) that is not otherwise classified • Plays a desired game either as a solo player or in competition with others
PREPARATORY METHODS AND TASKS—Methods and tasks that prepare the client for occupational performance, used as *part of a treatment session* in preparation for or concurrently with occupations and activities or provided to a client as a home-based engagement to support daily occupational performance.		
Preparatory methods	Modalities, devices, and techniques to prepare the client for occupational performance. Often preparatory methods are interventions that are "done to" the client without the client's active participation.	The practitioner • Administers physical agent modalities to decrease pain, assist with wound healing or edema control, or prepare muscles for movement • Provides massage • Performs manual lymphatic drainage techniques • Performs wound care techniques, including dressing changes
Splints	Construction and use of devices to mobilize, immobilize, and support body structures to enhance participation in occupations.	The practitioner • Fabricates and issues a splint or orthotic to support a weakened hand and decrease pain • Fabricates and issues a wrist splint to facilitate movement and enhance participation in household activities
Assistive technology and environmental modifications	Identification and use of assistive technologies (high and low tech), application of universal design principles, and recommends changes to the environment or activity to support the client's ability to engage in occupations. This preparatory method includes assessment, selection, provision, and education and training in use of devices.	The practitioner • Provides a pencil grip and slant board • Provides electronic books with text-to-speech software • Recommends visual supports (e.g., a social story) to guide behavior • Recommends replacing steps with an appropriately graded ramp • Recommends universally designed curriculum materials
Wheeled mobility	Use of products and technologies that facilitate a client's ability to maneuver through space, including seating and positioning, and that improve mobility, enhance participation in desired daily occupations, and reduce risk for complications such as skin breakdown or limb contractures.	The practitioner • Recommends, in conjunction with the wheelchair team, a sip-and-puff switch to allow the client to maneuver the power wheelchair independently and interface with an environmental control unit in the home

(Continued)

TABLE 6. TYPES OF OCCUPATIONAL THERAPY INTERVENTIONS

(Continued)

Category	Description	Examples
Preparatory tasks	Actions selected and provided to the client to target specific client factors or performance skills. Tasks involve active participation of the client and sometimes comprise engagements that use various materials to simulate activities or components of occupations. Preparatory tasks themselves may not hold inherent meaning, relevance, or perceived utility as stand-alone entities.	The client • Refolds towels taken from a clean linen cart to address shoulder range of motion • Participates in fabricated sensory environment (e.g., through movement, tactile sensations, scents) to promote alertness • Uses visual imagery and rhythmic breathing to promote rest and relaxation • Performs a home-based conditioning regimen using free weights • Does hand-strengthening exercises using therapy putty, exercise bands, grippers, and clothespins • Participates in an assertiveness training program to prepare for self-advocacy

EDUCATION AND TRAINING

Category	Description	Examples
Education	Imparting of knowledge and information about occupation, health, well-being, and participation that enables the client to acquire helpful behaviors, habits, and routines that may or may not require application at the time of the intervention session	The practitioner • Provides education regarding home and activity modifications to the spouse or family member of a person with dementia to support maximum independence • Educates town officials about the value of and strategies for making walking and biking paths accessible for all community members • Educates providers of care for people who have experienced trauma on the use of sensory strategies • Provides education to people with mental health issues and their families on the psychological and social factors that influence engagement in occupation
Training	Facilitation of the acquisition of concrete skills for meeting specific goals in a real-life, applied situation. In this case, *skills* refers to measurable components of function that enable mastery. Training is differentiated from education by its goal of enhanced performance as opposed to enhanced understanding, although these goals often go hand in hand (Collins & O'Brien, 2003).	The practitioner • Instructs the client in how to operate a universal control device to manage household appliances • Instructs family members in the use and maintenance of the father's power wheelchair • Instructs the client in the use of self range of motion as a preparatory technique to avoid joint contracture of wrist • Instructs the client in the use of a handheld electronic device and applications to recall and manage weekly activities and medications • Instructs the client in how to direct a personal care attendant in assisting with self-care activities • Trains parents and teachers to focus on a child's strengths to foster positive behaviors

ADVOCACY—Efforts directed toward promoting occupational justice and empowering clients to seek and obtain resources to fully participate in daily life occupations. The outcomes of advocacy and self-advocacy support health, well-being, and occupational participation at the individual or systems level.

Category	Description	Examples
Advocacy	Advocacy efforts undertaken by the practitioner.	The practitioner • Collaborates with a person to procure reasonable accommodations at a work site • Serves on the policy board of an organization to procure supportive housing accommodations for people with disabilities • Serves on the board of a local park district to encourage inclusion of children with disabilities in mainstream district sports programs when possible • Collaborates with adults who have serious mental illness to raise public awareness of the impact of stigma • Collaborates with and educates staff at federal funding sources for persons with disabling conditions
Self-advocacy	Advocacy efforts undertaken by the client, which the practitioner can promote and support.	• A student with a learning disability requests and receives reasonable accommodations such as textbooks on tape. • A grassroots employee committee requests and procures ergonomically designed keyboards for their work computers. • People with disabilities advocate for the use of universal design principles with all new public construction. • Young adults contact their Internet service provider to request support for cyberbullying prevention.

(Continued)

TABLE 6. TYPES OF OCCUPATIONAL THERAPY INTERVENTIONS
(Continued)

Category	Description	Examples
GROUP INTERVENTIONS—Use of distinct knowledge and leadership techniques to facilitate learning and skill acquisition across the life span through the dynamics of group and social interaction. Groups may also be used as a method of service delivery.		
Groups	Functional groups, activity groups, task groups, social groups, and other groups used on inpatient units, within the community, or in schools that allow clients to explore and develop skills for participation, including basic social interaction skills, tools for self-regulation, goal setting, and positive choice making.	• A group for older adults focuses on maintaining participation despite increasing disability, such as exploring alternative transportation if driving is no longer an option and participating in volunteer and social opportunities after retirement. • A community group addresses issues of self-efficacy and self-esteem as the basis for creating resiliency in preadolescent children at risk for being bullied. • A group in a mental health program addresses establishment of social connections in the community.

TABLE 7. ACTIVITY AND OCCUPATIONAL DEMANDS

Activity and occupational demands *are the components of activities and occupations that occupational therapy practitioners consider during the clinical reasoning process. Depending on the context and needs of the client, these demands can be deemed barriers to or supports for participation. Specific knowledge about the demands of activities and occupations assists practitioners in selecting activities for therapeutic purposes. Demands of the activity or occupation include the relevance and importance to the client, objects used and their properties, space demands, social demands, sequencing and timing, required actions and performance skills, and required underlying body functions and body structures.*

Type of Demand	Description	Examples
Relevance and importance to client	Alignment with the client's goals, values, beliefs, and needs and perceived utility	• Driving a car equates with independence. • Preparing a holiday meal connects with family tradition. • Voting is a rite of passage to adulthood.
Objects used and their properties	Tools, supplies, and equipment required in the process of carrying out the activity	• Tools (e.g., scissors, dishes, shoes, volleyball) • Supplies (e.g., paints, milk, lipstick) • Equipment (e.g., workbench, stove, basketball hoop) • Inherent properties (e.g., heavy, rough, sharp, colorful, loud, bitter tasting)
Space demands (related to the physical environment)	Physical environmental requirements of the activity (e.g., size, arrangement, surface, lighting, temperature, noise, humidity, ventilation)	• Large, open space outdoors for a baseball game • Bathroom door and stall width to accommodate wheelchair • Noise, lighting, and temperature controls for a library
Social demands (related to the social environment and virtual and cultural contexts)	Elements of the social environment and virtual and cultural contexts that may be required by the activity	• Rules of the game • Expectations of other participants in the activity (e.g., sharing supplies, using language appropriate for the meeting, appropriate virtual decorum)
Sequencing and timing	Process required to carry out the activity (e.g., specific steps, sequence of steps, timing requirements)	• *Steps to make tea:* Gather cup and tea bag, heat water, pour water into cup, let steep, add sugar. • *Sequence:* Heat water before placing tea bag in water. • *Timing:* Leave tea bag to steep for 2 minutes. • *Steps to conduct a meeting:* Establish goals for meeting, arrange time and location, prepare agenda, call meeting to order. • *Sequence:* Have people introduce themselves before beginning discussion of topic. • *Timing:* Allot sufficient time for discussion of topic and determination of action items.
Required actions and performance skills	Actions (performance skills—motor, process, and social interaction) required by the client that are an inherent part of the activity	• Feeling the heat of the stove • Gripping a handlebar • Choosing ceremonial clothes • Determining how to move limbs to control the car • Adjusting the tone of voice • Answering a question
Required body functions	"Physiological functions of body systems (including psychological functions)" (WHO, 2001, p. 10) required to support the actions used to perform the activity	• Mobility of joints • Level of consciousness • Cognitive level
Required body structures	"Anatomical parts of the body such as organs, limbs, and their components" that support body functions (WHO, 2001, p. 10) and are required to perform the activity	• Number of hands or feet • Olfactory or taste organs

TABLE 8. APPROACHES TO INTERVENTION

Approaches to intervention *are specific strategies selected to direct the process of evaluation and intervention planning, selection, and implementation on the basis of the client's desired outcomes, evaluation data, and evidence. Approaches inform the selection of practice models, frames of references, or treatment theories.*

Approach	Description	Examples
Create, promote (health promotion)	An intervention approach that does not assume a disability is present or that any aspect would interfere with performance. This approach is designed to provide enriched contextual and activity experiences that will enhance performance for all people in the natural contexts of life (adapted from Dunn, McClain, Brown, & Youngstrom, 1998, p. 534).	• Create a parenting class to help first-time parents engage their children in developmentally appropriate play • Provide a falls prevention class to a group of older adults at the local senior center to encourage safe mobility throughout the home
Establish, restore (remediation, restoration)	An intervention approach designed to change client variables to establish a skill or ability that has not yet developed or to restore a skill or ability that has been impaired (adapted from Dunn et al., 1998, p. 533).	• Restore a client's upper-extremity movement to enable transfer of dishes from the dishwasher into the upper kitchen cabinets • Develop a structured schedule, chunking tasks to decrease the risk of being overwhelmed when faced with the many responsibilities of daily life roles • Collaborate with a client to help establish morning routines needed to arrive at school or work on time
Maintain	An intervention approach designed to provide the supports that will allow clients to preserve the performance capabilities they have regained, that continue to meet their occupational needs, or both. The assumption is that without continued maintenance intervention, performance would decrease, occupational needs would not be met, or both, thereby affecting health, well-being, and quality of life.	• Provide ongoing intervention for a client with amyotrophic lateral sclerosis to address participation in desired occupations through provision of assistive technology • Maintain independent gardening for people with arthritis by recommending tools with modified grips, long-handled tools, seating alternatives, and raised gardens • Maintain safe and independent access for people with low vision by increasing hallway lighting in the home
Modify (compensation, adaptation)	An intervention approach directed at "finding ways to revise the current context or activity demands to support performance in the natural setting, [including] compensatory techniques . . . [such as] enhancing some features to provide cues or reducing other features to reduce distractibility" (Dunn et al., 1998, p. 533).	• Simplify task sequence to help a person with cognitive impairments complete a morning self-care routine • Consult with builders to design homes that will allow families to provide living space for aging parents (e.g., bedroom and full bath on the main floor of a multilevel dwelling) • Modify the clutter in a room to decrease a client's distractibility
Prevent (disability prevention)	An intervention approach designed to address the needs of clients with or without a disability who are at risk for occupational performance problems. This approach is designed to prevent the occurrence or evolution of barriers to performance in context. Interventions may be directed at client, context, or activity variables (adapted from Dunn et al., 1998, p. 534).	• Aid in the prevention of illicit chemical substance use by introducing self-initiated routine strategies that support drug-free behavior • Prevent social isolation of employees by promoting participation in after-work group activities • Consult with a hotel chain to provide an ergonomics educational program designed to prevent back injuries in housekeepers

TABLE 9. OUTCOMES

Outcomes *are the end result of the occupational therapy process; they describe what clients can achieve through occupational therapy intervention. The outcomes of occupational therapy can be described in two ways. Some outcomes are measurable and are used for intervention planning, monitoring, and discharge planning. These outcomes reflect the attainment of treatment goals that relate to engagement in occupation. Other outcomes are experienced by clients when they have realized the effects of engagement in occupation and are able to return to desired habits, routines, roles, and rituals. The examples listed specify how the broad outcome of health and participation in life may be operationalized and are not intended to be all inclusive.*

Category	Description	Examples
Occupational performance	Act of doing and accomplishing a selected action (performance skill), activity, or occupation (Fisher, 2009; Fisher & Griswold, 2014; Kielhofner, 2008) and results from the dynamic transaction among the client, the context, and the activity. Improving or enabling skills and patterns in occupational performance leads to engagement in occupations or activities (adapted in part from Law et al., 1996, p. 16).	See "Improvement" and "Enhancement," below.
Improvement	Outcomes targeted when a performance limitation is present. These outcomes reflect increased occupational performance for the person, group, or population.	• A child with autism playing interactively with a peer (person) • An older adult returning to a desired living situation in the home from a skilled nursing facility (person) • Decreased incidence of back strain in nursing personnel as a result of an in-service education program in body mechanics for carrying out job duties that require bending, lifting, and so forth (group) • Construction of accessible playground facilities for all children in local city parks (population)
Enhancement	Outcomes targeted when a performance limitation is not currently present. These outcomes reflect the development of performance skills and performance patterns that augment existing performance in life occupations.	• Increased confidence and competence of teenage mothers in parenting their children as a result of structured social groups and child development classes (person) • Increased membership in the local senior citizen center as a result of expanding social wellness and exercise programs (group) • Increased ability of school staff to address and manage school-age youth violence as a result of conflict resolution training to address bullying (group) • Increased opportunities for older adults to participate in community activities through ride-share programs (population)
Prevention	Education or health promotion efforts designed to identify, reduce, or prevent the onset and reduce the incidence of unhealthy conditions, risk factors, diseases, or injuries (AOTA, 2013b). Occupational therapy promotes a healthy lifestyle at the individual, group, community (societal), and governmental or policy level (adapted from AOTA, 2001).	• Appropriate seating and play area for a child with orthopedic impairments (person) • Implementation of a program of leisure and educational activities for a drop-in center for adults with severe mental illness (group) • Access to occupational therapy services in underserved areas regardless of cultural or ethnic background (population)
Health and wellness	Resources for everyday life, not the objective of living. For individuals, *health* is a state of physical, mental, and social well-being, as well as a positive concept emphasizing social and personal resources and physical capacities (WHO, 1986). Health for groups and populations includes these individual aspects but also includes social responsibility of members to the group or population as a whole. *Wellness* is "an active process through which individuals [or groups or populations] become aware of and make choices toward a more successful existence" (Hettler, 1984, p. 1117). Wellness is more than a lack of disease symptoms; it is a state of mental and physical balance and fitness (adapted from *Taber's Cyclopedic Medical Dictionary*, 1997, p. 2110).	• Participation by a person with a psychiatric disability in an empowerment and advocacy group to improve services in the community (person) • Implementation of a company-wide program for employees to identify problems and solutions regarding the balance among work, leisure, and family life (group) • Decreased incidence of childhood obesity (population)

(Continued)

TABLE 9. OUTCOMES

(Continued)

Category	Description	Examples
Quality of life	Dynamic appraisal of the client's life satisfaction (perceptions of progress toward goals), hope (real or perceived belief that one can move toward a goal through selected pathways), self-concept (the composite of beliefs and feelings about oneself), health and functioning (e.g., health status, self-care capabilities), and socioeconomic factors (e.g., vocation, education, income; adapted from Radomski, 1995).	• Full and active participation of a deaf child from a hearing family during a recreational activity (person) • Residents being able to prepare for outings and travel independently as a result of independent living skills training for care providers (group) • Formation of a lobby to support opportunities for social networking, advocacy activities, and sharing of scientific information for stroke survivors and their families (population)
Participation	Engagement in desired occupations in ways that are personally satisfying and congruent with expectations within the culture.	• A person recovering the ability to perform the essential duties of his or her job after a flexor tendon laceration (person) • A family enjoying a vacation while traveling cross-country in their adapted van (group) • All children within a state having access to school sports programs (population)
Role competence	Ability to effectively meet the demands of roles in which the client engages.	• An individual with cerebral palsy being able to take notes or type papers to meet the demands of the student role (person) • Implementation of job rotation at a factory that allows sharing of higher demand tasks to meet the demands of the worker role (group) • Improved accessibility of polling places to all people with disabilities to meet the demands of the citizen role (population)
Well-being	Contentment with one's health, self-esteem, sense of belonging, security, and opportunities for self-determination, meaning, roles, and helping others (Hammell, 2009). *Well-being* is "a general term encompassing the total universe of human life domains, including physical, mental, and social aspects" (WHO, 2006, p. 211).	• A person with amyotrophic lateral sclerosis being content with his ability to find meaning in fulfilling the role of father through compensatory strategies and environmental modifications (person) • Members of an outpatient depression and anxiety support group feeling secure in their sense of group belonging and ability to help other members (group) • Residents of a town celebrating the groundbreaking of a school during reconstruction after a natural disaster (population)
Occupational justice	Access to and participation in the full range of meaningful and enriching occupations afforded to others, including opportunities for social inclusion and the resources to participate in occupations to satisfy personal, health, and societal needs (adapted from Townsend & Wilcock, 2004).	• An individual with an intellectual disability serving on an advisory board to establish programs offered by a community recreation center (person) • Workers having enough break time to have lunch with their young children in their day care center (group) • Increased sense of empowerment and self-advocacy skills for people with persistent mental illness, enabling them to develop an antistigma campaign promoting engagement in the civic arena (group) and alternative adapted housing options for older adults to age in place (population)

References

Accreditation Council for Occupational Therapy Education. (2012). 2011 Accreditation Council for Occupational Therapy Education (ACOTE®) standards. *American Journal of Occupational Therapy, 66,* S6–S74. http://dx.doi.org/10.5014/ajot.2012.66S6

American Heritage dictionary of the English language (4th ed.). (2003). Retrieved from http://www.thefreedictionary.com/framework

American Occupational Therapy Association. (1979). *Occupational therapy product output reporting system and uniform terminology for reporting occupational therapy services.* (Available from American Occupational Therapy Association, 4720 Montgomery Lane, PO Box 31220, Bethesda, MD 20824-1220; pracdept@aota.org)

American Occupational Therapy Association. (1989). *Uniform terminology for occupational therapy* (2nd ed.). (Available from American Occupational Therapy Association, 4720 Montgomery Lane, PO Box 31220, Bethesda, MD 20824-1220; pracdept@aota.org)

American Occupational Therapy Association. (1994). Uniform terminology for occupational therapy (3rd ed.). *American Journal of Occupational Therapy, 48,* 1047–1054. http://dx.doi.org/10.5014/ajot.48.11.1047

American Occupational Therapy Association. (2001). Occupational therapy in the promotion of health and the prevention of disease and disability statement. *American Journal of Occupational Therapy, 55,* 656–660. http://dx.doi.org/10.5014/ajot.55.6.656

American Occupational Therapy Association. (2002a). Broadening the construct of independence [Position Paper]. *American Journal of Occupational Therapy, 56,* 660. http://dx.doi.org/10.5014/ajot.56.6.660

American Occupational Therapy Association. (2002b). Occupational therapy practice framework: Domain and process. *American Journal of Occupational Therapy, 56,* 609–639. http://dx.doi.org/10.5014/ajot.56.6.609

American Occupational Therapy Association. (2006). Policy 1.44: Categories of occupational therapy personnel. In *Policy manual* (2007 ed., pp. 33–34). Bethesda, MD: Author.

American Occupational Therapy Association. (2008). Occupational therapy practice framework: Domain and process (2nd ed.). *American Journal of Occupational Therapy, 62,* 625–683. http://dx.doi.org/10.5014/ajot.62.6.625

American Occupational Therapy Association. (2009). Guidelines for supervision, roles, and responsibilities during the delivery of occupational therapy services. *American Journal of Occupational Therapy, 63,* 797–803. http://dx.doi.org/10.5014/ajot.63.6.797

American Occupational Therapy Association. (2010). Standards of practice for occupational therapy. *American Journal of Occupational Therapy, 64*(Suppl.), S106–S111. http://dx.doi.org/10.5014/ajot.2010.64S106

American Occupational Therapy Association. (2011). *Definition of occupational therapy practice for the AOTA Model Practice Act.* Retrieved from http://www.aota.org/-/media/Corporate/Files/Advocacy/State/Resources/PracticeAct/Model%20Definition%20of%20OT%20Practice%20%20Adopted%2041411.ashx

American Occupational Therapy Association. (2013a). Guidelines for documentation of occupational therapy. *American Journal of Occupational Therapy, 67*(Suppl.), S32–S38. http://dx.doi.org/10.5014/ajot.2013.67S32

American Occupational Therapy Association. (2013b). Occupational therapy in the promotion of health and well-being. *American Journal of Occupational Therapy, 67*(Suppl.), S47–S59. http://dx.doi.org/10.5014/ajot.2013.67S47

American Occupational Therapy Association. (2013c). Telehealth. *American Journal of Occupational Therapy, 67*(Suppl.), S69–S90. http://dx.doi.org/10.5014/ajot.2013.67S69

Americans With Disabilities Act of 1990, Pub. L. 101–336, 42 U.S.C. § 12101.

Ayres, A. J. (1972). *Sensory integration and learning disorders.* Los Angeles: Western Psychological Services.

Ayres, A. J. (2005). *Sensory integration and the child.* Los Angeles: Western Psychological Services.

Bandura, A. (1986). *Social foundations of thought and action: A social cognitive theory.* Englewood Cliffs, NJ: Prentice Hall.

Bedell, G. M. (2012). Measurement of social participation. In V. Anderson & M. H. Beauchamp (Eds.), *Developmental social neuroscience and childhood brain insult: Theory and practice* (pp. 184–206). New York: Guilford Press.

Bergen, D. (Ed.). (1988). *Play as a medium for learning and development: A handbook of theory and practice.* Portsmouth, NH: Heinemann.

Boyt Schell, B. A., Gillen, G., & Scaffa, M. (2014a). Glossary. In B. A. Boyt Schell, G. Gillen, & M. Scaffa (Eds.), *Willard and Spackman's occupational therapy* (12th ed., pp. 1229–1243). Philadelphia: Lippincott Williams & Wilkins.

Boyt Schell, B. A., Gillen, G., & Scaffa, M. (Eds.). (2014b). *Willard and Spackman's occupational therapy* (12th ed.). Philadelphia: Lippincott Williams & Wilkins.

Chisholm, D., & Boyt Schell, B. A. (2014). Overview of the occupational therapy process and outcomes. In B. A. Boyt Schell, G. Gillen, & M. Scaffa (Eds.), *Willard and Spackman's occupational therapy* (12th ed., pp. 266–280). Philadelphia: Lippincott Williams & Wilkins.

Christiansen, C. H., & Baum, M. C. (Eds.). (1997). *Occupational therapy: Enabling function and well-being.* Thorofare, NJ: Slack.

Christiansen, C., Baum, M. C., & Bass-Haugen, J. (Eds.). (2005). *Occupational therapy: Performance, participation, and well-being.* Thorofare, NJ: Slack.

Christiansen, C. H., & Hammecker, C. L. (2001). Self care. In B. R. Bonder & M. B. Wagner (Eds.), *Functional performance in older adults* (pp. 155–175). Philadelphia: F. A. Davis.

Christiansen, C. H., & Townsend, E. A. (2010). *Introduction to occupation: The art and science of living* (2nd ed.). Cranbury, NJ: Pearson Education.

Clark, F. A. (2000). The concept of habit and routine: A preliminary theoretical synthesis. *OTJR: Occupation, Participation and Health, 20,* 123S–137S.

Clark, F., Jackson, J., Carlson, M., Chou, C. P., Cherry, B. J., Jordan-Marsh, M., . . . Azen, S. P. (2012). Effectiveness of a lifestyle intervention in promoting the well-being of independently living older people: Results of the Well Elderly 2 Randomised Controlled Trial. *Journal of Epidemiology and Community Health, 66,* 782–790. http://dx.doi.org/10.1136/jech.2009.099754

Cohn, E. S. (2001). Parent perspectives of occupational therapy using a sensory integration approach. *American Journal of Occupational Therapy, 55,* 285–294. http://dx.doi.org/10.5014/ajot.55.3.285

Cohn, E. S., Miller, L. J., & Tickle-Degnen, L. (2000). Parental hopes for therapy outcomes: Children with sensory modulation disorders. *American Journal of Occupational Therapy, 54,* 36–43. http://dx.doi.org/10.5014/ajot.54.1.36

Cole, B., & McLean, V. (2003). Therapeutic relationships redefined. *Occupational Therapy in Mental Health, 19,* 33–56. http://dx.doi.org/10.1300/J004v19n02_03

Collins, J., & O'Brien, N. P. (2003). *Greenwood dictionary of education.* Westport, CT: Greenwood Press.

Crepeau, E. (2003). Analyzing occupation and activity: A way of thinking about occupational performance. In E. Crepeau, E. Cohn, & B. A. Boyt Schell (Eds.), *Willard and Spackman's occupational therapy* (10th ed., pp. 189–198). Philadelphia: Lippincott Williams & Wilkins.

Davidson, L., Shahar, G., Lawless, M. S., Sells, D., & Tondora, J. (2006). Play, pleasure, and other positive life events: "Non-specific" factors in recovery from mental illness. *Psychiatry, 69,* 151–163.

Dickie, V., Cutchin, M., & Humphry, R. (2006). Occupation as transactional experience: A critique of individualism in occupational science. *Journal of Occupational Science, 13,* 83–93. http://dx.doi.org/10.1080/14427591.2006.9686573

Doucet, B. M., & Gutman, S. A. (2013). Quantifying function: The rest of the measurement story. *American Journal of Occupational Therapy, 67,* 7–9. http://dx.doi.org/10.5014/ajot.2013.007096

Dunlea, A. (1996). An opportunity for co-adaptation: The experience of mothers and their infants who are blind. In R. Zemke & F. Clark (Eds.), *Occupational science: The evolving discipline* (pp. 227–342). Philadelphia: F. A. Davis.

Dunn, W. (2000). Habit: What's the brain got to do with it? *OTJR: Occupation, Participation and Health, 20*(Suppl. 1), 6S–20S.

Dunn, W., McClain, L. H., Brown, C., & Youngstrom, M. J. (1998). The ecology of human performance. In M. E. Neistadt & E. B. Crepeau (Eds.), *Willard and Spackman's occupational therapy* (9th ed., pp. 525–535). Philadelphia: Lippincott Williams & Wilkins.

Dunton, W. R. (1934). The need for and value of research in occupational therapy. *Occupational Therapy and Rehabilitation, 13,* 325–328.

Esdaile, S. A., & Olson, J. A. (2004). *Mothering occupations: Challenge, agency, and participation.* Philadelphia: F. A. Davis.

Fiese, B. H. (2007). Routines and rituals: Opportunities for participation in family health. *OTJR: Occupation, Participation and Health, 27,* 41S–49S.

Fiese, B. H., Tomcho, T. J., Douglas, M., Josephs, K., Poltrock, S., & Baker, T. (2002). A review of 50 years of research on naturally occurring family routines and rituals: Cause for celebration. *Journal of Family Psychology, 16,* 381–390. http://dx.doi.org/10.1037/0893-3200.16.4.381

Fisher, A. (2006). Overview of performance skills and client factors. In H. Pendleton & W. Schultz-Krohn (Eds.), *Pedretti's occupational therapy: Practice skills for physical dysfunction* (pp. 372–402). St. Louis, MO: Mosby/Elsevier.

Fisher, A. G. (2009). *Occupational Therapy Intervention Process Model: A model for planning and implementing top-down, client-centered, and occupation-based interventions.* Fort Collins, CO: Three Star Press.

Fisher, A. G., & Griswold, L. A. (2014). Performance skills: Implementing performance analyses to evaluate quality of occupational performance. In B. A. Boyt Schell, G. Gillen, & M. Scaffa (Eds.), *Willard and Spackman's occupational therapy* (12th ed., pp. 249–264). Philadelphia: Lippincott Williams & Wilkins.

Gillen, G., & Boyt Schell, B. (2014). Introduction to evaluation, intervention, and outcomes for occupations. In B. A. Boyt Schell, G. Gillen, & M. Scaffa (Eds.), *Willard and Spackman's occupational therapy* (12th ed., pp. 606–609). Philadelphia: Lippincott Williams & Wilkins.

Gitlin, L. N., & Corcoran, M. A. (2005). *Occupational therapy and dementia care: The Home Environmental Skill-Building Program for individuals and families.* Bethesda, MD: AOTA Press.

Gitlin, L. N., Corcoran, M. A., Winter, L., Boyce, A., & Hauck, W. W. (2001). A randomized controlled trial of a home environmental intervention to enhance self-efficacy and reduce upset in family caregivers of persons with dementia. *Gerontologist, 41,* 15–30. http://dx.doi.org/10.1093/geront/41.1.4

Gitlin, L. N., Winter, L., Burke, J., Chernett, N., Dennis, M. P., & Hauck, W. W. (2008). Tailored activities to manage neuropsychiatric behaviors in persons with dementia and reduce caregiver burden: A randomized pilot study. *American Journal of Geriatric Psychiatry, 16,* 229–239.

Gitlin, L. N., Winter, L., Corcoran, M., Dennis, M. P., Schinfeld, S., & Hauck, W. W. (2003). Effects of the Home Environmental Skill-Building Program on the caregiver–care recipient dyad: 6-month outcomes from the Philadelphia REACH Initiative. *Gerontologist, 43,* 532–546. http://dx.doi.org/10.1093/geront/43.4.532

Glass, T. A., de Leon, C. M., Marottoli, R. A., & Berkman, L. F. (1999). Population based study of social and productive activities as predictors of survival among elderly Americans. *British Medical Journal, 319,* 478–483. http://dx.doi.org/10.1136/bmj.319.7208.478

Graff, M. J., Vernooij-Dassen, M. J., Thijssen, M., Dekker, J., Hoefnagels, W. H., & Olderikkert, M. G. (2007). Effects of community occupational therapy on quality of life, mood, and health status in dementia patients and their caregivers: A randomized controlled trial. *Journals of Gerontology, Series A: Biological Sciences and Medical Sciences, 62,* 1002–1009. http://dx.doi.org/10.1093/gerona/62.9.1002

Graham, F., Rodger, S., & Ziviani, J. (2013). Effectiveness of occupational performance coaching in improving children's and mothers' performance and mothers' self-competence. *American Journal of Occupational Therapy, 67,* 10–18. http://dx.doi.org/10.5014/ajot.2013.004648

Gutman, S. A., Mortera, M. H., Hinojosa, J., & Kramer, P. (2007). Revision of the *Occupational Therapy Practice Framework*. *American Journal of Occupational Therapy, 61,* 119–126. http://dx.doi.org/10.5014/ajot.61.1.119

Hagedorn, R. (2000). *Tools for practice in occupational therapy: A structured approach to core skills and processes.* Edinburgh: Churchill Livingstone.

Hakansson, C., Dahlin-Ivanoff, S., & Sonn, U. (2006). Achieving balance in everyday life. *Journal of Occupational Science, 13,* 74–82. http://dx.doi.org/10.1080/14427591.2006.9686572

Hammell, K. W. (2009). Self-care, productivity, and leisure, or dimensions of occupational experience? Rethinking occupational "categories." *Canadian Journal of Occupational Therapy, 76,* 107–114. http://dx.doi.org/10.1177/000841740907600208

Hettler, W. (1984). Wellness—The lifetime goal of a university experience. In J. D. Matarazzo, S. M. Weiss, J. A. Herd, N. E. Miller, & S. M. Weiss (Eds.), *Behavioral health: A handbook of health enhancement and disease prevention* (pp. 1117–1124). New York: Wiley.

Hildenbrand, W. C., & Lamb, A. J. (2013). Health Policy Perspectives—Occupational therapy in prevention and wellness: Retaining relevance in a new health care world. *American Journal of Occupational Therapy, 67,* 266–271. http://dx.doi.org/10.5014/ajot.2013.673001

Hinojosa, J., & Blount, M.-L. (2009). Occupation, purposeful activities, and occupational therapy. In J. Hinojosa & M.-L. Blount (Eds.), *The texture of life: Purposeful activities in context of occupation* (3rd ed., pp. 1–19). Bethesda, MD: AOTA Press.

Hinojosa, J., Kramer, P., Royeen, C. B., & Luebben, A. (2003). The core concepts of occupation. In P. Kramer, J. Hinojosa, & C. B. Royeen (Eds.), *Perspectives in human occupation: Participation in life* (pp. 1–17). Philadelphia: Lippincott Williams & Wilkins.

Hooper, B., & Wood, W. (2014). The philosophy of occupational therapy: A framework for practice. In B. A. Boyt Schell, G. Gillen, & M. Scaffa (Eds.), *Willard and Spackman's occupational therapy* (12th ed., pp. 35–46). Philadelphia: Lippincott Williams & Wilkins.

Individuals With Disabilities Education Improvement Act of 2004, Pub. L. 108–446, 20 U.S.C. § 1400 et seq.

Jackson, J. (1998a). Contemporary criticisms of role theory. *Journal of Occupational Science, 5,* 49–55. http://dx.doi.org/10.1080/14427591.1998.9686433

Jackson, J. (1998b). Is there a place for role theory in occupational science? *Journal of Occupational Science, 5,* 56–65. http://dx.doi.org/10.1080/14427591.1998.9686434

Jackson, J., Carlson, M., Mandel, D., Zemke, R., & Clark, F. (1998). Occupation in lifestyle redesign: The Well Elderly Study occupational therapy program. *American Journal of Occupational Therapy, 52,* 326–336. http://dx.doi.org/10.5014/ajot.52.5.326

James, A. B. (2008). Restoring the role of independent person. In M. V. Radomski & C. A. Trombly Latham (Eds.), *Occupational therapy for physical dysfunction* (pp. 774–816). Philadelphia: Lippincott Williams & Wilkins.

Kielhofner, G. (2008). *The model of human occupation: Theory and application* (4th ed.). Philadelphia: Lippincott Williams & Wilkins.

Koome, F., Hocking, C., & Sutton, D. (2012). Why routines matter: The nature and meaning of family routine in the context of adolescent mental illness. *Journal of Occupational Science, 19,* 312–325. http://dx.doi.org/10.1080/14427591.2012.718245

Larson, E., & Zemke, R. (2003). Shaping the temporal patterns of our lives: The social coordination of occupation. *Journal of Occupational Science, 10,* 80–89. http://dx.doi.org/10.1080/14427591.2003.9686514

Law, M., Baum, M. C., & Dunn, W. (2005). *Measuring occupational performance: Supporting best practice in occupational therapy* (2nd ed.). Thorofare, NJ: Slack.

Law, M., Cooper, B., Strong, S., Stewart, D., Rigby, P., & Letts, L. (1996). Person–Environment–Occupation Model: A transactive approach to occupational performance. *Canadian Journal of Occupational Therapy, 63,* 9–23. http://dx.doi.org/10.1177/000841749606300103

Law, M., Polatajko, H., Baptiste, W., & Townsend, E. (1997). Core concepts of occupational therapy. In E. Townsend (Ed.), *Enabling occupation: An occupational therapy perspective* (pp. 29–56). Ottawa, ON: Canadian Association of Occupational Therapists.

Magasi, S., & Hammel, J. (2004). Social support and social network mobilization in African American woman who have experienced strokes. *Disability Studies Quarterly, 24*(4). Retrieved from http://dsq-sds.org/article/view/878/1053

Meyer, A. (1922). The philosophy of occupational therapy. *Archives of Occupational Therapy, 1,* 1–10.

Moreira-Almeida, A., & Koenig, H. G. (2006). Retaining the meaning of the words *religiousness* and *spirituality:* A commentary on the WHOQOL SRPB group's "A Cross-Cultural Study of Spirituality, Religion, and Personal Beliefs as Components of Quality of Life" (62: 6, 2005, 1486–1497). *Social Science and Medicine, 63,* 843–845. http://dx.doi.org/10.1016/j.socscimed.2006.03.001

Mosey, A. C. (1996). *Applied scientific inquiry in the health professions: An epistemological orientation* (2nd ed.). Bethesda, MD: American Occupational Therapy Association.

Moyers, P. A.; American Occupational Therapy Association. (1999). The guide to occupational therapy practice. *American Journal of Occupational Therapy, 53,* 247–322. http://dx.doi.org/10.5014/ajot.53.3.247

Moyers, P. A., & Dale, L. M. (2007). *The guide to occupational therapy practice* (2nd ed.). Bethesda, MD: AOTA Press.

Nelson, D., & Jepson-Thomas, J. (2003). Occupational form, occupational performance, and a conceptual framework for therapeutic occupation. In P. Kramer, J. Hinojosa, & C. B. Royeen (Eds.), *Perspectives in human occupation: Participation in life* (pp. 87–155). Philadelphia: Lippincott Williams & Wilkins.

Nilsson, I., & Townsend, E. (2010). Occupational justice—Bridging theory and practice. *Scandinavian Journal of Occupational Therapy, 17,* 57–63. http://dx.doi.org/10.3109/11038120903287182

Nurit, W., & Michal, A. B. (2003). Rest: A qualitative exploration of the phenomenon. *Occupational Therapy International, 10,* 227–238. http://dx.doi.org/10.1002/oti.187

Olson, J. A. (2004). Mothering co-occupations in caring for infants and young children. In S. A. Esdaile & J. A. Olson

March/April 2014, Volume 68(Supplement 1)

(Eds.), *Mothering occupations* (pp. 28–51). Philadelphia: F. A. Davis.

Parham, L. D., & Fazio, L. S. (Eds.). (1997). *Play in occupational therapy for children.* St. Louis, MO: Mosby.

Peloquin, S. M. (2003). The therapeutic relationship: Manifestations and challenges in occupational therapy. In E. B. Crepeau, E. S. Cohn, & B. A. Boyt Schell (Eds.), *Willard and Spackman's occupational therapy* (10th ed., pp. 157–170). Philadelphia: Lippincott Williams & Wilkins.

Pierce, D. (2001). Untangling occupation and activity. *American Journal of Occupational Therapy, 55,* 138–146. http://dx.doi.org/10.5014/ajot.55.2.138

Polatajko, H., & Mandich, A. (2004). *Enabling occupation in children: The Cognitive Orientation to Daily Occupational Performance (CO–OP) approach.* Ottawa, ON: CAOT Publications.

Polatajko, H. J., Mandich, A., & Martini, R. (2000). Dynamic performance analysis: A framework for understanding occupational performance. *American Journal of Occupational Therapy, 54,* 65–72. http://dx.doi.org/10.5014/ajot.54.1.65

Puchalski, C., Ferrell, B., Virani, R., Otis-Green, S., Baird, P., Bull, J., . . . Sulmasy, D. (2009). Improving the quality of spiritual care as a dimension of palliative care: The report of the Consensus Conference. *Journal of Palliative Medicine, 12,* 885–904. http://dx.doi.org/10.1089/jpm.2009.0142

Radomski, M. V. (1995). There is more to life than putting on your pants. *American Journal of Occupational Therapy, 49,* 487–490. http://dx.doi.org/10.5014/ajot.49.6.487

Rand, K. L., & Cheavens, J. S. (2009). Hope theory. In S. J. Lopez & C. R. Snyder (Eds.), *The Oxford handbook of positive psychology* (2nd ed., pp. 323–334). Oxford, England: Oxford University Press.

Reed, K. L. (2005). An annotated history of the concepts used in occupational therapy. In C. H. Christiansen, M. C. Baum, & J. Bass-Haugen (Eds.), *Occupational therapy: Performance, participation, and well-being* (3rd ed., pp. 567–626). Thorofare, NJ: Slack.

Rogers, J. C., & Holm, M. B. (1994). Assessment of self-care. In B. R. Bonder & M. B. Wagner (Eds.), *Functional performance in older adults* (pp. 181–202). Philadelphia: F. A. Davis.

Sandqvist, G., Akesson, A., & Eklund, M. (2005). Daily occupations and well-being in women with limited cutaneous systemic sclerosis. *American Journal of Occupational Therapy, 59,* 390–397. http://dx.doi.org/10.5014/ajot.59.4.390

Segal, R. (2004). Family routines and rituals: A context for occupational therapy interventions. *American Journal of Occupational Therapy, 58,* 499–508. http://dx.doi.org/10.5014/ajot.58.5.499

Shumway-Cook, A., & Woollacott, M. H. (2007). *Motor control: Translating research into clinical practice* (3rd ed.). Philadelphia: Lippincott Williams & Wilkins.

Slagle, E. C. (1924). A year's development of occupational therapy in New York State hospitals. *Modern Hospital, 22,* 98–104.

Spencer, J., Davidson, H., & White, V. (1997). Help clients develop hopes for the future. *American Journal of Occupational Therapy, 51,* 191–198. http://dx.doi.org/10.5014/ajot.51.3.191

Taber's cyclopedic medical dictionary. (1997). Philadelphia: F. A. Davis.

Taylor, R. R., & Van Puymbroeck, L. (2013). Therapeutic use of self: Applying the intentional relationship model in group therapy. In J. C. O'Brien & J. W. Solomon (Eds.), *Occupational analysis and group process* (pp. 36–52). St. Louis, MO: Elsevier.

Townsend, E., & Wilcock, A. A. (2004). Occupational justice and client-centred practice: A dialogue in progress. *Canadian Journal of Occupational Therapy, 71,* 75–87. http://dx.doi.org/10.1177/000841740407100203

Trombly, C. A. (1995). Occupation: Purposefulness and meaningfulness as therapeutic mechanisms (Eleanor Clarke Slagle Lecture). *American Journal of Occupational Therapy, 49,* 960–972. http://dx.doi.org/10.5014/ajot.49.10.960

Uniform Data System for Medical Rehabilitation. (1996). *Guide for the Uniform Data Set for Medical Rehabilitation (including the FIM instrument).* Buffalo, NY: Author.

Unruh, A. M. (2004). Reflections on: "So . . . what do you do?" Occupation and the construction of identity. *Canadian Journal of Occupational Therapy, 71,* 290–295. http://dx.doi.org/10.1177/000841740407100508

Wilcock, A. A. (2006). *An occupational perspective of health* (2nd ed.). Thorofare, NJ: Slack.

Wilcock, A. A., & Townsend, E. A. (2014). Occupational justice. In B. A. Boyt Schell, G. Gillen, & M. Scaffa (Eds.), *Willard and Spackman's occupational therapy* (12th ed., pp. 541–552). Philadelphia: Lippincott Williams & Wilkins.

World Federation of Occupational Therapists. (2012). *Definition of occupation.* Retrieved from http://www.wfot.org/aboutus/aboutoccupationaltherapy/definitionofoccupationaltherapy.aspx

World Health Organization. (1986, November 21). *The Ottawa Charter for Health Promotion (First International Conference on Health Promotion, Ottawa).* Retrieved from http://www.who.int/healthpromotion/conferences/previous/ottawa/en/print.html

World Health Organization. (2001). *International classification of functioning, disability and health.* Geneva: Author.

World Health Organization. (2006). *Constitution of the World Health Organization* (45th ed.). Retrieved from http://www.afro.who.int/index.php?option=com_docman&task=doc_download&gid=19&Itemid=2111WHO 2006

Zemke, R. (2004). Time, space, and the kaleidoscopes of occupation (Eleanor Clarke Slagle Lecture). *American Journal of Occupational Therapy, 58,* 608–620. http://dx.doi.org/10.5014/ajot.58.6.608

Zemke, R., & Clark, F. (1996). *Occupational science: An evolving discipline.* Philadelphia: F. A. Davis.

Authors

THE COMMISSION ON PRACTICE:

Deborah Ann Amini, EdD, OTR/L, CHT, FAOTA,
Chairperson, 2011–2014

Kathy Kannenberg, MA, OTR/L, CCM,
Chairperson-Elect, 2013–2014

Stefanie Bodison, OTD, OTR/L

Pei-Fen Chang, PhD, OTR/L

Donna Colaianni, PhD, OTR/L, CHT

Beth Goodrich, OTR, ATP, PhD

Lisa Mahaffey, MS, OTR/L, FAOTA

Mashelle Painter, MEd, COTA/L

Michael Urban, MS, OTR/L, CEAS, MBA, CWCE

Dottie Handley-More, MS, OTR/L,
SIS Liaison

Kiel Cooluris, MOT, OTR/L,
ASD Liaison

Andrea McElroy, MS, OTR/L,
Immediate-Past ASD Liaison

Deborah Lieberman, MHSA, OTR/L, FAOTA,
AOTA Headquarters Liaison

for

THE COMMISSION ON PRACTICE

Deborah Ann Amini, EdD, OTR/L, CHT, FAOTA,
Chairperson

Adopted by the Representative Assembly 2013DecCO11

Note. This document replaces the 2008 *Occupational Therapy Practice Framework: Domain and Process* (2nd ed.).

Copyright © 2014 by the American Occupational Therapy Association. Published in the *American Journal of Occupational Therapy, 68*(Suppl. 1), S1–S48. http://dx.doi.org/10.5014/ajot.2014.682006

Acknowledgments

The Commission on Practice (COP) expresses sincere appreciation to all those who participated in the development of the *Occupational Therapy Practice Framework: Domain and Process.*

In addition to those named below, the COP wishes to thank everyone who has contributed to the dialogue, feedback and concepts presented in the document. Sincerest appreciation is extended to Madalene Palmer for all her support and to AOTA's policy and regulatory affairs staff. Further appreciation and thanks is extended to Mary Jane Youngstrom, MS, OTR, FAOTA; Susanne Smith Roley, OTD, OTR/L, FAOTA; Anne G. Fisher, PhD, OTR, FAOTA; and Deborah Pitts, PhD, OTR/L, BCMH, CPRP.

The COP wishes to acknowledge the authors of the second edition of this document: Susanne Smith Roley, MS, OTR/L, FAOTA, *Chairperson (2005–2008);* Janet V. DeLany, DEd, OTR/L, FAOTA; Cynthia J. Barrows, MS, OTR/L; Susan Brownrigg, OTR/L; DeLana Honaker, PhD, OTR/L, BCP; Deanna Iris Sava, MS, OTR/L; Vibeke Talley, OTR/L; Kristi Voelkerding, BS, COTA/L, ATP; Deborah Ann Amini, MEd, OTR/L, CHT, FAOTA, *SIS Liaison;* Emily Smith, MOT, *ASD Liaison;* Pamela Toto, MS, OTR/L, BCG, FAOTA, *Immediate-Past SIS Liaison;* Sarah King, MOT, OTR, *Immediate-Past ASD Liaison;* and Deborah Lieberman, MHSA, OTR/L, FAOTA, *AOTA Headquarters Liaison;* With contributions from M. Carolyn Baum, PhD, OTR/L, FAOTA; Ellen S. Cohn, ScD, OTR/L, FAOTA; Penelope A. Moyers Cleveland, EdD, OTR/L, BCMH, FAOTA; and Mary Jane Youngstrom, MS, OTR, FAOTA.

The COP also wishes to acknowledge the authors of the first edition of this document: Mary Jane Youngstrom, MS, OTR, FAOTA, *Chairperson (1998–2002);* Sara Jane Brayman, PhD, OTR, FAOTA, *Chairperson-Elect (2001–2002);* Paige Anthony, COTA; Mary Brinson, MS, OTR/L, FAOTA; Susan Brownrigg, OTR/L; Gloria Frolek Clark, MS, OTR/L, FAOTA; Susanne Smith Roley, MS, OTR; James Sellers, OTR/L; Nancy L. Van Slyke, EdD, OTR; Stacy M. Desmarais, MS, OTR/L, *ASD Liaison;* Jane Oldham, MOTS, *Immediate-Past ASCOTA Liaison;* Mary Vining Radomski, MA, OTR, FAOTA, *SIS Liaison;* and Sarah D. Hertfelder, MEd, MOT, OTR, FAOTA, *National Office Liaison.*

Appendix A. Glossary

A

Activities

Actions designed and selected to support the development of performance skills and performance patterns to enhance occupational engagement.

Activities of daily living (ADLs)

Activities oriented toward taking care of one's own body (adapted from Rogers & Holm, 1994). ADLs also are referred to as *basic activities of daily living (BADLs)* and *personal activities of daily living (PADLs)*. These activities are "fundamental to living in a social world; they enable basic survival and well-being" (Christiansen & Hammecker, 2001, p. 156; see Table 1).

Activity analysis

Analysis of "the typical demands of an activity, the range of skills involved in its performance, and the various cultural meanings that might be ascribed to it" (Crepeau, 2003, p. 192).

Activity demands

Aspects of an activity or occupation needed to carry it out, including relevance and importance to the client, objects used and their properties, space demands, social demands, sequencing and timing, required actions and performance skills, and required underlying body functions and body structures (see Table 7).

Adaptation

Occupational therapy practitioners enable participation by modifying a task, the method of accomplishing the task, and the environment to promote engagement in occupation (James, 2008).

Advocacy

Efforts directed toward promoting occupational justice and empowering clients to seek and obtain resources to fully participate in their daily life occupations. Efforts undertaken by the practitioner are considered advocacy, and those undertaken by the client are considered self-advocacy and can be promoted and supported by the practitioner (see Table 6).

Analysis of occupational performance

The step in the evaluation process in which the client's assets and problems or potential problems are more specifically identified through assessment tools designed to observe, measure, and inquire about factors that support or hinder occupational performance and in which targeted outcomes are identified (see Exhibit 2).

Assessments

"Specific tools or instruments that are used during the evaluation process" (American Occupational Therapy Association [AOTA], 2010, p. S107).

B

Body functions

"Physiological functions of body systems (including psychological functions)" (World Health Organization [WHO], 2001, p. 10; see Table 2).

Body structures

"Anatomical parts of the body, such as organs, limbs, and their components" that support body functions (WHO, 2001, p. 10; see Table 2).

C

Client

Person or persons (including those involved in the care of a client), group (collective of individuals, e.g., families, workers, students, or community members), or population (collective of groups or individuals living in a similar locale—e.g., city, state, or country—or sharing the same or like concerns).

Client-centered care (client-centered practice)

Approach to service that incorporates respect for and partnership with clients as active participants in the therapy process. This approach emphasizes clients' knowledge and experience, strengths, capacity for choice, and overall autonomy (Boyt Schell et al., 2014a, p. 1230).

Client factors

Specific capacities, characteristics, or beliefs that reside within the person and that influence performance in occupations. Client factors include values, beliefs, and spirituality; body functions; and body structures (see Table 2).

Clinical reasoning

"Process used by practitioners to plan, direct, perform, and reflect on client care" (Boyt Schell et al., 2014a, p. 1231). The term *professional reasoning* is sometimes used and is considered to be a broader term.

Collaborative approach

Orientation in which the occupational therapy practitioner and client work in the spirit of egalitarianism and mutual participation. Collaboration involves encouraging clients to describe their therapeutic concerns, identify their own goals, and contribute to decisions regarding therapeutic interventions (Boyt Schell et al., 2014a).

Context

Variety of interrelated conditions within and surrounding the client that influence performance, including cultural, personal, temporal, and virtual contexts (see Table 5).

Co-occupation

Occupation that implicitly involves two or more people (Boyt Schell et al., 2014a, p. 1232).

Cultural context

Customs, beliefs, activity patterns, behavioral standards, and expectations accepted by the society of which a client is a member. The cultural context influences the client's identity and activity choices (see Table 5).

D

Domain

Profession's purview and areas in which its members have an established body of knowledge and expertise.

E

Education

- *As an occupation:* Activities involved in learning and participating in the educational environment (see Table 1).

- *As an intervention:* Activities that impart knowledge and information about occupation, health, well-being, and participation, resulting in acquisition by the client of helpful behaviors, habits, and routines that may or may not require application at the time of the intervention session (see Table 6).

Engagement in occupation

Performance of occupations as the result of choice, motivation, and meaning within a supportive context and environment.

Environment

External physical and social conditions that surround the client and in which the client's daily life occupations occur (see Table 5).

Evaluation

"Process of obtaining and interpreting data necessary for intervention. This includes planning for and documenting the evaluation process and results" (AOTA, 2010, p. S107).

G

Goal

Measurable and meaningful, occupation-based, long-term or short-term aim directly related to the client's ability and need to engage in desired occupations (AOTA, 2013a, p. S35).

Group

Collective of individuals (e.g., family members, workers, students, community members).

Group intervention

Skilled knowledge and use of leadership techniques in various settings to facilitate learning and acquisition by clients across the life span of skills for participation, including basic social interaction skills, tools for self-regulation, goal setting, and positive choice making, through the dynamics of group and social interaction. Groups may be used as a method of service delivery (see Table 6).

H

Habilitation

Health care services designed to assist people in acquiring, improving, minimizing the deterioration of, compensating for an impairment of, or maintaining (partially or fully) skills, function, or performance for participation in occupation and daily life activities (AOTA policy staff, personal communication, December 17, 2013).

Habits

"Acquired tendencies to respond and perform in certain consistent ways in familiar environments or situations; specific, automatic behaviors performed repeatedly, relatively automatically, and with little variation" (Boyt Schell et al., 2014a, p. 1234). Habits can be useful, dominating, or impoverished and can either support or interfere with performance in areas of occupation (Dunn, 2000; see Table 4).

Health

"State of complete physical, mental, and social well-being, and not merely the absence of disease or infirmity" (WHO, 2006, p. 1).

Health promotion

"Process of enabling people to increase control over, and to improve, their health. To reach a state of complete physical, mental, and social well-being, an individual or group must be able to identify and realize aspirations, to satisfy needs, and to change or cope with the environment" (WHO, 1986).

Hope

"Perceived ability to produce pathways to achieve desired goals and to motivate oneself to use those pathways" (Rand & Cheavens, 2009, p. 323).

I

Independence

"Self-directed state of being characterized by an individual's ability to participate in necessary and preferred occupations in a satisfying manner irrespective of the amount or kind of external assistance desired or required" (AOTA, 2002a, p. 660).

Instrumental activities of daily living (IADLs)

Activities that support daily life within the home and community and that often require more complex interactions than those used in ADLs (see Table 1).

Interdependence

"Reliance that people have on one another as a natural consequence of group living" (Christiansen & Townsend, 2010, p. 419). "Interdependence engenders a spirit of social inclusion, mutual aid, and a moral commitment and responsibility to recognize and support difference" (Christiansen & Townsend, 2010, p. 187).

Interests

"What one finds enjoyable or satisfying to do" (Kielhofner, 2008, p. 42).

Intervention

"Process and skilled actions taken by occupational therapy practitioners in collaboration with the client to facilitate engagement in occupation related to health and participation. The intervention process includes the plan, implementation, and review" (AOTA, 2010, p. S107; see Table 6).

Intervention approaches

Specific strategies selected to direct the process of interventions on the basis of the client's desired outcomes, evaluation data, and evidence (see Table 8).

L

Leisure

"Nonobligatory activity that is intrinsically motivated and engaged in during discretionary time, that is, time not committed to obligatory occupations such as work, self-care, or sleep" (Parham & Fazio, 1997, p. 250; see Table 1).

M

Motor skills

"Occupational performance skills observed as the person interacts with and moves task objects and self around the task environment" (e.g., activity of daily living [ADL] motor skills, school motor skills; Boyt Schell et al., 2014a, p. 1237; see Table 3).

O

Occupation

Daily life activities in which people engage. Occupations occur in context and are influenced by the interplay among client factors, performance skills, and performance patterns. Occupations occur over time; have purpose, meaning, and perceived utility to the client; and can be observed by others (e.g., preparing a meal) or be known only to the person involved (e.g., learning through reading a textbook). Occupations can involve the execution of multiple activities for completion and can result in various outcomes. The *Framework* identifies a broad range of occupations categorized as activities of daily living, instrumental activities of daily living, rest and sleep, education, work, play, leisure, and social participation (see Table 1).

Occupational analysis

See *activity analysis.*

Occupational demands

See *activity demands.*

Occupational identity

"Composite sense of who one is and wishes to become as an occupational being generated from one's history of occupational participation" (Boyt Schell et al., 2014a, p. 1238).

Occupational justice

"A justice that recognizes occupational rights to inclusive participation in everyday occupations for all persons in society, regardless of age, ability, gender, social class, or other differences" (Nilsson & Townsend, 2010, p. 58). Access to and participation in the full range of meaningful and enriching occupations afforded to others, including opportunities for social inclusion and the resources to participate in occupations to satisfy personal, health, and societal needs (adapted from Townsend & Wilcock, 2004).

Occupational performance

Act of doing and accomplishing a selected action (performance skill), activity, or occupation (Fisher, 2009; Fisher & Griswold, 2014; Kielhofner, 2008) that results from the dynamic transaction among the client, the context, and the activity. Improving or enabling skills and patterns in occupational performance leads to engagement in occupations or activities (adapted in part from Law et al., 1996, p. 16).

Occupational profile

Summary of the client's occupational history and experiences, patterns of daily living, interests, values, and needs (see Exhibit 2).

Occupational therapy

Therapeutic use of everyday life activities (occupations) with individuals or groups for the purpose of enhancing or enabling participation in roles, habits, routines, and rituals in home, school, workplace, community, and other settings. Occupational therapy practitioners use their knowledge of the transactional relationship among the person, his or her engagement in valued occupations, and the context to design occupation-based intervention plans that facilitate change or growth in client factors (values, beliefs, and spirituality; body functions, body structures) and performance skills (motor, process, and social interaction) needed for successful participation. Occupational therapy practitioners are concerned with the end result of participation and thus enable engagement through adaptations and modifications to the environment or objects within the environment when needed. Occupational therapy services are provided for habilitation, rehabilitation, and promotion of health and wellness for clients with disability- and non–disability-related needs. These services include acquisition and preservation of occupational identity for those who have or are at risk for developing an illness, injury, disease, disorder, condition, impairment, disability, activity limitation, or participation restriction (adapted from AOTA, 2011).

Organization

Entity composed of individuals with a common purpose or enterprise, such as a business, industry, or agency.

Outcome

End result of the occupational therapy process; what clients can achieve through occupational therapy intervention (see Table 9).

P

Participation

"Involvement in a life situation" (WHO, 2001, p. 10).

Performance patterns

Habits, routines, roles, and rituals used in the process of engaging in occupations or activities; these patterns can support or hinder occupational performance (see Table 4).

Performance skills

Goal-directed actions that are observable as small units of engagement in daily life occupations. They are learned and developed over time and are situated in specific contexts and environments (Fisher & Griswold, 2014; see Table 3).

Person

Individual, including family member, caregiver, teacher, employee, or relevant other.

Personal context

"Features of the individual that are not part of a health condition or health status" (WHO, 2001, p. 17). The personal context includes age, gender, socioeconomic and educational status and may also include membership in a group (i.e., volunteers, employees) or population (i.e., members of a society; see Table 5).

Physical environment

Natural and built nonhuman surroundings and the objects in them. The natural environment includes geographic terrain, plants, and animals, as well as the sensory qualities of the natural surroundings. The built environment includes buildings, furniture, tools, and devices (see Table 5).

Play

"Any spontaneous or organized activity that provides enjoyment, entertainment, amusement, or diversion" (Parham & Fazio, 1997, p. 252; see Table 1).

Population

Collective of groups of individuals living in a similar locale (e.g., city, state, country) or sharing the same or like characteristics or concerns.

Preparatory methods and tasks

Methods and tasks that prepare the client for occupational performance, used either as part of a treatment session in preparation for or concurrently with occupations and activities or as a home-based engagement to support daily occupational performance. Often preparatory methods are interventions that are done to clients without their active participation and involve modalities, devices, or techniques.

Prevention

Education or health promotion efforts designed to identify, reduce, or prevent the onset and reduce the incidence of unhealthy conditions, risk factors, diseases, or injuries (AOTA, 2013b).

Process

Way in which occupational therapy practitioners operationalize their expertise to provide services to clients. The occupational therapy process includes evaluation, intervention, and targeted outcomes; occurs within the purview of the occupational therapy domain; and involves collaboration among the occupational therapist, occupational therapy assistant, and client.

Process skills

"Occupational performance skills [e.g., ADL process skills, school process skills] observed as a person (1) selects, interacts with, and uses task tools and materials; (2) carries out individual actions and steps; and (3) modifies performance when problems are encountered" (Boyt Schell et al., 2014a, p. 1239; see Table 3).

Q

Quality of life

Dynamic appraisal of life satisfaction (perception of progress toward identified goals), self-concept (beliefs and feelings about oneself), health and functioning (e.g., health status, self-care capabilities), and socioeconomic factors (e.g., vocation, education, income; adapted from Radomski, 1995).

R

Reevaluation

Reappraisal of the client's performance and goals to determine the type and amount of change that has taken place.

Rehabilitation

Rehabilitation services are provided to persons experiencing deficits in key areas of physical and other types of function or limitations in participation in daily life activities. Interventions are designed to enable the achievement and maintenance of optimal physical, sensory, intellectual, psychological, and social functional levels. Rehabilitation services provide tools and techniques needed to attain desired levels of independence and self-determination.

Rituals

Sets of symbolic actions with spiritual, cultural, or social meaning contributing to the client's identity and reinforcing values and beliefs. Rituals have a strong affective component (Fiese, 2007; Fiese et al., 2002; Segal, 2004; see Table 4).

Roles

Sets of behaviors expected by society and shaped by culture and context that may be further conceptualized and defined by the client (see Table 4).

Routines

Patterns of behavior that are observable, regular, and repetitive and that provide structure for daily life. They can be satisfying and promoting or damaging. Routines require momentary time commitment and are embedded in cultural and ecological contexts (Fiese et al., 2002; Segal, 2004; see Table 4).

S

Self-Advocacy

Advocating for oneself, including making one's own decisions about life, learning how to obtain information to gain an understanding about issues of personal interest or importance, developing a network of support, knowing one's rights and responsibilities, reaching out to others when in need of assistance, and learning about self-determination.

Service delivery model

Set of methods for providing services to or on behalf of clients.

Social environment

Presence of, relationships with, and expectations of persons, groups, and populations with whom clients have contact (e.g., availability and expectations of significant individuals, such as spouse, friends, and caregivers; see Table 5).

Social interaction skills

"Occupational performance skills observed during the ongoing stream of a social exchange" (Boyt Schell et al., 2014a, p. 1241; see Table 3).

Social participation

"Interweaving of occupations to support desired engagement in community and family activities as well as those involving peers and friends" (Gillen & Boyt Schell, 2014, p. 607) or involvement in a subset of activities that involve social situations with others (Bedell, 2012) and that support social interdependence (Magasi & Hammel, 2004). Social participation can occur in person or through remote technologies such as telephone calls, computer interaction, and video conferencing (see Table 1).

Spirituality

"Aspect of humanity that refers to the way individuals seek and express meaning and purpose and the way they experience their connectedness to the moment, to self, to others, to nature, and to the significant or sacred" (Puchalski et al., 2009, p. 887; see Table 2).

T

Task

What individuals do or have done (e.g., drive, bake a cake, dress, make a bed; A. Fisher, personal communication, December 16, 2013).

Temporal context

Experience of time as shaped by engagement in occupations. The temporal aspects of occupations that "contribute to the patterns of daily occupations" include "rhythm . . . tempo . . . synchronization . . . duration . . . and sequence" (Larson & Zemke, 2003, p. 82; Zemke, 2004, p. 610). The temporal context includes stage of life, time of day, duration and rhythm of activity, and history (see Table 5).

Transaction

Process that involves two or more individuals or elements that reciprocally and continually influence and affect one another through the ongoing relationship (Dickie, Cutchin, & Humphry, 2006).

V

Values

Acquired beliefs and commitments, derived from culture, about what is good, right, and important to do (Kielhofner, 2008); principles, standards, or qualities considered worthwhile or desirable by the client who holds them (Moyers & Dale, 2007).

Virtual context

Environment in which communication occurs by means of airwaves or computers in the absence of physical contact. The virtual context includes simulated, real-time, or near-time environments such as chat rooms, email, video conferencing, and radio transmissions; remote monitoring via wireless sensors; and computer-based data collection (see Table 5).

W

Well-being

"General term encompassing the total universe of human life domains, including physical, mental, and social aspects" (WHO, 2006, p. 211).

Wellness

"Perception of and responsibility for psychological and physical well-being as these contribute to overall satisfaction with one's life situation" (Boyt Schell et al., 2014a, p. 1243).

Work

"Labor or exertion; to make, construct, manufacture, form, fashion, or shape objects; to organize, plan, or evaluate services or processes of living or governing; committed occupations that are performed with or without financial reward" (Christiansen & Townsend, 2010, p. 423).

Appendix B. Preparation and Qualifications of Occupational Therapists and Occupational Therapy Assistants

Who Are Occupational Therapists?

To practice as an occupational therapist, the individual trained in the United States

- Has graduated from an occupational therapy program accredited by the Accreditation Council for Occupational Therapy Education (ACOTE®) or predecessor organizations;
- Has successfully completed a period of supervised fieldwork experience required by the recognized educational institution where the applicant met the academic requirements of an educational program for occupational therapists that is accredited by ACOTE or predecessor organizations;
- Has passed a nationally recognized entry-level examination for occupational therapists; and
- Fulfills state requirements for licensure, certification, or registration.

Educational Programs for the Occupational Therapist

These include the following:

- Biological, physical, social, and behavioral sciences
- Basic tenets of occupational therapy
- Occupational therapy theoretical perspectives
- Screening, evaluation, and referral
- Formulation and implementation of an intervention plan
- Context of service delivery
- Management of occupational therapy services (master's level)
- Leadership and management (doctoral level)
- Scholarship
- Professional ethics, values, and responsibilities.

The fieldwork component of the program is designed to develop competent, entry-level, generalist occupational therapists by providing experience with a variety of clients across the lifespan and in a variety of settings. Fieldwork is integral to the program's curriculum design and includes an in-depth experience in delivering occupational therapy services to clients, focusing on the application of purposeful and meaningful occupation and/or research, administration, and management of occupational therapy services. The fieldwork experience is designed to promote clinical reasoning and reflective practice, to transmit the values and beliefs that enable ethical practice, and to develop professionalism and competence in career responsibilities. Doctoral-level students also must complete a doctoral experiential component designed to develop advanced skills beyond a generalist level.

Who Are Occupational Therapy Assistants?

To practice as an occupational therapy assistant, the individual trained in the United States

- Has graduated from an occupational therapy assistant program accredited by ACOTE or predecessor organizations;
- Has successfully completed a period of supervised fieldwork experience required by the recognized educational institution where the applicant met the academic requirements of an educational program for occupational therapy assistants that is accredited by ACOTE or predecessor organizations;
- Has passed a nationally recognized entry-level examination for occupational therapy assistants; and
- Fulfills state requirements for licensure, certification, or registration.

Educational Programs for the Occupational Therapy Assistant

These include the following:

- Biological, physical, social, and behavioral sciences
- Basic tenets of occupational therapy
- Screening and assessment
- Intervention and implementation
- Context of service delivery
- Assistance in management of occupational therapy services
- Scholarship
- Professional ethics, values, and responsibilities.

The fieldwork component of the program is designed to develop competent, entry-level, generalist occupational therapy assistants by providing experience with a variety of clients across the lifespan and in a variety of settings. Fieldwork is integral to the program's curriculum design and includes an in-depth experience in

Note. The majority of this information is taken from ACOTE (2012).

delivering occupational therapy services to clients, focusing on the application of purposeful and meaningful occupation. The fieldwork experience is designed to promote clinical reasoning appropriate to the occupational therapy assistant role, to transmit the values and beliefs that enable ethical practice, and to develop professionalism and competence in career responsibilities.

Regulation of Occupational Therapy Practice

All occupational therapists and occupational therapy assistants must practice under federal and state law. Currently, 50 states, the District of Columbia, Puerto Rico, and Guam have enacted laws regulating the practice of occupational therapy.

Specialized Knowledge and Skills Papers

Specialized Knowledge and Skills in Adult Vestibular Rehabilitation for Occupational Therapy Practice

Introduction

People with impairments of the vestibular system often have subtle problems that have profound ramifications for their ability to engage in daily life tasks and activities at home and to participate in society outside the home. Vestibular impairment often restricts an individual's ability to participate in everyday occupations, affecting not only that individual but also significant others, including family members, friends, coworkers, and caregivers. Occupational therapy facilitates increased independence in daily life tasks and participation in work and social occupations. For these reasons, occupational therapy is an appropriate intervention for clients needing vestibular rehabilitation to decrease symptoms and increase independence in all aspects of their lives. Thus, vestibular rehabilitation is within the scope of practice for occupational therapists and occupational therapy assistants[1] who have specialized knowledge and skills in this area. This document provides an understanding of the essential knowledge and skills needed by practitioners working with individuals with vestibular impairments and will be of interest to payers, practitioners, or consumers who wish to know more about occupational therapy practice using vestibular rehabilitation techniques.

People with vestibular disorders may present with symptoms including vertigo, oscillopsia, nausea, disequilibrium, spatial disorientation, visual motion sensitivity, decreased dynamic visual acuity, decreased concentration, and decreased skill in dual task performance. Spatial orientation deficits and disequilibrium may be manifested as head and body tilt while sitting or standing, perception of tilt while sitting or standing, veering or drifting to the side while walking or steering a vehicle, or a sense of not knowing which way is up. These problems may result in fear of falling. These symptoms may affect occupational performance and can result in social withdrawal and depression. For example, visual motion sensitivity may cause disequilibrium, vertigo, nausea, and disorientation, leading to slower or more awkward performance of self-care skills, decreased participation in social activities, and decreased ability to perform home management tasks outside of the home, such as grocery shopping. Vertigo, disequilibrium, and other symptoms may interfere with job skills as they cause difficulty standing, reaching, walking, turning the head to scan the environment, or making social gestures with the head such as nodding.

Definition

The term *vestibular rehabilitation* refers to intervention to decrease symptoms and increase independence, safety, and participation in people with specific disorders of the peripheral vestibular apparatus, the central vestibular pathways, and age-related disequilibrium. Interventions include, but are not limited to, exercise and activity programs to reduce vertigo and oscillopsia, repositioning interventions for positional vertigo, exercises and activities to improve standing and walking balance during activities, and safety

---

[1]*Occupational therapists* are responsible for all aspects of occupational therapy service delivery and are accountable for the safety and effectiveness of the occupational therapy service delivery process. *Occupational therapy assistants* deliver occupational therapy services under the supervision of and in partnership with an occupational therapist (AOTA, 2004).

training at home and at work. A client receiving occupational therapy including vestibular rehabilitation techniques may also receive occupational therapy using other interventions. For example, a client with a head injury may also receive perceptual, motor, or life skills training.

Vestibular rehabilitation is used to treat the sequelae of specific medical conditions, and provides an alternative or adjunct to pharmacologic and surgical intervention by the physician. Clients who receive vestibular rehabilitation have specific medical conditions that can be demonstrated with objective diagnostic tests or otherwise medically determined. Most people who are referred for vestibular rehabilitation are adults. They have a wide variety of health conditions including, but not limited to, benign paroxysmal positional vertigo (BPPV); acute, chronic, and recurrent labyrinthitis; vestibular neuronitis; some autoimmune disorders; postconcussion vertigo; postoperative vertigo; Ménierè's disease; bilateral vestibular weakness or total vestibular loss due to ototoxicity; presbystasis or disequilibrium of aging; some cases of strokes, some cases of multiple sclerosis, some cases of Parkinson's disease, some Parkinsonian syndromes, and some cases of migraine.

Although the focus of this document is on adult vestibular rehabilitation, we note that the same or similar vestibular impairments may occur in children. The literature has few papers on the efficacy of vestibular rehabilitation in children. These disorders are difficult to diagnose because children may not be able to describe their symptoms and because, for technical reasons, young children cannot always be tested with standard objective diagnostic tests. Vestibular disorders that occur in childhood that may respond to vestibular rehabilitation include childhood paroxysmal vertigo, which may be related to migraine; BPPV; labyrinthitis; vestibular neuronitis; bilateral impairment due to ototoxicity; some autoimmune disorders; and congenital malformations of the inner ear. In pediatric vestibular rehabilitation, treatment activities must be age appropriate.

Knowledge and Skills for Entry-Level and Advanced Practitioners

Clients with vestibular disorders have a complex combination of physiological and psychological problems. The effects of vestibular impairments are subtle and pervasive. Many people with these problems are not able to describe the sensations they have or the motions that elicit vertigo or disequilibrium. Therefore, rehabilitation of most individuals with vestibular impairments requires skills beyond entry-level competence. The specialized nature of this intervention requires specific, advanced-level knowledge. Intervention may require specific techniques that focus directly on the vestibular impairment. Advanced skills build on earlier competencies in knowledge, performance, critical reasoning, interpersonal abilities, and ethical reasoning and additional competencies developed during independent study of the literature, continuing education coursework, and additional practice.

An in-depth understanding of the structure and function of the vestibular system, visual/vestibular/proprioceptive interactions, and the principles of motor control is essential when providing vestibular rehabilitation. Occupational therapy entry-level education provides a foundation in functional anatomy, neuroscience, and motor control that assists the practitioner in understanding the types of complex problems experienced by clients with vestibular impairments. Practitioners need further training, however, to address the subtle problems of clients with these disorders. Advanced-level skills are necessary for evaluation of the deficits and specific manipulations that alter vestibular function. This knowledge and these skills are not provided to occupational therapists at the entry level. Appendix 1 outlines the basic science knowledge necessary for advanced practice.

Occupational therapists use knowledge of vestibular system anatomy and physiology when determining underlying problems that affect occupational performance. An individual's central nervous system uses information about head movement to help control four classes of behavior: (a) postural reflexes for control of balance, (b) vestibulo-ocular reflexes to stabilize gaze so the individual can see clearly, (c) coding of spatial coordinates for object orientation and navigation, and (d) some autonomic responses to prepare for "fight-or-flight" behavior. Appendix 2 outlines the applied science knowledge necessary for advanced practice.

The occupational therapist must be highly skilled at evaluating the consequences of subtle vestibular deficits, such as balance disturbances due to head movements while sitting, standing, walking, reaching, and performing transfers between positions. Understanding the potential impact of vestibular impairment on participation in healthy occupations requires knowledge of the effect of vestibular impairment on the life of the person. See Appendices 3–8 for specific examples of how vestibular impairments impact performance in occupation (AOTA, 2002).

Refined skills in activity analysis are essential for evaluation of and intervention planning for these clients. The occupational therapist uses knowledge of body structure and function in conjunction with observation and activity analysis when evaluating subtle decrements in performance during typical daily activities. At the entry level, occupational therapists and occupational therapy assistants are familiar with the location of the vestibular labyrinth and know that the symptoms of vestibular disorders include vertigo, poor balance, and fear of falling. Their use of the occupational profile helps to determine which tasks elicit those symptoms. They are able to determine if clients would benefit from adaptive safety equipment; to recommend equipment appropriate for the home; and to educate clients about other safety concerns, such as appropriate clothing and shoes. They also are able to evaluate many activities of daily living directly to determine if training is needed and provide training when necessary. Appendix 9 outlines the essential evaluation skills for the advanced practitioner. Appendix 10 outlines specific information on intervention using vestibular rehabilitation methods.

Occupation therapy practitioners who do vestibular rehabilitation may seek reimbursement through Medicare and other third-party payers. Examples of possible *Current Procedural Technology (CPT)* codes include, but are not limited to, codes for neuromuscular reeducation of movement, balance, coordination, and/or posture for sitting and/or standing activities (97112); manual therapy (97140); and therapeutic activities to improve functional performance (97530) (American Medical Association, 2006).

The occupational therapist assumes the ultimate responsibility for the delivery of occupational therapy services, including evaluation of the person and development of the intervention plan. The advanced occupational therapist may delegate certain selected interventions to an entry-level occupational therapist or to an occupational therapy assistant who has demonstrated service competency in those interventions. All practitioners should know when and how to refer clients to other health professionals when needed, including but not limited to: specialty physicians, certified driving rehabilitation specialists, psychologists, physical therapists, audiologists, and social workers.

Brief Review of the Research Literature

Vestibular rehabilitation in occupational therapy practice is supported by the literature, although considerable research remains to be done. This section is not an exhaustive review of the research but gives an overview of the research on vestibular impairment and vestibular rehabilitation that is relevant to occupational therapy. Suggested readings not cited here are listed in the "Additional Reading" list.

In the first paper describing the use of exercises for vertigo, Cawthorne (1944) indicated that some patients with postconcussion vertigo are rendered "helpless and immobile," preceding later work by occupational therapists and their collaborators showing that patients with disorders that cause vertigo have significantly reduced independence in activities of daily living (Cohen, 1992; Cohen, Ewell, & Jenkins, 1995; Cohen & Jerabek, 1999; Cohen & Kimball, 2000; Cohen, Kimball, & Adams, 2000; Cohen, Wells, Kimball, & Owsley, 2003; Farber, 1989; Morris, 1991).

In Cooksey's first paper describing vestibular rehabilitation exercises (Cooksey, 1945), he mentioned the need for teamwork by rehabilitation staff, including occupational therapists. Cooksey specifically noted the role of occupational therapy in the early resumption of purposeful activity. In his 1946 paper, Cooksey indicated that purposeful activity should be incorporated into the daily exercise program for these patients. Structured, purposeful activity is an effective treatment modality for reducing vertigo, improving balance, and increasing independence in activities of daily living (Cohen, Kane-Wineland, Miller, & Hatfield, 1995; Cohen, Miller, Kane-Wineland, & Hatfield, 1995). Vertigo habituation exercises are also effective in decreasing symptoms, improving spatial orientation skills, and increasing independence and ability to perform purposeful activity that involves repetitive head movements (Cohen & Kimball, 2002, 2003, 2004b, 2004c). Thus, exercises and purposeful activities may be components of a successful rehabilitation program for many patients with vertigo. For a critical review of more recent studies on vertigo habituation treatments and other issues, see Cohen's 2006 review paper.

A series of studies has shown that patients with vestibular disorders also have high rates of anxiety and other psychosocial problems (Eagger, Luxon, Davies, Coelho, & Ron, 1992; Yardley & Hallam, 1996; Yardley, Luxon, & Haacke, 1994; Yardley & Putman, 1992). Many of these kinds of problems might be appropriate for intervention by occupational therapists, combining our understanding of physical and psychosocial disorders.

Patients with benign paroxysmal positional vertigo are best treated with passive maneuvers of the head that are thought to reposition otoconial particles that have become displaced from one compartment to another. Occupational therapists and their collaborators have been in the forefront of investigators showing that these repositioning maneuvers are effective treatments (Cohen & Jerabek, 1999; Cohen Kimball, 2004a, 2005; Macias, Lambert, Massingale, Ellensohn, & Fritz, 2000; Steenerson & Cronin, 1996; Steenerson, Cronin, & Marbach, 2005).

Appendixes

The following Appendixes outline the basic knowledge needed to understand and treat vestibular disorders, the effects of vestibular disorders on occupational performance, and the types of interventions occupational therapists use. The appendices are not exhaustive. Further knowledge of specific conditions may be needed in some circumstances, particularly when clients have more than one diagnosis or health condition. Also, by the nature of growth in clinical skills, the division between entry-level and advanced knowledge is somewhat fluid as the practitioner learns more and advances in clinical knowledge and skill. Furthermore, the knowledge base listed here is not absolute. Research in basic and applied science continues to expand the available knowledge base. Therefore, practitioners continue to read the literature, attend continuing education courses, and otherwise engage in activities to maintain and improve their knowledge and understanding of intervention in this area, to support their evidence-based practice.

Vestibular disorders decrease the ability to be independent in many activities of daily living. In general, tasks that require rapid or repeated head movements, tasks that require good postural control, especially while standing or walking, and tasks that require good spatial orientation may be affected. Clients who have fallen or who are at risk for falls may severely restrict their movements and may actually increase their risk of falling as a result. These people often cease participation in exercise programs for strengthening, cardiovascular conditioning, weight loss, or bone health. In a few rare instances, avoiding motions or positions that elicit vertigo may even mean delaying necessary surgical procedures due to potential discomfort during postoperative bed rest.

Clients with vestibular impairments often require more time to complete routine self-care skills. They may need to adapt the environment for safety or change the way in which they perform some tasks (e.g., to sit rather than stand or to hold an object for safety while standing). They may need to reduce the amount of extraneous stimulation in the environment during task performance since divided attention becomes

Appendix 1. Basic Science Knowledge for Vestibular Rehabilitation

Detailed knowledge of the structure of the ear and vestibular labyrinth, including semicircular canals, otoliths, and vestibular nerve

Detailed knowledge of the physiology of the vestibular labyrinth, including basic understanding of the inertial mechanisms of the semicircular canals and otoliths

Understanding of central vestibular projections, including vestibular nuclei, vestibulocerebellar projections, vestibulospinal projections, vestibulo-ocular projections, and vestibulocortical projections

Understanding of multisensory interactions, including visual, vestibular, haptic, and proprioceptive

Understanding of vestibulo-autonomic interactions

Manifestations of the vestibular influence on postural control (e.g., vestibulopostural responses)

Manifestations of vestibuloocular control (e.g., vestibuloocular reflex)

Understanding of other eye movements and oculomotor responses: saccades, smooth pursuit, optokinetic responses, fixation/suppression, and interaction of vestibulo-ocular reflex with other eye movements

Manifestations of vestibular influence on spatial orientation: vertical orientation and path integration

Manifestations of vestibulo-autonomic responses

Appendix 2. Applied Science Knowledge for Vestibular Rehabilitation

Familiarity with symptoms of vestibular disorders: vertigo and oscillopsia, balance deficits, path integration impairments, autonomic signs, cognitive problems, psychosocial problems, hearing loss, and auditory/perceptual illusions on rare occasions

Familiarity with principles of objective diagnostic tests: low-frequency sinusoidal tests of the vestibuloocular reflex, bithermal caloric tests, vestibular-evoked myogenic potentials, Dix-Hallpike and side-lying tests, and computerized dynamic posturography. Advanced practitioners should be familiar with the standard techniques for recording eye movements, including electrooculography/electronystagmography and infrared videooculography. Advanced practitioners should also be familiar with related oculomotor tests and auditory screening tests.

Familiarity with peripheral vestibular disorders: Labyrinthitis/vestibular neuronitis; acute, self-limiting, recurrent, and chronic benign paroxysmal positional vertigo, Ménierè's disease, perilymph fistula, acoustic neuroma, Tullio's phenomenon, ototoxicity, and other causes of bilateral vestibular impairment

Familiarity with central vestibular disorders: presbystasis, cerebellopontine angle tumor, Arnold Chiari malformation, medulloblastoma, migraine, multiple sclerosis, Parkinson's disease and the Parkinsonian syndromes, lateral medullary syndrome and other cerebrovascular accidents, traumatic brain injury, and vertebrobasilar insufficiency

Familiarity with systemic disorders: diabetes, autoimmune disorders, especially those causing connective tissue disorders

Understanding of relevant physician subspecialties: otology/neurotology and otoneurology

Understanding of cognitive strategies and problems in dual- and multitask performance

more difficult, so they may require reduced noise, less visual clutter, or fewer tasks requiring simultaneous attention. Therefore, they may become less efficient when performing tasks.

Many clients deliberately constrain their lives, becoming less active within and outside the home. So, they may abandon activities that they consider to be nonessential and reduce their participation in essential tasks. Many people stop driving or drive only within their neighborhoods and avoid highway driving. They may even change jobs to reduce travel or to avoid other job-related requirements that elicit vertigo or disequilibrium. Many people with vestibular disorders stop socializing or attending worship services because they are embarrassed by their ataxic gaits and do not want to give the appearance of intoxication. Some clients, who have vertigo when they bow during required prayers or who are unable to kneel while praying, may feel spiritually bereft. These problems can affect relationships with family, friends, and coworkers. Even the most understanding spouses may become upset when intimate sexual activity is interrupted by vertigo, quiet time together while taking a walk is made unpleasant due to repeated stumbling or drifting back and forth, and the affected individual may no longer be able to participate in shared sports or other exercise activities. See Appendixes 3–8 for further examples.

Specific evaluation and intervention skills are used in vestibular rehabilitation. The occupational therapy practitioner who works in this specialty must be familiar with the evaluation skills in Appendix 9 and the intervention skills in Appendix 10.

Appendix 3. Examples of Impact on Activities of Daily Living

Eating: Leaning across a table to pass something

Bathing: Bending to reach the legs, feet, perineal area, closing eyes to wash hair

Toileting: Bending to wipe, bending to pull garments up or down, maintaining balance while standing to urinate (males), twisting to reach toilet paper if behind toilet

Transferring: Sit-to-stand transfers from toilet, other seats

Grooming and hygiene: Bending the head forward to groom hair or brush teeth

Taking medication: Bending the head back to swallow medication

Sexual activity: Being in the superior position and weight shifting or moving the head rapidly; stability on water bed or other positioning furniture

Sleep: Head movements during sleep, changing sleeping positions, or maintaining the head in certain positions during sleep will elicit vertigo and cause waking, possibly nausea, and disequilibrium while groggy

Instrumental Activities of Daily Living

Meal preparation, cleaning, other home management skills: Bending down, looking into high or low cabinets or shelves, and tasks that require repetitive head movements may all elicit symptoms. Task performance may be compromised or the task may be abandoned altogether.

Gardening, yard work: Tasks may be performed less efficiently or abandoned; falls may occur on uneven ground.

Vehicle care: Car washing and changing oil and filters may be difficult or impossible.

Child, elder, and pet care: Tasks that involve picking up and carrying loads, bending rapidly, performing or assisting in transfers, diaper changing, cleaning up messes on floor

Community mobility: Driving will be more difficult, especially under conditions of reduced visibility, and may be abandoned or performed only for limited errands.

Shopping: Navigating stores, carrying packages, bending to pick up items, scanning shelves for items will be more difficult and may be abandoned.

Safety: Ascending/descending fire escapes and stairs, dim areas with only emergency lighting

Play, leisure, social participation, religious activities: Visual motion sensitivity, difficulty kneeling, navigating in crowds, vertigo elicited by repetitive head movements or bending the head down; activities and rituals may be severely restricted or abandoned.

Work, either paid employment or volunteer jobs: Symptoms elicited by a wide range of tasks will cause reduced efficiency and sometimes total inability to perform some jobs, depending on task demands.

Appendix 4. Examples of Performance Skills Affected by Vestibular Impairments

Posture: Standing balance is impaired in most people with vestibular impairments. People may tilt the head and/or body off the vertical. They may have difficulty attaining and maintaining upright standing. This skill is particularly difficult when visual cues are absent or decreased. Static head and trunk posture while seated are sometimes impaired; dynamic sitting balance may also be impaired.

Mobility: Mobility skills are manifested as veering toward one side while walking, ataxic gait, and falling or stumbling, particularly on uneven surfaces. Load compensation skills are impaired. Clients may need to use light touch to improve orientation and stability.

Coordination: Dual-task performance skill is decreased.

Energy: Routine tasks take more energy than usual, and endurance is decreased.

Appendix 5. Examples of Performance Patterns Affected by Vestibular Impairments

Habits: Skill components of habits may be disrupted, and performance efficiency may be reduced, increasing the cognitive load and increasing the difficulty of performing habitual skills that were previously easy to perform (e.g., basic activities of daily living may have to be performed with modifications).

Routines: Due to effects on performance skills, routines are less efficient and may need to be changed or abandoned altogether (e.g., hair washing may require supervision for safety and may take too long in the morning before work, so the client's morning and evening routines may be changed).

Roles: Some roles may be reduced or even abandoned, with consequent detrimental economic and psychosocial effects (e.g., clients with Ménierè's disease may have to leave their jobs).

Appendix 6. Examples of Context Affected by Vestibular Impairments

Physical: The physical environment may require modifications for safety (e.g., installing bathroom grab bars), or the home environment may require significant change (e.g., removing throw rugs, changing lighting patterns).

Social: Misunderstanding of symptoms and problems by family, friends, and significant others may lead to hard feelings, reduced participation in socialization, changes in preferred social environments. These problems may occur due to decreased self-confidence, fear of falling, and a history of falls.

Spiritual: Falls, vertigo, decreased concentration, and decreased ability in dual task performance, which all lead to decreased performance in vocational and vocational activities and decreased participation in the community, can cause decreased sense of self-worth, self-doubt, and decreased joy in life.

Virtual: Visual motion sensitivity may lead to avoidance of virtual environments.

Appendix 7. Examples of Activity Demands Affected by Vestibular Impairments

Timing: Tasks may take longer than before.

Space demands: Lighting, flooring, and support surfaces may have to be changed.

Social demands: Reduced social interaction per task may be required due to reduced tolerance for auditory and visual noise.

Required bodily functions: Reduced function of vestibulo-ocular reflex, vestibulospinal reflex, and reduced spatial orientation skills all affect functional performance.

Appendix 8. Examples of Client Factors Affected by Vestibular Impairments

Mental functions: Reduced attention skills, reduced ability for dual task performance

Sensory functions: Reduced vestibular function, sometimes reduced auditory function

Neuromuscular functions: Reduced postural control, reduced dynamic visual acuity, impaired gait

Vestibular labyrinth: In some instances, structural abnormalities in the physical labyrinth may be present, but these features cannot be observed; they may only be inferred.

Appendix 9. Occupational Therapy Evaluation Skills for Vestibular Rehabilitation

Detailed occupational and health histories relevant to symptoms

Objective clinical tests involving the vestibuloocular reflex head thrusts, Dix-Hallpike and sidelying maneuvers, and other tests of positional vertigo in lateral and anterior canals

Tests of path integration skill

Oculomotor tests: saccades, pursuit, optokinetic nystagmus, vergence, visual/vestibuloocular reflex interaction, evaluation of spontaneous nystagmus

Standardized and nonstandardized tests of standing and walking balance, including Clinical Test of Sensory Organization on Balance, Functional Reach, Berg Balance Scale, Get Up and Go/ Timed Up and Go, Dynamic Gait Index, expert observation of other gait and balance skills including stair climbing, subtle gait deficits, and weight-shifting deficits

Qualitative self-evaluations of ADL independence: Activities-Specific Balance Confidence scale, Dizziness Handicap Inventory, and Vestibular Disorders Activities of Daily Living scale

Tests of dynamic visual acuity and oscillopsia

Measures to evaluate vertigo: head shaking, repetitive activities

Cognitive and psychosocial assessments: qualitative assessments and self-report on scales

Evaluation of independence in activities of daily living, including subtle changes and problems

Home, work, and driving safety

Appendix 10. Occupational Therapy Intervention Skills for Vestibular Rehabilitation

Repositioning treatments for benign paroxysmal positional vertigo, including canalith repositioning, liberatory maneuvers, log-rolling maneuvers, Brandt Daroff exercises, other repositioning exercises and activities

Vertigo habituation exercises and activity programs

Gaze stabilization exercises and activities, including eye–head coordination tasks

Balance therapy: exercises and activities for "static" standing, weight shifting, and balance control; exercises and activities for "dynamic" balance control during translation through space, leading to independence in dual task performance and safety during obstacle avoidance tasks

Home and work safety, including environmental modifications for lighting, flooring, modification of work area

Training in mobility skills on the bed; transfers to and from the floor, in the home, and in the external environment for falls prevention (e.g., use of a ladder, elevator, escalator, stairs, opening door, transfers to and from automobile, and functional mobility through visually challenging environments and environments with challenging support surfaces)

Knowledge of community and online resources for patient information

Patient education about condition, symptoms

Specific to Ménierè's disease patients: in coordination with nursing, work on meal-planning skills if dietary restriction is recommended by the physician

In coordination with audiology, for patients with hearing loss, recommend communication and functional devices for telephone, alarm clock, and other devices for which sound is important; recommendations for modification of work and other tasks, as needed, for hearing loss

Recommendation of assistive devices for balance and safety during standing, walking, carrying objects, and other activities of daily living

Task modification to reduce cognitive load during dual- and multitask performance; dual-task performance training

Glossary

Benign paroxysmal positional vertigo
A common disorder of the vestibular system characterized by vertigo elicited by head movements in the pitch plane and characterized by a positive response on the Dix–Hallpike maneuver.

Disequilibrium
Poor balance.

Labyrinthitis
Inflammation or disease of the vestibular labyrinth of the inner ear.

Ménière's disease
A disorder of the inner ear affecting both the auditory and vestibular systems. It is characterized by sensorineural hearing loss on at least one occasion, two or more spontaneous episodes of vertigo lasting at least 20 minutes, and tinnitus or aural fullness in the affected ear. Nystagmus is present during an attack (Committee on Hearing and Equilibrium, American Academy of Otolaryngology—Head and Neck Surgery, 1995).

Neurotologist
An otolaryngologist who specializes in ear and inner-ear disorders, including vestibular disorders.

Nystagmus
A stereotyped combination of repetitive slow- and fast-phase eye movements. The slow phase, usually difficult to observe with the naked eye, represents compensatory vestibulo-ocular or optokinetic responses; the fast phase represents rapid saccades that reset the position of the globe in the eye socket.

Optokinetic responses
Conjugate eye movements used to follow a full-field moving visual stimulus (i.e., when the entire visual scene moves around the person).

Oscillopsia
The illusion of object motion during head movement.

Otolaryngologist
A physician who specializes in ear, nose, and throat disorders.

Otoneurologist
A neurologist who specializes in vestibular and auditory disorders.

Presbystasis
Disequilibrium of aging. This diagnosis excludes known causes of balance problems, such as central neurologic conditions, peripheral vestibular impairments, or peripheral neuropathies that affect the lower extremities (e.g., diabetic neuropathies).

Pursuit
Also known as *smooth pursuit*. Conjugate eye movements are used to follow a discrete moving visual stimulus.

Saccades
Conjugate eye movements in which the eyes move for one of three reasons: (1) as the quick phase of nystagmus, to reset the position of the globe in the eye socket; (2) for gaze error correction (i.e., to catch up with a visual stimulus that is moving too fast for pursuit movements); and (3) volitional movements to look around a stationary visual environment. Saccades are the only volitional eye movements that we are able to generate. (You are using saccades to read this page.)

Spatial orientation
Awareness of one's position relative to gravity and the environment.

Vergence
Disconjugate eye movements used to make the eyes move toward or away from each other, in order to focus on an object.

Vertigo
The illusion of self-motion (e.g., spinning, falling).

Vestibular rehabilitation
The use of activities and exercise to treat vertigo, balance problems, functional limitations, and disability caused by impairments in the vestibular system.

Vestibular system
The sensory system with receptors in the vestibular labyrinth of the inner ear. It detects head motion and contributes to control of posture, eye movements, and spatial orientation. The brain pathways include the vestibular portion of Cranial Nerve VIII; the vestibular nuclei; the parts of the cerebellum that receive and process vestibular signals; the projections from the vestibular nuclei that descend in the spinal cord via the vestibulospinal tracts; the projections from the vestibular nuclei that ascend in the medial longitudinal fasciculus to Cranial Nerves III, IV, and VI to control the vestibulo-ocular reflex; and the smaller projections that ascend from the vestibular nuclei to the thalamus and related nuclei with further small projections to the vestibular cortex.

References

American Medical Association. (2006). *Current procedural terminology* (2006 ed.). Chicago: Author.

American Occupational Therapy Association. (2002). Occupational therapy practice framework: Domain and process. *American Journal of Occupational Therapy, 56*, 609–639.

American Occupational Therapy Association. (2004). Guidelines for supervision, roles, and responsibilities during the delivery of occupational therapy services. *American Journal of Occupational Therapy, 58*, 663–667.

Cawthorne, T. (1944). The physiological basis for head exercises. *Journal of the Chartered Society of Physiotherapy, 29*, 106–107.

Cohen, H. (1992). Vestibular rehabilitation reduces functional disability. *Otolaryngology—Head and Neck Surgery, 107*, 638–643.

Cohen, H. S. (2006). Disability and rehabilitation in the dizzy patient. *Current Opinion in Neurology, 19*, 49–54.

Cohen, H., Ewell, L. R., & Jenkins, H. A. (1995). Disability in Ménière's disease. *Archives of Otolaryngology, 121*, 29–33.

Cohen, H. S., & Jerabek, J. (1999). Effectiveness of liberatory maneuvers for benign paroxysmal positional vertigo of the posterior canal. *Laryngoscope, 109*, 584–590.

Cohen, H., Kane-Wineland, M., Miller, L. V., & Hatfield, C. L. (1995). Occupation and visual/vestibular interaction in vestibular rehabilitation. *Otolaryngology—Head and Neck Surgery, 112*, 526–532.

Cohen, H. S., & Kimball, K. T. (2000). Development of the Vestibular Disorders Activities of Daily Living Scale. *Archives of Otolaryngology, 126*, 881–887.

Cohen, H. S., & Kimball, K. T. (2002). Improvements in path integration after vestibular rehabilitation. *Journal of Vestibular Research, 12,* 47–51.

Cohen, H. S., & Kimball, K. T. (2003). Increased independence and decreased vertigo after vestibular rehabilitation. *Otolaryngology—Head and Neck Surgery, 128,* 560–566.

Cohen, H. S., & Kimball, K. T. (2004a). Treatment variations on the Epley maneuver for benign paroxysmal positional vertigo. *American Journal of Otolaryngology, 25,* 33–37.

Cohen, H. S., & Kimball, K. T. (2004b). Changes in a repetitive head movement task after vestibular rehabilitation. *Clinical Rehabilitation, 18,* 125–131.

Cohen, H. S., & Kimball, K. T. (2004c). Decreased ataxia and improved balance after vestibular rehabilitation. *Otolaryngology—Head and Neck Surgery, 130,* 418–425.

Cohen, H. S., & Kimball, K. T. (2005). Effectiveness of treatments for benign paroxysmal positional vertigo of the posterior canal. *Otology and Neurotology, 26,* 1034–1040.

Cohen, H. S., Kimball, K. T., & Adams, A. (2000). Application of the Vestibular Disorders Activities of Daily Living Scale. *Laryngoscope, 110,* 1204–1209.

Cohen, H., Miller, L. V., Kane-Wineland, M., & Hatfield, C. L. (1995). Case Report—Vestibular rehabilitation with graded occupations. *American Journal of Occupational Therapy, 49,* 362–367.

Cohen, H. S., Wells, J., Kimball, K. T., & Owsley, C. (2003). Driving disability in dizziness. *Journal of Safety Research, 34*(4), 361–369.

Committee on Hearing and Equilibrium, American Academy of Otolaryngology—Head and Neck Surgery. (1995). Guidelines for the diagnosis and evaluation of therapy in Ménière's disease. *Otolaryngology—Head and Neck Surgery, 113,* 181–185.

Cooksey, F. S. (1945). Physical medicine. *Practitioner, 155,* 300–305.

Cooksey, F. S. (1946). Rehabilitation in vestibular injuries. *Proceedings of the Royal Society of Medicine, 39,* 273–278.

Eagger, S., Luxon, L. M., Davies, R. A., Coelho, A., & Ron, M. A. (1992). Psychiatric morbidity in clients with peripheral vestibular disorder: A clinical and neuro-otological study. *Journal of Neurology, Neurosurgery, and Psychiatry, 55,* 383–387.

Farber, S. D. (1989). Living with Ménière's disease: An occupational therapist's perspective. *American Journal of Occupational Therapy, 43,* 341–343.

Macias, J. D., Lambert, K. M., Massingale, S., Ellensohn, A., & Fritz, J. A. (2000). Variables affecting treatment in benign paroxysmal positional vertigo. *Laryngoscope, 110,* 1921–1924.

Morris, P. A. (1991). A habituation approach to treating vertigo in occupational therapy. *American Journal of Occupational Therapy, 45,* 556–558.

Steenerson, R. L., & Cronin, G. W. (1996). Comparison of the canalith repositioning procedure and vestibular habituation training in forty patients with benign paroxysmal positional vertigo. *Otolaryngology—Head and Neck Surgery, 1214,* 61–64.

Steenerson, R. L., Cronin, G. W., & Marbach, P. M. (2005). Effectiveness of treatment techniques in 932 cases of benign paroxysmal positional vertigo. *Laryngoscope, 115,* 226–231.

Yardley, L., & Hallam, R. S. (1996). Psychosocial aspects of balance and gait disorders. In A. M. Bronstein, T. Brandt, & M. Woollacott (Eds.), *Clinical disorders of balance, posture and gait* (pp. 251–267). London: Arnold.

Yardley, L., Luxon, L. M., & Haacke, N. P. (1994). A longitudinal study of symptoms, anxiety, and subjective well-being in clients with vertigo. *Clinical Otolaryngology and Allied Sciences, 19*, 109–116.

Yardley, L., & Putman, J. (1992). Quantitative analysis of factors contributing to handicap and distress in vertiginous clients: A questionnaire study. *Clinical Otolaryngology and Allied Sciences, 17*, 231–236.

Additional Reading

Aw, S. T., Halmagyi, G. M., Black, R. A., Curthoys, I. S., Yavor, R. A., & Todd, M. J. (1999). Head impulses reveal loss of individual semicircular canal function. *Journal of Vestibular Research, 9*, 173–180.

Baloh, R. W., Furman, J. M. R., Halmagyi, M., & Allum, J. H. J. (1995). Recent advances in clinical neurotology. *Journal of Vestibular Research, 5*, 231–252.

Baloh, R. W., & Halmagyi, G. M. (Eds.). (1996). *Disorders of the vestibular system.* New York: Oxford University Press.

Baloh, R. W., & Honrubia, V. (1990). *Clinical neurophysiology of the vestibular system* (2nd ed.). Philadelphia: F. A. Davis.

Black, R. A., Halmagyi, G. M., Thurtell, M. J., Todd, M. J., & Curthoys, I. S. (2005). The active head-impulse test in unilateral peripheral vestibulopathy. *Annals of Neurology, 62*, 290–293.

Brandt, T. (1998). *Vertigo: Its multisensory syndromes.* Berlin: Springer-Verlag.

Brandt, T., Steddin, S., & Daroff, R. B. (1994). Therapy for benign paroxysmal positioning vertigo, revisited. *Neurology, 44*, 796–800.

Bronstein, A. M., Brandt, T., & Woollacott, M. (Eds.). (1996). *Clinical disorders of balance, posture and gait.* London: Arnold/Hodder Headline PLC.

Campbell, A. J., Robertson, M. C., La Grow, S. J., Kerse, N. M., Sanderson, G. F., Jacobs, R. J., et al. (2005, October). Randomised controlled trial of prevention of falls in people aged 75 with severe visual impairment: The VIP trial. *British Medical Journal, 331*(7520), 817. Retrieved March 21, 2006, from http://bmj.bmjjournals.com/cgi/reprint_abr/331/7520/817

Cawthorne, T. (1946). Vestibular injuries. *Proceedings of the Royal Society of Medicine, 39*, 270–273.

Chronister, K. M. (2003). Divided attention: The role that cognition plays in fall prevention programs has been overlooked. *Rehab Management, 16*, 30, 32–33.

Chronister, K. (2004). Cognition: The missing link in fall-prevention programs. *Rehab Management, 9*, 11–14.

Clemson, L., Cumming, R. G., Kendig, H., Swann, M., Heard, R., & Taylor, K. (2004). The effectiveness of a community-based program for reducing the incidence of falls in the elderly: A randomized trial. *Journal of the American Geriatric Society, 52*, 1487–1494.

Cohen, H. (1994). Vestibular rehabilitation improves daily life function. *American Journal of Occupational Therapy, 48*, 919–925.

Cohen, H. (1998). *Special senses 2: The vestibular system. Neuroscience for rehabilitation.* Philadelphia: Lippincott Williams & Wilkins.

Cohen, H. S. (2000). Vertigo and balance disorders: Vestibular rehabilitation. *Occupational Therapy Practice, 5*, 14–18.

Cohen, H. S. (2004). Vestibular rehabilitation and stroke. In G. Gillen & A. Burkhardt (Eds.), *Stroke rehabilitation: A function-based approach* (2nd ed., pp. 164–171). St. Louis, MO: Mosby.

Cohen, H. S. (in press). Disability in vestibular disorders. In S. J. Herdman (Ed.), *Vestibular rehabilitation* (3rd ed). Philadelphia: F. A. Davis.

Cohen, H., Blatchly, C. A., & Gombash, L. L. (1993). A study of the clinical test of sensory interaction and balance. *Physical Therapy, 73,* 346–351.

Cohen, H., Friedman, E. M., Lai, D., Duncan, N., Pellicer, M., & Sulek, M. (1997). Balance in children with otitis media with effusion. *International Journal of Pediatric Oto-Rhino-Laryngology, 42,* 107–115.

Cohen, H. S., & Gavia, J. A. (1998). A task for assessing vertigo elicited by repetitive head movements. *American Journal of Occupational Therapy, 52,* 644–649.

Cohen, H., Heaton, L. G., Congdon, S. L., & Jenkins, H. A. (1996). Changes in sensory organization test scores with age. *Age and Ageing, 25,* 39–44.

Cohen, H. S., Kimball, K. T., & Stewart, M. G. (2004). Benign paroxysmal positional vertigo and co-morbid conditions. *ORL—Journal of Oto-Rhino-Laryngology and Related Specialties, 66,* 11–15.

Cohen, H., Rubin, A. M., & Gombash, L. L. (1991). The team approach to intervention of the dizzy client. *Archives of Physical Medicine and Rehabilitation, 73,* 703–708.

Colebatch, J. G. (2001). Vestibular evoked potentials. *Current Opinion in Neurology, 14,* 21–26.

Colebatch, J. G., Halmagyi, G. M., & Skuse, N. F. (1994). Myogenic potentials generated by a click-evoked vestibulocollic reflex. *Journal of Neurology, Neurosurgery, and Psychiatry, 57,* 190–107.

Cronin, G. W. (1990). Vestibular rehab enhances patient's quality of life. *Advance for Occupational Therapists, 6*(43), 2.

Crowe, T. K., Deitz, J. C., Richardson, P. K., & Atwater, S. W. (1990). Interrater reliability of the Pediatric Clinical Test of Sensory Interaction for Balance. *Physical and Occupational Therapy in Pediatrics, 10,* 1–27.

Cumming, R. G., Thomas, M., Szonyi, G., Frampton, G., Salkeld, G., & Clemson, L. (2001). Adherence to occupational therapist recommendations for home modifications for falls prevention. *American Journal of Occupational Therapy, 55,* 641–648.

Davison, J., Bond, J., Dawson, P., Steen, I. N., & Kenny, R. A. (2005). Patients with recurrent falls attending accident and emergency benefit from multifactorial intervention—A randomized controlled trial. *Age and Ageing, 34,* 162–168.

De la Meilleure, G., Dehaene, I., Depondt, M., Damman, W., Crevits, L., & Vanhooren, G. (1996). Benign paroxysmal positional vertigo of the horizontal canal. *Journal of Neurology, Neurosurgery, and Psychiatry, 60,* 68–71.

Dix, M. R. (1974). Intervention of vertigo. *Physiotherapy, 60,* 380–384.

Dix, M. R. (1976). The physiological basis and practical value of head exercises in the intervention of vertigo. *Practitioner, 217,* 919–924.

Dix, M. R. (1984). Rehabilitation of vertigo. In M. R. Dix & J. D. Hood (Eds.), *Vertigo* (pp. 467–479). Chichester, NY: Wiley.

Fife, T. D., Tusa, R. J., Furman, J. M., Zee, D. S., Frohman, E., Baloh, R. W., et al. (2000). Assessment: Vestibular testing techniques in adults and children. Report of the Therapeutics and Technology Assessment Subcommittee of the American Academy of Neurology. *Neurology, 55,* 1431–1441.

Gottshall, K., Gray, N., & Drake, A. I. (2005). A unique collaboration of female medical providers within the United States Armed Forces: Rehabilitation of a marine with post-concussive vestibulopathy. *Work, 24,* 381–386.

Halmagyi, G. M., & Curthoys, I. A. (1988). A clinical sign of canal paresis. *Archives of Neurology, 45,* 737–739.

Hecker, H. C., Haug, C. O., & Herndon, J. W. (1974). Intervention of the vertiginous client using Cawthorne's vestibular exercises. *Laryngoscope, 84,* 2065–2072.

Hillman, E. J., Bloomberg, J. J., McDonald, V. P., & Cohen, H. S. (1999). Dynamic visual acuity while walking in normal and labyrinthine-deficient clients. *Journal of Vestibular Research, 9,* 49–57.

Honrubia, V., Bell, T. S., Harris, M. R., Baloh, R. W., & Fisher, L. M. (1996). Quantitative evaluation of dizziness characteristics and impact on quality of life. *American Journal of Otology, 17,* 595–602.

Horak, F. B., Shumway-Cook, A., Crowe, T. K., & Black, F. O. (1988). Vestibular function and motor proficiency of children with impaired hearing, or with learning disability and motor impairments. *Developmental Medicine and Child Neurology, 30,* 64–79.

Jacobson, G. P., & Newman, C. W. (1990). The development of the Dizziness Handicap Inventory. *Archives of Otolaryngology, 116,* 424–427.

Jacobson, G. P., Newman, C. W., & Kartush, J. M. (1993). *Handbook of balance function testing.* St. Louis, MO: Mosby/YearBook.

Konnur, M. K. (2000). Vertigo and vestibular rehabilitation. *Postgraduate Medicine, 46,* 222–223.

McCabe, B. F. (1970). Labyrinthine exercises in the intervention of diseases characterized by vertigo: Their physiologic basis and methodology. *Laryngoscope, 80,* 1429–1433.

Medeiros, I. R. T., Bittar, R. S. M., Pedalini, E. B., Lorenzi, M. C., Formigoni, L. G., et al. (2005). Vestibular rehabilitation therapy in children. *Otology and Neurotology, 26,* 699–703.

Myers, A. M., Powell, L. E., Maki, B. E., Holliday, P. J., Brawley, L. R., & Sherk, W. (1996). Psychological indicators of balance confidence: Relationship to actual and perceived abilities. *Journal of Gerontology: Medical Science, 51A,* M37–M43.

Norré, M. E., & De Weerdt, W. (1979). Vestibular habituation training: Technique and first results—Preliminary report. *Acta Oto-Rhino-Laryngologica Belgica, 33,* 347–364.

Parnes, L. S., & Sindwani, R. (1997). Impact of vestibular disorders on fitness to drive: A consensus of the American Neurotology Society. *American Journal of Otology, 18,* 79–85.

Rine, R. M., Braswell, J., Fisher, D., Joyce, K., Kalar, K., & Shaffer, M. (2004). Improvement of motor development and postural control following intervention in children with sensorineural hearing loss and vestibular impairment. *International Journal of Pediatric Oto-Rhino-Laryngology, 68,* 1141–1148.

Sherlock, J. (1996). Getting into balance. *Rehab Management, 9,* 33–38.

Shumway-Cook, A., & Horak, F. B. (1986). Assessing the influence of sensory interaction on balance. *Physical Therapy, 66,* 1548–1550.

Shumway-Cook, A., & Horak, F. B. (1989). Vestibular rehabilitation: An exercise approach to managing symptoms of vestibular dysfunction. *Seminars in Hearing, 10,* 196–208.

Sindwani, R., & Parnes, L. S. (1997). Reporting of vestibular clients who are unfit to drive: Survey of Canadian otolaryngologists. *Journal of Otolaryngology, 26,* 104–111.

Steultjens, E. M. J., Dekker, J., Bouter, L. M., Jellma, S., Bakker, E. B., & van den Ende, C. H. M. (2004). Occupational therapy for community dwelling elderly people: A systematic review. *Age and Ageing, 33,* 453–460.

Uneri, A., & Turkdogan, D. (2003). Evaluation of vestibular functions in children with vertigo attacks. *Archives of Disease in Childhood, 88,* 510–511.

Whitney, S. L., Poole, J. L., & Cass, S. P. (1998). A review of balance instruments for older adults. *American Journal of Occupational Therapy, 52,* 666–671.

Wilson, V. J., & Melvill Jones, G. (1979). *Mammalian vestibular physiology.* New York: Plenum.

Wilson, V. J., & Melvill Jones, G. (1985). *Adaptive mechanisms of gaze control.* New York: Plenum.

Yardley, L. (1994). Prediction of handicap and emotional distress in clients with recurrent vertigo: Symptoms, coping strategies, control beliefs, and reciprocal causation. *Social Science and Medicine, 39,* 573–581.

Yardley, L., Burgneau, J., Nazareth, I., & Luxon, L. (1998). Neuro-otological and psychiatric abnormalities in a community sample of people with dizziness: A blind, controlled investigation. *Journal of Neurology, Neurosurgery and Psychiatry, 65,* 679–684.

Other Information Resources

American Academy of Otolaryngology—Head and Neck Surgery
One Prince Street
Alexandria, VA 22314-3357
703-836-4444
www.entnet.org
This group is the professional organization for otolaryngologists, including neurotologists. To find a neurotologist in your area, see the "Find an ENT" link. See also useful patient information brochures.

Anatomical Chart Company
Lippincott Williams & Wilkins
www.lww.com/anatomicalchart/
They produce good charts and three-dimensional models of the vestibular labyrinth.

Journal of Vestibular Research
Eye and Ear Institute
203 Lothrop Street, Suite 500
Pittsburgh, PA 15213
e-mail: jvr@upmc.edu
Web address: www.jvr-web.org
This journal specializes in publishing research on basic and clinical vestibular sciences, including research on vestibular rehabilitation and balance disorders.

National Institute on Deafness and Other Communication Disorders (NIDCD)
National Institutes of Health
31 Center Drive, MSC 2320
Bethesda, MD 20892-2320
800-241-1044
www.nidcd.nih.gov
The NIH funds much of the biomedical and biobehavioral research in this country. The NIDCD, an institute of the NIH, funds research on balance and vestibular function, including research on vestibular rehabilitation. See their Web page for free patient information brochures and a tutorial for patients with balance problems.

Vestibular Disorders Association
PO Box 4467
Portland OR 97208
Telephone: 800-837-8428
Telephone in Oregon: 503-229-7705
e-mail: veda@vestibular.org
Web address: www.vestibular.org
This patient advocacy group has useful information for patients about a variety of vestibular disorders.
They also maintain a resource list of health care professionals who specialize in care of people with vestibular disorders.

Authors
Helen S. Cohen, EdD, OTR, FAOTA, *Chairperson*
Ann Burkhardt, OTD, OTR/L, BCN, FAOTA
Gaye W. Cronin, OTD, OTR
Mary Jo McGuire, MS, OTR, FAOTA

for

The Commission on Practice
Susanne Smith Roley, MS, OTR/L, FAOTA, *Chairperson*

Adopted by the Representative Assembly 2006C405

Reviewed by the Commission on Practice September 2010

Note. This document replaces the 2000 document *Specialized Knowledge and Skills in Adult Vestibular Rehabilitation for Occupational Therapy Practice,* previously published in the *American Journal of Occupational Therapy, 55,* 661–665.

Specialized Knowledge and Skills in Feeding, Eating, and Swallowing for Occupational Therapy Practice

Introduction

Occupational therapy's long-standing expertise in activities of daily living includes involvement in the feeding, eating, and swallowing performance of individuals across the life span (American Occupational Therapy Association [AOTA], 2002). Both occupational therapists and occupational therapy assistants[1] provide essential services in the comprehensive management of feeding, eating, and swallowing problems. These problems can be wide ranging and may include physical difficulty (e.g., bringing food to the mouth), processing food in the mouth (e.g., motor or sensory deficits), dysphagia, psychosocially based eating disorders (e.g., food obsessions, maladaptive eating habits), dysfunction related to cognitive impairments (e.g., understanding nutrition or food preparation), surgical intervention, and neurological impairments, as well as positioning problems that affect feeding, eating, and swallowing. Interventions focused on occupations of daily living include facilitating an individual's ability to participate in feeding and eating activities that are valued and meaningful to that person, such as learning to eat independently, joining friends for lunch, or feeding a child. Occupational therapists and occupational therapy assistants possess the education, experience, knowledge, and skills necessary in the evaluation and intervention of feeding, eating, and swallowing problems. Physical, cognitive, social, emotional, and cultural elements of feeding, eating, and swallowing are considered in evaluation and intervention.

The purpose of this document is to describe the knowledge and skills that are necessary for occupational therapists and occupational therapy assistants to provide comprehensive feeding, eating, and swallowing management and services. It provides information on occupational therapists' and occupational therapy assistants' roles in feeding, eating, and swallowing; outlines advanced-level knowledge and skills; and defines feeding-, eating-, and swallowing-related terms.

Occupational Therapy's Role in Feeding, Eating, and Swallowing Management

Feeding, Eating, and Swallowing

Feeding and eating occur within the social environment and often include family members and caregivers as part of the process. Thus, when occupational therapy practitioners address feeding, eating, and swallowing concerns, the collaboration with and involvement of family members and caregivers as well as other professionals is paramount.

Feeding, eating, and swallowing are complex activities that require effective, coordinated function of the motor, sensory, and cognitive systems. In recent years, the complexity of occupational therapy services to address these issues has grown. Feeding, eating, and swallowing services now are often provided to clients who have complicated, specialized problems and who may be medically fragile. In addition,

---

[1]*Occupational therapists* are responsible for all aspects of occupational therapy service delivery and are accountable for the safety and effectiveness of the occupational therapy service delivery process. *Occupational therapy assistants* deliver occupational therapy services under the supervision of and in partnership with an occupational therapist (AOTA, 2004).

new technologies are increasingly available for evaluation and intervention of swallowing or dysphagia management. Thus, in a variety of situations, occupational therapists and occupational therapy assistants demonstrate baseline knowledge in feeding, eating, and swallowing and may provide advanced-level knowledge and skills in the field of dysphagia management.

Feeding, eating, and swallowing are interdependent activities, and definitions of each term overlap in literature sources. For purposes of this paper, broad definitions are noted. *Feeding* is the term used to describe "the process of setting up, arranging, and bringing food [or fluid] from the plate or cup to the mouth; sometimes called self-feeding" (AOTA, 2006a). *Eating* is defined as "the ability to keep and manipulate food or fluid in the mouth and swallow it; eating and swallowing are often used interchangeably" (AOTA, 2006a). Feeding and eating, essential to human functioning for nourishment of the body, is a form of social interaction and is involved in many facets of a person's culture—from leisure to professional activities. *Swallowing* involves a complicated act in which food, fluid, medication, or saliva is moved from the mouth through the pharynx and esophagus into the stomach (AOTA, 2006a). Thus, feeding, eating, and swallowing are strongly influenced by psychosocial, cultural, and environmental factors. As part of the evaluation and intervention process, occupational therapists and occupational therapy assistants under the supervision of an occupational therapist consider comprehensive management of feeding, eating, and swallowing problems; adaptive feeding equipment ranging from modified utensils to sophisticated feeding equipment (e.g., the Winsford Feeder); the physical and sensory difficulty of bringing food, liquid, or medication to the mouth; sensory processing issues in the mouth (e.g., oral defensiveness); management of mechanical devices for feeding; dysphagia; psychosocially based eating disorders (e.g., anorexia, bulimia); behaviorally based eating disorders (e.g., selective eating); dysfunction related to cognitive impairments, neurological impairments, or surgical intervention; and positioning problems that affect feeding, eating, and swallowing.

Feeding, eating, and swallowing are within the domain and scope of practice for occupational therapy. Occupational therapists and occupational therapy assistants have the knowledge and skills necessary to take a lead role in the evaluation and intervention of feeding, eating, and swallowing problems. Further, occupational therapists have the entry-level knowledge and skills to evaluate oral and pharyngeal swallowing function.

Occupational Therapy Services

Occupational therapy practitioners[2] use their knowledge and skills to provide services over a broad range of ages, medical conditions, and social or cultural situations. For many clients, feeding, eating, and swallowing issues are quite complex. For instance, in populations with complicated feeding problems such as post-surgical cancer patients, patients in intensive care units, or young infants, the interplay of medical and developmental factors is complex and requires advanced-level knowledge to provide safe and effective service. As foundational skills in understanding impairments in feeding, eating, and swallowing, occupational therapists and occupational therapy assistants receive education in the structure and function of the human body, including the biological and physical sciences (e.g., anatomy, physiology, neuroanatomy, kinesiology), human development throughout the life span, and human behavior, including the behavioral and social sciences (Accreditation Council for Occupational Therapy Education, 2006). They develop clinical-reasoning skills to consider the interplay of physical, cognitive, environmental, and sociocultural factors in providing effective services for feeding, eating, and swallowing dysfunction.

As part of therapeutic services, occupational therapists are trained to conduct comprehensive evaluations, which include selecting, administering, and interpreting assessment measures. They also develop specific intervention plans and provide therapeutic interventions.

---

[2]When the term *occupational therapy practitioner* is used in this document, it refers to both occupational therapists and occupational therapy assistants (AOTA, 2006b).

The occupational therapist assumes the ultimate responsibility for the delivery of occupational therapy services. Occupational therapy assistants are trained to provide services under the supervision of and in collaboration with an occupational therapist (AOTA, 2004). During the evaluation process, occupational therapy assistants may gather data and administer selected assessment tools or measures for which they have demonstrated competence.

During intervention, both occupational therapists and occupational therapy assistants select, administer, and adapt activities that support the intervention plan developed by the occupational therapist. Practitioners must always adhere to state and agency regulatory laws when providing services across these continua of care. Reimbursement for services may be available through various sources, including legislation (e.g., Individuals With Disabilities Education Act, Medicare), private insurance, Medicaid, and private pay. Information on specific entry-level knowledge and skills occupational therapists and occupational therapy assistants should have to serve clients with feeding, eating, and swallowing dysfunction can be found in Appendix A.

For both occupational therapists and occupational therapy assistants, the progression from entry-level knowledge and skills to advanced-level knowledge and skills is individualized. Although practitioners exit their academic program with the basic knowledge and skills to provide occupational therapy services to clients with feeding, eating, and swallowing dysfunction, over time they may develop additional individualized expertise such as in the area of dysphagia. Occupational therapy practitioners ensure advanced competence in feeding, eating, and swallowing by maintaining and documenting competence in practice, education, and research and by participating in professional development, educational activities, and critical examination of available evidence (AOTA, 2005a). In addition, higher level knowledge, skills, and clinical reasoning are developed through experience.

The practitioner's acquisition of advanced-level knowledge and skills as related to intervention with people with feeding, eating, and swallowing difficulties is individualized; thus, a practitioner may possess differing levels of expertise in a wide variety of skill areas and populations served by occupational therapy. For example, an occupational therapist with advanced-level skills in feeding with premature infants may possess only entry-level skills in assessing swallowing function in a client who has had a cerebral vascular accident resulting in hemiplegic weakness. It is the ethical responsibility of occupational therapists and occupational therapy assistants to ensure that they are competent in the services they provide and that they continually seek out new knowledge and techniques that apply to their clinical practice (AOTA, 2005a).

Supervision Considerations

The amount of supervision provided to an occupational therapist or occupational therapy assistant in the area of feeding, eating, and swallowing should directly relate to their training and experience and state practice acts. Occupational therapy assistants and entry-level occupational therapists should seek supervision and mentoring from a more experienced occupational therapist or an occupational therapist with advanced knowledge and skills in feeding, eating, and swallowing. The occupational therapist and occupational therapy assistant also may supervise other nonlicensed health care aides providing feeding and eating assistance to clients (AOTA, 2004). Most state practice acts mandate the frequency and duration for supervision for entry-level occupational therapists, occupational therapy assistants, and nonlicensed health care aides. The occupational therapist has the primary role in evaluation and intervention planning; the occupational therapy assistant collaborates with the occupational therapist in the provision of specific interventions (AOTA, 2004, 2005b). Occupational therapy assistants who hold an AOTA specialty certification in feeding, eating, and swallowing may have a more active role in collaborating in the evaluation process and in making intervention decisions. However, it is implicit that these tasks are carried out under the supervision of an occupational therapist. The supervising occupational therapist must be experienced in feeding, eating, and swallowing disorders or seek consultation from an occupational therapist who has such experience.

Knowledge and Skills

The progression from entry-level knowledge and skills to advanced-level knowledge and skills is individualized for each occupational therapist and occupational therapy assistant. Although practitioners exit their academic program with the basic knowledge and skills to provide occupational therapy services to clients with feeding, eating, and swallowing dysfunction, over time they may develop additional individualized expertise, such as in the area of dysphagia. Entry-level knowledge and skills for both occupational therapists and occupational therapy assistants, as supported by the 2006 Standards (Accreditation Council of Occupational Therapy Education, 2006), are delineated in Appendix A. The advanced-level knowledge and skills necessary to provide a continuum of services in the area of feeding, eating, and swallowing are delineated in Appendix B. These advanced-level skills build on existing knowledge, performance skills, critical reasoning, interpersonal abilities, and ethical reasoning.

Appendix A.
Entry-Level Knowledge and Skills Assessment

Occupational Therapists and Occupational Therapy Assistants Will Have Entry-Level Knowledge and Skills to Assess:

Context	Occupational Therapist	Occupational Therapy Assistant *(Based on the Establishment of Service Competency and Supervision by an Occupational Therapist)*
Cultural components that affect feeding: utensils, food types, meanings/symbolism of food, mealtime practices and rituals, dietary restrictions	✓	✓
Attitudes and values of client, family or caregivers, and friends toward feeding and mealtime	✓	✓
Settings where feeding/eating take place	✓	✓
Social opportunities during mealtime that support or interfere with social interaction	✓	✓
Aspects of the client's developmental status/life phase that support or interfere with eating/feeding	✓	—
Effect of medical condition/disability status on feeding performance	✓	—
Factors in the environment that support or interfere with feeding/eating (e.g., foods, seating, time, feeders)	✓	—
Pre-Oral Phase		
Role of appetite and hunger sensation	✓	✓
Tactile and proprioceptive qualities of food and equipment in both the hands and the mouth	✓	✓
Ability to see/locate food/drink/utensils	✓	✓
Ability to appreciate smell—pleasant/noxious	✓	✓
Need for use of auditory cues (verbal cues, utensils hitting plate)	✓	✓
Ability to achieve a position of proximal postural control that allows upper-extremity and oral function for eating	✓	✓
Nature of communication during feeding/mealtime	✓	✓
Feeding experience as satisfactory to self	✓	✓

✓ = able to perform the task
— = does not perform the task

(Continued)

Appendix A.
Entry-Level Knowledge and Skills Assessment *(cont.)*

Occupational Therapists and Occupational Therapy Assistants Will Have Entry-Level Knowledge and Skills to Assess:

Pre-Oral Phase *(continued)*	Occupational Therapist	Occupational Therapy Assistant *(Based on the Establishment of Service Competency and Supervision by an Occupational Therapist)*
Ability to bring food to mouth as supported or prevented by factors such as figure ground, depth perception, spatial relations, and motor planning	✓	—
Neuromotor components that support or interfere with adequate positioning	✓	—
Upper-extremity function and hand manipulation adequate for self-feeding	✓	—
Influence of motor activity involved in bringing food to mouth	✓	—
Ability to orient mouth to receive food (timing, positioning of structures)	✓	—
Initiation of eating as supported/prevented by level of alertness/arousal, orientation to task, recognition, and memory	✓	—
Persistence with feeding that is supported/prevented by level of arousal, attention span, initiation of activity, memory, and sequencing	✓	—
Carryover of skill to future feeding tasks is supported/ prevented by level of memory, learning, and generalization	✓	—
Factors that influence the willingness or unwillingness to eat (self-image, self-esteem, caregiver, family, feeder interaction, eating history, dying)	✓	—
Oral Phase		
Behaviors or reports that indicate pain or discomfort in the oral area	✓	✓
Behaviors that interfere with the oral phase (spitting foods, pocketing foods, refusing to swallow)	✓	✓
Level of awareness/sensation in the oral–motor area	✓	—
Level of reception and perception of tactile (texture), temperature, proprioception, and gustatory qualities of food and utensils	✓	—
Factors supporting/interfering with secretion management	✓	—

(Continued)

Appendix A.
Entry-Level Knowledge and Skills Assessment *(cont.)*

Occupational Therapists and Occupational Therapy Assistants Will Have Entry-Level Knowledge and Skills to Assess:

Oral Phase *(continued)*	Occupational Therapist	Occupational Therapy Assistant *(Based on the Establishment of Service Competency and Supervision by an Occupational Therapist)*
Respiratory control factors that permit safe and efficient bolus manipulation (mouth breathers, Adult Respiratory Distress Syndrome, bronchopulmonary dysplasia), chronic obstructive pulmonary disease, cardiopulmonary compromise	✓	—
Structural or neuromotor factors (reflexes, range of motion, muscle tone, strength, endurance) that support or interfere with oral–motor function	✓	—
Level of coordinated movements (praxis) of oral structures (cheeks, lips, jaw, tongue, palate, teeth) with or without foods	✓	—
Oral structures' ability to work together to contain, form, and propel the bolus	✓	—
Bolus manipulation supported/compromised by memory, attention span, orientation, and problem solving	✓	—
Speed of the oral phase adequate to support sufficient oral intake	✓	—
Pharyngeal Phase		
Behaviors, reports, or symptoms that indicate pain or discomfort localized to the pharyngeal area	✓	—
Presence of signs and symptoms indicating possible pharyngeal dysfunction or clinical signs indicating possible aspiration (e.g., coughing, choking, tachypnea)	✓	—
Esophageal Phase		
Behaviors, reports, or symptoms that indicate pain or discomfort in the esophageal area	✓	—
Presence of refluxed material from the stomach into the esophagus, pharynx, or oral cavity	✓	—

Occupational Therapists and Occupational Therapy Assistants Will Have Entry-Level Knowledge and Skills to:

Instrumentation		
Understand formal instrumentation used by therapists or other professionals to evaluate the oral, pharyngeal, and esophageal phase of the swallow, including, but not limited to, videofluoroscopy, ultrasonography, fiberoptic endoscopy, scintigraphy, and manometry	✓	—

(Continued)

271

Appendix A.
Entry-Level Knowledge and Skills Assessment *(cont.)*

Occupational Therapists and Occupational Therapy Assistants Will Have Entry-Level Knowledge and Skills to:

Discharge Planning *(Discharge Planning is Addressed Throughout the Intervention Process)*	**Occupational Therapist**	**Occupational Therapy Assistant** *(Based on the Establishment of Service Competency and Supervision by an Occupational Therapist)*
Collaborate with client, family, caregivers, and team members to formulate discharge needs	✓	—
Provide appropriate referrals, follow-up plans, and reevaluation related to discharge needs	✓	—
Develop and document discharge and follow-up programs and resources in accordance with discharge environment	✓	—
Provide for educational needs related to feeding, eating, and swallowing management and establishment of proficiency of recommendations with client and family	✓	—
Implement discharge and follow-up plan with client, family, caregivers, and team members to promote transition to discharge environment and integration of intervention management techniques	✓	—
Terminate intervention when client has achieved maximum benefit from services	✓	—

Entry-Level Knowledge and Skills Intervention

Occupational Therapists and Occupational Therapy Assistants Will Have Entry-Level Knowledge and Skills to:

Context	**Occupational Therapist**	**Occupational Therapy Assistant** *(Based on the Establishment of Service Competency and Supervision by an Occupational Therapist)*
Consider cultural practices in selecting foods, utensils, and mealtime setting	✓	✓
Provide environmental modifications to promote appetite and feeding/eating performance (e.g., location, timing, seating, lighting)	✓	✓
Use eating/feeding activities appropriate for developmental status/life phase	✓	✓
Facilitate social interactions that support feeding performance	✓	✓
Plan intervention within the context of person's medical condition, particularly considering specific restrictions and limitations, expected progression, and outcome	✓	—

(Continued)

Appendix A.
Entry-Level Knowledge and Skills Intervention *(cont.)*

Occupational Therapists and Occupational Therapy Assistants Will Have Entry-Level Knowledge and Skills to:

Pre-Oral Phase	Occupational Therapist	Occupational Therapy Assistant *(Based on the Establishment of Service Competency and Supervision by an Occupational Therapist)*
Facilitate olfactory stimulation	✓	✓
Provide verbal or physical cues	✓	✓
Use sensitization and desensitization techniques	✓	✓
Facilitate oral hygiene	✓	✓
Facilitate visual–perceptual activity and body schema awareness	✓	✓
Increase awareness on affected/neglected side	✓	✓
Facilitate strategies to minimize visual field deficits and enhance acuity	✓	✓
Modify environment to enhance attention	✓	✓
Help client/caregiver to develop problem-solving methods	✓	✓
Use communicative strategies to increase participation in feeding	✓	✓
Use techniques to attain and maintain optimal level of arousal	✓	✓
Provide appropriate positioning and seating equipment	✓	✓
Provide nonnutritive oral stimulation, techniques, and/or exercises	✓	✓
Facilitate upper-extremity control and hand function (dexterity, strength, coordination)	✓	✓
Facilitate oral–motor control through exercises, play, and games	✓	✓
Improve self-esteem to increase engagement in self-feeding	✓	✓
Structure mealtime habits	✓	✓
Implement nutritional recommendations	✓	✓
Manipulate feeding schedule to facilitate hunger	✓	—
Select, modify, and establish set-up of mealtime equipment	✓	—
Facilitate postural control	✓	—
Fabricate upper-extremity orthotics	✓	—
Use behavior modification	✓	—

(Continued)

Appendix A.
Entry-Level Knowledge and Skills Intervention *(cont.)*

Occupational Therapists and Occupational Therapy Assistants Will Have Entry-Level Knowledge and Skills to:

Oral Phase	Occupational Therapist	Occupational Therapy Assistant (Based on the Establishment of Service Competency and Supervision by an Occupational Therapist)
Provide nonnutritive oral stimulation and exercises (jaw, lip, cheeks, tongue)	✓	✓
Use desensitization techniques	✓	✓
Maintain appropriate position during mealtime (facilitate stability or movement)	✓	✓
Time the introduction of food to facilitate coordinated respiration	✓	✓
Facilitate placement of food in mouth and use of utensils	✓	✓
Use verbal, written, tactile cues to initiate, maintain, and follow through (chew, swallow) with feeding/eating task	✓	✓
Provide an environmental modification program	✓	✓
Facilitate oral compensatory strategies for altered sensation, structure, or function	✓	—
Select and modify equipment for feeding	✓	—
Grade or alter qualities of bolus (e.g., texture, taste, temperature)	✓	—
Provide a behavior modification program	✓	—
Pharyngeal Phase		
Facilitate head and neck positioning for swallowing (e.g., chin tuck, head turns)	✓	—
Facilitate compensatory swallow techniques	✓	—
Esophageal Phase		
Modify position before, during, and after feeding task	✓	—
Refer to gastrointestinal service when appropriate	✓	—

Appendix B.
Advanced-Level Knowledge and Skills

Occupational Therapist	Occupational Therapy Assistant
I. *Eating function*—The occupational therapist with advanced-level knowledge and skills has built upon foundational knowledge of the eating process, thus enhancing the depth and specificity of evaluation and intervention. The occupational therapist has developed	I. *Eating function*—The occupational therapy assistant with advanced-level knowledge and skills has built upon foundational knowledge of the eating process for the purpose of providing more comprehensive intervention. The occupational therapy assistant has developed
A. Extensive knowledge of anatomy and physiology of the phases of eating for the purpose of assessing structural, neuromotor, and sensory factors that support or interfere with function and of determining intervention strategies	A. Advanced knowledge of anatomy and physiology of the phases of eating
1. Pre-oral phase	1. Pre-oral phase
2. Oral phase	2. Oral phase
3. Pharyngeal phase	3. Pharyngeal phase
4. Esophageal phase	4. Esophageal phase
B. Extensive knowledge of airway functions, including protective responses and respiratory control factors that affect swallowing and eating.	B. Advanced knowledge of airway functions, including protective responses and respiratory control factors that affect swallowing and eating.
II. *Specialized client populations and settings*—The occupational therapist with advanced-level knowledge and skills has gained extensive knowledge and experience in the feeding, eating, and swallowing needs of specific client populations or clients in specific settings. The increased depth of knowledge allows the occupational therapist to provide services to clients who are more medically fragile or whose problems/ needs are more complex than those addressed by entry-level therapists. By developing expertise with specific client populations, occupational therapists with advanced-level knowledge and skills not only provide services that represent "best practice" but also contribute to the development of new and innovative approaches to evaluation and intervention for that population. Areas of expertise that may be developed include	II. *Specialized client populations and settings*—The occupational therapy assistant with advanced-level knowledge and skills has gained extensive knowledge and experience in the feeding, eating, and swallowing needs of specific client populations or clients in specific settings. The increased depth of knowledge allows the occupational therapy assistant with advanced-level knowledge and skills to provide services to clients who are more medically fragile or whose problems/ needs are more complex than those addressed by the occupational therapy assistant with entry-level knowledge and skills. Areas of expertise that may be developed include
A. Specific medical diagnoses	A. Specific medical diagnoses
1. In-depth knowledge of diagnosis, including potential impact on feeding, eating, and swallowing	1. In-depth knowledge of diagnosis, including potential impact on feeding, eating, and swallowing
2. Common medications used and their interaction with the feeding, eating, and swallowing process; advising regarding oral administration of medications (e.g., crushing meds, through nasogastric tube, changing to liquid suspension)	2. Common medications used and their interaction with the feeding, eating, and swallowing process
3. Dietary needs or restrictions	3. Dietary needs or restrictions
4. Specialized equipment that may be used and can affect feeding, eating, and swallowing (e.g., tracheostomy tubes, ventilators, feeding tubes)	4. Specialized equipment that may be used and can affect feeding, eating, and swallowing (e.g., tracheostomy tubes, ventilators, feeding tubes)
B. Specialized settings such as general intensive care units and neonatal intensive care units (AOTA, 1993)	B. Specialized settings such as intensive care units (AOTA, 1993)

(Continued)

275

Appendix B.
Advanced-Level Knowledge and Skills *(cont.)*

Occupational Therapist	Occupational Therapy Assistant
C. Specific developmental, social, or cultural factors	C. Specific developmental, social, or cultural factors
1. In-depth knowledge of age-related expectations, such as feeding processes in infants and children and the effects of aging on feeding	1. In-depth knowledge of age-related expectations, such as feeding processes in children and the effects of aging on feeding
2. Extensive knowledge of particular cultural groups and the influence of their custom on eating, particularly for persons with feeding, eating, and swallowing problems	2. Extensive knowledge of particular cultural groups and the influence of their custom on eating, particularly for persons with feeding, eating, and swallowing problems
3. Extensive knowledge of social or emotional factors that can influence feeding	3. Extensive knowledge of social or emotional factors that can influence feeding
III. *Instrumental evaluation*—The occupational therapists with advanced-level knowledge and skills may develop the following skills for instrumental evaluations relevant to their area of practice. These assessment techniques require specialized formal training and equipment. They may include, but are not limited to, videofluoroscopy, cervical auscultation, ultrasonography, fiberoptic endoscopy, scintigraphy, manometry, electromyography, and manofluorography.	III. *Instrumental evaluation*—The occupational therapy assistants with advanced-level knowledge and skills may develop the following skills for those instrumental evaluations relevant to their area of practice.
A. Knowledge and application of instrumental techniques, including purpose, indications for use, limitations, reliability, and validity	A. Knowledge of the instrumentation techniques, including purpose, indications for use, limitations, reliability, and validity
B. Ability to recommend appropriate instrumental evaluation	B. Ability to assist the occupational therapist in carrying out the assessment
C. Collaboration with other professionals in carrying out the instrumental evaluation and interpretation of data	
D. Ability to independently carry out the assessment, including interpretation of data and implementation of recommendations	
E. Ability to use results effectively in evaluation and intervention	
IV. *Specialized interventions*—Occupational therapists with advanced-level knowledge and skills have knowledge and skills of all existing intervention procedures in their specialty area and can provide the clinical judgment and rationale for selection of any procedure being used. They are aware of new interventions and potential applications from other fields. Skills may be developed in using specialized interventions that include, but are not limited to	IV. *Specialized interventions*—Occupational therapy assistants who have advanced-level knowledge and skills of specialized intervention procedures in their specialty area in order to implement intervention recommendations made by the occupational therapist. Skills may be developed in implementing specialized interventions that include, but are not limited to
A. Interventions to facilitate oral performance, improve pharyngeal swallow, and potentially reduce the risk of aspiration, if present. Use of these interventions is based on the results of instrumental evaluation of function, with safety to the client as a primary concern. Examples include	A. Interventions to improve pharyngeal swallow and esophageal function. Use of these interventions is based on results of instrumental evaluation of function by the occupational therapist. Examples Include
1. Compensatory swallowing techniques/strategies	1. Compensatory swallowing techniques
2. Thermal or tactile stimulation	2. Thermal or tactile stimulation
3. Grading or altering the bolus size/texture/changing consistency of liquids/route of administering medications orally	3. Grading or altering the bolus size/texture
4. Specialized positioning	4. Specialized positioning

Appendix B.
Advanced-Level Knowledge and Skills *(cont.)*

Occupational Therapist	Occupational Therapy Assistant
B. Enteral feeding 1.Knowledge of purpose, types, indications, limitations, and precautions 2.Ability to integrate enteral feeding systems into occupational therapy intervention plan 3.Ability to make recommendations regarding use of or need for enteral feeding systems C. Oral appliances (prosthodontics) 1.Knowledge of purpose, indications, limitations, and pre-cautions 2.Ability to fabricate or collaborate on fabrication 3.Client training and education	B. Enteral feeding 1.Knowledge of purpose, types, indications, limitations, and precautions C. Oral appliances (prosthodontics) 1.Knowledge of purpose, indications, limitations, and pre-cautions
V. *Training and education*—Occupational therapists who have advanced-level knowledge and skills that should be disseminated to others. Through formal and informal methods, occupational therapists with advanced-level knowledge and skills should provide training and education to other occupational therapists, occupational therapy assistants, students, staff members, and professionals from related fields.	V. *Training and education*—Occupational therapy assistants with advanced-level knowledge and skills provide training and education to clients, family, and staff members, in collaboration with an occupational therapist.

Definitions—Common Terminology

Adaptive feeding equipment
Equipment used to support optimal feeding performance and to compensate for associated deficits related to coordination, strength, praxis, range of motion, or positioning.

Airway protection
Methods designed to prevent accidental loss of food, medications, or liquids into the airway while eating or drinking.

Aspiration
The entry of secretions, fluids, food, or any foreign substance below the vocal cords and into the lungs; may result in aspiration pneumonia, which may be fatal.

Bolus
The mass of food or liquid that is orally processed and swallowed.

Cervical auscultation
A method of assessing the pharyngeal swallow by listening to stereotypical sounds using the stethoscope.

Chin tuck
An intervention strategy where the head is flexed (chin tucked downward toward the chest) during the swallow allowing the anterior structures of the pharynx posteriorly resulting in a smaller entrance to the larynx; this strategy reduces the chance of food or liquid to fall into the airway.

Clearing techniques
Strategies used to clear the mouth or pharynx of food or liquid residue.

Clinical evaluation

The observation of feeding, eating, and swallowing, including client/caregiver interaction, positioning, food consistencies, method of intake, food preferences, oral structures, oral–motor patterns, tone, tactile responses, strength, fatigue, time required for mealtime activities, oral reflexes, sucking, coordination, labial, lingual, velar, facial, mandibular, dentition.

Clinical feeding, eating, and swallowing evaluation

A comprehensive evaluation, not including instrumentation, that examines the client's ability to feed, eat, and initiate the swallowing process; also referred to as "bedside dysphagia evaluation."

Cranial nerves

Nerves that provide motor and sensory innervation to the head and neck.

Diet liberalization

The relaxation of standards of accepted diets as ways to treat illness or decrease symptoms related to dsyphagia.

Double/multiple swallows

A swallow strategy whereby two or more attempts are used to swallow the food, medications, or liquid.

Dysphagia

Difficulty with any stage of swallowing (oral, pharyngeal, esophageal); dysfunction in any stage or process of eating; includes any difficulty in the passage of food, liquid, or medicine during any stage of swallowing that impairs the client's ability to swallow independently or safely.

Eating

"…the ability to keep and manipulate food or fluid in the mouth and swallow it; eating and swallowing are often used interchangeably" (AOTA, 2006a).

Eating disorders

Dysfunction in eating and nutrition related to complex biological, psychological, and sociocultural factors that may result in a life-threatening illness, such as anorexia and bulimia nervosa.

Effortful/hard swallows

A swallow strategy whereby the tongue muscles are volitionally contracted with increased effort while swallowing; results in the base of the tongue moving posteriorly during the pharyngeal swallow, which helps to clear food material from the valleculae during swallow.

Electromyography (EMG)

A procedure by which skeletal muscles are electrically stimulated and changes in electrical activity are recorded. Paralysis of the pharyngeal constrictors and vocal cords can be determined.

Enteral feeding

Feedings that use the intestinal tract for absorption of nutrients; often called gastrostomy tube feedings.

Esophageal phase

The phase of swallowing in which the bolus travels through the esophagus into the stomach.

Esophageal state function

Includes upper esophagus/cricopharyngeal function, esophageal motility.

Feeding

"…the process of setting up, arranging, and bringing food [or fluid] from the plate or cup to the mouth; sometimes called self-feeding" (AOTA, 2006a).

Feeding, eating, and swallowing history

Includes medical diagnoses, past medical history, food allergies, gastrointestinal disorders, current medications, developmental level (as appropriate), nutritional status, neurological status, respiratory status, pertinent diagnostic studies, feeding history including progression of solids and liquids, alternate/supplemental feeding interventions, positioning, cognition, behavior, communication, eating habits/patterns, methods of feeding, dietary restrictions.

Fiberoptic endoscopic evaluation of swallowing (FEES)
Process of passing a flexible fiberoptic endoscope through the nose and positioning it to observe structures and function of the swallowing mechanism to include the nasopharynx, oropharynx, and hypopharynx. The procedure is also known as fiberoptic endoscopic examination of swallowing and videoendoscopic swallowing study.

Food and liquid consistencies
Includes thin liquids, nectar-thick liquids, honey-thick liquids, puree, chopped, soft, solid food consistencies.

Gastrostomy tube
A tube placed surgically or endoscopically into the stomach through which fluids and nutrition are provided.

Graded tactile pressure
Includes deep touch, light touch, sustained touch, pulsing touch, symmetrical touch, asymmetrical touch.

Grading/altering bolus
Manipulation of the food or liquid to change its properties related to temperature, size, or texture.

Instrumental assessment
An assessment of swallowing using radiological or imaging procedures; may include but is not limited to modified barium swallow, fiberoptic endoscopy, ultrasound, scintigraphy, electromyography, and manometry.

Jejunostomy tube
A tube placed into the jejunum of the small intestine during surgery through which enteral feedings are provided.

Manofluorography
Simultaneous videofluoroscopy and manometry by which oropharyngeal and esophageal pressure and bolus information are recorded. This procedure is also known as pharyngeal manofluorography and videomanometry.

Manometry
A procedure by which the strength, timing, and sequencing of pressure events in the esophagus are measured by a catheter with pressure transducers. Alone, it is an ineffective tool for the diagnosis of oropharyngeal dysphagia (Bastian, 1998).

Mendelsohn maneuver
A swallowing technique to facilitate prolonged laryngeal elevation during the swallow; results in keeping the upper esophageal sphincter open longer to allow passage of the bolus.

Nasogastric tube
A tube used to provide feedings directly into the stomach through a tube inserted in the nose into the stomach.

National Dysphagia Diet (NDD)
From the National Dysphagia Diet Task Force (2000) of the American Dietetic Association, these diet levels aim to establish standard terminology and practice applications of dietary texture modification in dysphagia management. Diet levels include the following:

> *NDD Level I:* Dysphagia–Pureed (homogenous, very cohesive, pudding-like, requiring very little chewing ability)

NDD Level II: Dysphagia–Mechanical Altered (cohesive, moist, semisolid foods, requiring some chewing)

NDD Level III: Dysphagia–Advanced (soft foods that require more chewing ability)
- Regular: All foods allowed
- Proposed levels of liquid viscosity are:
  –Thin
  –Nectar-like
  –Honey-like
  –Spoon-thick

Oral phase
The phase of swallow in which the bolus of food or liquid is propelled to the pharynx by the tongue.

Oral preparatory phase
The phase of swallowing during which the bolus of food or liquid is masticated by the teeth and gums and manipulated by the lips, cheek, and tongue to create a bolus of appropriate texture for swallowing; this phase also allows for sensory appreciation of bolus qualities.

Oral reflexes
Abnormal and primitive reflexes include hyperactive gag, tonic bite, tongue thrust, jaw jerk, rooting, sucking.

Oral stage function
Includes bolus intake and containment, bolus formation, bolus transit and clearing time, velar function, behavioral components, base of tongue contact to pharyngeal wall, residue post swallow.

Orogastric tube
Used to lavage or decompress the stomach; it must be removed prior to assessment.

Penetration
The entry of secretions, fluids, food, medications, or any foreign substance into the laryngeal vestibule at or above the level of the true vocal cords.

Pharyngeal phase
The phase of swallow when the swallowing response is initiated.

Pharyngeal state function
Includes nasopharyngeal insufficiency and reflux, vallecular function, pyriform sinus function, epiglottal function, timing of swallow response, initiation of pharyngeal swallow, timing of clearance, pharyngeal competence, pharyngeal wall residue, laryngeal elevation, laryngeal penetration, or aspiration risk.

Pleasure/recreational feedings
Meals or snacks that provide enjoyment and stimulation but that are not depended on to provide nutrition.

Pocketing
Retention of food between the teeth and cheek.

Pre-oral phase
The process in which food, medication, or drink is brought to the mouth either by the person engaged in eating or by the feeder.

Presentation
Includes temperature, texture, size, placement, utensil choice, flavor, rate, method of delivery.

Prosthodontics

Prosthetic appliances used to facilitate oral and/or pharyngeal function either inside or outside of the oral cavity. May also be used for cosmesis.

Reflux

Reflux of food, medication, liquids, and gastric juice from the stomach into the esophagus; also called gastroesophageal reflux disease (GERD).

Scintigraphy

A procedure by which a radioactive bolus is monitored during and after ingestion to assess and measure bolus transit and aspiration (Bastian, 1998).

Secretion management

The ability to retain, manipulate, and swallow one's own saliva.

Self-feeding

The process of setting up, arranging, and bringing food from the plate or cup to the mouth; sometimes just referred to as feeding.

Silent aspiration

Aspiration that occurs without coughing or overt choking, indicating motor and/or sensory deficits (if present) that inhibit protective responses.

Supraglottic swallow

A swallowing technique used for airway protection where the client is told to take a breath and hold it while swallowing and then coughs after the swallow; results in the voluntary closure of the vocal folds before, during, and after the swallow.

Swallowing

A complicated act where food, fluid, medication, or saliva is moved from the mouth through the pharynx and esophagus into the stomach (AOTA, 2006a).

Therapeutic feedings

Controlled delivery of food, medication, or liquid used to facilitate therapeutic outcomes to improve feeding, eating, and swallowing ability; not used as a primary source of nutrition or hydration.

Thickening agent

Substances used to increase the viscosity of liquids.

Total parenteral nutrition

A formula providing nutrients through an intravenous tube.

Ultrasonography

The use of high frequency sound waves to provide ultrasonic images of the upper digestive tract structures and motilities, bolus transit, and vallecular stasis. It is not effective to detect penetration or aspiration (Bastian, 1998).

Upper aerodigestive tract

The combined organs and tissues of the respiratory tract and the upper part of the digestive tract (including the lips, nose, mouth, tongue, pharynx, larynx, upper trachea, and upper esophagus).

VitalStim

A Food and Drug Administration (FDA)–cleared method to promote swallowing through the application of neuromuscular electrical stimulation to the swallowing muscles to strengthen and re-educate muscles and to facilitate motor control/function of the swallowing mechanism.

References

Accreditation Council for Occupational Therapy Education. (2006). *ACOTE standards and interpretive guidelines*. Retrieved September 19, 2006, from http://www.aota.org/nonmembers/area13/docs/acotestandards806.pdf

American Occupational Therapy Association. (1993). Occupational therapy roles. *American Journal of Occupational Therapy, 47*, 1087–1099.

American Occupational Therapy Association. (2002). Occupational therapy practice framework: Domain and process. *American Journal of Occupational Therapy, 56*, 609–639.

American Occupational Therapy Association. (2004). Guidelines for supervision, roles, and responsibilities during the delivery of occupational therapy services. *American Journal of Occupational Therapy, 58*, 663–667.

American Occupational Therapy Association. (2005a). Occupational therapy code of ethics. *American Journal of Occupational Therapy, 59*, 639–642.

American Occupational Therapy Association. (2005b). Standards of practice for occupational therapy. *American Journal of Occupational Therapy, 59*, 663–665.

American Occupational Therapy Association. (2006a). *AOTA specialty certification in feeding, eating, and swallowing: 2007 candidate handbook—Occupational therapists* [PDF, available from http://www.aota.org/memservices/certappprogram/cr_login.aspx]. Bethesda, MD: Author.

American Occupational Therapy Association. (2006b). Policy 1.44: Categories of occupational therapy personnel. *American Journal of Occupational Therapy, 60*, 683–684.

Bastian, R. W. (1998). Contemporary diagnosis of the dysphagic patient. In R. L. Plant & G. L. Schectiter (Eds.), The otolaryngologic clinics of North America. *Dysphagia in Children, Adults, and Geriatrics, 31*, 489–506.

National Dysphagia Diet Task Force. (2000). *National dysphagia diet: Standardization for optimal care*. Washington, DC: American Dietetic Association.

World Health Organization. (2001). *International classification of functioning, disability and health (ICF)*. Geneva, Switzerland: Author.

Selected Readings

Adult Eating and Dysphagia Treatment

Bastian, R. W. (1998). Contemporary diagnosis of the dysphagic patient. In R. L. Plant & G. L. Schectiter (Eds.), The otolaryngologic clinics of North America. *Dysphagia in Children, Adults, and Geriatrics, 31*, 489–506.

Groher, M. E. (1997). *Dysphagia: Diagnosis and management* (3rd ed.). Boston: Butterworth-Heinemann.

Healthy People 2010. Retrieved March 5, 2007, from http://www.cdc.gov/nchs/datawh/nchsdefs/ healthypeople2010.htm

Joint Commission on Accreditation of Healthcare Organizations. (2007). Retrieved March 5, 2007, from www.jointcommission.org

Note. This list of selected readings is not meant to be exhaustive but to suggest current resources for library building pertinent to eating and dysphagia treatment. Key words that are helpful in accomplishing a literature review search of this topic may include *dysphagia, feeding, eating, swallowing disorders, deglutition disorders,* and *dysphagia rehabilitation.*

Langmore, S. E., & Miller, R. M. (1994). Behavioral treatment for adults with oropharyngeal dysphagia. *Archives of Physical Medicine and Rehabilitation, 75*, 1154–1159.

Logemann, J. A. (1998). *Evaluation and treatment of swallowing disorders* (2nd ed.). Austin, TX: Pro-Ed.

Logsdon, B. (2002). Cultivating competence. *Advance for Directors in Rehabilitation, 11*(10), 71–73.

Neumann, S. (1993). Swallowing therapy with neurologic clients: Results of direct and indirect therapy methods in 66 clients suffering from neurological disorders. *Dysphagia, 8*, 150–153.

Neumann, S., Bartolome, D., Buchholz, D., & Prosiegal, M. (1995). Swallowing therapy of neurologic patients: Correlation of outcome with pretreatment variables and therapeutic methods. *Dysphagia, 10*, 1–5.

Clinical Dysphagia Assessment

Avery-Smith, W., Dellarosa, D. M., & Rosen, A. B. (1992). Clinical assessment of dysphagia in adults. *Occupational Therapy Practice, 3*(2), 51–58.

Avery-Smith, W., Rosen, A. B., & Dellarosa, D. (1997). *Dysphagia evaluation protocol*. San Antonio, TX: Therapy Skill Builders.

Depippo, K. L., Holas, M. A., & Reding, M. J. (1994). The Burke Dysphagia Screening Test: Validation of its use in patients with stroke. *Archives of Physical Medicine and Rehabilitation, 75*, 1284–1286.

Fleming, S. M., & Weaver, A. W. (1986). Index of dysphagia: A tool for identifying deglutition problems. *Dysphagia, 1*, 206–208.

Hardy, E. (1995). *Bedside evaluation of dysphagia*. Bisbee, AZ: Imaginart.

Hopper, P., & Holme, S. (1999). The role of fiberoptic endoscopy in dysphagia rehabilitation. *Journal of Head Trauma Rehabilitation, 5*, 475–485.

Leopold, N. A., & Kagel, M. C. (1997). Dysphagia—Ingestion or deglutition: A proposed paradigm. *Dysphagia, 12*, 202–206.

Shanley, C., & O'Loughlin, G. (2000). Dysphagia among nursing home residents: An assessment and management protocol. *Journal of Gerontology in Nursing, 26*(8), 35–48.

Eating Disorders

Bouley, B., & Sadik, C. (1992). Inpatient treatment of eating disorders within a cognitive–behavioral framework. *Occupational Therapy Practice, 3*(2), 1–11.

Giles, G. M. (1985). Anorexia nervosa and bulimia: An activity-oriented approach. *American Journal of Occupational Therapy, 39*, 510–517.

Martin, J. E. (1998). *Eating disorders, food, and occupational therapy*. London: Whurr.

Instrumental Dysphagia Assessment

Bastian, R. (1993). The videoendoscopic swallowing study: An alternative and partner to the videofluoroscopic swallowing study. *Dysphagia, 8*, 359–367.

Broniatowski, M. (1998). Fiberoptic endoscopic evaluation of dysphagia and videofluoroscopy. *Dysphagia, 13*, 22–23.

Langmore, S. E., Schatz, K., & Olsen, N. (1988). Fiberoptic endoscopic examination of swallowing safety: A new procedure. *Dysphagia, 2*, 216–219.

Leder, S. B., Sasaki, C. T., & Burrell, M. I. (1998). Fiberoptic endoscopic evaluation of dysphagia to identify silent aspiration. *Dysphagia, 13,* 19–21.

Logemann, J. A. (1993). *Manual for the videofluoroscopic study of swallowing* (2nd ed.). Austin, TX: Pro-Ed.

Perlman, A. L. (1993). Electromyography and the study of oropharyngeal swallowing. *Dysphagia, 8,* 351–355.

Silverman, K. H. (1994). The use of scintigraphy in the management of patients with pulmonary aspiration. *Dysphagia, 9,* 107–115.

Pediatric Eating and Dysphagia Treatment

Arvedson, J. C., & Brodsky, L. (1993). *Pediatric swallowing and feeding: Assessment and management.* San Diego, CA: Singular.

Backes, L., Deitz, J., Price, R., Glass, R., & Hays, R. (1994). The effect of oral support on sucking efficiency in pre-term infants. *American Journal of Occupational Therapy, 48,* 490–498.

Carruth, B. R., & Skinner, J. D. (2002). Feeding behaviors and other motor development in healthy children (2–24 months). *Journal of the American College of Nutrition, 21*(2), 88–96.

Clark, G. (1993). Oral–motor and feeding issues. In C. Royeen (Ed.), *AOTA Self-Study Series: Classroom applications for school-based practice.* Bethesda, MD: American Occupational Therapy Association.

Glass, R. P., & Wolf, L. S. (1994). Global perspective on feeding assessment in the neonatal intensive care unit. *American Journal of Occupational Therapy, 48,* 487–489.

Mathisen, B., Worrall, L., Masel, J., Wall, C., & Shepherd, R.W. (1999). Feeding problems in infants with gastro-oesophageal reflux disease: A controlled study. *Journal of Paediatrics and Child Health, 35*(2), 163–169.

Morris, S., & Klein, M. (2000). *Pre-feeding skills* (2nd ed.). San Antonio, TX: Therapy Skill Builders.

Nelson, C. A., Meek, M. M., & Moore, J. C. (1994). *Head–neck treatment issues as a base for oral–motor function.* Albuquerque, NM: Clinician's View.

Rogers, B. (2004). Feeding method and health outcomes of children with cerebral palsy. *Journal of Pediatrics, 145*(Suppl.2).

Schwarz, S. M. (2003). Feeding disorders in children with developmental disabilities. *Infants and Young Children, 16,* 317–330.

Sullivan, P. B., & Rosenbloom, L. (1996). *Feeding the disabled child.* London: Mac Keith Press.

Tuchman, D. N., & Walter, R. S. (1994). *Disorders of feeding and swallowing in infants and children: Pathophysiology, diagnosis, and treatment.* San Diego, CA: Singular.

Waterman, E. T., Koltai, P. J., Downey, J. C., & Cacace, A. T. (1992). Swallowing disorders in a population of children with cerebral palsy. *International Journal of Pediatric Otorhinolaryngology, 24,* 63–71.

Wolf, L. S., & Glass, R. P. (1992). *Feeding and swallowing disorders in infancy: Assessment and management.* San Antonio, TX: Therapy Skill Builders.

Miscellaneous

Mody, M., & Nagai, J. (1990). A multidisciplinary approach to the development of competency standards and appropriate allocation for patients with dysphagia. *American Journal of Occupational Therapy, 44,* 369–372.

Authors

This paper was originally authored in 2000 by the Eating and Feeding Task Force: Gloria Frolek Clark, MS, OTR/L, FAOTA *(Chairperson)*; Wendy Avery-Smith, MS, OTR; Lynn S. Wold, MA, OTR; Paige Anthony, COTA; and Suzanne E. Holm, MA, OTR, BCN.

In 2005–2006, the paper was revised and updated by Gloria Frolek Clark, MS, OTR/L, FAOTA *(Coordinator)* and

The AOTASB Feeding and Swallowing Specialty Certification Panel:

Pam Roberts, MSHA, OTR/L, CPHQ, FAOTA, *Chairperson*
Marcia S. Cox, MHS, OTR/L
Suzanne E. Holm, MA, OTR, BCN
Sharon T. Kurfuerst, MEd, OTR/L
Amy K. Lynch, MS, OTR/L
Linda Miller Schuberth, MA, OTR/L

for

The Commission on Practice
Susanne Smith Roley, MS, OTR/L, FAOTA, *Chairperson*

Adopted by the Representative Assembly 2007C76

Note. This document replaces the 2000 document *Specialized Knowledge and Skills for Eating and Feeding in Occupational Therapy Practice,* previously published and copyrighted in 2000 by the American Occupational Therapy Association and reprinted in 2003 (*American Journal of Occupational Therapy, 57,* 660–678).

Specialized Knowledge and Skills of Occupational Therapy Educators of the Future

Introduction

In 2006, the American Occupational Therapy Association (AOTA) articulated a *Centennial Vision* statement for the profession as it nears its 100th anniversary. This statement affirms that

> We envision that occupational therapy is a powerful, widely recognized, science-driven, and evidence-based profession with a globally connected and diverse workforce meeting society's occupational needs. (AOTA, 2007)

This vision reflects the long-standing commitment of the profession to serve society in ways that are relevant and forward-thinking. As social concerns evolve, occupational therapy practitioners must understand the occupational implications of broad contextual issues that affect health and well-being directly and indirectly. Global effort to deal with climate change, for example, are causing downward economic pressures on middle-class living standards, thus altering daily routines, limiting occupational opportunities, increasing chronic health conditions, and reducing access to health care (Kawachi & Wamala, 2006). Occupational therapy practitioners need not only know how to respond to evolving social needs; they need to do so quickly, creatively, and proactively.

Occupational therapy education is critical to the achievement of this vision in 2017 and beyond. The constellation of skills and attitudes occupational therapy practitioners must possess are the result of their inherent abilities and motivations refined into long-standing dispositions through a deliberate educational process. Indeed, occupational therapy education embodies the aspirations for the kind of society we wish to see. To talk about the purpose of the profession is also to talk about the purpose of occupational therapy education, as it is here where these aspirations are nurtured and shaped.

Use of This Document

Occupational therapy is essentially an educative profession. Occupational therapy practitioners are skilled at analyzing limitations that may result in diminished occupational participation and designing therapeutic programs through which people learn new skills or re-learn skills lost to illness, injury, or contextual constraints. While to some degree all occupational therapy practitioners are educators, this document focuses on recognized roles related to education in the profession (Academic Program Director, Academic Faculty, Academic Fieldwork Coordinator, and Fieldwork Educator). The purpose is to articulate the attributes practitioners should possess in such roles in order to have an enduring legacy in the fulfillment of the *Centennial Vision* and beyond. These attributes are described in the language of possibility, including the characteristics of innovator/visionary, scholar/explorer, leader, integrator, and mentor. Because the embodiment of these attributes is developmental, they are described in a continuum of experience from novice, intermediate, and advanced practitioner.

The context surrounding the educator will determine which attributes are most needed and/or appropriate. While all professionals will demonstrate some aspects of the attributes, not everyone is expected to achieve the advanced level in all the attributes. Indeed, because of experience, available opportunities, and personal curiosities and strengths, an educator will likely demonstrate some attributes at the novice level while demonstrating others at the intermediate and advanced levels. Therefore, the purpose of this document is not to identify rigid standards of performance but rather to serve as a guide of desired attributes toward which an educator may aspire in order to contribute to the fulfillment of the *Centennial Vision* and beyond.

It is recommended that this document be used as an aid in the articulation of the professional development plans of faculty. Such plans are essential in their growth and are required by the Accreditation Council for Occupational Therapy Education (ACOTE) for all program directors and faculty who teach two or more courses (ACOTE, 2006, Standard A.5.2).

Desired attributes include the following:

- *Innovator/Visionary:* Someone who embraces new directions, is forward-thinking, projecting into the future. This person thinks outside of the traditional confines of the profession to predict and propose how to meet future societal needs. A visionary can see past traditional boundaries to new possibilities at all levels of personal and societal life.

- *Scholar/Explorer:* A scholar/explorer is someone who seeks, uses, and produces knowledge and effectively disseminates new findings to internal and external audiences. These individuals use a critical, theoretically grounded, and systematic approach in their scholarly endeavors to produce outcomes that inform and address societal needs.

- *Leader:* Someone who analyzes past, present, and future trends and develops solutions to problems or strategies for taking advantage of opportunities by collaborating, inspiring, and influencing people to create a desired future.

- *Integrator:* Someone who seeks and finds divergent information, perceives meaningful relationships, and makes connections through analysis to create a new, more coherent understanding.

- *Mentor:* A trusted role model who inspires, encourages, influences, challenges, and facilitates the growth and development of others' goals and aspirations. This involves a collaborative process that may be between peers, colleagues, experienced and inexperienced individuals, practitioners and academicians, and others. The mentor may function in various roles such as educator, tutor, coach, counselor, encourager, consultant, etc.

As stated earlier, the embodiment of these attributes is developmental, and not all tributes are likely to be developed at the same time nor needed equally. An educator can demonstrate an attribute at a novice level while demonstrating another at an advanced level. In this document, *novice* performance is understood as beginning expertise, as when a person has had limited experience in an area and therefore has limited familiarity with the associated knowledge or its application. *Intermediate* performance is understood as consistent demonstration of and attribute in specific situations as a result of prior experience in those situations. Finally, *advanced* performance is understood as the ability to demonstrate an attribute in multiple situations, including some in which a person has no prior experience. Advanced performance denotes a high level of expertise.

In Tables 1–5, each attribute is represented, summarizing how it might be demonstrated in each educator role. It is assumed that the incumbent in a role has met or exceeded occupational therapy practitioner competencies described in the *Standards for Continuing Competence* (AOTA, 2005). The attributes are general statements and specific characteristics may not apply to all situations.

References

Accreditation Council for Occupational Therapy Education. (2006). *Standards and interpretive guidelines.* Available at http://www.aota.org/Educate/Accredit/StandardsReview/guide/42369.aspx

American Occupational Therapy Association. (2005). Standards for continuing competence. *American Journal of Occupational Therapy, 59,* 661–662.

American Occupational Therapy Association. (2007). AOTA's *Centennial Vision* and executive summary. *American Journal of Occupational Therapy, 61,* 613–614.

Kawachi, I., & Wamala, S. (2006). *Globalization and health.* New York: Oxford University Press.

Authors
Commission on Education:
René Padilla, PhD, OTR/L, FAOTA, *Chairperson*
Andrea Bilics, PhD, OTR/L
Judith C. Blum, MS, OTR/L
Paula C. Bohr, PhD, OTR/L, FAOTA
Jennifer C. Coyne, COTA/L
Jyothi Gupta, PhD, OTR/L
Linda Musselman, PhD, OTR, FAOTA
Linda Orr, MPA, OTR/L
Abbey Sipp, *ASD Liaison*
Patricia Stutz-Tanenbaum, MS, OTR
Neil Harvison, PhD, OTR/L , *AOTA Staff Liaison*

Adopted by the Representative Assembly 2009FebCS112

Note. This document replaces the following documents: *Role Competencies for a Professional-Level Program Director in an Academic Setting, 2003M167; Role Competencies for a Program Director in an Occupational Therapy Assistant Academic Setting, 2005C239; Role Competencies for a Professional-Level Occupational Therapist Faculty Member in an Academic Setting, 2003M168; Role Competencies for a Faculty Member in an Occupational Therapy Assistant Academic Setting, 2005C240; Role Competencies for an Academic Fieldwork Coordinator, 2003M169;* and *Role Competencies for a Fieldwork Educator, 2005M284.*

Table 1.
Innovator/Visionary

Experience	Academic Program Director	OT/OTA Faculty Member	Academic Fieldwork Coordinator	Fieldwork Educator
Novice	1. Analyzes the current curriculum to reflect the future needs of the program, profession, and society. 2. Analyzes institutional needs in order to identify new ways that the program can fulfill the institution's mission. 3. Develops curriculum that challenges and prepares students to identify and fulfill innovative practice roles.	1. Demonstrates the ability to prepare ethical and competent practitioners for both traditional and emerging practice settings. 2. Develops plan to maintain self abreast of the breadth and depth of knowledge of the profession in order to incorporate such knowledge in student learning. 3. Assists with the development of new learning processes that can enhance learning opportunities for students in the program. 4. Develops a plan of continued proficiency in emerging pedagogy through investigation, and formal and informal education.	1. Embraces new approaches for fieldwork, including in non-OT practice settings, international fieldwork, diverse settings. 2. Projects an exemplary curricular model representing the OT/OTA academic program.	1. Embraces new approaches for fieldwork in traditional or emerging practice settings. 2. Implements a model fieldwork program that reflects the curricular design of the academic program. 3. Uses innovation within own fieldwork setting to enhance student learning experience during fieldwork.
Intermediate	1. Projects future trends and societal needs of the profession and appropriately adapts the curriculum, including both the academic and fieldwork components. 2. Establishes a management plan that guides student development in the OT program and facilitates faculty development within the OT unit and the college/university community.	1. Proposes and implements nontraditional learning environments that facilitate development of competent and ethical professionals. 2. Participates in college-/university-wide committees and assists in propelling the institution forward in the future in order to meet projected societal needs. 3. Embraces the use and development of course materials and experiences that are innovative and non-traditional.	1. Proposes strategies that facilitate linkages between academic program curriculum and fieldwork practice opportunities. 2. Proposes strategies to support client centered, meaningful, occupation-based, and evidence-based outcomes of the OT process during fieldwork experiences.	1. Proposes strategies that facilitate collaborative partnerships between academic program curricula and fieldwork practice opportunities. 2. Proposes strategies to support client-centered, meaningful, occupation-based, and evidence-based outcomes of the OT process during fieldwork experiences.

Table 1.

Innovator/Visionary *(cont.)*

Experience	Academic Program Director	OT/OTA Faculty Member	Academic Fieldwork Coordinator	Fieldwork Educator
Intermediate		4. Assesses and predicts the effectiveness of new learning processes to enhance learning opportunities for students in the program.		3. Promotes innovation among fieldwork educators in OT as well as other disciplines in own and other related settings to enhance student learning experiences and interdisciplinary collaboration.
Advanced	1. Anticipates future directions of the profession in meeting societal needs by exploring new possibilities for strategic planning and identifying factors related to funding, resources, etc. 2. Identifies opportunities to engage with the community to promote OT as a profession in order to serve society's evolving needs. 3. Identifies new ways of applying the use of occupation that will lead to societal growth, prosperity and social justice.	1. Proposes innovative solutions and designs innovative strategies to address predicted future trends in education, practice, and research. 2. Proposes, builds, and sustains novel integrative collaborations across disciplines.	1. Predicts future directions for fieldwork environments in emerging practice areas and propose fieldwork opportunities for students. 2. Innovates strategies for providing fieldwork in emerging practice areas 3. Anticipates and prepares for the direction of legal and health care policy that influences fieldwork and designs strategies for compliance.	1. Predicts future directions of practice and fieldwork in emerging environments and develops fieldwork opportunities for students. 2. Consults with other fieldwork educators and sites to develop creative learning experiences for students. 3. Innovates strategies for providing fieldwork in emerging practice areas. 4. Anticipates and prepares for the direction of legal and health care policy that influences fieldwork and designs strategies for compliance.

(Continued)

Table 2.
Scholar/Explorer

Experience	Academic Program Director	OT/OTA Faculty Member	Academic Fieldwork Coordinator	Fieldwork Educator
Novice	1. Possesses requisite knowledge and skills to design and conduct independent research relevant to OT practice and education and to disseminate results. 2. Recognizes the importance of scholarship within the academic community in general and within own educational institution in particular. 3. Designs a curriculum that meets accreditation standards relating to the scholarly role and skills of entry-level practitioners. 4. Actively engages in scholarly activities within area of expertise. 5. Creates a scholarly environment in which faculty and students have substantive resources and infrastructure necessary for productive scholarship.	1. Effectively critiques and uses new research literature and educational materials that will promote critical thinking, evidence-based practice, and lifelong learning in preparing future practitioners. 2. Critically integrates theory and research evidence into practice and facilitates that process in learners. 3. Models behaviors that demonstrate the importance of scholarship to learners and practitioners. 4. Initiates research inquiry within contextually determined expectations, either independently or with a mentor.* 5. Initiates the processes to develop a line of inquiry for research.* *May not always be possible for faculty in an OTA program.*	1. Effectively critiques and utilizes new research literature and educational materials that will promote critical thinking, evidence-based practice, and lifelong learning in preparing future practitioners. 2. Facilitates fieldwork educators' ability to effectively critique and use new research literature and educational materials that will promote critical thinking, evidence-based practice, and lifelong learning in preparing future practitioners. 3. Critically integrates theory and research evidence into practice and facilitates that process in fieldwork educators. 4. Facilitates integration and agreement of the academic philosophy and curriculum design within the fieldwork site. 5. Identifies questions about the fieldwork learning experiences for future research. 6. Facilitates best practices in using scholarship of teaching and learning in practice settings.	1. Critically evaluates current research to reflect best practice in teaching and practice. 2. Engages in systematic literature reviews to support and enhance practice. 3. Recognizes scholarly role in client service provision and program evaluation. 4. Models engagement in evidence-based practice specific to setting and populations served. 5. Seeks current evidence and information regarding effective fieldwork education and educational methodologies. 6. Translates practice knowledge into learning modes appropriate for fieldwork students. 7. Identifies questions about the fieldwork learning experiences for future research. 8. Monitors and interprets fieldwork student learning outcomes and effectiveness of student fieldwork program. 9. Coordinates with the Academic Fieldwork Coordinator to monitor and interpret student fieldwork learning outcomes.

Table 2.
Scholar/Explorer *(cont.)*

Experience	Academic Program Director	OT/OTA Faculty Member	Academic Fieldwork Coordinator	Fieldwork Educator
Intermediate	1. Coordinates active research agenda within the occupational therapy program. 2. Facilitates interdisciplinary collaboration and cooperation in research.	1. Contributes to the production of new findings and educational materials that add to the knowledge base of the profession. 2. Actively cultivates knowledge, skills, and interests in students by incorporating evidence from research into practice. 3. Conducts scholarship independently and begins to identify a coherent line(s) of inquiry.* 4. Successfully advises and guides students and practitioners in research.* 5. Disseminates findings in a public format such as presentations and publications. 6. Seeks opportunities to serve as a reviewer, editor, or publisher of scholarly work to internal and external audiences. *May not always be possible for faculty in an OTA program.*	1. Synthesizes new research literature and educational materials that will promote critical thinking, evidence-based practice, and lifelong learning in preparing future practitioners. 2. Conducts workshops and training programs to facilitate fieldwork educators' ability to use evidence in fieldwork education. 3. Plans and engages in the scholarship of teaching and learning regarding fieldwork education. 4. Collaborates with fieldwork educators and faculty to conduct research regarding fieldwork.	1. Designs evidence-based practice learning opportunities for fieldwork students to enhance understanding of the OT process. 2. Contributes to the breadth and body of knowledge through collaborative research projects. 3. Generates a clinical research agenda in collaboration with clinical and academic colleagues. 4. Collaborates with Academic Fieldwork Coordinator and faculty to conduct research regarding fieldwork.
Advanced	1. Provides national leadership in the development of and/or implementation of scholarship that further establishes foundational knowledge and efficacy of occupational therapy interventions.	1. Develops collaborative opportunities in research and scholarly work with other faculty. 2. Effectively produces and disseminates new findings within and outside of the profession.	1. Creates and disseminates new resources for fieldwork educators and Academic Fieldwork Coordinators to incorporate best practices in fieldwork education through student–fieldwork educator collaboration.	1. Models for students the importance of practitioner scholarship by engaging in independent and/or collaborative research projects and program evaluation.

(Continued)

Table 2.
Scholar/Explorer *(cont.)*

Experience	Academic Program Director	OT/OTA Faculty Member	Academic Fieldwork Coordinator	Fieldwork Educator
Advanced	2. Contributes to and/or leads national dialogue concerning the advancement of OT theory and practice through research and scholarship.	3. Establishes a well-defined scholarly agenda or lines of inquiry. 4. Provides leadership in advancing the profession's knowledge base. 5. Uses innovative methodologies to identify, analyze, and effectively address the changing needs of society at the local, national, or global levels. 6. Establishes a national or international reputation or recognition as an expert in their area of inquiry.	2. Conducts research with other Academic Fieldwork Coordinator and fieldwork educators 3. Uses research evidence to inform professional educational policy.	2. Engages in multisite research.

Table 3.
Leader

Experience	Academic Program Director	OT/OTA Faculty Member	Academic Fieldwork Coordinator	Fieldwork Educator
Novice	1. Uses management and leadership skills related to finance, planning, policy, marketing, public relations, and legal issues in order to meet accreditation standards and fulfill the program and institutional missions within an increasingly challenging educational environment. 2. Uses excellent interpersonal skills and demonstrates the ability to relate to diverse groups, constituencies, and organizations. 3. Takes responsibility for the assessment process for specific and overall program evaluation to enable the individual faculty to assess, diagnose, and apply interventions necessary to ensure quality.	1. Facilitates student development toward leadership roles. 2. Models ethical and professional behavior to facilitate the transition from student to clinician, advocate, and future fieldwork educator. 3. Assesses course materials, objectives, and educational experiences to promote optimal learning for students. 4. Develops plan of continued competency in leadership skills as related to role of teaching. 5. Participates with faculty in identifying trends that may influence future student learning and preparation.	1. Takes responsibility to develop systems to manage data for record keeping, fieldwork contract agreements, confidential student health records, and so on to ensure compliance with standards and legal requirements of local, state, and federal jurisdictions. 2. Develops a working relationship between the institution and fieldwork sites to facilitate ongoing collaborative partnerships to support education and practice. 3. Assists and monitors students in the development of their successful transition from the academic to the fieldwork portion of the educational program. 4. Evaluates the ongoing effectiveness of the fieldwork program, including student performance and fieldwork site integration of academic curricular design.	1. Critically reviews site-specific fieldwork program to ensure that quality learning experiences reflect best practice. 2. Advocates for department-wide participation in fieldwork education. 3. Facilitates student's transition into practice.
Intermediate	1. Forms strategic alliances with critical constituent groups within and outside the program's organization that can assist and promote the program's goals.	1. Seeks and obtains leadership role as representative from OTA/OT/OS department on institution-wide committees and organizations where collaboration occurs between various disciplines of study.	1. Analyzes current and future trends in OT practice to develop fieldwork settings to reflect emerging practice.	1. Modifies site-specific fieldwork objectives to ensure that high-quality learning experiences reflect best practice.

(Continued)

Table 3.
Leader *(cont.)*

Experience	Academic Program Director	OT/OTA Faculty Member	Academic Fieldwork Coordinator	Fieldwork Educator
	2. Builds and maintains systems that ensure that the program operates in concert with the mission of the institution and the mission of the academic unit in which the program is housed. 3. Seeks and accepts institutional leadership roles.	2. Analyzes past, present, and future trends to integrate practice, theory, literature, and research for instruction in evidence-based practice. 3. Collaborates with other faculty members on scholarship/research activities related to the advancement of occupational therapy, occupational science, teaching, and outcomes assessment.	2. Develops or explores innovative strategies of supervision for students in emerging practice areas. 3. Collaborates with other clinical coordinators within the institution to streamline policies and procedures with regard to student placements in fieldwork.	2. Educates colleagues and develops networks and programs to ensure fieldwork excellence. 3. Participates in knowledge generation by contributing to local, regional, and/or national fieldwork discussion/dialogues. 4. Participates in national initiatives that are collaborative efforts between educational institutions and fieldwork sites (e.s. backpack awareness month).
Advanced	1. Applies the processes of advancement (philanthropy), including identifying, cultivating, and securing gifts through the matching of potential donors with well-articulated needs. 2. Seeks and accepts leadership roles within the community as well as within state, national, and international associations.	1. Proposes innovative solutions and designs innovative strategies to address predicted future trends in education, practice, and research. 2. Proposes, builds, and sustains novel integrative collaborations across disciplines.	1. Develops national and international fieldwork student exchanges, placements, and programs. 2. Provides national and global leadership in the development of fieldwork education. 3. Develops and evaluates the ongoing effectiveness and quality of national and international fieldwork education. 4. Seeks and fully embraces the leadership role in the education of regional fieldwork consortiums.	1. Develops national models for fieldwork education in collaboration with other Fieldwork Educators and Academic Feildwork Coordinators across disciplines. 2. Shares innovative models of fieldwork supervision on a state, national, and international levels. 3. Seeks leadership roles in regional, national, and international fieldwork education.

Table 4.
Integrator

Experience	Academic Program Director	OT/OTA Faculty Member	Academic Fieldwork Coordinator	Fieldwork Educator
Novice	1. Forms strategic alliances with critical constituent groups within and outside the program's organization that can assist and promote the program's goals.	1. Develops a plan to continue proficiency in teaching through investigation, continuing education, and self-investigation. 2. Meets diverse learning needs of students and faculty. 3. Creates learning environments that facilitate the development of culturally sensitive, competent, and ethical professionals. 4. Independently seeks, selectively chooses relevant resources from OT and other disciplines, and disseminates information to promote advanced understanding in a variety of areas. 5. Develops a strategic plan for professional development that combines teaching, scholarship, and service.	1. Seeks close collaboration with fieldwork educators to facilitate student fieldwork learning and align clinical fieldwork program with curriculum design/outcomes. 2. Facilitates partnerships between program faculty and fieldwork educators. 3. Supports communication, collaboration, and connections between students and fieldwork educators to support the selection, matching, and scheduling of appropriate fieldwork experiences. 4. Designs culturally sensitive fieldwork programs and fieldwork objectives. Advocates for interdisciplinary fieldwork learning opportunities. 5. Collaborates with fieldwork educators and faculty to facilitate congruence of curriculum design and best practice.	1. Seeks close collaboration with academic programs to facilitate student fieldwork learning and align clinical fieldwork program with curriculum design/outcome. 2. Develops and/or modifies clinical fieldwork manual/objectives to reflect national standards and academic fieldwork objectives. 3. Collaborates with Academic Fieldwork Coordinator to ensure integration of curriculum design into the practice setting. 4. Designs culturally sensitive fieldwork programs and fieldwork objectives. 5. Facilitates collaborative learning among fieldwork students within the profession and across disciplines.
Intermediate	1. Integrates increasingly diverse sources of information in order to define problems, explore solutions, and formulate appropriate decisions that result in effective management of the academic unit to meet its mission.	1. Develops a framework from which to practice using divergent resources. 2. Demonstrates progress of professional development plan that combines teaching, scholarship, and service.	1. Analyzes current trends to create new fieldwork opportunities. 2. Facilitates development of Academic Fieldwork Advisory Panels that integrate diverse perspectives from the community.	1. Serves on Academic Fieldwork Advisory Panels. 2. Actively facilitates interdisciplinary fieldwork learning opportunities.

(Continued)

Table 4.
Integrator (cont.)

Experience	Academic Program Director	OT/OTA Faculty Member	Academic Fieldwork Coordinator	Fieldwork Educator
Intermediate		3. Forms strategic alliances across disciplines to advance the profession.		3. Develops and/or modifies fieldwork student manual/objectives to reflect national standards and academic fieldwork objectives. 4. Functions as a practice resource for Academic Fieldwork Coordinators to enhance fieldwork collaboration and academic outcomes. 5. Models cultural sensitivity when designing fieldwork programs and fieldwork objectives.
Advanced	1. Fosters ongoing relationships among educators, researchers, and practitioners that address the needs of both the profession and society. 2. Creatively collaborates with consumers, interdisciplinary educators, and researchers to meet the increasingly complex needs of national and global communities. 3. Effectively utilizes various venues, such as regulatory bodies, nongovernmental organizations, legislatures, and other bodies such as the World Health Organization or the Centers for Disease Control and Prevention in order to promote the health and well-being of people through occupation.	1. Collaborates with diverse disciplines for information synthesis and dissemination. 2. Articulates and represents the role of OT in emerging areas of practice at the local, national, and international levels. 3. Creatively collaborates with consumers, interdisciplinary educators, and researchers to meet the increasingly complex needs of national and global communities. 4. Effectively uses various venues, such as regulatory bodies, nongovernmental organizations, legislatures, and other internationally recognized agencies in order to promote the health and well-being through occupation.	1. Bridges the gap between OT/OTA practitioner needs (evidence-based practice) and resources available through OT/OTA academic program and student fieldwork experiences. 2. Enhances relationships with regional/national/international fieldwork committees. 3. Creatively contributes to a national/ international understanding of the importance of fieldwork education by facilitating meaningful relationships and networking among practitioners, students, and educators.	1. Contributes to a more coherent understanding of health care service provision and a national fieldwork student network. 2. Develops/contributes to interdisciplinary experimental learning modules. 3. Serves on regional/national/international fieldwork committees. 4. Creatively contributes to a national and international understanding of the importance of fieldwork education by facilitating meaningful relationships and networking among practitioners, students, and educators.

298

Table 5.
Mentor

Experience	Academic Program Director	OT/OTA Faculty Member	Academic Fieldwork Coordinator	Fieldwork Educator
Novice	1. Serves as a model to mentor diverse faculty, students, alumni, and occupational therapy practitioners in their area of expertise. 2. Facilitates mentoring relationships within the academic institution. 3. Models professional and ethical behavior within the academic setting. 4. Instills in students the professional responsibility of seeking and offering mentoring relationships. 5. Analyzes personal and professional goals and acquires resources necessary to attain professional growth.	1. Demonstrates a competent and positive attitude that results in the mentoring of students in professional development in scholarship, research, and/or service. 2. Develops and fosters trusting relationships with practitioners interested in transitioning from practice into academia. 3. Identifies a variety of tangible and intangible resources that can enhance the professional growth of self and others. 4. Analyzes personal and professional goals and acquires resources necessary to attain professional growth. 5. Encourages potential students to develop relationships with OT/OTA practitioners, alumni, students, and faculty prior to entering the profession. 6. Facilitates the inclusion of a diverse community of faculty and students through the mentoring process.	1. Coaches and guides students to engage in appropriate professional and fieldwork education activities. 2. Creates a collaborative process between academic faculty and fieldwork educators. 3. Serves as a model and consultant for fieldwork educators to facilitate development of quality fieldwork programs. 4. Facilitates the growth of practitioners and fieldwork educators for implementing best practice principles during fieldwork education. 5. Analyzes personal and professional goals and acquires resources necessary to attain professional growth. 6. Encourages potential students to develop relationships with occupational therapy practitioners, students, alumni, and faculty prior to entering the profession. 7. Facilitates the inclusion of a diverse community of faculty and students through the mentoring process. 8. Serves as a model representative of the academic program locally and regionally.	1. Mentors students prior to and during fieldwork by functioning as a model. 2. Serves as a model to mentor diverse individuals and occupational therapy practitioners in their area of expertise. 3. Encourages potential students to develop relationships with occupational therapy practitioners, students, and faculty prior to entering the profession. 4. Analyzes personal and professional goals and acquires resources necessary to attain professional growth.

(Continued)

Table 5.
Mentor *(cont.)*

Experience	Academic Program Director	OT/OTA Faculty Member	Academic Fieldwork Coordinator	Fieldwork Educator
Intermediate	1. Develops innovative strategies for negotiating creative, constructive, and ethical solutions to address interpersonal and academic issues within a complex environment. 2. Develops resources, policies and procedures/ guidelines for faculty that can be used to facilitate progressively higher levels of responsibility at the department, university, community, and professional levels. 3. Uses a variety of methods and technology to expand mentoring relationships beyond the academic institution and the community it serves. 1. Anticipates and facilitates	1. Identifies individuals or groups in need of mentoring who would otherwise not seek mentorship and encourages them to develop mentoring relationships to maximize their potential. 2. Participates in mentoring or coaching of junior faculty through constructive feedback and role modeling of work with students, practitioners, and peers. 3. Effectively mentors and functions as faculty advisor for student organizations. 4. Inspires others to serve as mentor to students, alumni, practitioners, and faculty. 5. Actively contributes to the accomplishment of long-term expectations and outcomes of mentor relationships necessary for own personal and professional growth. 6. Uses a variety of methods and technology to expand mentoring relationships beyond the academic institution and the community it serves.	1. Collaborates with fieldwork educators to promote effective and innovative learning opportunities for students. 2. Tutors and coaches non-OT fieldwork educators in their development as supervisors and their implementation of fieldwork experiences reflecting OT practice. 3. Models and facilitates development of innovative strategies to obtain excellence within the constraints of the fieldwork practice environment. 4. Coaches students, fieldwork educators, and Academic Fieldwork Coordinators to negotiate and problem solve challenging fieldwork dilemmas. 5. Creates effective resources reflecting current trends and emerging practice areas to sustain excellence in fieldwork education. 6. Influences the development of innovative programs to bridge the gap between fieldwork and didactic content into a cohesive curriculum design. 7. Uses a variety of methods and technology to expand mentoring relationships beyond existing fieldwork education network.	1. Identifies a variety of tangible and intangible resources that can be used to enhance the professional growth of self and others. 2. Recruits and guides inexperienced OT/OTA staff to develop in the role as a fieldwork educator. 3. Models excellence as a fieldwork educator and fieldwork site coordinator. 4. Models excellence and commitment to the tenets of the profession using occupational-based and evidence-based practice during the OT process. 5. Develops mentorship programs within the facility that reflect and promote interdisciplinary and intradisciplinary fieldwork excellence. 6. Uses a variety of methods and technology to expand mentoring relationships beyond the fieldwork site. 7. Develops innovative strategies for negotiating creative, constructive, and ethical solutions to address interpersonal and practice issues within a complex environment. 8. Serves as role model for other fieldwork educators.

Table 5.

Mentor *(cont.)*

Experience	Academic Program Director	OT/OTA Faculty Member	Academic Fieldwork Coordinator	Fieldwork Educator
Advanced	the development of future mentoring relationships within and outside the educational program to meet the needs of the profession and society. 2. Facilitates intra- and interdisciplinary mentoring relationships for faculty, students, alumni, and practitioners. 3. Models advocacy and acts as a change agent to fulfill the occupational and social justice vision of the profession both nationally and globally. 4. Identifies and addresses professional and societal trends that may present new ethical challenges for the profession and society. 5. Inspires others to develop new strategies and paradigms in response to societal issues.	1. Creates and shares networks, resources, and opportunities for growth of mentees at the national and international levels. 2. Develops and sustains programs across disciplines and geographical regions to foster mentees' successful performance in scholarship, teaching, and practice. 3. Models advocacy and acts as a change agent to fulfill the occupational and social justice vision of the profession both nationally and globally. 4. Develops innovative strategies for facilitating connections among students, educators, alumni, practitioners, and other colleagues for unusual, challenging, and/or complex mentee needs or situations. 5. Anticipates and develops mentoring opportunities and programs designed to address disparities in health care, social injustices, issues within the profession, and society. 6. Develops innovative strategies for negotiating creative, constructive, and ethical solutions to address interpersonal and academic issues within a complex environment.	1. Models the creation of innovative fieldwork training programs globally to anticipate and meet the needs of the profession in the future. 2. Facilitates national and international networks among academic fieldwork coordinators to collectively and systematically address fieldwork issues. 3. Develops innovative strategies for negotiating creative, constructive, and ethical solutions that address interpersonal and academic issues within a complex environment. 4. Develops and sustains programs across disciplines and geographical regions to foster mentees' successful performance in scholarship, teaching, and practice. 5. Anticipates and develops mentoring opportunities and programs designed to address disparities in health care, social injustices, issues within the profession, and society. 6. Models advocacy and acts as a change agent to fulfill the occupational and social justice vision of the profession both nationally and globally.	1. Consults on the development of new fieldwork programs, supporting at other fieldwork sites, settings, and practice areas. 2. Develops national and international programs of mentorship excellence that connect students, practitioners, fieldwork educators, and academic fieldwork coordinators. 3. Anticipates and develops mentoring opportunities and programs designed to address disparities in health care, social injustices, issues within the profession, and society. 4. Models advocacy and act as a change agent to fulfill the occupational and social justice vision of the profession both nationally and globally.

Specialized Knowledge and Skills for Occupational Therapy Practice in the Neonatal Intensive Care Unit

Purpose

The purpose of this paper is to provide a reference for occupational therapists on the advanced knowledge and skills necessary to practice in a neonatal intensive care unit (NICU). Occupational therapy practice with infants in the NICU and their families is high risk and specialized, only appropriate for occupational therapists with advanced knowledge and skills in neonatal care.

Introduction

Occupational therapy philosophy and education provide the foundation for this profession to make a valuable contribution to neonatal practice (American Occupational Therapy Association [AOTA], 2004b). Specialized knowledge of neonatal medical conditions and developmental variability and abnormality in infants cared for in the NICU is essential to safe, effective practice. The therapist must recognize the complex medical needs and vulnerabilities of acutely ill or premature infants. These infants frequently are physiologically fragile and easily compromised by environmental conditions. Interactions and therapeutic interventions that may appear innocuous can trigger physiologic instability in an infant and can be life threatening. In fact, protecting the fragile neonate from excessive or inappropriate sensory aspects of the environment is often a more urgent priority than direct interventions or interactions with the infant. Occupational therapy approaches, such as sensory integration and neurodevelopmental intervention, are applicable within the NICU setting. However, these approaches may need to be modified according to the infant's medical status, physiological homeostasis, and developmental and family needs.

The special needs of families whose infants are in the NICU also must be recognized. The infant's medical status and uncertain outcome, the highly technical environment of the NICU, separation from parents, and potential maternal complications after labor and delivery may contribute to family stress or crisis. These situations often alter the parent–infant attachment process, which is essential to optimal infant developmental outcomes. Families are best served by an occupational therapist who is not only knowledgeable about infant needs, but also sensitive to family circumstances, priorities, concerns, and cultural beliefs. The occupational therapist must seek ways to establish supportive, collaborative, and therapeutic relationships with family members in order to foster the infant's optimal development.

The social and physical aspects of the environment can be stressful to both the infant and the family. All persons who interact with the infant constitute the social environment. The physical environment is composed of inanimate elements and properties (e.g., lighting, sound, bedding, equipment). The occupational therapist must understand the interplay of the social and physical features of the NICU and the way in which this interplay influences the infant, family, and staff members. This knowledge is used as a basis for the occupational therapy evaluation and contributes to effective intervention strategies.

Working within the social and physical bounds of the NICU environment, an important role of the occupational therapist is to assist each family to foster optimal infant development, including the encouragement of developmentally appropriate occupations, sensorimotor processes, and neurobehavioral organization. This must occur while considering the often fragile medical and physiological status of the infant. Through direct observation, intervention, consultation, education, and research, the occupational therapist collaborates with others to provide the infant with the most effective and appropriate social and physical environment.

The occupational therapist working in the NICU must have a basic knowledge of occupational therapy, pediatric experience, and specialized knowledge and skills related to the complex needs of high-risk infants, their families, and the NICU environment. Basic occupational therapy education includes knowledge of biological sciences, disease processes, mental health, and typical and atypical child and adult family development. Occupational therapy's domain of concern, encompassing the interaction among the biological, developmental, and social–emotional aspects of human function as expressed in daily activities and occupations, makes it particularly suited to address the needs of the developing infant and family (AOTA, 2002). The occupational therapy method of activity analysis and adaptation to achieve a functional outcome is valuable in promoting "goodness of fit" (i.e., the match between the infant's capabilities and the physical and social environment), as there is often a mismatch between the NICU environment, parental expectations, and the infant's capabilities.

Experience in pediatric occupational therapy is essential for practice in the NICU. This experience provides a perspective on the continuum of typical and atypical child development and on the significance of the family in the child's life. Experience in pediatric occupational therapy affords the practitioner opportunities for development of the critical thinking skills necessary for evaluation and intervention to promote competent occupational performance and emotional well-being of children and their families. Therefore, the therapist interested in practicing in the NICU should have experience in the following areas: pediatric occupational therapy with infants and young children, longitudinal follow-up of infants treated in the NICU, and collaboration with families.

In addition to basic occupational therapy education and pediatric experience, the occupational therapist working in the NICU requires advanced knowledge and skills to provide complex interventions to critically ill neonates and their families. These interventions require continuous evaluation and a dynamic approach to intervention planning. They also require knowledge of grief reactions, social structures, attachment, medical procedures, and other issues relating to the health and well-being of the family unit. Intervention in the NICU context is not a recommended area of practice for occupational therapy assistants because such knowledge and skills are beyond the scope of their practice. Since practice in the NICU requires advanced-level expertise and clinical reasoning, this area of practice also is not recommended for entry-level occupational therapists or occupational therapists who do not have the pediatric experience described above. Extensive continuing education; mentoring by an occupational therapist experienced in neonatal care; and graded, closely supervised, mentored practice are recommended for any occupational therapist entering neonatal practice. Supervision often is required until the therapist demonstrates competency in working with infants and their families in the NICU environment (AOTA, 2004a).

The specialized knowledge required for practice in the NICU includes familiarity with relevant medical conditions, procedures, and equipment; an understanding of the individualized developmental abilities and vulnerabilities of infants; an understanding of theories of neonatal neurobehavioral organization; working knowledge of family systems, early social–emotional development, infant mental health, and NICU ecology; and an understanding of multidisciplinary team collaboration. Most importantly, the NICU therapist must have a clear understanding of the manner in which these factors interact to influence behavior. The occupational therapist develops the necessary skills through continuing education and supervised mentored clinical experience in evaluation and intervention specific to the NICU. Neonatal practice requires advanced clinical reasoning skills. These skills include the flexibility to recognize and respond to unfamiliar situations and nuances of behavior, the ability to anticipate future directions of intervention, and the ability to perceive the clinical condition as a whole. The occupational therapist in the NICU applies these competencies with regard to the infant; the infant's family and caregivers; and the NICU environment, including staff. Specifically, the occupational therapist in the NICU designs an individualized intervention plan in collaboration with the family and others that incorporates the family's priorities and NICU contexts along with the individualized needs of the infant. This requires understanding the occupations and activities valued by families and the NICU culture; defining what factors limit each infant's participation or engagement in those occupations and activities; identifying factors that would constitute readiness for engagement in occupations and activities; and finally, delineating what physical and/or social environmental supports will maximize participation for both the infant and the family in the short term and in the long term.

Maintenance of clinical competency and an evidence-based approach to practice are both vitally important in the rapidly changing field of neonatology. Clinical competence can be sustained through regular supervision or a mentoring relationship, participation in peer study groups, reflective process, and formal and informal continuing education. An evidence-based approach to practice necessitates ongoing critical review of the relevant research, literature, and clinical tools available in this rapidly changing field of practice. An occupational therapy practitioner is knowledgeable about evidence-based research and applies it ethically and appropriately to the occupational therapy process (AOTA, 2005b).

Knowledge and Skills: The Infant, Family, and NICU Environment

The following information identifies the knowledge and skills needed to function as an occupational therapist in the NICU. This information is organized under the three main areas of occupational therapy concern described previously: the infant, the family, and the NICU environment.

The Infant

To be competent, the occupational therapist has to have an in-depth understanding of approaches to evaluation and intervention, including use of a developmentally supportive consultative model of service delivery. These approaches are presented in the literature specific to occupational therapy, neonatology, psychology, and infant and family studies. In addition, the therapist has to have a thorough understanding of medical factors and the potential risks they pose to normal fetal and infant growth and development. The therapist must understand and critically analyze this information within the context of occupational therapy practice and the specific philosophy of the NICU in which the occupational therapist works. The therapist develops an evaluation plan that includes use of appropriate standardized tools, parent or caregiver interviews, and observations of infant adaptation to the social and physical environments. The occupational therapist, in conjunction with the family and medical caregivers, then develops appropriate intervention strategies, individually suited to each infant and family.

For clarity in this paper, infant behavior is discussed separately from family and environmental concerns. However, in program implementation, the infant is assessed and treated within the context of the family and the NICU environment.

The following is a comprehensive outline of the essential knowledge base that an occupational therapist must possess for working with NICU infants.

I. Medical knowledge base as the foundation for understanding infant behavior

    A. General information

        1. Medical terminology and abbreviations used in the NICU

        2. Basic principles, uses, and potential complications of the medical equipment and procedures, including precautions and implications for the therapist and infant

        3. Medical complications frequently encountered, including pathophysiology, risks, precautions, and prognoses associated with specific conditions.

    B. Specific knowledge

        1. NICU equipment

        2. Diagnostic procedures

        3. Medical procedures

        4. Nursing procedures and routines

        5. Respiratory support

        6. Thermoregulatory support

        7. Nutritional support

        8. Medication effects

        9. Infection control

        10. Institution-specific policies and procedures.

II. Factors that may influence infant and child development

    A. Prenatal

        1. Maternal and fetal complications during pregnancy

        2. Genetic disorders, congenital anomalies, syndromes, isolated defects

        3. Teratogens (e.g., licit and illicit drug exposure, radiation, environmental contaminates)

        4. Infectious diseases (e.g., rubella, cytomegalovirus, herpes, toxoplasmosis, HIV)

        5. Social risk factors (e.g., poverty, inadequate support, stress, environmental toxins).

    B. Perinatal

        1. Maternal complications during delivery

        2. Neonatal complications during delivery

        3. Gestational age and birth weight.

    C. Postnatal conditions and complications

        1. Respiratory

        2. Cardiovascular

        3. Neurologic

        4. Sensory

        5. Orthopedic

        6. Gastrointestinal

        7. Metabolic

        8. Hemolytic

        9. Dermatologic

        10. Infectious disease

        11. Iatrogenic complications.

III. Knowledge of the developmental course, abilities, and vulnerabilities of infants in the NICU

   A. Differences in body structure and body functions, developmental progression, variations, deviations, and abnormalities in infants in relation to preterm, term, or postterm birth and/or prenatal, perinatal, or postnatal factors

      1. Infant neurobehavioral organization

         a. Physiologic (e.g., cardiorespiratory)

         b. States of arousal

         c. Regulatory abilities
            Sleep and waking states
            Circadian rhythms
            Typical and atypical patterns
            Self-regulation
            External regulation
            Medication effects/side effects

         d. Neurosocial (e.g., attention, interaction).

      2. Sensory development and processing of sensory information

         a. Sequential developmental progression in utero and adaptations to the extra-uterine environment

         b. Thresholds for stimulation within the sensory systems: tactile, vestibular, proprioceptive, visual, auditory, olfactory, gustatory

         c. Responses: arousal, attention, modulation, transition, range, decompensation

         d. Sensory acuity.

      3. Motor function

         a. Neuromotor development, including, but not limited to, muscle tone, posture, quality of movement, reflexes and reactions, and motor control

         b. Biomechanical factors, including, but not limited to, active and passive range of motion, strength, and orthopedic status.

      4. Social–emotional development

         a. Early communicative cues

         b. Self-regulation of interaction

         c. Initial formation of attachment relationships

         d. Temperament.

   B. Emerging competencies in infant occupation

      1. General factors that influence participation in daily life activities

         a. Postconceptional age and weight

         b. Physical and developmental maturation

         c. Physiological status and medical conditions

         d. Neurobehavioral organization

    e. Sensory processing

    f. Biomechanical and neuromotor function

    g. Social interaction

    h. Physical environment

    i. Social environment.

2. Specific activities

    a. Ability to cope with and participate in caregiving

        (1) Feeding process

            (a) Modes (e.g., breast, bottle, tube)

            (b) Function (e.g., ability to meet nutritional needs, physiologic cost, endurance)

            (c) Oral–motor mechanism (e.g., structure, function, quality)

            (d) Maturation of mechanical and neural control of sucking, swallowing, and breathing

            (e) Relationship among nutritive and non-nutritive sucking, respiration, and oxygenation

            (f) Positioning and handling

            (g) Feeding readiness cues

            (h) Physiologic issues, such as metabolic and neurologic

            (i) Competency of the infant as a partner

            (j) Relationship with primary caregivers

            (k) Tolerance of oral–facial and intraoral sensations.

        (2) Bathing

        (3) Dressing and diapering

        (4) Medical routines and procedures.

    b. Engaging in nurturing interactions

        (1) Skin-to-skin holding (kangaroo care)

        (2) Physical and social dialogue

        (3) Feeding.

    c. Interrelationship between medical and developmental domains

        (1) Present conditions

        (2) Future implications.

IV. Knowledge of evolving developmental approaches in the NICU

    A. Historical and current perspectives

        1. Supplemental stimulation

        2. Reduced stimulation

        3. Environmental neonatology

4. Individualized developmental care

5. Family-centered care

6. Relationship-based approach.

B. Modification and integration of current pediatric occupational therapy frames of reference (e.g., sensory integration, neurodevelopmental therapy, coping, dynamic systems).

V. Specific skills related to occupational therapy with infants in the NICU, including the ability to

A. Instruct, consult, and communicate with caregivers

B. Use NICU equipment appropriately and safely, including understanding of the purpose, basic operation, settings, and precautions of all relevant equipment

C. Conduct appropriate assessments

1. Determine appropriate timing of infant assessments on the basis of the infant's medical and physiological status, postconceptional age, and NICU and family routines

2. Select and administer formal and informal assessment procedures that are appropriate for postconceptional age and medical condition and that identify developmental abilities, vulnerabilities, and limitations in daily life activities and occupations as they are influenced by medical status and

   a. Neurobehavioral organization

   b. Sensory development and processing

   c. Motor function

   d. Pain

   e. Daily activity (e.g., feeding)

   f. Social–emotional development.

3. Assess the effects of physical environment, caregiving practices, positioning, and nurturance on the infant's neurobehavioral organization, sensory, motor, and medical status.

D. Formulate an individualized therapeutic intervention plan that supports the infant's current level of function and facilitates optimal social–emotional, physical, cognitive, and sensory development of the infant within the context of the family and the NICU

1. Determine appropriate timing of infant interventions on the basis of the infant's medical and physiological status, postconceptional age, and NICU and family bedside routines

2. Modify sensory aspects of physical environment according to infant sensory threshold

3. Participate with the infant and caregivers in occupational therapy interventions that reinforce the role of the family as the constant in the life of the infant and support the individual infant's medical and physiological status in order to

   a. Enhance infant neurobehavioral organization

   b. Facilitate social participation

   c. Promote optimal infant neuromotor functioning and engagement in daily life activities

   d. Promote developmentally appropriate motor function and engagement in daily life activities through the use of biomechanical techniques, when appropriate

   e. Facilitate well-organized infant behavior through adaptation of infant daily life activities.

E. Continuously observe and critically analyze subtle infant responses to the intervention program and modify as needed

F. Collaborate with family, NICU staff, and other persons who potentially may have an impact on infant well-being to

1. Create and maintain individualized developmental care plans

2. Incorporate the occupational therapy program into NICU routines

3. Modify intervention and discharge plans considering anticipated infant outcome.

G. Provide documentation that is objective, interpretive, thorough, and concise

H. Formulate discharge and follow-up plans in coordination with the interdisciplinary team and community resources to meet the developmental needs of the infant and family.

The Family

Parents and other family members are acknowledged to be the most important and consistent influence in the infant's life. Their occupational roles as primary caregivers and nurturers constantly need to be recognized and reaffirmed. Typically, parents are mediators of the infant's affective, sensory, and motor experiences. When an infant is hospitalized in the NICU immediately after birth, parents are not always able to play this mediation role. The bi-directional attachment process, which begins at delivery and in which both infant and parent play a part, can be disrupted. Since attachment provides a foundation for the infant's future development and independent function, its promotion is an important consideration for the occupational therapist. Therefore, the occupational therapist collaborates with family members, on-site and off-site, to facilitate the infant's optimal development, promote the parents' occupational roles, support parent–infant attachment, and ensure a successful transition from hospital to home and community.

The following outline summarizes the knowledge base that would enable an occupational therapist to provide services in the NICU from a family-centered perspective.

I. Knowledge of the family as a basis for collaboration

A. Family systems

1. Family structure, occupational roles, cultural identification, beliefs, values, and practices

2. Family resources: Sources and allocation (e.g., time, money, energy, social–emotional support)

3. Family adaptation: Adjustment to adding a new family member, adjustment to stressful situations

4. Needs, culture, and roles of family members, including siblings.

B. Adult learning styles

1. Individual differences in learning

2. Relationship between emotional state and learning capacities

3. Changes in parental focus during NICU course.

C. Parent–infant interactions: progression and individual differences

1. Parents' role in the infant's early social–emotional development

2. Attachment as an ongoing two-way process between parents and infant, including the importance of attachment to later developmental function and the influence of hospitalization on parents and infants on the attachment process

   3. Development of synchronous interactions

   4. Importance of parents' learning to accurately observe, interpret, and respond to their infant's unique cues.

   D. The transition of the infant from hospital to home and community

      1. Possible stresses and difficulties inherent in the transition process for the infant and each family member

      2. Knowledge of community resources and local, state, and federal guidelines and services.

II. Specific skills related to occupational therapy with families of infants in the NICU. The occupational therapist

   A. Identifies family hopes, dreams, expectations, attitudes, knowledge, strengths, priorities, preferred communication styles, and skills regarding daily care, play, and other interactions with the infant

   B. Identifies family members' learning styles

   C. Assists parents in feeling comfortable with their infant and as parents to a new family member

   D. Guides family members in observing and interpreting their infant's behavior and in adapting their own behaviors in response to the infant's cues to elicit appropriate sensory, motor, and social responses

      1. During daily life activities

      2. During interactions involving exploration, attention, and orientation

      3. While engaged in nurturing interactions.

   E. Recognizes and acknowledges the infant's contribution and strengths in others' lives

   F. Fosters successful parent–infant interactions via mutual problem solving, anticipatory guidance, modeling of behaviors, didactic and experiential education, and modification of the infant's environment

   G. Integrates family observations and priorities in formulating occupational therapy intervention recommendations

   H. Interprets and discusses occupational therapy evaluation findings in collaboration with the family

   I. Adapts intervention approaches according to family culture, changing emotions, needs, and resources that may be influenced by the infant's changing medical status or other circumstances

   J. Formulates and implements a discharge and follow-up plan with the family and other team members to ensure a smooth transition to the community, integrating occupational therapy goals into the overall goals and priorities of the family.

The NICU Environment

The neonate who is born prematurely or acutely ill is not well-adapted to the stressful and technologically complex environment of the NICU. This mismatch between the infant and the environment may have a deleterious effect on the infant's medical and developmental outcomes. Therefore, a primary intervention goal in the NICU is to provide the best match or fit between the infant and the NICU environment. Adapting or structuring the environment to enhance function is a well-accepted occupational therapy approach. However, this first requires knowledge of the various components of the environment as well as their interplay. The occupational therapist assesses the environment and collaborates with others to shape the infant's physical and social environment to provide a milieu of developmentally supportive care. The following competencies are essential:

I. Knowledge of the unique sensory properties of the NICU and their relationship to each infant's neurobehavioral organization

   A. *Tactile:* Timing, intensity, texture, handling for medical and nursing procedures, parent interaction

   B. *Proprioceptive–vestibular:* Timing, intensity, handling for medical and nursing procedures, parent interaction

   C. *Olfactory and gustatory experiences specific to the NICU* (timing, quality, intensity)

   D. *Auditory:* Intensity, duration, timing, animate versus inanimate

   E. *Visual:* Timing, ambient and focal light intensity, contents of visual field.

II. Knowledge of the social environment and its relationship to each infant's neurobehavioral organization, including interactions and relationships among

   A. Parents and infant

   B. Extended family members and infant

   C. Staff members and infant

   D. Parents and staff members

   E. Occupational therapist, parents, staff, and infant.

III. Knowledge of the physical environment and its relationship to each infant's maturation and behavioral organization

   A. Medical equipment and procedures as described under the medical knowledge base section

   B. Frequency, timing, duration, quality, and intensity of sensory input from medical equipment and procedures

   C. Sensory input from equipment, procedures, and staff activities that is disruptive to the infant's neurobehavioral organization.

IV. Knowledge of the NICU culture

   A. The NICU's specific philosophy of care, including its particular orientation toward acute and chronic care of infants

   B. The team members' roles, functions, attitudes, and positions in the organizational structure of the individual NICU

   C. The influence of NICU stressors (e.g., census changes and subsequent staffing patterns)

   D. Communication patterns and structure, both formal and informal, among staff members and between family and staff members

   E. Spoken and unspoken rules of behavior

   F. The effect of the physical and social environments on staff performance and morale

   G. Hospital administrative policies (e.g., confidentiality).

V. Specific skills related to occupational therapy in assessing and adapting the environment. The occupational therapist

   A. Assesses the sensory aspects of the NICU physical and social environments and its effect on infant well-being

B. Develops intervention strategies in collaboration with the family, NICU staff, and other team members to adapt the environment in order to foster optimal infant development and family interactions

1. Communicates with all levels of staff to establish rapport and develop team commitment to developmental and family goals

2. Integrates occupational therapy goals into the infant's medical priorities and the NICU setting.

C. Develops and implements strategies to influence philosophy and practice of developmental and family-centered care within the NICU

D. Assesses the effect of intervention strategies and revises the plan accordingly.

VI. Knowledge of structures that support occupational therapy practice in the NICU

The occupational therapist position exists within the NICU structure. The following knowledge and skills are needed to ensure integration of occupational therapy services into the NICU setting for optimal infant-family outcomes:

A. Ability to articulate the role and function of occupational therapists in the NICU to demonstrate their value and effectiveness

B. Ability to use relevant research literature to support occupational therapy practice in the NICU

C. Knowledge of the hospital's structure, mission, strategic plan, and fiscal priorities as they relate to both NICU and occupational therapy programs

D. Ability to identify and access sources of administrative and fiscal support to maintain occupational therapy services in the NICU

E. Knowledge of the larger local, state, and national health and social service systems as they influence policy and fiscal support for occupational therapy services in the NICU and early intervention services

F. Ability to identify sources of administrative and fiscal support for the practice of occupational therapy within the NICU from the community and the health care system at large

G. Knowledge of confidentiality guidelines (e.g., HIPAA).

Professional and Personal Characteristics Necessary for Occupational Therapists Practicing in the NICU

The NICU, as a critical care area, necessitates certain professional and personal characteristics. These characteristics include the following:

1. Ability to synthesize information from multiple sources, including research findings, and judiciously apply it to the NICU

2. Ability to observe the infant and environment for prolonged periods, without intervening, and to identify and understand subtle nuances of behavior and physiology

3. Interest in and ability to bring about changes in the infant's social and physical environments through direct intervention with the infant and family, consultation and collaboration with other team members, and implementation of policies and procedures at the organizational level

4. Understanding of one's interpersonal communication skills and style and the ability to modify them in response to family and staff behavior, learning styles, and needs

5. Commitment to seek ongoing knowledge, education, and peer consultation in this field

6. Ability to provide formal and informal educational programs for the hospital and the community

7. Insight into one's professional knowledge and skills

8. Ability to value, communicate, and collaborate with other NICU team members, community-based early intervention programs, and other resources

9. Understanding of and ability to articulate one's values and attitudes about

   a. The rights and responsibilities of families

   b. Relationships between cultural or religious beliefs and medical management decisions

   c. Working with infants who ultimately may not survive

   d. Working with infants who may have severe and permanent disabilities

   e. Working with families whose values, attitudes, behaviors, and life circumstances differ from one's own

   f. Allocating limited fiscal, personnel, and technological resources to sustain life.

10. Understanding of the *AOTA Code of Ethics* (2005a) as it applies to the NICU.

Definitions

Activity
"[T]he performance of a task or action by an individual" (World Health Organization [WHO], 2001, p. 10).

Activity Limitations
"[D]ifficulties an individual may have in executing activities" (WHO, 2001, p. 10).

Attachment
"A bond between an infant and a caregiver, usually its mother. Attachment is generally formed within the context of a family, providing the child with the necessary feelings of safety and nurturing at a time when the infant is growing and developing. This relationship between the infant and his caregiver serves as a model for all future relationships" (Gale, 2005).

Body Functions
"[T]he physiological or psychological functions of body systems" (including psychological functions; WHO, 2001, p. 10).

Body Structures
"[A]natomical parts of the body, such as organs, limbs, and their components" (WHO, 2001, p. 10).

Bonding
See *Attachment*.

Clinical Reasoning Skills in Occupational Therapy
The process by which occupational therapists individualize and modify treatment. It includes not only the application of theory to practice, but also the treatment of the meaning of illness as experienced by the individual and family (Mattingly, 1991).

Environmental Factors
"[T]he physical, social, and attitudinal environment in which people live and conduct their lives" (WHO, 2001, p. 10).

Environmental Neonatology

The study of environment of newborn special care facilities and its impact on the medical and developmental status of at-risk infants (Gottfried & Gaiter, 1985).

Family

A unit composed of individuals who are linked by shared kinship, function, and/or responsibilities and who identify themselves in a common relationship (Crockenberg, Lyons-Ruth, & Dickson, 1993).

Family-Centered Care

A constellation of philosophies, attitudes, and approaches to the care of children with special health and developmental needs that recognizes that the family is the constant in the child's life and that parent–professional partnerships are essential to effective and high-quality service delivery (Dunst, Trivette, & Deal, 1988; Institute for Family-Centered Care, 1990).

Goodness-of-Fit

"When the properties of the environment and its expectations and demands are in accord with the organism's own capacities, characteristics, and style of behaving" (Chess & Thomas, 1999, p. 3).

Impairments

"[P]roblems in body function or structure such as a significant deviation or loss" (WHO, 2001, p. 10).

Infant Mental Health

"Infant" refers to children under 3 years of age. "Mental" includes social–emotional and cognitive domains. "Health" refers to the well-being of young children and families (Fraiberg, 1980). A multidisciplinary intervention approach for the "early identification of risk and treatment to reduce the likelihood of serious developmental failure and relationship disturbance" (Weatherston, 2002, p. 1).

Medical Caregivers

House staff involved in the care of infants in the NICU. Although personnel may vary between institutions, medical caregivers typically include nurses, physicians (e.g., neonatologists, attending physicians, residents, interns), therapists, pharmacists, nutritionists, and other personnel (adapted from U. S. National Library of Medicine, 2005).

Neurobehavioral Organization

An interrelationship among infant central nervous system integrity and maturation, behaviors, and the caregiving environment. The interrelationship is expressed in terms of self-regulation and mutual regulation of autonomic, motoric, state, and interactional functions (Als, 1982).

Neurosocial

The ability to interact as the nervous system matures in preterm infants. There are three developmental stages of neurosocial development: turning in, coming out, and reciprocity (Gorski, Davidson, & Brazelton, 1979).

NICU

Neonatal intensive care unit. Newborn Nurseries are designated as Basic (Level I), Specialty (Level II), or Subspecialty (Level III) on the basis of their responsibilities and the availability of special service. Basic Neonatal Care Nurseries (*Level I*) provide postnatal care to healthy newborn infants and are equipped to provide resuscitation and to stabilize ill newborn infants until they can be transferred to a neonatal intensive care facility. Specialty Care Nurseries (*Level II*) "provide care to infants who are moderately ill with problems that are expected to resolve rapidly or who are recovering from serious illness" after receiving subspecialty care. Subspecialty Nurseries (*Level III*) provide care to infants who are extremely premature, are critically ill, or require surgical management (American Academy of Pediatrics & American College of Obstetricians and Gynecologists, 2004, p. 134).

Participation

"[I]nvolvement in a life situation" (WHO, 2001, p. 10).

Participation Restrictions

"[P]roblems an individual may experience in involvement in life situations" (WHO, 2001, p. 10).

Physiologic Instability

Refers to a lack of balance or equilibrium within the autonomic nervous system. Signs of physiologic instability may include changes in cardiorespiratory status (heart rate, respiratory rate, decreased oxygen saturation), color changes (pale, dusky, mottled, flushed), or visceral cues (yawning, sneezing, gagging, spitting up, hiccupping, having bowel movement). Conversely, an infant with physiologic stability will be calm with stable color and vital signs (Als, 1986).

Regulatory Abilities

The infant's capacity to modulate or modify his or her own state of arousal and neurobehavioral organization (Als, 1982).

Relationship-Based Approach

An approach that is "guided by a neurodevelopmental framework for understanding preterm infants and depends on the capacities of professionals to collaborate with one another and with families in support of the infants medical, developmental, and emotional well being" (Als & Gilkerson, 1997, p. 178).

References

Als, H. (1982). Toward a synactive theory of development: Promise for the assessment of infant individuality. *Infant Mental Health Journal, 3,* 229–243.

Als, H. (1986). A synactive model of neonatal behavioral organization: Framework for the assessment of neurobehavioral development in the premature infant and for the support of infants and parents in the neonatal intensive care environment. *Physical and Occupational Therapy in Pediatrics, 6*(3/4), 3–53.

Als, H., & Gilkerson, L. (1997). The role of relationship-based developmentally supportive newborn intensive care in strengthening outcome of preterm infants. *Seminars in Perinatology, 21,* 178–189.

American Academy of Pediatrics, & American College of Obstetricians and Gynecologists. (2004). *Guidelines for perinatal care* (5th ed.). Elk Grove Village, IL: Author

American Occupational Therapy Association. (2002). Occupational therapy practice framework: Domain and process. *American Journal of Occupational Therapy, 56,* 609–639.

American Occupational Therapy Association. (2004a). Guidelines for supervision, roles, and responsibilities during the delivery of occupational therapy services. *American Journal of Occupational Therapy, 58,* 663–677.

American Occupational Therapy Association. (2004b). Scope of practice. *American Journal of Occupational Therapy, 58,* 673–677.

American Occupational Therapy Association. (2005a). Occupational therapy code of ethics (2005). *American Journal of Occupational Therapy, 59,* 639–642.

American Occupational Therapy Association. (2005b). Standards of practice for occupational therapy. *American Journal of Occupational Therapy, 59,* 663–665.

Chess, F., & Thomas, A. (1999). *Goodness of fit: Clinical applications from infancy through adult life.* Philadelphia: Brunner/Mazel.

Crockenberg, S., Lyons-Ruth, K., & Dickson, S. (1993). The family context of infant mental health: II. Infant development in multiple family relationships. In C. H. Zeanah (Ed.), *Handbook of infant mental health* (pp. 38–55). New York: Guilford.

Dunst, C. J., Trivette, C. M., & Deal, A. G. (1988). *Enabling and empowering families: Principles and guidelines for practice.* Cambridge, MA: Brookline Books.

Fraiberg, S. (1980). *Clinical studies in infant mental health.* New York: Basic Books.

Gale, T. (2005). *The Gale encyclopedia of children's health: Infancy through adolescence.* Farmington Hills, MI: Thomson Gale.

Gorski, P., Davidson, M. E., & Brazelton, T. B. (1979). Stages of behavioral organization in the high-risk neonate: Theoretical–clinical considerations. *Seminars in Perinatology, 3,* 61–73.

Gottfried, A. W., & Gaiter, J. L. (1985). *Infant stress under intensive care.* Baltimore: University Park Press.

Institute for Family-Centered Care. (1990). *Association for the care of children's health.* Washington, DC: Author.

Mattingly, C. (1991). What is clinical reasoning? *American Journal of Occupational Therapy, 45,* 979–996.

U.S. National Library of Medicine. (2005, December 13). *MedlinePlus medical encyclopedia.* Retrieved January 11, 2006, from http://www.nlm.nih.gov/medlineplus/ency/article/007241.htm

Weatherston, D. J. (2002). Introduction to the infant mental health program. In J. J. Shirilla & D. J. Weatherston (Eds.), *Case studies in infant mental health: Risk, resiliency, and relationships* (pp. 1–13). Washington, DC: ZERO to THREE.

World Health Organization. (2001). *International classification of functioning, disability, and health (ICF).* Geneva, Switzerland: Author.

Related Readings

Als, H., Duffy, F. H., McAnulty, G. B., Rivkin, M. J., Vajapeyam, S., Mulkern, R. V., et al. (2004). Early experience alters brain function and structure. *Pediatrics, 113,* 846–857.

Als, H., Gilkerson, L., Duffy, F. H., McAnulty, G. B., Buehler, D. M., VanderBerg, K., et al. (2003). A three-center randomized controlled trial of individualized developmental care for very low birth weight infants: Medical, neurodevelomental, parenting, and caregiving effects. *Journal of Developmental and Behavioral Pediatrics, 24,* 399–408.

Anzalone, M. E. (1994). Occupational therapy in neonatology: What is our ethical responsibility? *American Journal of Occupational Therapy, 48,* 563–566.

Browne, J. V. (2003). New perspectives on premature infants and their parents. *ZERO to THREE, 24*(2), 4–12.

Buehler, D., Als, H., Duffy, F., McAnulty, G., & Liederman, J. (1995). Effectiveness of individualized developmental care for low-risk preterm infants: Behavioral and electrophysiologic evidence. *Pediatrics, 96,* 923–932.

Carter, B. S. (2003). Collaborative decision making in the NICU: When life is uncertain, satisfice. *ZERO to THREE, 24*(2), 21–25.

Holloway, E. (1998). Relationship-based occupational therapy in the neonatal intensive care unit. In J. Case-Smith (Ed.), *Pediatric occupational therapy and intervention* (pp. 111–126). Boston: Butterworth-Heinemann.

Holloway, E. (in press). Fostering early parent–infant playfulness in the neonatal intensive care unit. In L. D. Parham & L. S. Fazio (Eds.), *Play in occupational therapy for children* (2nd ed.). St. Louis, MO: Mosby.

Hunter, J. G. (2005). Neonatal intensive care unit. In J. Case-Smith, (Ed.), *Occupational therapy with children* (5th ed., pp. 688–770). St. Louis, MO: Elsevier/Mosby**.**

Johnson, B. H., Abraham, M. R., & Parrish, R. N. (2004). Designing the neonatal intensive care until for optimal family involvement. *Clinics in Perinatology, 31,* 353–383.

McGrath, J. M., & Conliffe-Torres, S. (1996). Integrating family-centered developmental assessment and intervention into routine care in the neonatal intensive care unit. *Nursing Clinics of North America, 31,* 367–368.

Meyer, E. C., Lester, B. M., Boukydis, C. F. Z., & Bigsby, R. (1998). Family-based intervention with high-risk infants and their families. *Journal of Clinical Psychology in Medical Settings, 5,* 49–69.

Talmi, A., & Harmon, R. J. (2003). Relationships between preterm infants and their parents: Disruption and development. *ZERO to THREE, 24*(2), 13–20.

Vergara, E., & Bigsby, R. (2004). *Developmental and therapeutic interventions in the NICU.* Baltimore: Paul H. Brookes.

Authors

Revised by the 2005 Neonatal Intensive Care Unit Task Force
Elsie Vergara, ScD, OTR, FAOTA, *Chairperson*
Marie Anzalone, ScD, OTR, FAOTA
Rosemarie Bigsby, ScD, OTR, FAOTA
Delia Gorga, PhD, OTR, FAOTA
Elise Holloway, MPH, OTR
Jan Hunter, MA, OTR
Ginny Laadt, PhD, OTR/L
Susan Strzyzewski, MEd, OTR

for

The Commission on Practice
Susanne Smith Roley, MS, OTR/L, FAOTA, *Chairperson*

Adopted by the Representative Assembly 2006C404

Reviewed by the Commission on Practice July 2010

Note. This document replaces the 2000 document *Specialized Knowledge and Skills for Occupational Therapy Practice in the Neonatal Intensive Care Unit,* previously published in the *American Journal of Occupational Therapy, 54,* 641–648.

Specialized Knowledge and Skills in Mental Health Promotion, Prevention, and Intervention in Occupational Therapy Practice

Purpose

The purpose of this document is to describe the specialized knowledge and skills for entry-level occupational therapy practice in the promotion of mental health and the prevention and intervention of mental health problems, including mental illness. The foundations of occupational therapy are rooted firmly in psychiatry. The profession brings a habilitation and rehabilitation perspective to mental health services in keeping with increased emphasis on recovery and functionality directed toward participation in daily life occupations. The American Occupational Therapy Association (AOTA) supports the inclusion of the profession of occupational therapy as a core mental health profession in the *U.S. Code of Federal Regulations* and as a qualified mental health profession as defined by state statute and regulation (AOTA, 2006a).

In addition to intervention for persons with mental illness, occupational therapy practitioners contribute to the promotion of *mental health,* which refers to a positive state of functioning reflected in the presence of four characteristics: (1) positive affective or emotional state (e.g., subjective sense of well-being, feeling happy); (2) positive psychological and social function (e.g., self-acceptance, fulfilling relationships, self control); (3) productive activities; and (3) resilience in the face of adversity and the ability to cope with life stressors (U.S. Department of Health and Human Services, 1999; World Health Organization [WHO], 2004). A public health approach to mental health has been advocated by WHO (2001), which emphasizes the promotion of mental health as well as the prevention of and intervention for mental illness. As such, this document focuses on the knowledge and skills that substantiate occupational therapy's role in mental health promotion, prevention, and intervention.

Both occupational therapists and occupational therapy assistants are educated to provide services that support mental and physical health, rehabilitation, and recovery-oriented approaches. Occupational therapy practitioners[1] serve people throughout their life course in institutional, outpatient, home, school, and other community settings. Entry-level occupational therapists must have at least a master's degree but also may enter the profession with a clinical doctorate degree. Occupational therapy assistants enter the field at the associate's-degree level.

Intended for internal and external audiences, this document specifies the knowledge, reasoning, and performance skills necessary for competent and ethical occupational therapy practice in mental health promotion, prevention and intervention.

---

[1]When the term *occupational therapy practitioner* is used in this document, it refers to both occupational therapists and occupational therapy assistants (AOTA, 2006b). *Occupational therapists* are responsible for all aspects of occupational therapy service delivery and are accountable for the safety and effectiveness of the occupational therapy service delivery process. *Occupational therapy assistants* deliver occupational therapy services under the supervision of and in partnership with an occupational therapist (AOTA, 2009).

Introduction

The roots of occupational therapy are grounded in psychiatry. The moral treatment movement sought to replace the brutality and idleness of earlier treatment for disorders of the mind with kindness and "occupation" (Gordon, 2009, p. 203). In the early 20th century, the founders and early writers in occupational therapy created a body of literature that supported the value of occupation in the healing of mind and body (Gordon, 2009, p. 205). In 1922, Adolph Meyer acknowledged the importance of "work and play and rest and sleep" in his desire to address a therapeutic approach that healed the mind and improved the human condition for those with mental illness (as cited in Gordon, 2009, p. 207).

"Occupational therapy is founded on the understanding that engaging in occupations structures everyday life and contributes to health and well-being" (AOTA, 2008, p. 628). The term *occupation* is defined as "activities that people engage in throughout their daily lives to fulfill their time and give life meaning" (p. 672). The goals of occupational therapy are twofold: (1) to promote mental health and well-being in all persons with and without disabilities and (2) to restore, maintain, and improve function and quality of life for people at risk for or affected by mental illness. Occupational therapy practitioners support "health and participation in life through engagement in occupation" (p. 627).

Through the use of everyday activities, occupational therapy practitioners promote mental health and support functioning in people with or at risk of experiencing a range of mental health disorders, including psychiatric, behavioral, and substance abuse. Occupational therapy facilitates full participation in valued occupations in one's home, school, workplace, and community. As in all occupational therapy practice, services in mental health are client-centered. The client may be an individual or group of individuals, an organization, or a population. Occupational therapists work with clients to determine their wants and needs. Together, they determine the factors that are either barriers or supports to healthy participation in daily life activities. Occupational therapy assistants work under the supervision of and in partnership with occupational therapists (AOTA, 2009) to implement the plan and to assist the team with ongoing evaluation of success and need for change in the intervention strategies.

Through the clinical reasoning process, occupational therapy practitioners select and apply different theoretical perspectives and approaches informed by evidence. These perspectives and approaches are drawn primarily from occupational therapy and occupational science but also from other fields and areas of practice such as physical and psychiatric rehabilitation, psychology, school mental health, sociology, psychiatry, neuropsychiatry, and anthropology. This clinical reasoning process guides occupational therapy evaluation and intervention.

Although there is overlap in knowledge, skills, and attitudes with other professions, occupational therapy offers a unique contribution to mental health service provision. The profession holds a firm belief in the inherent need of all humans to engage in occupations, which are central to fulfilling meaningful life roles, engaging with one's environment, improving and sustaining health and well-being, and allowing full participation in society (Wilcock, 2007). Occupational therapy practitioners are educated to select and use evaluations and interventions that not only promote mental health but also address physical, sensory, and cognitive function affecting clients' abilities to participate in daily life while considering their interests, values, habits, and roles.

The profession recognizes and emphasizes the complex interplay among the individual variables, the activity demands, and the environmental demands. Occupational therapy practitioners are skilled in analyzing, adapting, or modifying the task or environment to support goal attainment and optimal engagement in occupation so that clients can develop and maintain healthy ways of living in their home, workplace, and community.

Using This Document

Health care, education, community, and mental health services stakeholders (e.g., clients, family members, policymakers, mental health practitioners of all disciplines) may use the document

- As a resource to advocate for inclusion of and coverage for occupational therapy as a core mental health service,

- To assist in articulating occupational therapy's contribution to the promotion of mental health in all persons, and

- To assist in articulating occupational therapy's contribution to mental illness prevention and intervention by promoting successful participation in a meaningful array of occupations that foster emotional well-being.

Occupational therapy practitioners and educators may use the document to

- Guide mental health curriculum and fieldwork development;

- Educate others on the mental health practice knowledge and skills that occupational therapy practitioners have in common with other core mental health practitioners;

- Educate others on occupational therapy's vital and unique contribution to mental health services; and

- Engage clients and family members in discussions about how occupational therapy practice supports mental health promotion, prevention, and intervention to assist individuals and groups in developing and meeting their goals that promote health and participation in daily life.

To facilitate its usefulness, this document is organized into two sections. Section 1, "Core Mental Health Professional Knowledge and Skills," describes knowledge and skills that occupational therapy practitioners share with other core mental health professionals. A deeper understanding of occupational therapy's approach to mental health services can be gleaned by reviewing Section 2, "Specific Occupational Therapy Knowledge and Skills Applied to Mental Health Promotion, Prevention, and Intervention," which describes mental health knowledge and skills specific to occupational therapy practice. Both sections help readers differentiate entry-level occupational therapy and occupational therapy assistant knowledge and skills.

The core mental health knowledge and skills of occupational therapy practitioners have been organized into four domains: (1) Foundations, (2) Evaluation and Intervention, (3) Professional Role and Service Outcomes, and (4) Mental Health Systems. Occupational therapists use and apply skills and knowledge from each domain to promote mental health and help persons with or at risk for psychiatric, substance abuse, and behavior disorders develop and maintain successful and satisfying ways of living in their home, work, and community. Occupational therapy assistants possess knowledge and skills to deliver services in each domain under the supervision of and in partnership with occupational therapists.

- *Foundations*—Occupational therapy practitioners are knowledgeable about how mental illnesses affect the ability to successfully participate in everyday occupations and what skills, compensatory strategies, or accommodations are needed to mitigate this impact. The are knowledgeable about (1) the promotion of positive mental health through competency enhancement (e.g., skill development, task adaptations, environmental supports, participation in meaningful occupations); (2) prevention of mental illness using risk reduction efforts (e.g., relaxation strategies with early signs of anxiety; establishing habits and routines that support adequate sleep, time for relationships, physical activity, and task accomplishment); and (3) intervention strategies to minimize symptoms experienced with the presence of mental illness (e.g., therapeutic task groups, relaxation strategies) provide an essential contribution to mental health services systems. Occupational therapy interventions promote successful participation in everyday occupations, allowing people to remain engaged and to re-engage in fulfilling, meaningful, and contributory roles. The foundation for this knowledge comes from occupational therapy; occupational science; and other fields of study such as physical and psychiatric rehabilitation, psychology, school mental health, sociology, psychiatry, neuropsychiatry, and anthropology.

- *Evaluation and intervention*—Occupational therapists are qualified to use relevant screening and assessment procedures to identify strengths, needs, problems, and concerns regarding a person's occupational engagement and successful performance of their daily life tasks. Further, therapists determine specific occupational performance issues and selected environmental and contextual factors that support and hinder performance. Occupational therapy assistants can assist with this evaluation process. Occupational therapy mental health interventions are based on assessment/ evaluation results, developmental and life stage knowledge, and theoretical concepts of occupation. Interventions can be provided on an individual or group basis as in direct care or education or can be provided via consultation to populations of people to promote mental health and to address mental ill health.

- *Professional role and service outcomes*—Occupational therapy practitioners are educated to partner with consumers of mental health services, families and other natural support persons, individual practitioners, interdisciplinary teams, and community stakeholders to enhance service outcomes. To do this, practitioners learn to value multiple perspectives in addition to that of occupational therapy. In addition, occupational therapists are trained in the process of program evaluation, the knowledge and tools necessary to measure outcomes of occupational therapy intervention, and the context of the application of outcome measurement to mental health practice. They also are responsible for developing mechanisms to ensure the quality and effectiveness of service provision along with client satisfaction.

- *Mental health systems*—Occupational therapists have an understanding of how systems influence mental health services delivery, support mental health and the prevention of mental illness, and facilitate or inhibit people's ability to be full participants in their communities. Disability, health care, education, workforce, welfare, shelter, legal, criminal justice, housing, and social and familial systems all affect people with or at risk for psychiatric conditions. Occupational therapists are educated to analyze the interaction between and among systems, contexts, persons, populations, and occupations. Therapists use this knowledge to meet the participation needs of individuals as well as others within their communities (e.g., schools, employers, landlords, families).

References

American Occupational Therapy Association. (2006a). AOTA's statement on mental health practice. FAQ: *School mental health*. Retrieved January 10, 2010, from http://www.aota.org/Practitioners/Practice Areas/MentalHealth/Highlights/36364.aspx

American Occupational Therapy Association. (2006b). Policy 1.44: Categories of occupational therapy personnel. In *Policy manual* (2007 ed., pp. 33–34). Bethesda, MD: Author.

American Occupational Therapy Association. (2008). Occupational therapy practice framework: Domain and process (2nd ed.). *American Journal of Occupational Therapy, 62,* 625–683.

American Occupational Therapy Association. (2009). Guidelines for supervision, roles, and responsibilities during the delivery of occupational therapy services. *American Journal of Occupational Therapy, 63,* 797–803.

American Psychiatric Association. (2000). *Diagnostic and statistical manual of mental disorders* (4th ed., text. rev.). Washington, DC: American Psychiatric Association.

Gordon, D. M. (2009). The history of occupational therapy. In E. Crepeau, E. Cohn, & B. Schell (Eds.), *Willard and Spackman's occupational therapy* (11th ed., pp. 202–215). Philadelphia: Lippincott Williams & Wilkins.

U.S. Department of Health and Human Services. (1999). *Mental health: A report of the Surgeon General—Executive summary.* Rockville, MD: Author.

Wilcock, A. (2007). *An occupational perspective on health* (2nd ed.). Thorofare, NJ: Slack.

World Health Organization. (2001). *International classification of functioning, disability, and health (ICF).* Geneva, Switzerland: Author.

World Health Organization. (2004). *Promoting mental health: Concepts, emerging evidence, practice* (Summary report). Geneva, Switzerland: Author.

Authors

This document is based on a charge from the 2007 Representative Assembly and the work of the Mental Health Competencies Ad Hoc Committee. The Ad Hoc Committee along with the COP developed this work into a Knowledge and Skills Paper.

Katherine A. Burson, MS, OTR/L, CPRP, *Ad Hoc Committee Chairperson*
Cynthia Barrows, MS, OTR/L, CPRP
Cathy Clark, MS, OTR/L
Jyothi Gupta, PhD, OT(C), OTR/L
Jamie Geraci, MS, OTR/L
Lisa Mahaffey, MS, OTR/L
Penelope Moyers Cleveland, EdD, OTR/L, BCMH, FAOTA, *AOTA Board Liaison to the Ad Hoc Committee*

for

The Commission on Practice
Janet DeLany, DEd, OTR/L, FAOTA, *Chairperson*

Adopted by the Representative Assembly 2010CApr15

Section 1. Core Mental Health Professional Knowledge and Skills

The entry-level occupational therapy practitioners in mental health have these knowledge and skills in common with all other core mental health professionals:

X = competent at entry level

A = able to assist at entry level

KX = competent at entry level to analyze and integrate knowledge to make judgments about occupational therapy service provision

KA – competent at entry level to demonstrate knowledge and apply it to occupational therapy practice

		OT	OTA
Evaluation and Intervention			
Knowledge of			
1.	Influence of neurophysiological changes, environmental factors, and contexts on mental health and the development of psychiatric conditions.	KX	KA
2.	Historical and current perspectives on mental health and its promotion, mental illness and its treatments, including the consumer/survivor/ex-patient movement and concepts of recovery.	KX	KA
3.	Current *Diagnostic and Statistical Manual of Mental Disorders* taxonomy (American Psychiatric Association, 2000) with regard to psychiatric diagnosis, etiology, symptoms, impairments, clinical course, and prognosis.	KX	KA
4.	Common comorbidities with mental illnesses (e.g., diabetes, COPD, obesity, substance abuse, ADHD, autism spectrum disorders).	KX	KA
5.	Psychiatric medications and their actions and side effects.	KX	KA
6.	Non-discipline-specific, evidence-based practices and service delivery models (e.g., assertive community treatment, illness management and recovery, supported employment, permanent supportive housing, school mental health, cognitive–behavioral therapy, social and emotional learning (SEL), positive behavioral interventions and supports (PBIS).	KX	KA
Performance Skills			
7.	Assess mental health status (e.g., affect, cognitive competency, insight, comprehension, impulse control, suicide risk) and factor findings in all phases of evaluation and intervention.	X	A
8.	Establish rapport and promote behavioral change in clients by selecting therapeutic counseling and communication strategies (e.g., therapeutic use of self, communication of hope, ethical and interpersonal boundaries, motivational interviewing, active listening, limit setting, group process, conflict resolution).	X	A
9.	Prevent, manage, and/or facilitate the resolution of crisis for individuals and groups by comparing and selecting effective counseling techniques and interventions (e.g., crisis prevention and management, conflict resolution, strategies for dealing with problem behaviors, psychopathological behaviors, psychiatric emergencies).	X	A
10.	Perform comprehensive and targeted functional assessments using evidence-informed approaches and tools.	X	A
11.	Establish medical necessity for rehabilitation services directed toward functional impairments associated with psychiatric conditions by articulating how symptoms and underlying neuropsychiatric conditions interfere with performance of daily life tasks.	X	A

	OT	OTA
12. Design and execute individual and group intervention approaches used in mental health practice, including but not limited to those below: I. Cognitive–behavior therapy II. Psychoeducation III. Psychodynamic approach IV. Behavioral approaches V. Social and emotional learning VI. Recovery models VII. Resiliency models VIII. Psychosocial rehabilitation IX. Skills training X. Biopsychosocial XI. Dialectic behavioral therapy XII. Motivational stages of change.	X	A

Reasoning Skills

	OT	OTA
13. Evaluate human development and behaviors throughout the life course, including how the time and/or the life stage of the emergence of mental illness influence development and the capacity to function as a member of society.	X	A
14. Integrate client-centered and recovery-oriented approaches in collaborating with clients to facilitate goal development and attainment.	X	X
15. Identify and evaluate one's own values, attitudes, and beliefs toward individuals with psychiatric conditions and their potential impact on a person's potential for recovery.	X	X
16. Evaluate the influence of culture, diversity, socioeconomics, and values on a person's experience of mental health challenges, their view of mental health treatment, and their experience of and potential for recovery.	X	A
17. Critique current medical and psychological intervention approaches associated with common psychiatric diagnoses, including the impact of medication side effects on functioning.	X	A
18. Synthesize relevant theories and models that guide intervention and delivery of mental health services, in different settings.	X	A

Professional Role and Service Outcomes

Knowledge of

	OT	OTA
19. Mental health practice roles that an occupational therapist or occupational therapy assistant can assume, such as case manager, group facilitator, community support worker, qualified mental health professional, consultant, program developer, and advocate.	KX	KA
20. Mental health disciplines and professions (e.g., psychology, social work, nursing, psychiatry, mental health technicians, therapeutic recreation, art therapy, music therapy, peer support, rehabilitation counseling, occupational therapy) and the issues involved in both role differentiation and role collaboration.	KX	KA
21. Methodologies for measuring individual, program, and systems outcomes in mental health practice.	KX	KA
22. Methods and principles used to conduct needs assessments and generate practical recommendations.	KX	KA

Performance Skills

	OT	OTA
23. Demonstrate skill in writing medical documentation and behavioral objectives.	X	X
24. Demonstrate basic skills in program development and consultation, supervision, management, administration, quality improvement, outcome measurement, and advocacy related to mental health services.	X	A

(Continued)

(cont.)

	OT	OTA
Reasoning Skills		
25. Synthesize and evaluate perspectives of collaborating disciplines to maximize client outcomes.	X	A
26. Synthesize and incorporate key factors into consultation and program planning and development, including determining client expectations, understanding the purpose of the organization, understanding of systems, desired and expected outcomes, culture and willingness to change, resources available to client or organization, and regulations and laws governing the organization.	X	A
27. Critique barriers to implementation of programs and interventions.	X	A
Mental Health Systems		
Knowledge of		
28. Legislation, policies, procedures, and related legal and ethical issues that influence mental health service delivery (e.g., involuntary treatment, insurance parity, advance directives, confidentiality, school mental health).	KX	KA
29. Payment systems relevant to mental health practice settings.	KX	KX
30. Diverse mental health service delivery contexts (e.g., schools, hospitals, community-based centers, shelters, prisons, institutes for mental disease).	KX	KA
31. Mental health stakeholder groups (e.g., consumers, family members, at-risk populations, employers, mental health care providers, community programs, advocacy groups, legislators, third-party payers).	KX	KA
32. Agencies and standards that influence mental health and rehabilitation service delivery (e.g., SAMHSA, RSA, CMS, state Medicaid agency, Center for School Mental Health, state mental health authority, state vocational rehabilitation agency, private insurance, standards of practice, state licensure, certification, JCAHO, CARF, confidentiality).	KX	KA
Performance Skills		
33. Access relevant information to ensure service delivery and documentation complies with current applicable standards (e.g., state mental health acts, HIPAA, confidentiality acts, licensure laws, CARF, JCAHO, President's New Freedom Commission Report, criminal justice acts).	X	A
34. Engage in activities to transform mental health service delivery systems to be consumer-driven, family-driven, and community-focused.	X	X
Reasoning Skills		
35. Critique social, economic, policy, and system factors that affect the health, well-being, and participation of persons with serious mental illnesses (e.g., poverty, housing, education, unemployment, estrangement from family, inadequate insurance, lack of integration between/among service systems).	X	A
36. Evaluate the dynamic interactions between/among an individual, family, community, and social systems and their impact on a person's mental health.	X	A
37. Integrate the consumer/survivor/ex-patient movement and its implications for mental health services and systems of care.	X	X

Note. CARF = Commission on Accreditation of Rehabilitation Facilities. CMS = Centers for Medicare and Medicaid Services. COPD = chronic obstructive pulmonary disease. HIPAA = Health Insurance Portability and Accountability Act of 1996 (P.L. 104-191). JCAHO = Joint Commission on the Accreditation of Healthcare Organizations. OT = occupational therapist. OTA = occupational therapy assistant. RSA = Rehabilitation Services Administration. SAMHSA = Substance Abuse and Mental Health Services Administration.

Section 2. Specific Occupational Therapy Knowledge and Skills Applied to Mental Health Promotion, Prevention, and Intervention Practice

Led by their firm belief in the inherent drive of all humans to engage in meaningful and purposeful occupations and also the influence of occupational engagement on health and recovery from psychiatric conditions, occupational therapy practitioners use occupation and an understanding of the variables that influence a person's ability to successfully engage in occupations (everyday activities) to engage clients in achieving their occupational participation recovery goals.

X = competent at entry level

A = able to assist at entry level

KX = competent at entry level to analyze and integrate knowledge to make judgments about occupational therapy service provision

KA = competent at entry level to demonstrate knowledge and apply it to occupational therapy practice

		OT	OTA
Foundations			
Knowledge of			
38.	Occupational therapy practices for medical, physical/somatic, intellectual, learning, and other nonpsychiatric disabling conditions.	KX	KA
Performance Skills			
39.	Evaluate the relationship between/among health, well-being, and participation in daily life activities throughout the life course for individuals at risk for or with mental health challenges.	KX	KA
40.	Analyze activities, occupations, contexts, and environmental characteristics to determine those that challenge or support the client's interests, skills, and performance.	KX	KA
Reasoning Skills			
41.	Evaluate and select occupational therapy theories, frames of references, and intervention models of practice to design and deliver occupational therapy services in various practice settings in order to promote mental health, prevent mental illness, and intervene with the presence of diagnosed psychiatric conditions.	X	A
42.	Assess and determine how to guide the transactional interactions among persons with or at risk for psychiatric conditions, environment, and activity to influence engagement in occupations, participation, and health of clients.	X	A
Evaluation and Intervention			
Knowledge of			
43.	Role of occupational therapy in the evaluation and intervention processes persons with or at risk for psychiatric conditions and the promotion of mental health in all individuals with or without disabilities.	KX	KA
44.	Impact of mental health on the ability to engage in everyday occupations (e.g., ADLs, IADLs, education, work, play, leisure and social participation, sleep/rest).	KX	KA
45.	Impact of psychiatric conditions and medication side effects on performance skills (e.g., sensory–perceptual, motor and praxis, emotional regulation, cognitive, communication and social skills) and performance patterns (e.g., habits, routines, roles, rituals) within relevant contexts and environments.	KX	KA
46.	Influence of a client's values, beliefs, spirituality, sense of efficacy, and experience of mental health challenges on the meaningfulness of occupations.	KX	KA
47.	Assessment tools and methods to evaluate occupational engagement and the impact of mental and physical impairments on performance skills (e.g., sensory–perceptual, motor and praxis, emotional regulation, cognitive, communication and social skills) and performance patterns (e.g., habits, routines, roles, rituals).	KX	KA

(Continued)

(cont.)

	OT	OTA
48. Environmental supports for and barriers to occupational performance and environmental modification strategies to enable participation at home, school, community, and work.	KX	KA
49. Cognitive skills training and adaptive strategies.	KX	KA
50. Sensory processing and modulation skill development and adaptive strategies.	KX	KA
51. Strategies and environmental accommodations used to compensate for performance skill and pattern challenges commonly associated with psychiatric conditions.	KX	KA
52. Learning styles and a variety of teaching methods that can be adapted to accommodate challenges commonly associated with psychiatric conditions.	KX	KA

Performance Skills

	OT	OTA
53. Develop an occupational profile using client-centered strategies to gather information about a client's occupational history and experiences, life roles, interests, needs, and concerns about performance in areas of occupation and identifying strengths and limitations.	X	A
54. Incorporate knowledge of co-occurring medical and somatic conditions into the evaluation and intervention process to facilitate engagement in meaningful and necessary occupations.	X	A
55. Evaluate client's performance in ADLs, IADLs, sleep and rest, education, work, play/leisure, and social participation using standardized and nonstandardized procedures.	X	A
56. Evaluate client's performance skills that support and interfere with participation in meaningful life roles using standardized and nonstandardized procedures. Performance skills include • Motor and praxis skills • Sensory–perceptual skills • Emotional regulation skills • Cognitive skills • Communication and social skills.	X	A
57. Evaluate a client's performance patterns that support and interfere with participation in meaningful life roles using standardized and nonstandardized procedures. Performance patterns include habits, routines, roles, and rituals.	X	A
58. Evaluate client factors that may affect performance in areas of occupation using standardized and nonstandardized procedures. Client factors include a client's values, beliefs, and spirituality; body functions (e.g., cardiovascular, pulmonary) and body structures (e.g., bones, organs).	X	A
59. Observe, measure, and inquire about the physical and social/interpersonal environmental influences on engagement in occupation through formal and informal evaluation procedures.	X	A
60. Establish medical necessity for rehabilitation services directed toward functional impairments associated with psychiatric conditions by discerning and articulating the relationship between/among functional impairments, occupational engagement, and the performance skills and patterns affected by the mental health challenges.	X	A
61. Collaborate with clients to determine targeted outcomes specific to that individual's personal vision of recovery.	X	X
62. In collaboration with clients, develop intervention plans to help clients complete tasks related to life roles such as developing of skills, habits, and routines for work or school; obtaining and preparing meals for self or others; maintaining home or apartment; and participating in healthy social and leisure occupations as determined from the evaluation.	X	A
63. Apply a variety of approaches used in mental health practice, such as but not limited to, those listed in Item 12 above, in individual and group interventions to enable occupational performance and participation.	X	A
64. Enable clients to explore a variety of interests and begin to develop competencies to support increased participation in meaningful occupations.	X	X
65. Develop intervention sessions using activities to teach and practice new skills and when possible develop actual opportunity to engage in needed tasks such as work or school tasks.	X	X

	OT	OTA
66. Design and implement individual and group interventions that support development of cognitive, sensory regulation, social, and communication skills requisite for role performance.	X	A
67. Teach clients to understand the role of their sensory system in regulating their level of alertness and how to use different sensory tools to increase or decrease their level of alertness so they can focus on and participate successfully in their chosen activities.	X	A
68. Teach clients to understand their cognitive strengths and challenges and to make use of strategies and treatments that optimize occupational performance.	X	A
69. Develop modifications to tasks and environments to compensate for cognitive, sensory, interpersonal, and communication challenges, and increase successful/effective participation in life roles.	X	A
70. Select and communicate to clients, relevant support systems, and other professionals best evidence that supports intervention choices.	X	A
71. Select appropriate teaching methods (e.g., handouts; schedules; organizational charts; visual, auditory, and tactile cueing systems; grading of activity; chunking) to address client needs with respect to culture, learning style, and current abilities.	X	A
Reasoning Skills		
72. Synthesize information from different theoretical perspectives, models of practice, frames of reference, and evidenced-based practices from occupational therapy, physical and psychiatric rehabilitation, psychology, sociology, psychiatry, school mental health, and neuropsychiatry to select relevant assessment tools and guide the evaluation and intervention processes.	X	A
73. Determine need to refer clients for additional evaluation or services to specialists internal and external to the profession.	X	X
74. Analyze the environmental and contextual factors that support or hinder a person's ability to participate in meaningful and productive roles and occupations.	X	A
75. Determine the effects of medical treatment side effects (e.g., psychiatric medications, ECT) on participation in occupation: ADLs, IADLs, rest and sleep, education, work, play and leisure, and social participation.	X	A
76. Identify and analyze historical barriers to occupational participation that result in inability to develop an occupational identity or in loss of occupational identity.	X	A
77. Synthesize information gathered from the evaluation of a person's strengths, skills, abilities, preferences, goals, challenges, needs, and environments, as well as information from activity analysis to create effective interventions to enable occupational performance at home, school, and workplace.	X	A
78. Anticipate barriers to participation due to aging, physical disabilities, medical conditions and illnesses, and problem solve to maximize participation.	X	A
79. Synthesize intervention and support needs with appropriate resources to maximize participation in desired occupations.	X	A
80. Formulate most effective intervention to enable occupational participation (e.g., skills training, adaptation of task, modification of environment).	X	A
81. Determine how environmental supports and barriers influence participation in meaningful and productive roles in one's community and facilitate reducing barriers.	X	A
82. Explain the clinical reasoning process behind the occupational therapy procedures or care processes in a way that is understandable and usable for the client, other professionals, and funding sources.	X	A

(Continued)

(cont.)

		OT	OTA
83.	Select appropriate means to explain the importance of participation and its relationship to recovery for people with or at risk for psychiatric conditions in a way that is understandable and relevant to clients, team members, and third-party payers.	X	X
	Professional Role and Service Outcomes		
	Knowledge of		
84.	AOTA Code of Ethics, applicable licensure laws, AOTA Scope of Practice, and AOTA Standards of Practice as they pertain to mental health practice.	KX	KX
85.	Different practice roles that occupational therapy practitioners may assume in mental health practice.		
	i. Direct intervention aimed at changing the functional participation of a client using a variety of approaches such as promoting health, restoring or maintaining function, modifying the environment or activity, or preventing disability		
	ii. Education of caregivers and staff aimed at imparting knowledge and information that results in improved health and improved ability to perform and participate in desired occupations		
	iii. Consultation aimed at improving occupational participation goals for the client.	KX	KA
86.	Practice scopes of occupational therapy and other mental health disciplines and professions (e.g., psychology, social work, nursing, psychiatry, mental health technicians, therapeutic recreation, art therapy, music therapy, peer support, rehabilitation counseling).	KX	KA
87.	Funding sources for occupational therapy services in different mental health service delivery systems.	KX	KX
88.	Strategies to evaluate occupation-based outcomes in mental health service delivery systems and client satisfaction with occupational therapy services.	KX	KA
	Performance Skills		
89.	Build respectful relationships and select effective strategies to work with persons with a variety of skills, abilities, and experiences (e.g., paraprofessionals, professionals, consumers, family members) to make successful changes in the organization.	X	X
90.	Clarify how occupational therapy interventions support and compliment interventions of other providers.	X	X
91.	Conduct needs assessment to determine when OT services may benefit a partial or full mental health system that does not currently utilize occupational therapy.	X	A
92.	Partner with consumers, family members, and other mental health professionals/disciplines in the development, implementation, and evaluation of mental health and occupational therapy services.	X	A
93.	Select and use standardized procedures and tools to organize, collect, compile, analyze, synthesize, and interpret quantitative and qualitative occupational performance practice outcomes and client satisfaction data, summarizing findings into comprehensive, objective reports.	X	A
94.	Design ongoing processes for quality improvement based on functional outcomes.	X	A
95.	Design and implement needs assessments that determine best occupation-based practices for individuals with or at risk for psychiatric conditions, factoring in setting, population characteristics, and funding.	X	A
96.	Frame consultation within the regulations and structure of the organization.	X	A
97.	Operationalize administrative and occupational therapy process changes that target improved outcomes for occupational therapy intervention and client satisfaction in mental health practice settings.	X	A

	OT	OTA
Reasoning Skills		
98. Appraise the priority outcomes for an individual or groups of individuals receiving occupational therapy services in a mental health context.	X	A
99. Infer the role of recovery in promoting occupational engagement for people with psychiatric conditions.	X	X
100. Critique, discern, and interpret the applicability of qualitative and/or quantitative outcome and satisfaction measurements and methods when evaluating services directed toward persons with or at risk for psychiatric conditions.	X	A
101. Choose interventions that fit the values and abilities of those providing and receiving care.	X	A
102. Discern and critique factors that affect change for clients with or at risk for psychiatric conditions.	X	A
103. Discern and critique factors that facilitate/hinder provision of occupational therapy services in settings that serve people with or at risk for psychiatric conditions.	X	A
104. Justify administrative changes in the provision of occupational therapy services that will promote positive outcomes for clients in settings that serve people with or at risk for psychiatric conditions.	X	A
105. Compare and contrast occupational therapy outcome measures with outcome measures related to the recovery model in mental health practice.	X	A
106. Integrate health insurance language and mental health recovery language with *Occupational Therapy Practice Framework* (AOTA, 2008).	X	A
Mental Health Systems		
Knowledge of		
107. Different environments and contexts in which occupational therapy practitioners have a role in mental health promotion, prevention, and intervention (e.g., psychiatric settings, schools, residential facilities, jails).	KX	KA
108. Systems (e.g., organizations, entitlements, community programs) to be accessed that enable occupational participation and performance.	KX	KA
Performance Skills		
109. Use relationships with advocacy organizations and persons with the lived experience of mental illness to understand challenges with occupational engagement and performance, such as what these persons have identified as most and least helpful in regaining, maintaining, and improving their ability to engage fully and meaningfully in desired occupations (e.g., roles, activities).	X	X
110. Facilitate clients' access to support systems (e.g., family, associations, friends, organizations) to enhance recovery.	X	X
111. Recommend reasonable changes/accommodations that can be made to policies, procedures, and practices to improve occupational engagement, participation, and performance of populations served.	X	A
112. Locate and access information about a system's goals, priorities, or needs.	X	X
113. Choose methods to explain the role of occupational therapy to various mental health stakeholder groups that relate to stakeholders' system, goals, priorities, or needs (see Item 31 for example stakeholder groups).	X	A
114. Discern actual and potential consumer and family member leadership roles within mental health service systems (e.g., programs, agencies, organizations, private and public payer systems).	X	A

(Continued)

(cont.)

	OT	OTA
115. Use evidence to help organizations understand how the regulations with which they must comply influence occupational participation of persons with or at risk for psychiatric conditions.	X	A
116. Obtain and synthesize information about third-party payer coverage for occupational therapy services directed toward the remediation and restoration of functional impairments caused by mental illnesses (example payers include private insurance, Medicaid, Medicare, vocational rehabilitation, state board of education).	X	A
Reasoning Skills		
117. Differentiate and critique mental health services and service delivery systems that are consumer-driven and community-focused from those that are more staff-driven and mental health setting–focused.	X	X
118. Differentiate and critique "recovery," "resiliency," and "strengths-based" planning, interventions, and programs from those that are problem-based or deficit-based.	X	X
119. Discern and create means by which occupational therapy practitioners partner with consumers and family members to develop consumer-driven and family-driven care for individuals and programs.	X	A
120. Evaluate the interactions between/among individuals, family, community, and other social systems (e.g., schools, faith-based organizations, police, long-term-care facilities, group homes, one-stop centers, vocational rehabilitation systems) and their impact on occupational participation and mental health.	X	A
121. Discern how changes in policies, procedures, and practices in various systems may enhance or deter occupational performance and participation for persons with or at risk for mental health challenges/conditions (example systems include family, community agency or program, mental health care, medical care, education/schools, employment/employer, social security, disability).	X	A

Note. ADLs = activities of daily living. AOTA = American Occupational Therapy Association. ECT = electroconvulsive therapy. IADLs = instrumental activities of daily living. OT = occupational therapist. OTA = occupational therapy assistant.

Position Papers

Complementary and Alternative Medicine

The American Occupational Therapy Association (AOTA) asserts that complementary and alternative medicine (CAM) may be used responsibly by occupational therapists and occupational therapy assistants as part of a comprehensive approach to enhance engagement in occupation by people, organizations, and populations to promote their health and participation in life (AOTA, 2005; Giese, Parker, Lech-Boura, Burkhardt, & Cook, 2003). Occupational therapy is a holistic, client-centered practice that acknowledges the importance of context and environment in framing a client's occupational needs, desires, and priorities (AOTA, 2008). Because CAM is a culturally sensitive system used by nearly 40% of adults and 12% of children in the United States (Barnes, Bloom, & Nahin, 2008), it is important to acknowledge the ethical and pragmatic issues surrounding the use of CAM in occupational therapy practice. This position paper defines the appropriate use of CAM by occupational therapy practitioners[1] within the scope of occupational therapy practice.

Use

The U.S. Department of Health and Human Services reports that CAM is used in the United States by persons who are "seeking ways to improve their health and well-being or to relieve symptoms associated with chronic, even terminal, illnesses or the side effects of conventional treatments for them" (Barnes et al., 2008). CAM interventions most often are used for treatment of pain conditions by non-poor women ages 30–69 with significant levels of education beyond high school (Barnes et al., 2008). Similar to the holistic nature of occupational therapy practice, practitioners who use CAM also address the influence of the contexts on health status and collaborate with clients who demonstrate a desire for personal control over health outcomes (Cheung, Wyman, & Halcon, 2007). Clients who are living with and adjusting to life with chronic conditions such as back pain or a traumatic event such as domestic abuse may combine the holistic nature of CAM approaches with other intervention approaches to improve their ability to participate in occupations they need and want to perform.

Definition

The National Center for Complementary and Alternative Medicine (NCCAM) of the National Institutes of Health has identified five domains of CAM practice and defines *complementary and alternative medicine* as "a group of diverse medical and health care systems, practices, and products that are not presently considered to be part of conventional medicine" (NCCAM, 2010). The five domains of CAM practice are (1) alternative medical systems, (2) mind–body interventions, (3) biologically based treatments, (4) manipulative and body-based methods, and (5) energy therapies. By definition, *alternative medicine* is practiced *in place of* conventional medicine, while *complementary interventions* are accessed *in conjunction with* allopathic medical practices.

---

[1] When the term *occupational therapy practitioner* is used in this document, it refers to both occupational therapists and occupational therapy assistants (AOTA, 2006). *Occupational therapists* are responsible for all aspects of occupational therapy service delivery and are accountable for the safety and effectiveness of the occupational therapy service delivery process. *Occupational therapy assistants* deliver occupational therapy services under the supervision of and in partnership with an occupational therapist (AOTA, 2009).

The definition of CAM is dynamic. Practices contained within the definition of CAM change as clinical evidence supports their inclusion with conventional health practices, and novel approaches emerge (AOTA, 2005; Giese et al., 2003). The term *integrative medicine* is used for combined treatments from conventional medicine and CAM for which there is high-quality scientific evidence of safety and effectiveness (NCCAM, 2008).

Research

The NCCAM was established by Congress in 1998 through Title VI, Section 601, of the Omnibus Consolidated and Emergency Appropriations Act of 1999 (P.L. 105-277) as the federal government's lead agency for scientific research on CAM. The NCCAM mission is to investigate promising CAM products and practices with neutrality and scientific rigor to determine their safety and effectiveness, to train CAM researchers, and to provide information about CAM to professionals and the general public (NCCAM, 2008). Since its inception, the NCCAM has funded more than 1,200 research projects at scientific institutions across the United States and internationally.

The NCCAM has proposed a framework for setting research priorities that consists of four pillars: (1) scientific promise, (2) extent and nature of practice and use, (3) amenability to rigorous scientific inquiry, and (4) potential to change health practices (NCCAM, 2009). Key priority areas are currently non-mineral, non-vitamin, natural products and mind–body interventions such as yoga, tai chi, qi gong, guided imagery, meditation, deep-breathing exercises, and progressive relaxation (NCCAM, 2009). Studies to support the integration of CAM and conventional medicine, to encourage insurance coverage for CAM therapies, and to develop practice and referral guidelines are needed in addition to research about the safety and efficacy of CAM practices (Coulter & Khorsan, 2008; Herman, D'Huyvetter, & Mohler, 2006).

Access to information about CAM practices has been enhanced by a collaborative project between the National Library of Medicine and the NCCAM. These two government agencies have created *CAM on PubMed* (see http://nccam.nih.gov/research/camonpubmed/), a search option that automatically limits research citations to a CAM subset from the MEDLINE database and additional life science journals.

Use Within the Scope of Occupational Therapy Practice

Occupational therapy values engagement in occupations and promotes the health and participation of people, organizations, and populations through engagement in occupation (AOTA, 2008). *Occupations* are "activities . . . of everyday life, named, organized, and given value and meaning by individuals and a culture" (Law, Polatajko, Baptiste, & Townsend, 1997, p. 29). Occupations encompass activities of daily living (ADLs), instrumental activities of daily living, rest and sleep, education, work, play, leisure, and social participation (AOTA, 2008).

Occupational therapy practitioners may utilize CAM in the delivery of occupational therapy services when they are used as preparatory methods or purposeful activities to facilitate the ability of clients to engage in their daily life occupations. CAM approaches have been utilized in occupational therapy for several years and include but are not limited to guided imagery, massage, myofascial release, meditation, and behavioral relaxation training (AOTA, 1998; Brachtesende, 2005; Lindsay, Fee, Michie, & Heap, 1994; Scott, 1999). Yoga postures also have been used prior to engagement in ADLs to reduce reliance on pain medication and to promote relaxation for restorative sleep (Brachtesende, 2005).

Occupational therapy practitioners need to respect the use of CAM as part of the client's occupational performance habits, routines, or rituals and to understand that CAM practices may be embedded within particular cultures (Cassidy, 1998a, 1998b). In a study of patients with cardiac conditions in Hong Kong, the use of qi gong as a method for reducing stress added psychological benefit to the reduction of blood pressure when compared to progressive relaxation training alone (Hui, Wan, Chan, & Yung, 2006).

By collaborating with the client in the selection and application of specific CAM interventions, the occupational therapy practitioner supports and respects the client's autonomy and reasoned participation in decision-making. Outcome studies about engagement in occupation continue to be a priority for determining the efficacy and effectiveness of using CAM techniques during occupational therapy intervention.

To determine whether to use CAM in the delivery of occupational therapy services, occupational therapists must evaluate the client, develop an intervention based on the client's needs and priorities, and conduct outcomes measurement. The evaluation contributes to the understanding of the client's strengths, priorities, and current limitations in carrying out daily occupations. Evaluation and intervention address factors that influence the client's occupational performance, including how the client performs the daily life occupations, the demands of those occupations, and the contexts and environments within which those occupations are performed. As part of the evaluation and the intervention, the occupational therapy practitioner must determine whether the use of CAM is consistent with the client's cultural practices, priorities, and needs; is safe to use; and is an appropriate approach to facilitate the ability of the client to participate in daily life occupations and to promote health and participation. Selected assessments are used to measure the effectiveness of the outcomes of occupational therapy services and guide future therapeutic interventions with the client. The occupational therapy practitioner must measure whether the use of CAM results in positive outcomes for improving occupational performance.

Ethical Considerations, Continuing Competency, and Standards of Practice

The *Occupational Therapy Code of Ethics and Ethics Standards (2010)* (AOTA, 2010a) mandates safe and competent practice, holding occupational therapy practitioners responsible for maintenance of high standards of competence. Occupational therapy practitioners need to maintain continuing competency in CAM approaches just as they do with other areas of practice. Using CAM approaches may require additional training, competency examinations, certification, and regulatory knowledge (AOTA, 2010b). The use of specific CAM approaches may be subject to federal, state, and often local municipal regulations that govern practice, advertising, ethics, professional terminology, and training (AOTA, 2010c). It is the responsibility of occupational therapy practitioners to know and comply with applicable laws and regulations associated with the use of CAM approaches during occupational therapy intervention. Occupational therapy practitioners must abide by state regulations when billing for occupational therapy services that incorporate the use of CAM. Practitioners must distinguish between the incorporation of CAM techniques into occupational therapy practice and the use of CAM as a salutatory method that is separate from occupational therapy practice (AOTA, 2007, 2008).

Issues of client safety and health care worker safety are salient to all areas of occupational therapy practice. The use of CAM requires attention to client safety in consumer decision-making, client interventions, and professional education and training. The risks and benefits of CAM used in occupational therapy should be communicated to clients as standard practice in a client-centered, evidence-based approach to service provision.

Payment for Services

The NCCAM (2008) reports that U.S. adults annually spend $34 billion out-of-pocket on CAM products and services. CAM services, although often paid for privately, increasingly are covered by insurance companies and health maintenance organizations (Astin, Pelletier, Marie, & Haskell, 2000; Cleary-Guida, Okvat, Oz, & Ting, 2001; Wolsko, Eisenberg, Davis, Ettner, & Phillips, 2002). Factors that influence third-party payers to include selected CAM in health care policies include cost-effectiveness, consumer demand, demonstrated clinical efficacy, and state mandate (Pelletier & Astin, 2002; Pelletier, Astin, & Haskell, 1999).

Summary

Occupational therapy practitioners facilitate proficient and meaningful engagement in the significant occupations of life. CAM practices, systems, and products may be appropriately incorporated into occupational therapy practice to encourage a client's engagement in meaningful occupations. Scientific studies are needed to validate the safety and efficacy of CAM methods within occupational therapy practice. Advanced-level training and continuing education are important to acquire the knowledge and skill to utilize CAM methods, to address the concerns for patient safety and informed consent, and to meet the rigors of regulatory requirements.

References

American Occupational Therapy Association. (1998). OT perspective: Complementary care survey results. *OT Week, 12*(48), 4.

American Occupational Therapy Association. (2005). Complementary and alternative medicine (CAM). *American Journal of Occupational Therapy, 59,* 653–655.

American Occupational Therapy Association. (2006). Policy 1.41. Categories of occupational therapy personnel. In *Policy manual* (2009 ed.). Bethesda, MD: Author.

American Occupational Therapy Association. (2007). *Definition of occupational therapy practice for the AOTA Model Practice Act.* (Available from the State Affairs Group, American Occupational Therapy Association, 4720 Montgomery Lane, Bethesda, MD 20814)

American Occupational Therapy Association. (2008). Occupational therapy practice framework: Domain and process (2nd ed.). *American Journal of Occupational Therapy, 62,* 625–683.

American Occupational Therapy Association. (2009). Guidelines for supervision, roles, and responsibilities during the delivery of occupational therapy services. *American Journal of Occupational Therapy, 63,* 173–179.

American Occupational Therapy Association. (2010a). Occupational therapy code of ethics and ethics standards (2010). *American Journal of Occupational Therapy, 64*(Suppl.), S17–S26.

American Occupational Therapy Association. (2010b). Standards for continuing competence. *American Journal of Occupational Therapy, 64*(Suppl.), S103–S105.

American Occupational Therapy Association. (2010c). Standards of practice for occupational therapy. *American Journal of Occupational Therapy, 64*(Suppl.), S106–S111.

Astin, J. A., Pelletier, K. R., Marie, A., & Haskell, W. L. (2000). Complementary and alternative medicine use among elderly persons: One-year analysis of a Blue Shield Medicare supplement. *Journals of Gerontology Series A: Biological Sciences and Medical Sciences, 55*(1), M4–M9.

Barnes, P. M., Bloom, B., & Nahin, R. (2008, December 10). Complementary and alternative medicine use among adults and children: United States, 2007. *CDC National Health Statistics Report.* Retrieved January 6, 2010, from http://nccam.nih.gov/news/camstats/2007/

Brachtesende, A. (2005). Using complementary and alternative medicine in occupational therapy. *OT Practice, 10*(11), 9–13.

Cassidy, C. M. (1998a). Chinese medicine users in the United States. Part I: Utilization, satisfaction, medical plurality. *Journal of Alternative and Complementary Medicine, 4*(1), 17–27.

Cassidy, C. M. (1998b). Chinese medicine users in the United States. Part II: Preferred aspects of care. *Journal of Alternative and Complementary Medicine, 4*(2), 189–202.

Cheung, C. K., Wyman, J. F., & Halcon, L. L. (2007). Use of complementary and alternative therapies in community-dwelling older adults. *Journal of Alternative and Complementary Medicine, 13*(9), 997–1006.

Cleary-Guida, M. B., Okvat, H. A., Oz, M. C., & Ting, W. (2001). A regional survey of health insurance coverage for complementary and alternative medicine: Current status and future ramifications. *Journal of Alternative and Complementary Medicine, 7,* 269–273.

Coulter, I. D., & Khorsan, R. (2008). Is health services research the Holy Grail of complementary and alternative medicine research? *Alternative Therapies in Health and Medicine, 14*(4), 40–45.

Giese, T., Parker, J. A., Lech-Boura, J., Burkhardt, A., & Cook, A. (2003). *The role of occupational therapy in complementary and alternative medicine* [White Paper, adopted by the AOTA Board of Directors June 22, 2003]. (Available from American Occupational Therapy Association, 4720 Montgomery Lane, Bethesda, MD 20814)

Herman, P. M., D'Huyvetter, K., & Mohler, M. J. (2006). Are health services research methods a match for CAM? *Alternative Therapies in Health and Medicine, 12*(3), 78–83.

Hui, P. M., Wan, M., Chan, W. K., & Yung, P. M. (2006). An evaluation of two behavioral rehabilitation programs, qigong versus progressive relaxation, in improving the quality of life in cardiac patients. *Journal of Alternative and Complementary Medicine, 12*(4), 373–378.

Law, M., Polatajko, H., Baptiste, W., & Townsend, E. (1997). Core concepts of occupational therapy. In E. Townsend (Ed.), *Enabling occupation: An occupational therapy perspective* (pp. 29–56). Ottawa, ON: Canadian Association of Occupational Therapists.

Lindsay, W. R., Fee, M., Michie, A., & Heap, I. (1994). The effects of cue control relaxation on adults with severe mental retardation. *Research in Developmental Disabilities, 15,* 425–437.

National Center for Complementary and Alternative Medicine. (2008). *Overview of NCCAM.* Retrieved January 6, 2010, from http://nccam.nih.gov/news/events/grants08/slides2.htm

National Center for Complementary and Alternative Medicine. (2009). *NCCAM priority setting—Framework and other considerations.* Retrieved January 6, 2010, from http://plan.nccam.nih.gov/ index.cfm?-module=paper2

National Center for Complementary and Alternative Medicine. (2010). *What is complementary and alternative medicine?* Retrieved January 6, 2010, from http://www.nccam.nih.gov/health/whatiscam/

Omnibus Consolidated and Emergency Appropriations Act of 1999, P.L. 105-277, Title VI, Section 601.

Pelletier, K. R., & Astin, J. A. (2002). Integration and reimbursement of complementary and alternative medicine by managed care and insurance providers: 2000 update and cohort analysis. *Alternative Therapies in Health and Medicine, 8*(1), 38–39, 42, 44.

Pelletier, K. R., Astin, J. A., & Haskell, W. L. (1999). Current trends in the integration and reimbursement of complementary and alternative medicine by managed care organizations (MCOs) and insurance providers: 1998 update and cohort analysis. *American Journal of Health Promotion, 4,* 125–133.

Scott, A. H. (1999). Wellness works: Community service health promotion groups led by occupational therapy students. *American Journal of Occupational Therapy, 53,* 566–574.

Wolsko, P. M., Eisenberg, D. M., Davis, R. B., Ettner, S. L., & Phillips, R. S. (2002). Insurance coverage, medical conditions, and visits to alternative medicine providers: Results of a national survey. *Archives of Internal Medicine, 162,* 281–287.

Additional Reading

Bausell, R. B., Lee, W. L., & Berman, B. M. (2001). Demographic and health-related correlates to visits to complementary and alternative medical providers. *Medical Care, 9,* 190–196.

Burkhardt, A., & Parker, J. (1998, November 26). OT perspective: Complementary care survey results. *OT Week, 12*(48), 4.

Carlson, J. (2003). *Complementary therapies and wellness: Practice essentials for holistic healthcare.* Upper Saddle River, NJ: Prentice Hall.

Eisenberg, D. M., Davis, R. B., Ettner, S. L., Appel, S., Wilkey, S., Van Rompay, M., et al. (1998). Trends in alternative medicine use in the United States, 1990–1997: Results of a follow-up national survey. *JAMA, 280,* 1569–1575.

Eisenberg, D. M., Kessler, R. C., Van Rompay, M. I., Kaptchuk, T. J., Wilkey, S. A., Appel, S., et al. (2001). Perceptions about complementary therapies relative to conventional therapies among adults who use both: Results from a national survey. *Annals of Internal Medicine, 13,* 344–351.

Kaboli, P. J., Doebbeling, B. N., Saag, K. G., & Rosenthal, G. E. (2001). Use of complementary and alternative medicine by older patients with arthritis: A population-based study. *Arthritis and Rheumatology, 45,* 398–403.

Ni, H., Simile, C., & Hardy, A. M. (2002). Utilization of complementary and alternative medicine by United States adults: Results from the 1999 National Health Interview Survey. *Medical Care, 40,* 353–358.

Rakel, D. P., Guerrera, M. P., Bayles, B. P., Desai, F. J., & Ferrara, E. (2008). CAM education: Promoting a salutogenic focus in health care. *Journal of Alternative and Complementary Medicine, 14*(1), 87–93.

Author

Terry Giese, MBA, OT/L, FAOTA

for

The Commission on Practice

Janet V. DeLany, DEd, MSA, OTR/L, FAOTA, *Chairperson*

Adopted by the Representative Assembly Coordinating Council (RACC) for the Representative Assembly

Revised by the Commission on Practice 2011

Note. This revision replaces the 2005 document *Complementary and Alternative Medicine*, previously published and copyrighted in 2005 by the American Occupational Therapy Association in the *American Journal of Occupational Therapy, 59,* 653–655.

Complex Environmental Modifications

The American Occupational Therapy Association (AOTA) asserts that the evaluation and provision of complex adaptations and modifications to environments where people complete daily life occupations is within the scope of occupational therapy practice. Occupational therapists and occupational therapy assistants[1] routinely work with individuals and populations who are at risk for limitations in occupational performance and participation as a result of obstacles within their home, work, school, or community environments.

AOTA further asserts that occupational therapy practitioners,[2] by virtue of their academic training, knowledge, and expertise, can provide solutions to challenges affecting occupational performance and participation in daily life activities of all types that affect individuals across the life course. Furthermore, occupational therapy practitioners are distinctly qualified to be members of interdisciplinary teams composed of professionals in fields such as architecture, construction, city planning, and disability services. Occupational therapy practitioners offer both high- and low-technology equipment options and suggestions for structural alterations, modifications, and space enhancements that provide clients across the life course with access, safety, and efficiency in function.

This document provides a description of complex environmental modifications (CEMs) and highlights the role of occupational therapy practitioners as providers of service within this area. It is intended for internal and external audiences and to inform consumers, health care providers, educators, payers, referral sources, and policymakers about the distinctive skill set and contributions that occupational therapy brings to CEMs. Occupational therapy practitioners recognize the influence of environments (physical and social) and contexts (cultural, personal, temporal, and virtual) on human performance and occupational participation (AOTA, 2014b); this paper focuses primarily on the physical environment.

Complex Environmental Modifications

CEMs are alterations, modifications, or creations of new spaces to meet the needs of an individual, family, group, or community to preserve or facilitate optimal participation in daily life. CEM interventions can include, but are not limited to, a combination of structural changes, assistive technologies (AT), and services. CEMs are differentiated from services in which more basic, simpler, low-tech solutions are adequate to improve function. Examples of more basic solutions may include a tub transfer bench, rug removal, and adapted door knobs.

In addition to the recognition that the modifications to environments can be complex (e.g., installation of home automation systems) is the understanding that the environment itself may offer complex challenges. For example, a complex modification is to create a fully accessible kitchen in a home that not only was built

---

[1]*Occupational therapists* are responsible for all aspects of occupational therapy service delivery and are accountable for the safety and effectiveness of the occupational therapy service delivery process. *Occupational therapy assistants* deliver occupational therapy services under the supervision of and in partnership with an occupational therapist (AOTA, 2014a).

[2]When the term *occupational therapy practitioner* is used in this document, it refers to both occupational therapists and occupational therapy assistants (AOTA, 2006).

in the 1800s but also, because of its historical designation, requires the modifications to meet the guidelines set forth by the town's historic commission.[3]

Role of Occupational Therapy in Complex Environmental Modifications

As interdisciplinary team members, occupational therapy practitioners working in this area provide expertise in the core knowledge of human function and occupational participation, AT, and specialized products. In addition, occupational therapy practitioners bring a distinct perspective through their knowledge of human development, the impact of physical and cognitive changes through the life course, and knowledge of community resources. With advanced study, occupational therapy practitioners enhance their knowledge in the areas of construction, architecture, structural design, and legislative guidelines.

The occupational therapy perspective in the area of CEMs combines an understanding of the impact of the environment[4] and context[5] on a person's occupational performance.[6] Occupational therapists conduct evaluations and provide consultation, and practitioners provide intervention, training, education, and advocacy to individuals and groups, caregivers, and employers to remove environmental barriers and support occupational performance.

The occupational therapy process involves completion of a comprehensive, client-focused evaluation of the person and the environment and the process of engagement from the perspective of occupational participation. On the basis of the results of the evaluation and in conjunction with the client, the occupational therapist identifies and recommends environmental modifications and AT with a focus on the outcomes of client safety, satisfaction, and participation in desired daily occupations. In addition, the occupational therapy practitioner may manage funding and installation of technologies and modifications as well as the training of clients in their use. Details of the occupational therapy process relevant to CEMs include

- *Evaluation:* Information gathering about the client's occupational performance within his or her physical and social environments and contexts to determine the impact of client factors,[7] performance skills,[8] performance patterns,[9] and occupational participation;

- *Intervention:* Eliminating environmental barriers via a combination of environmental modifications, AT, specialized products, and resources; matching the complex environmental modification or AT with the client's current level of executive functioning to ensure successful occupational performance; and

- *Outcomes:* The results of the interventions, including increased performance, increased ease of use and adaptation of the environment or AT, decreased caregiver burden, and increased participation in daily

---

[3]Historic homes also engage another level of regulatory standards that are not within the scope of this document to address.

[4]"The term *environment* refers to the external physical and social conditions that surround the client and in which the client's daily life occupations occur" (AOTA, 2014b, p. S28). *Physical environment* refers to the "natural . . . and built . . . surroundings in which daily life occupations occur" (p. S8). The *social environment* is constructed by the "presence of, relationships with, and expectations of persons, groups, and populations with whom clients have contact" (p. S9).

[5]The term *context* refers to a variety of interrelated conditions that are within and surrounding the client that influence performance, including cultural, personal, temporal, and virtual contexts (AOTA, 2014b, p. S9).

[6]*Occupational performance* is the act of doing and accomplishing a selected action (performance skill), activity, or occupation (Fisher, 2009; Fisher & Griswold, 2014; Kielhofner, 2008) that results from the dynamic transaction among the client, the context and environment, and the activity (AOTA, 2014b, p. S43).

[7]*Client factors* are specific capacities, characteristics, or beliefs that reside within the individual and that influence performance in occupations (AOTA, 2014b).

[8]*Performance skills* are goal-directed actions that are observable as small units of engagement in daily life occupations. They are learned and developed over time and are situated in specific contexts and environments (Fisher & Griswold, 2014).

[9]*Performance patterns* are the habits, routines, roles, and rituals used in the process of engaging in occupations or activities that can support or hinder occupational performance (AOTA, 2014a).

life (Dooley & Hinojosa, 2004; Graff et al., 2006; Hendriks et al., 2008; Heywood, 2005; Mann, Ottenbacher, Fraas, Tomita, & Granger, 1999; Petersson, Kottorp, Bergstrom, & Lilja, 2009).

Examples of services provided by occupational therapy practitioners in the area of CEMs include

- Interventions that require knowledge of AT, environmental modifications, and community resources to ensure that the solutions will meet the client's immediate and future needs;

- Modifications that expand beyond consumer-grade and marketed adaptations such as grab bars, ramps, and AT found at retail and medical equipment stores;

- Modifications for clients with significant changes in function due to injury or disability or those with progressive or chronic conditions such as diabetes, asthma, and obesity;

- Consultation on projects requiring additional knowledge and experience such as remodeling and construction of new homes, work environments, and community spaces, including plan review;

- Consultation on projects that include a general contractor, designer, or architect or modifications requiring building permits; and

- Advocacy for the needs of clients requiring modifications to home and community environments through interfacing with government agencies, payment sources, and community planners.

Client-centered environmental modification interventions provided by an occupational therapy practitioner reduce functional challenges in performing daily living activities, minimize environmental barriers, and enhance perceived quality of life (Szanton et al., 2011). Evidence supports occupational therapy interventions to reduce falls (Campbell et al., 2005; Clemson et al., 2004; Davison, Bond, Dawson, Steen, & Kenny, 2005; Nikolaus & Bach, 2003), promote increased participation in activities of daily living (ADLs); Fänge & Iwarsson, 2005; Gitlin, Miller, & Boyce, 1999; Gitlin et al., 2006; Graff et al., 2006; Petersson et al., 2009; Stark, 2004; Stark, Landsbaum, Palmer, Somerville, & Morris, 2009), increase satisfaction in occupational performance (Graff, Vernooij-Dassen, Hoefnagels, Dekker, & de Witte, 2003; Petersson, Lilja, Hammel, & Kottorp, 2008; Stark et al., 2009), and promote safe performance of caregiving (Dooley & Hinojosa, 2004). Furthermore, occupational therapy interventions directed at the caregiver reduced decline in self-care of family members (Gitlin, Corcoran, Winter, Boyce, & Hauck, 2001), thus decreasing cost of care and delaying institutionalization (Wilson, Mitchell, Kemp, Adkins, & Mann, 2009), as well as increased perceived quality of life (Szanton et al., 2011).

Significance to Society

In 2001, the World Health Organization (WHO), in the *International Classification of Functioning, Disability and Health* (*ICF*), described the ability of individuals to participate in life situations as a core component of addressing health and disability. According to the *ICF,* life situations in which participation occurs are identified as learning and applying knowledge; performing general tasks and demands; communication; mobility; self-care; domestic life; interpersonal interactions and relationships; and major life areas, including work, school, community, and social and civic life (Law, 2002; WHO, 2001). These areas of daily living and the view of the human as an occupational being whose level of ability is not a reflection of infirmity but of participation is found throughout the occupational therapy literature and is a grounding tenet of the *Occupational Therapy Practice Framework* (AOTA, 2010a, 2014b; Wood et al., 2000).

Addressing concerns related to participation is the driving force behind the occupational therapy profession's focus on creating spaces for living, working, playing, sleeping, learning, addressing self-care needs, and being involved in the community that are accessible and provide ample opportunities for the level of participation desired by each individual. Occupational therapy practitioners provide services and recommend products to enable consumers and caregivers to live as independently and safely as possible while considering functional limitations and progressive issues of illness, disability, or age-related decline

(AOTA, 2014b; Siebert, Smallfield, & Stark, 2014). Occupational therapy services are provided across the spectrum of ages and settings, as well as during transition from one setting to another. There is a demand for services to be provided to consumers not only to assist with maintaining health and wellness but also to allow for successful aging in place and community participation. CEMs are one means of removing barriers to daily functioning and maintaining independence and quality of life for both consumers and their caregivers.

In addition, supporting older adults and persons with disabilities who wish to live independently and participate in their chosen communities (Bayer & Harper, 2000; Houser, Fox-Grage, & Ujvari, 2012; Lipman, 2012; Redfoot & Houser, 2010) is believed not only to enhance quality of life but also to contain health care costs. Occupational therapy practitioners consulting with clients, their caregivers, builders, designers, and other involved professionals can ensure the most appropriate, evidence-based, safe, and accessible residential design; choice of specialized products; and ergonomically appropriate installation from the design and building team.

Practitioner Qualifications, Professional Development, and Ethical Considerations

Occupational therapy practitioners providing CEMs must assess their own competency and ensure that they are able to safely and effectively recommend, obtain, and install appropriate modifications. To this end, occupational therapy practitioners must adhere to the *Occupational Therapy Code of Ethics (2015)* (AOTA, 2015) and the *Standards of Practice for Occupational Therapy* (AOTA, 2010b) and must abide by federal and state regulations to ensure their competencies as practitioners and the well-being of their clients.

Occupational therapy practitioners choosing to pursue CEM as an area of practice can gain advanced experience through mentoring opportunities, continuing education courses, and review of national and international professional publications on this topic. To address the complex needs and challenges facing clients, additional occupational therapy knowledge and training are needed in the following areas: environmental or functional evaluations, accessible building guidelines, universal design, AT and architectural products and their installation, ergonomic design, and advocacy.

Summary

The goal of occupational therapy is to promote health, well-being, and participation in life through engagement in occupation (AOTA, 2014b). Occupational therapy practitioners bring a distinct skill set to CEMs, addressing needs through a holistic and client-centered approach and providing environmental interventions that facilitate client safety, independence, and participation in daily life occupations within an environment. This skill set supports interprofessional collaboration for best client outcomes. Design, construction, architectural, city planning, and disability providers are increasingly aware of the benefits of working with occupational therapy practitioners. In addition, consumers are seeking the services of occupational therapy practitioners in building and renovating environments to increase accessibility, participation, independence, and safety.

References

American Occupational Therapy Association. (2006). Policy 1.44: Categories of occupational therapy personnel. In *Policy manual* (2013 ed., pp. 32–33). Bethesda, MD: Author.

American Occupational Therapy Association. (2010a). Occupational therapy's perspective on the use of environments and contexts to support health and participation in occupations. *American Journal of Occupational Therapy, 64,* S57–S69. http://dx.doi.org/10.5014/ajot.2010.64S57

American Occupational Therapy Association. (2010b). Standards of practice for occupational therapy. *American Journal of Occupational Therapy, 64,* S106–S111. http://dx.doi.org/10.5014/ajot.2010.64S106

American Occupational Therapy Association. (2014a). Guidelines for supervision, roles, and responsibilities during the delivery of occupational therapy services. *American Journal of Occupational Therapy, 68*(Suppl. 3), S16–S22. http://dx.doi.org/10.5014/ajot.2014/686S03

American Occupational Therapy Association. (2014b). Occupational therapy practice framework: Domain and process (3rd ed.). *American Journal of Occupational Therapy, 68*(Suppl. 1), S1–S48. http://dx.doi.org/10.5014/ajot.2014.682006

American Occupational Therapy Association. (2015). Occupational therapy code of ethics (2015). *American Journal of Occupational Therapy, 69*(Suppl. 3), 6913410030. http://dx.doi.org/10.5014/ajot.2015.696S03

Bayer, A.-H., & Harper, L. (2000). *Fixing to stay: A national survey on housing and home modification issues* (AARP Research Report). Retrieved from http://assets.aarp.org/rgcenter/il/home_mod.pdf

Campbell, A. J., Robertson, M. C., La Grow, S. J., Kerse, N. M., Sanderson, G. F., Jacobs, R. J., . . . Hale, L. A. (2005). Randomised controlled trial of prevention of falls in people aged ≥ 75 with severe visual impairment: The VIP trial. *BMJ, 322,* 697–701. http://dx.doi.org/10.1136/bmj.38601.447731.55

Clemson, L., Cumming, R. G., Kendig, H., Swann, M., Heard, R., & Taylor, K. (2004). The effectiveness of a community-based program for reducing the incidence of falls in the elderly: A randomized trial. *Journal of the American Geriatrics Society, 52,* 1487–1494. http://dx.doi.org/10.1111/j.1532-5415.2004.52411.x

Davison, J., Bond, J., Dawson, P., Steen, I. N., & Kenny, R. A. (2005). Patients with recurrent falls attending accident and emergency benefit from multifactorial intervention—A randomised controlled trial. *Age and Ageing, 34,* 162–168. http://dx.doi.org/10.1093/ageing/afi053

Dooley, N. R., & Hinojosa, J. (2004). Improving quality of life for persons with Alzheimer's disease and their family caregivers: Brief occupational therapy intervention. *American Journal of Occupational Therapy, 58,* 561–569. http://dx.doi.org/10.5014/ajot.58.5.561

Fänge, A., & Iwarsson, S. (2005). Changes in ADL dependence and aspects of usability following housing adaptation—A longitudinal perspective. *American Journal of Occupational Therapy, 59,* 296–304. http://dx.doi.org/10.5014/ajot.59.3.296

Fisher, A. G. (2009). *Occupational Therapy Intervention Model: A model for planning and implementing top-down, client-centered, and occupation-based interventions.* Fort Collins, CO: Three Star Press.

Fisher, A. G., & Griswold, L. A. (2014). Performance skills: Implementing performance analyses to evaluate quality of occupational performance. In B. A. Boyt Schell, G. Gillen, & M. Scaffa (Eds.), *Willard and Spackman's occupational therapy* (12th ed., pp. 249–264). Philadelphia: Lippincott Williams & Wilkins.

Gitlin, L. N., Corcoran, M., Winter, L., Boyce, A., & Hauck, W. W. (2001). A randomized, controlled trial of a home environmental intervention: Effect on efficacy and upset in caregivers and on daily function of persons with dementia. *Gerontologist, 41,* 4–14. http://dx.doi.org/10.1093/geront/41.1.4

Gitlin, L. N., Miller, K. S., & Boyce, A. (1999). Bathroom modifications for frail elderly renters: Outcomes of a community-based program. *Technology and Disability, 10,* 141–149.

Gitlin, L. N., Winter, L., Dennis, M. P., Corcoran, M., Schinfeld, S., & Hauck, W. W. (2006). A randomized trial of a multicomponent home intervention to reduce functional difficulties in older adults. *Journal of the American Geriatrics Society, 54,* 809–816. http://dx.doi.org/10.1111/j.1532-5415.2006.00703.x

Graff, M. J. L., Vernooij-Dassen, M. J. F. J., Hoefnagels, W. H. L., Dekker, J., & de Witte, L. P. (2003). Occupational therapy at home for older individuals with mild to moderate cognitive impairments and their primary caregivers: A pilot study. *OTJR: Occupation, Participation and Health, 23,* 155–164. http://dx.doi.org/10.1177/153944920302300403

Graff, M. J., Vernooij-Dassen, M. J., Thijssen, M., Dekker, J., Hoefnagels, W. H., & Rikkert, M. G. (2006). Community based occupational therapy for patients with dementia and their care givers: Randomised controlled trial. *BMJ, 333,* 1196. http://dx.doi.org/10.1136/bmj.39001.688843.BE

Hendriks, M. R., Bleijlevens, M. H., van Haastregt, J. C., Crebolder, H. F., Diederiks, J. P., Evers, S. M., . . . van Eijk, J. T. (2008). Lack of effectiveness of a multidisciplinary fall-prevention program in elderly people at risk: A randomized, controlled trial. *Journal of the American Geriatrics Society, 56,* 1390–1397. http://dx.doi.org/10.1111/j.1532-5415.2008.01803.x

Heywood, F. (2005). Adaptation: Altering the house to restore the home. *Housing Studies, 20,* 531–547. http://dx.doi.org/10.1080/02673030500114409

Houser, A., Fox-Grage, W., & Ujvari, K. (2012). *Across the states: Profiles of long-term services and supports* (9th ed.). Washington, DC: AARP Public Policy Institute. Retrieved from http://www.aarp.org/content/dam/aarp/research/public_policy_institute/ltc/2012/across-the-states-2012-executive-summary-AARP-ppi-ltc.pdf

Kielhofner, G. (2008). *The human occupation: Theory and application* (4th ed.). Philadelphia: Lippincott Williams & Wilkins.

Law, M. (2002). Participation in the occupations of everyday life. *American Journal of Occupational Therapy, 56,* 640–649. http://dx.doi.org/10.5014/ajot.56.6.640

Lipman, B. (2012). *Housing an aging population: Are we prepared?* Washington, DC: Center for Housing Policy. Retrieved from http://www.nhc.org/media/files/AgingReport2012.pdf

Mann, W. C., Ottenbacher, K. J., Fraas, L., Tomita, M., & Granger, C. V. (1999). Effectiveness of assistive technology and environmental interventions in maintaining independence and reducing home care costs for the frail elderly: A randomized controlled trial. *Archives of Family Medicine, 8,* 210–217. http://dx.doi.org/10.1001/archfami.8.3.210

Nikolaus, T., & Bach, M. (2003). Preventing falls in community-dwelling frail older people using a home intervention team (HIT): Results from the Randomized Falls–HIT trial. *Journal of the American Geriatrics Society, 51,* 300–305. http://dx.doi.org/10.1046/j.1532-5415.2003.51102.x

Petersson, I., Kottorp, A., Bergstrom, J., & Lilja, M. (2009). Longitudinal changes in everyday life after home modifications for people aging with disabilities. *Scandinavian Journal of Occupational Therapy, 16,* 78–87. http://dx.doi.org/10.1080/11038120802409747

Petersson, I., Lilja, M., Hammel, J., & Kottorp, A. (2008). Impact of home modification services on ability in everyday life for people ageing with disabilities. *Journal of Rehabilitation Medicine, 40,* 253–260. http://dx.doi.org/10.2340/16501977-0160

Redfoot, D., & Houser, A. (2010). *More older people with disabilities living in the community: Trends from the National Long-Term Care Survey, 1984–2004.* Retrieved from http://assets.aarp.org/rgcenter/ppi/ltc/2010-08-disability.pdf

Siebert, C., Smallfield, S., & Stark, S. (2014). *Occupational therapy practice guidelines for home modifications.* Bethesda, MD: AOTA Press.

Stark, S. (2004). Removing environmental barriers in the homes of older adults with disabilities improves occupational performance. *OTJR: Occupation, Participation and Health, 24,* 32–40. http://dx.doi.org/10.1177/153944920402400105

Stark, S., Landsbaum, A., Palmer, J. L., Somerville, E. K., & Morris, J. C. (2009). Client-centred home modifications improve daily activity performance of older adults. *Canadian Journal of Occupational Therapy, 76,* 235–245.

Szanton, S. L., Thorpe, R. J., Boyd, C., Tanner, E. K., Leff, B., Agree, E., . . . Gitlin, L. N. (2011). Community aging in place, advancing better living for elders: A bio–behavioral–environmental intervention to improve function and health-related quality of life in disabled older adults. *Journal of the American Geriatrics Society, 59,* 2314–2320. http://dx.doi.org/10.1111/j.1532-5415.2011.03698.x

Wilson, D. J., Mitchell, J. M., Kemp, B. J., Adkins, R. H., & Mann, W. (2009). Effects of assistive technology on functional decline in people aging with a disability. *Assistive Technology: The Official Journal of RESNA, 21,* 208–217. http://dx.doi.org/10.1080/10400430903246068

Wood, W., Nielson, C., Humphry, R., Coppola, S., Baranek, G., & Rourk, J. (2000). A curricular renaissance: Graduate education centered on occupation. *American Journal of Occupational Therapy, 54,* 586–597. http://dx.doi.org/10.5014/ajot.54.6.586

World Health Organization. (2001). *International classification of functioning, disability and health.* Geneva: Author.

Authors

Marnie Renda, MEd, OTR/L, CAPS, ECHM

Shoshana Shamberg, MS, OTR/L, FAOTA

Debra Young, MEd, OTR/L, SCEM, ATP, CAPS

for

The Commission on Practice
Debbie Amini, EdD, OTR/L, CHT, FAOTA, *Chairperson*

Adopted by the Representative Assembly 2014NovCO44

Citation. American Occupational Therapy Association. (2015). Complex environmental modifications. *American Journal of Occupational Therapy, 69*(Suppl. 3), 6913410010. http://dx.doi.org/10.5014/ajot.2015.696S01

Importance of Interprofessional Education in Occupational Therapy Curricula

The American Occupational Therapy Association (AOTA) asserts that entry-level occupational therapy curricula should include interprofessional education (IPE) in which students have opportunities to learn and apply the knowledge and skills necessary for interprofessional collaborative practice. To achieve the goals of improved health outcomes and client experiences, along with reduced health care costs, practitioners must be prepared to contribute to interprofessional care teams (Earnest & Brandt, 2014). In the 21st century, clients' health and well-being will benefit when occupational therapy students are taught firsthand that interprofessional collaborations are essential in the health care arena and community-based systems of care. The purposes of this position paper are to describe the history of IPE, to provide evidence for the benefits of including IPE in professional curricula, to define key concepts and core competencies associated with IPE, to address implications of including IPE in entry-level occupational therapy curricula, and to provide resources for faculty.

Background

History of Interprofessional Education

IPE is not a new concept in health professions education. It has been attempted, reported on, and discussed since the 1970s. In a 1972 Institute of Medicine (IOM) report titled *Report of a Conference: Educating for the Health Team,* Pellegrino wrote,

> A major deterrent to fashion health care that is efficient, effective, comprehensive, and personalized is our lack of design for the *synergistic interrelationship* [emphasis added] of all who contribute to the patient's well-being.... We face a national challenge ... the development of educational programs aimed at preparing future professionals for interprofessional collaboration. (p. 4)

In the 1st decade of the 21st century, the IOM issued two significant reports that reexamined the U.S. health care system and health professions education. The first of these reports, *To Err Is Human: Building Safer Health Systems* (IOM, 2000), focused on improving patient safety. The second report, *Crossing the Quality Chasm: A New Health System for the 21st Century* (IOM, 2001), also focused on quality-related issues and recommendations for innovative redesign to improve care. Together, these reports added urgency in the development of interprofessional educational programs and interprofessional collaborative health care practice across the country.

One outcome of these reports was the establishment of the IOM's Committee on the Health Professions Education Summit. The members of the committee met to discuss and develop strategies for better preparing health care professionals to practice in the 21st-century health system. Specifically, the committee addressed strategies for "restructuring clinical education to be consistent with the six national quality aims of ... safety, effectiveness, patient-centeredness, timeliness, efficiency, and equity ... across the continuum of education for the allied health, medical, nursing, and pharmacy professions" (IOM, 2003, p. 20). National efforts in many arenas of health care professions education and practice have progressed and culminated in the 2012 establishment of the National Center for Interprofessional Practice and Education (2015) at the University of Minnesota. The need for integration and coordination of health care delivery in dealing with the rising incidence of chronic diseases, the complexity of the health care system, and the use of technology in health care are the driving forces behind the current IPE movement (Page et al., 2009).

Interprofessional Education, Occupational Therapy, and Accreditation

Interprofessional education is defined as "occasions when students from two or more professions learn about, from, and with each other to improve collaboration and the quality of care" (Centre for the Advancement of Interprofessional Education [CAIPE], 2002). The ultimate goal of IPE is improving patient-centered care, a goal resonant with the core values of occupational therapy (AOTA, 2015). Client-centered practice focuses on the occupational needs of individuals, families, and communities to improve their health and well-being through participation in meaningful occupations (AOTA, 2014; Townsend, Brintell, & Staisey, 1990). Similarly, IPE focuses on the needs of individuals, families, and communities to improve their quality of care, health outcomes, and well-being (Barr & Low, 2011). Collaborating with clients and factoring their input into the decision-making process, a hallmark of client-centered care, is based on parity and inclusion. Similarly, in IPE all professions collaborate regardless of status and power. Just as client-centered occupational therapy values clients' individuality regardless of their differences, IPE respects individuality and diversity within and between the professions. The unique identity, expertise, and contributions of individual professions are recognized and valued in IPE (Barr & Low, 2011).

Developing and incorporating standards for IPE and interprofessional care into accreditation and certification criteria is one way to ensure integration into curricula (Allison, 2007, p. 567). In actuality, the impetus for curriculum redesign to include IPE has in many fields been the accrediting bodies for the various professions and the insurance industry (Zorek & Raehl, 2013). Occupational therapy accreditation standards appear to align with this trend. The Preamble of the 2011 Accreditation Council for Occupational Therapy Education (ACOTE®) Educational Standards states that a graduate from an ACOTE-accredited doctoral-, master's-, or associate-degree-level occupational therapy program must "be prepared to effectively communicate and work interprofessionally with those who provide care for individuals and/or populations in order to clarify each member's responsibility in executing components of an intervention plan" (ACOTE, 2012, pp. S6–S8). This is the first time an educational standard specific to IPE and interprofessional practice has appeared in this document. In addition, ACOTE Standard B.5.21 states that students will be able to "effectively communicate, coordinate, and work interprofessionally with those who provide services to individuals, organizations, and/or populations in order to clarify each member's responsibility in executing components of an intervention plan" (ACOTE, 2012, p. S48). Although ACOTE standards have only recently addressed IPE specifically, collaboration and communication with other professional team members and consumers in all phases of occupational therapy processes have been integral to the educational standards and the profession's ethics standards (AOTA, 2015) for decades. Principle 6 of the *Occupational Therapy Code of Ethics (2015)* (AOTA, 2015) speaks to fidelity as it relates to interprofessional relationships. Occupational therapy personnel are specifically called to

> promote collaborative actions and communication as a member of interprofessional teams to facilitate quality care and safety for clients [as well as] respect the practices, competencies, roles, and responsibilities of their own and other professionals to promote a collaborative environment reflective of interprofessional teams.

Key Concepts and Core Competencies

The definition of IPE has been expanded by the Institute of Medicine (2003), CAIPE (2002), and the World Health Organization (WHO) to "when students from two or more professions learn about, from, and with each other to enable effective collaboration and improve health outcomes" (WHO, 2010, p. 13). On the basis of this definition, students are required to interact with one another in learning activities that are authentic and that require the complex problem solving that involves the knowledge and skills of multiple professions. Reflection on the experiences is a critical component to improve on the collaborative process. The overall goal is to develop *interprofessionality*, defined as

> the process by which professionals reflect on and develop ways of practicing that provides an integrated and cohesive answer to the needs of the client/family/population. . . . [It] involves continuous interaction and knowledge sharing between professionals, organized to solve or explore a variety of education and care issues all while seeking to optimize the patient's participation. . . . Interprofessionality requires a paradigm shift, since interprofessional practice has unique characteristics in terms of values, codes of conduct, and ways of working. (D'Amour & Oandasan, 2005, p. 9)

IPE is paramount to promoting effective interprofessional practice and collaboration. Multidisciplinary becomes interprofessional when team members transcend their separate disciplinary perspective and weave together their unique perspectives, methods, and practice to overcome problems and perform their work collaboratively (Klein, 1990). Pellegrino (1972) stated,

> Each member of the team, while providing the group with the knowledge and skills of his or her disciplinary perspective, also strives to incorporate that perspective with those of others to create solutions to healthcare problems that transcend conventional discipline specific methods, procedures, and techniques. (p. 4)

Others who have written on the distinction between multidisciplinary and interprofessional practice have commented on the quality of communication and degree of collaboration between professional team members (Hirokawa, 1990) and the cohesive, collaborative decision making in team-oriented health care delivery (D'Amour & Oandasan, 2005).

The Interprofessional Education Collaborative (IPEC) published a report from an expert panel (IPEC Expert Panel, 2011) that is the landmark document for the delineation of core competencies for interprofessional practice and that guides a competency-based approach to IPE. This document describes four core competency areas for practice, the ultimate goal of which is to guide the development of interprofessional learning activities and "prepare all health professions students for *deliberatively working together*" (p. 3):

- Competency Domain 1: Values/Ethics for Interprofessional Practice

- Competency Domain 2: Roles/Responsibilities

- Competency Domain 3: Interprofessional Communication

- Competency Domain 4: Teams and Teamwork.

These core competencies for practice as applied to education can be effectively planned in education through a learning continuum of exposure → immersion → competency (as entry to practice), using tools of reflective learning and formative assessment (CAIPE, 2002).

Ultimately, IPE aims to create more effective systems of *interprofessional practice,* defined as a higher form of practice wherein health care professionals from different disciplines make up a team, unique to the individual client–patient, that works with the client to develop a unified decision (National Academies of Practice, 2012). IPP results in safer and more efficient delivery of health care (Guitard, Dubouloz, Savard, Metthé, & Brasset-Latulippe, 2010) as well as greater patient satisfaction (Howell, Wittman, & Bundy, 2012; Kent & Keating, 2013; Shiyanbola, Lammers, Randall, & Richards, 2012; Solomon & Risdon, 2011), thus validating the need to embed IPE into entry-level preparation for occupational therapy practitioners.

Assessing the Outcomes of Interprofessional Education

Positive outcomes associated with IPE have been documented at several levels from students to patient, client, and consumer. Assessments used in these studies have focused on measuring changes in attitudes, perceptions, behaviors, knowledge, skills, and abilities, although changes in student attitudes and perceptions are by far the most commonly assessed variables. In addition to positive changes in students' perception of health care teams and IPE, recent studies have noted that students who participate in IPE increase knowledge of their own professional roles, improve communication skills with people outside of their own profession, and develop critical skills necessary for working on interprofessional teams (Buff et al., 2014; Howell et al., 2012; Olson & Bialocerkowski, 2014; Solomon & Risdon, 2011). Some studies have noted that engagement in interprofessional learning may lead to health care providers who demonstrate higher levels of safety and more efficient delivery of medical care. Unfortunately, the literature that connects student participation in IPE and potential benefit to health service delivery or patient outcomes is limited (Knier, Stichler, Ferber, & Catterall, 2014; Shrader, Kern, Zoller, & Blue, 2013).

The Canadian Interprofessional Health Collaborative (CIHC) has published several interprofessional resources over the past few years, including an inventory of 128 IPE measurement tools (Lindqvist, Duncan, Shepstone, Watts, & Pearce, 2005). The majority of these assessments measure student attitudes (64 tools) versus knowledge, behavior, or patient or provider satisfaction. Of note, no psychometric information was found in 33% of the report's entries. Nevertheless, the IPE field's overall high regard for quantitative measurement is impressive and remains a focus for future studies.

The National Center for Interprofessional Practice and Education offers online access to a collection of assessments used for IPE and collaborative practice (IPECP) research (National Center for Interprofessional Practice and Education, 2013; available at https://nexusipe.org/measurement-instruments). The collection started with a review of the CIHC inventory but narrowed the assessments to those that focused on IPECP and variables specifically related to attitudes, behavior, knowledge, skills, abilities, organizational practice, patient satisfaction, and provider satisfaction. Table 1 outlines commonly used assessments organized using the National Center's outcome levels, all with adequate psychometrics for educational research.

Table 1. Commonly Used Outcome Measures in Interprofessional Education and Collaborative Practice

Name of Tool	Tool Description	Setting and Sample	Citation
Outcome Level 1: Attitudes			
Attitudes Toward Health Professionals Questionnaire (AHPQ)	20 items (1 for each profession) 2 components, caring and subservience, with visual analog scales	University in UK 160 students from 6 professional programs	Lindqvist et al. (2005)
Attitudes Toward Health Care Teams	3 subscales: Quality of Care/Process, Physician Centrality, and Cost of Care 20 items with 4-point Likert scales	Community and hospital settings in US 1,018 interdisciplinary geriatric health care teams	Heineman, Schmitt, Farrell, & Brallier (1999)
Attitudes Toward IP Learning in the Academic Setting	4 areas: campus resources and support, faculty, students, and curriculum/outcomes supporting IP learning 13 items with 5-point Likert scales	University in Canada 194 faculties from 4 health disciplines	Curran, Sharpe, & Forristall (2007)
Attitudes Toward Teamwork questionnaire (also applies to Outcome Levels 2 and 3)	Subscales: Orientation Toward Team Problem Solving, Problem-Solving Confidence, Team Preparedness, Attitude Toward Interdisciplinary Team, and Self-Efficacy 10 items each with 5- or 6-point Likert scales	University in US 410 alumni from 8 allied health disciplines	Lindqvist et al. (2005)
Group Environment Scale (GES)	10 subscales: Cohesion, Leader Support, Expressiveness, Independence, Task Orientation, Self-Discovery, Anger and Aggression, Order and Organization, Leader Control, and Innovation 9 items, each with true–false ratings	College in US 191 students	Salter & Junco (2007)

(Continued)

Table 1. Commonly Used Outcome Measures in Interprofessional Education and Collaborative Practice *(cont.)*

Name of Tool	Tool Description	Setting and Sample	Citation
Index of Interprofessional Team Collaboration for Expanded School Mental Health (IITC–ESMH) (also applies to Outcome Level 4)	4 subscales: Reflection on Process, Professional Flexibility, Newly Created Professional Activities, and Role Interdependence 26 items with 5-point Likert scales	Schools in US 436 members of IP health care teams	Mellin et al. (2010)
Professional Identity Scale	Strength of students' professional identity regarding readiness for IP learning 10 items with 5-point Likert scales	University in UK 933 students from various health disciplines	Hind et al. (2003)
Readiness for Interprofessional Learning Scale (RIPLS)	3 subscales: Teamwork and Collaboration, Negative and Positive Professional Identity, Roles and Responsibilities 19 items with 5-point Likert scales	University in UK 120 students from 8 health disciplines	Parsell & Bligh (1999)
Outcome Level 2: Knowledge, Skills, Abilities			
Interprofessional Delirium Knowledge Test (IDKT)	Delirium case study tool 4 areas: identification, causes, and management of delirium in terminally ill patients; psychosocial care of patient and family; roles of team members and contribution to patient care; and communication 5 open-ended questions scored with rubric	Palliative care unit in Canada 10 team members, volunteers, and students from 6 professions	Brajtman et al. (2008)
Attitudes Toward Teamwork questionnaire (also applies to Outcome Levels 1 and 3)	Subscales: Orientation Toward Team Problem Solving, Problem-Solving Confidence, Team Preparedness, Attitude Toward Interdisciplinary Team, and Self-Efficacy 10 items each with 5- or 6-point Likert scales	University in US 410 alumni from 8 allied health disciplines	Lindqvist et al. (2005)
Team Skills Scale (TSS)	17 items with 5-point Likert scales. Modified from original: 17 of the 20 items related interdisciplinary team skills were used. Remaining 3 attitudinal items examined individually.	Hospital in US 25 students from 4 disciplines	Robben et al. (2012)
Outcome Level 3: Behavior			
Attitudes Toward Teamwork questionnaire (also applies to Outcome Levels 1 and 2)	Subscales: Orientation Toward Team Problem Solving, Problem-Solving Confidence, Team Preparedness, Attitude Toward Interdisciplinary Team, and Self-Efficacy 10 items each with 5- or 6-point Likert scales	University in US 410 alumni from 8 allied health disciplines	Lindqvist et al. (2005)
Collaborative Practice Assessment Tool (CPAT)	8 domains: mission, meaningful purpose, goals; general relationships; team leadership; general role responsibilities and autonomy; communication and information exchange; community linkages and coordination of care; decision making and conflict management; and patient involvement. 57 items with 7-point Likert scales 3 open-ended questions on team's strengths, challenges, and help needed to improve collaborative practice	111 practice teams in Canada	Schroder et al. (2011)

(Continued)

Table 1. Commonly Used Outcome Measures in Interprofessional Education and Collaborative Practice *(cont.)*

Name of Tool	Tool Description	Setting and Sample	Citation
Interprofessional Collaboration Scale	Collaboration among multiple health professional groups 3 subscales: Communication, Accommodation, and Isolation (Nurse–Physician Relations Subscale of the Nursing Work Index and the subscales of the Attitudes Toward Health Care Teams Scale were used to measure the concurrent, convergent, and discriminant validity.)	Hospitals in Canada; number of sample not provided	Kenaszchuk , Reeves, Nicholas, & Zwarenstein (2010)
Outcome Level 4: Organizational Practice			
Index of Interprofessional Team Collaboration for Expanded School Mental Health (IITC–ESMH) (also applies to Outcome Level 1)	4 subscales: Reflection on Process, Professional Flexibility, Newly Created Professional Activities, and Role Interdependence 26 items with 5-point Likert scales	Schools in US 436 members of IP health care teams	Mellin et al. (2010)
Outcome Level 5: Patient Satisfaction			
Satisfaction With Treatment Team Planning Rating Scale (also applies to Outcome Level 6)	Patient satisfaction with treatment team planning 10 items with 4-point Likert scales	Inpatient psychiatric hospital in US 18 health professionals from 6 disciplines	Singh, Singh, Sabaawi, Myers, & Wahler (2006)
Outcome Level 6: Provider Satisfaction			
Satisfaction With Treatment Team Planning Rating Scale (also applies to Outcome Level 5)	Staff satisfaction with treatment team planning 10 items with 4-point Likert scales	Inpatient psychiatric hospital in US 18 health professionals from 6 disciplines	Singh et al. (2006)
Satisfaction Survey	Attitudes toward teamwork and teamwork abilities 12 items with 5-point Likert scales	University in Canada 137 professionals	Curran, Heath, Kearney, & Button (2010)

Note. IP = interprofessional.
Source. Arthur et al., 2012.

Designing, Implementing, and Sustaining Interprofessional Education

It is of the highest importance that occupational therapy educators teach students to build their interprofessional toolkit during their educational journey. This toolkit includes building trust, open communication, mutual respect, and professionalism, as well as the skills required for effective teamwork: conflict resolution, negotiation, and empathy. Creating an atmosphere and culture within occupational therapy curricula that emphasize being a team player and being client focused is well supported through IPE. When students demonstrate effective collaborative reciprocity within the educational environment, best practices of interprofessionalism in occupational therapy will follow.

As Greer and Clay (2010) asserted, "Developing and sustaining IPE requires a mammoth effort that incorporates institutional support, leadership, and shared vision and which transverses multiple divisions, units, schools, or colleges within and among educational systems" (p. 224). Once the goal of IPE is established, best methods for implementing the experience must be identified. It is important to assess the level of understanding of faculty, staff, and administration who are interested in collaborating in the IPE effort. Occupational therapy faculty initiating or supporting IPE activities may need to provide educational programming to ensure that everyone understands the importance of and reasons to engage in this educational component. This may be accomplished through campus workshops, webinars, reading groups, and attendance at a national conference on IPE.

The next step is to assess the strengths and opportunities both within and external to the institution that are in place to support one's efforts. These can range from students and alumni in the community or settings in which interprofessional collaboration and practice exist to resources within the division or the university at large. Perhaps the institution has an office or advisory board that can assist in community outreach. Figure 1 displays important factors to consider at all levels of the institution when planning to implement IPE as well as suggested resources.

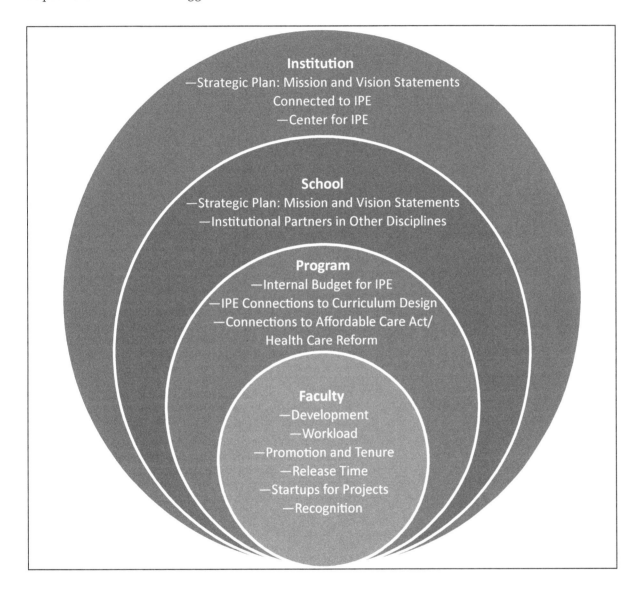

Figure 1. Institutional considerations and resources.

Note. IPE = interprofessional education.

A typical hierarchy of ease in implementation is to begin at the classroom level, then in-service learning and Level I fieldwork, and then campuswide experiences; however, depending on the balance of support available and the goals of the initiative, faculty may find a Level I fieldwork experience easier to carry out than a classroom experience. Level II fieldwork is certainly a place where students can put their interprofessional skills to the test, and it is recommended that all Level II fieldwork experiences have at least one assignment related to IPE and practice. Table 2 provides examples of IPE activities at all levels from classroom to community.

Table 2. Models of Interprofessional Education

Activity	Description
Institution	
Universitywide faculty IPE institute–training	IP faculty training about campuswide IP initiatives; engagement of faculty on IP teams to develop universitywide IP activities and new programs.
IPE Day	Planned by representative group of faculty from several disciplines (e.g., medicine, nursing, OT, pharmacy, physician assistant, physical therapy, social work). Each member has a coordinating responsibility: space, food, handouts, scheduling faculty facilitators, and so forth.
	Students from several disciplines are assigned to IP groups that meet in several classrooms across the campus and engage in activities addressing IP core competencies at the appropriate level. Faculty facilitators meet over lunch to receive instructions, and 2 or more (from different disciplines) are assigned to each room. Social activity with refreshments follows.
	Examples: Introduction to each discipline's educational curricula and scope of practice; case-study discussion emphasizing each profession's contributions and role.
Classroom	
OT faculty coteach with faculty from other professions; faculty jointly create and foster a collaborative learning environment or activity for students from 2 or more professions	OT students engage with students from other professions to conduct interviews with family and caregivers of people who have chronic conditions. The team of students considers the role of caregivers and how various professions can work collaboratively to assist patients and their caregivers with long-term and ongoing health care issues.
Sharing Knowledge and Skills: OTAs and PTAs: Adaptive Equipment and Gait Training	OTA students and PTA students teach each other. OTA students share, and provide simulations for, various pieces of adaptive equipment and explain their purpose(s) in daily activities. PTA students present case scenarios and rationale for gait training to increase problem solving and clinical reasoning behind the gait training process.
Community	
Service learning with 2 or more professions working together to engage in community-based programming	OT students work with students from dental medicine to develop school-based oral health programs for children with multiple disabilities.
Student-run free medical–therapy clinics for uninsured patients	OT students participate in student-run free clinics with other health professions including medicine, pharmacy, nursing, and physical therapy. These clinics provide free medical care and therapy services to uninsured and underserved patients while offering students an opportunity to translate their classroom learning directly to patient care in the form of experiential learning. As of 2014, 146 student-run free clinics are in existence, as tracked by the Society of Student-Run Free Clinics.
Cultivating Partnerships in the Garden: An IP Service Learning Experience; Quincy Gardening Club and OTA Students	Collaborative experiences between OTA and PTA, English, and forestry students, including • Modifications to gardening tools and garden terrain • Accessibility with raised garden beds • Restructuring of gardening tasks • Exploration of current market for adapted garden tools • Documentary of collaborative experience.

(Continued)

356

Table 2. Models of Interprofessional Education *(cont.)*

Activity	Description
Adaptive Equipment Project: An IP Learning Experience	Collaborative experience between OTA and engineering students, including • Creation of a piece of adaptive equipment intended for individuals with disabilities • Communication between students with different backgrounds and goals • Education of faculty, staff, and student body as well as the community.
Fieldwork—Level I	
Introduction to IP Collaborative Education and Practice *Learning outcomes:* • Understand the importance of good teamwork for the client's health and well-being. • Learn about another team professional's roles and job tasks.	Students ask fieldwork educator to assist in seeking out a non–OT professional at the fieldwork site. Student shadows the professional for 30 minutes and conducts a 15-minute interview based on the following: • Describe what you do during a typical day. • What is the best part of being a _____? • How do you see yourself working in tandem with OT practitioners? • How important is it to be a team player for the health and well-being of your clients? Student writes a reflection on • Whether, during the observation of the professional, he or she saw the professional use therapeutic use of self while communicating with clients. Explain. • What he or she learned about the professional's role in the care of clients and as a team member.
Synthesis and Application of IP Collaborative Education and Practice *Learning outcomes:* • Assess own IP collaborative practices, and use knowledge to effectively engage with peers. • Appraise the benefits and constraints on IP teamwork. • Actively engage with at least 1 other professional to ensure quality client care during the fieldwork experience.	Students read the IPEC Expert Panel's (2011) *Core Competencies for IP Collaborative Practice* before fieldwork. Students write a descriptive narrative about client care in relation to the following IP competencies: • Values/Ethics for IP Practice: Develop a trusting relationship with other team members • Roles/Responsibilities: Communicate one's roles and responsibilities • IP Communication: Listen actively, and encourage ideas and opinions of other team members • Teams and Teamwork: Share accountability with other professions.

(Continued)

Table 2. Models of Interprofessional Education *(cont.)*

Activity	Description
Fieldwork—Level II	
IP Collaborative Practice based on Educational Experiences *Learning outcomes:* • Effectively communicate and work IPly with those who provide services to individuals and groups to clarify each member's responsibility in executing an intervention plan.	On the basis of Level II fieldwork experiences, students write descriptive narratives of the following: • Identify non–OT professionals encountered on a frequent basis. • Discuss the level of collaboration between the above-named professionals and the OT staff during coordination of client care. • Discuss the format and frequency of communication between the OT staff and non–OT professionals as it relates to coordination of client care. • Discuss your level of confidence in effectively communicating with non–OT professionals as it relates to coordination of client care and explaining the basic tenets of OT. • Discuss a specific incident in which you directly collaborated or communicated with a non–OT professional in regard to client care or explanation of OT services. • List a specific component of a client's intervention plan that requires team collaboration.

Note. IP = interprofessional; IPE = interprofessional education; IPEC = Interprofessional Education Collaborative; OT = occupational therapy; OTA = occupational therapy assistant; PTA = physical therapy assistant.

Ways to ensure that IPE initiatives are sustainable include meeting with administration to discuss the stakes for IPE, which may include enhanced professional skills for graduates, improved standards of education, and opportunities for emergent practice and scholarship for faculty across the campus and within the community. One of the most productive means of ensuring the sustainability of IPE is to build a goal into the program's strategic plan in which each component of the educational experience has a measurable goal, identified strengths, and key stakeholders. Greer and Clay (2010) described a useful peer-reviewed instrument for assessing IPE in health care institutions that provides detailed insight into requirements for successfully implementing and sustaining IPE.

Ethical Considerations for Occupational Therapy Education and Practice

It is the professional and ethical responsibility of occupational therapy educators to provide students with opportunities to work and learn collaboratively during their professional education. Without opportunities to learn collaboratively as students, it is unlikely that occupational therapy practitioners will effectively work collaboratively in practice settings. Practice that is truly collaborative is aligned with health care reform efforts to benefit consumers with improved care and client experiences at reduced costs (IOM, 2003).

References

Accreditation Council for Occupational Therapy Education. (2012). 2011 Accreditation Council for Occupational Therapy Education (ACOTE®) standards. *American Journal of Occupational Therapy, 66,* S6–S74. http://dx.doi.org/10.5014/ajot.2012.66S6

Allison, S. (2007). Up a river! Interprofessional education and the Canadian healthcare professional of the future. *Journal of Interprofessional Care, 21,* 565–568. http://dx.doi.org/10.1080/13561820701497930

American Occupational Therapy Association. (2014). Occupational therapy practice framework: Domain and process (3rd ed.). *American Journal of Occupational Therapy, 68*(Suppl. 1), S1–S48. http://dx.doi.org/10.5014/ajot.2014.682006

American Occupational Therapy Association. (2015). Occupational therapy code of ethics (2015). *American Journal of Occupational Therapy, 69*(Suppl. 3), 6913410030. http://dx.doi.org/10.5014/ajot.2015.696S03

Barr, H., & Low, H. (2011). *Principles of interprofessional education.* London: Center for the Advancement of Interprofessional Education. Retrieved from http://caipe.org.uk/resources/principles-of-interprofessional-education/

Brajtman, S., Hall, P., Weaver, L., Higuchi, K., Allard, P., & Mullins D. (2008). An interprofessional educational intervention on delirium for health care teams: Providing opportunities to enhance collaboration. *Journal of Interprofessional Care, 22,* 658–660. http://dx.doi.org/10.1080/13561820802038732

Buff, S. M., Jenkins, K., Kern, D., Worrall, C., Howell, D., Martin, K., . . . Blue, A. (2014). Interprofessional service-learning in a community setting: Findings from a pilot study. *Journal of Interprofessional Care, 29,* 159–161.

Centre for the Advancement of Interprofessional Education. (2002). *CAIPE: Centre for the Advancement of Interprofessional Education.* Retrieved from http://caipe.org.uk/about-us/defining-ipe/

Curran, V. R., Heath, O., Kearney, A., & Button, P. (2010). Evaluation of an interprofessional collaboration workshop for post-graduate residents, nursing and allied health professionals. *Journal of Interprofessional Care, 24,* 315–318. http://dx.doi.org/10.3109/13561820903163827

Curran, V. R., Sharpe, D., & Forristall, J. (2007). Attitudes of health sciences faculty members towards interprofessional teamwork and education. *Medical Education, 41,* 892–896.

D'Amour, D., & Oandasan, I. (2005). Interprofessionality as the field of interprofessional practice and interprofessional education: An emerging concept. *Journal of Interprofessional Care, 19*(Suppl. 1), 8–20. http://dx.doi.org/10.1080/13561820500081604

Earnest, M., & Brandt, B. (2014). Aligning practice redesign and interprofessional education to advance Triple Aim outcomes. *Journal of Interprofessional Care, 28,* 497–500. http://dx.doi.org/10.3109/13561820.2014.933650

Greer, A. G., & Clay, M. C. (2010). Interprofessional education assessment and planning instrument for academic institutions. *Journal of Allied Health, 39,* 224–231.

Guitard, P., Dubouloz, C. J., Savard, J., Metthé, L., & Brasset-Latulippe, A. (2010). Assessing interprofessional learning during a student placement in an interprofessional rehabilitation university clinic in primary healthcare in a Canadian francophone minority context. *Journal of Research in Interprofessional Practice and Education, 1*(3). Retrieved from http://www.jripe.org/index.php/journal/article/viewArticle/26.

Heineman, G. D., Schmitt, M. H., Farrell, M. P., & Brallier, S. (1999). Development of an Attitudes Toward Health Care Teams Scale. *Evaluation of Health Professions, 22,* 123–142. http://dx.doi.org/10.1177/01632789922034202

Hind, M., Norman, I., Cooper, S., Gill, E., Hilton, R., Judd, P., & Jones, S. C. (2003). Interprofessional perceptions of health care students. *Journal of Interprofessional Care, 17,* 21–34. http://dx.doi.org/10.1080/1356182021000044120

Hirokawa, R. Y. (1990). The role of communication in group decision-making efficacy: A task-contingency perspective. *Small Group Research, 21,* 190–204. http://dx.doi.org/10.1177/1046496490212003

Howell, D., Wittman, P., & Bundy, M. (2012). Interprofessional clinical education for occupational therapy and psychology students: A social skills training program for children with autism spectrum disorders. *Journal of Interprofessional Care, 1,* 49–55. http://dx.doi.org/10.3109/13561820.2011.620186

Institute of Medicine. (2000). *To err is human: Building a safer health system.* Washington, DC: National Academies Press.

Institute of Medicine. (2001). *Crossing the quality chasm: A new health system for the 21st century.* Washington, DC: National Academies Press.

Institute of Medicine. (2003). *Health professions education: A bridge to quality.* Washington, DC: National Academies Press.

Interprofessional Education Collaborative Expert Panel. (2011). *Core competencies for interprofessional collaborative practice: Report of an expert panel.* Washington, DC: Interprofessional Education Collaborative.

Kenaszchuk, C., Reeves, S., Nicholas, D., & Zwarenstein, M. (2010). Validity and reliability of a multiple-group measurement scale for interprofessional collaboration. *BMC Health Service Research, 30,* 10–83. http://dx.doi.org/10.1186/1472-6963-10-83

Kent, F. M., & Keating, J. L. (2013). Patient outcomes from a student-led interprofessional clinic in primary care. *Journal of Interprofessional Care, 27,* 336–338. http://dx.doi.org/10.3109/13561820.2013.767226

Klein, J. (1990). *Interdisciplinarity: History, theory, and practice.* Detroit: Wayne State University Press.

Knier, S., Stichler, J. F., Ferber, L., & Catterall, K. (2014). Patients' perceptions of the quality of discharge teaching and readiness for discharge. *Rehabilitation Nursing, 40,* 30–39. http://dx.doi.org/10.1002/rnj.164

Lindqvist, S., Duncan, A., Shepstone L, Watts, F., & Pearce S. (2005). Development of the "Attitudes to Health Professionals Questionnaire" (AHPQ): A measure to assess interprofessional attitudes. *Journal of Interprofessional Care, 19,* 269–279. http://dx.doi.org/10.1080/13561820400026071

Mellin, A., Bronstein, L., Anderson-Butcher, D., Amorose, A. J., Ball, A., & Green, J. (2010). Measuring interprofessional team collaboration in expanded school mental health: Model refinement and scale development. *Journal of Interprofessional Care, 24,* 514–523. http://dx.doi.org/10.3109/13561821003624622

National Academies of Practice. (2012, March 26). *Toward interdisciplinary team development.* Retrieved May 2011 https://www.napractice.org/eweb/DynamicPage.aspx?Site=NAP2&WebCode=ArticleDetail&faq_key=a893ec43-74de-4c7e-8b29-7e09c04ae907

National Center for Interprofessional Practice and Education. (2013). *Measurement instruments.* Retrieved from https://nexusipe.org/measurement-instruments

National Center for Interprofessional Practice and Education. (2015). [Home page]. Retrieved from http://www.ahceducation.umn.edu/about/national-center-interprofessional-practice-and-education

Olson, R., & Bialocerkowski, A. (2014). Interprofessional education in allied health: A systematic review. *Medical Education, 48,* 236–246. http://dx.doi.org/10.1111/medu.12290

Page, R. L., Hume, A. L., Trujillo, J. M., Leader, W. G., Vardeny, O., Neuhauser, M. M.,. . . Cohen, L. J. (2009). Interprofessional education: Principles and application a framework for clinical pharmacy. *Pharmacotherapy, 29,* 879–879. http://dx.doi.org/10.1592/phco.29.7.879

Parsell, G., & Bligh, J. (1999). The development of a questionnaire to assess the readiness of health care students for interprofessional learning (RIPLS). *Medical Education, 33,* 95–100. http://dx.doi.org/10.1046/j.1365-2923.1999.00298.x

Pellegrino, E. (1972). Interdisciplinary education in the health professions: Assumptions, definitions, and some notes on teams. In *Report of a conference: Educating for the health team. Conference report of the Institute of Medicine* (pp. 4–18). Washington, DC: National Academy of Sciences.

Robben, S., Perry, M., van Nieuwenhuijzen, L., van Achterberg, T., Rikkert, M. O., Schers, H., . . . Melis, R. (2012). Impact of interprofessional education on collaboration attitudes, skills, and behavior among primary care professionals. *Continuing Education in Health Professions, 32,* 196–204. http://dx.doi.org/10.1002/chp.21145

Salter, D., & Junco, R. (2007). Measuring small-group environments: Validity study of scores from the Salter Environmental Type Assessment and the Group Environment Scale. *Educational and Psychological Measurement, 67,* 475–486. http://dx.doi.org/10.1177/0013164406292083

Schroder, C., Medves, J., Paterson, M., Byrnes, V., Chapman, C., O'Riordan, A., . . . Kelly, C. (2011). Development and pilot testing of the collaborative practice assessment tool. *Journal of Interprofessional Care, 25,* 189–195. http://dx.doi.org/10.3109/13561820.2010.532620

Shiyanbola, O. O., Lammers, C., Randall, B., & Richards, A. (2012). Evaluation of a student-led interprofessional innovative health promotion model for an underserved population with diabetes: A pilot project. *Journal of Interprofessional Care, 26,* 376–382. http://dx.doi.org/10.3109/13561820.2012.685117

Shrader, S., Kern, D., Zoller, J., & Blue, A. (2013). *Interprofessional teamwork skills as predictors of clinical outcomes in a simulated healthcare setting. Journal of Allied Health, 42,* e1–e6.

Singh, N. N., Singh, S. D., Sabaawi, M., Myers, R. E., & Wahler, R. G. (2006). Enhancing treatment team process through mindfulness-based mentoring in an inpatient psychiatric hospital. *Behavior Modification, 30,* 423–441. http://dx.doi.org/10.1177/0145445504272971

Solomon, P., & Risdon, C. (2011). Promoting interprofessional learning with medical students in home care settings. *Medical Teacher, 33,* e236–e241. http://dx.doi.org/10.3109/0142159X.2011.558534

Townsend, E., Brintell, S., & Staisey, N. (1990). Developing guidelines for client-centered occupational therapy practice. *Canadian Journal of Occupational Therapy, 57,* 69–76.

World Health Organization. (2010). *Framework for action on interprofessional education and collaborative practice.* Geneva: Author. Retrieved from http://whqlibdoc.who.int/hq/2010/WHO_HRH_HPN_10.3_eng.pdf

Zorek, J., & Raehl, C. (2013). Interprofessional education accreditation standards in the USA: A comparative analysis. *Journal of Interprofessional Care, 27,* 123–130. http://dx.doi.org/10.3109/13561820.2012.718295

Authors
Julie McLaughlin Gray, PhD, OTR/L, FAOTA
Patty Coker-Bolt, PhD, OTR/L, FAOTA
Jyothi Gupta, PhD, OTR/L, FAOTA
Angie Hissong, EdD, OTR/L, CMCP, CMMT
Kimberly D. Hartmann, PhD, OTR/L, FAOTA
Stephen B. Kern, PhD, OTR/L, FAOTA

for
The Commission on Education
Andrea Bilics, PhD, OTR/L, FAOTA, *Chairperson*
Tina DeAngelis, EdD, OTR/L
Jamie Geraci, MS, OTR/L
Michael Iwama, PhD, OT(C)
Julie Kugel, OTD, MOT, OTR/L
Julie McLaughlin Gray, PhD, OTR/L, FAOTA
Kate McWilliams
Maureen S. Nardella, MS, OTR/L
Renee Ortega, MA, COTA
Kim Qualls, MS, OTR/L
Tamra Trenary, OTD, OTR/L, BCPR
Neil Harvison, PhD, OTR/L, FAOTA, *AOTA Headquarters Liaison*

Adopted by the Representative Assembly 2015AprilA9

Copyright © 2015 by the American Occupational Therapy Association.

Citation. American Occupational Therapy Association. (2015). Importance of interprofessional education in occupational therapy curricula. *American Journal of Occupational Therapy, 69*(Suppl. 3), 6913141020. http://dx.doi.org/10.5014/ajot.2015.696S02

Fieldwork Level II and Occupational Therapy Students: A Position Paper

The purpose of this paper is to define the Level II fieldwork experience and to clarify the appropriate conditions and principles that must exist to ensure that interventions completed by Level II fieldwork students are of the quality and sophistication necessary to be clinically beneficial to the client. When appropriately supervised, adhering to professional and practice principles, and in conjunction with other regulatory and payer requirements, the American Occupational Therapy Association (AOTA) considers that students at this level of education are providing occupational therapy interventions that are skilled according to their professional education level of practice.

AOTA asserts that Level II occupational therapy fieldwork students may provide occupational therapy services under the supervision of a qualified occupational therapist in compliance with state and federal regulations. Occupational therapy assistant fieldwork students may provide occupational therapy services under the supervision of a qualified occupational therapist or occupational therapy assistant under the supervision of an occupational therapist in compliance with state and federal regulations.

Occupational therapy Level II fieldwork students are those individuals who are currently enrolled in an occupational therapy or occupational therapy assistant program accredited, approved, or pending accreditation by the Accreditation Council for Occupational Therapy Education (ACOTE®; 2012). At this point in their professional education, students have completed necessary and relevant didactic coursework that has prepared them for the field experience.

The fieldwork Level II experience is an integral and crucial part of the overall educational experience that allows the student an opportunity to apply theory and techniques acquired through the classroom and Level I fieldwork learning. Level II fieldwork provides an in-depth experience in delivering occupational therapy services to clients, focusing on the application of evidence-based purposeful and meaningful occupations, administration, and management of occupational therapy services. The experience provides the student with the opportunity to carry out professional responsibilities under supervision and to observe professional role models in the field (ACOTE, 2012).

The academic program and the supervising occupational therapy practitioner[1] are responsible for ensuring that the type and amount of supervision meet the needs of the student and ensure the safety of all stakeholders. The following General Principles represent the minimum criteria that must be present during a Level II fieldwork experience to ensure the quality of services being provided by the Level II student practitioner:

a. The student is supervised by a currently licensed or credentialed occupational therapy practitioner who has a minimum of 1 year of practice experience subsequent to initial certification and is adequately prepared to serve as a fieldwork educator.

---

[1]When the term *occupational therapy practitioner* is used in this document, it refers to both occupational therapists and occupational therapy assistants (AOTA, 2006).

b. Occupational therapy students will be supervised by an occupational therapist. Occupational therapy assistant students will be supervised by an occupational therapist or an occupational therapy assistant in partnership with the occupational therapist who is supervising the occupational therapy assistant (AOTA, 2009).

c. Supervision of occupational therapy and occupational therapy assistant students in fieldwork Level II settings will be of the quality and scope to ensure protection of consumers and provide opportunities for appropriate role modeling of occupational therapy practice.

d. The supervising occupational therapist and/or occupational therapy assistant must recognize when direct versus indirect supervision is needed and ensure that supervision supports the student's current and developing levels of competence with the occupational therapy process.

e. Supervision should initially be direct and in line of sight and gradually decrease to less direct supervision as is appropriate depending on the

- Competence and confidence of the student,

- Complexity of client needs,

- Number and diversity of clients,

- Role of occupational therapy and related services,

- Type of practice setting,

- Requirements of the practice setting, and

- Other regulatory requirements (ACOTE, 2012).

f. In all cases, the occupational therapist assumes ultimate responsibility for all aspects of occupational therapy service delivery and is accountable for the safety and effectiveness of the occupational therapy service delivery process involving the student. This also includes provision of services provided by an occupational therapy assistant student under the supervision of an occupational therapy assistant (AOTA, 2009).

g. In settings where occupational therapy practitioners are not employed,

1. Students should be supervised daily on site by another professional familiar with the role of occupational therapy in collaboration with an occupational therapy practitioner (see b above).

2. Occupational therapy practitioners must provide direct supervision for a minimum of 8 hours per week and be available through a variety of other contact measures throughout the workday. The occupational therapist or occupational therapy assistant (under the supervision of an occupational therapist) must have 3 years of practice experience to provide this type of supervision (ACOTE, 2012).

h. All state licensure policies and regulations regarding student supervision will be followed, including the ability of the occupational therapy assistant to serve as fieldwork educator.

i. Student supervision and reimbursement policies and regulations set forth by third-party payers will be followed.

j. If allowed by payment policies and applicable state and federal laws, occupational therapy services provided by students under the supervision of a qualified practitioner will be billed as services provided by the supervising licensed occupational therapy practitioner.

It is the professional and ethical responsibility of occupational therapy practitioners to be knowledgeable of and adhere to applicable state and federal laws and payer rules and regulations related to fieldwork education.

References

Accreditation Council for Occupational Therapy Education. (2012). Accreditation Council for Occupational Therapy Education (ACOTE®) standards. *American Journal of Occupational Therapy, 66*(6 Suppl.).

American Occupational Therapy Association. (2006). Policy 1.44: Categories of occupational therapy personnel. In *Policy manual* (2011 ed., pp. 33–34). Bethesda, MD: Author.

American Occupational Therapy Association. (2009). Guidelines for supervision, roles, and responsibilities during the delivery of occupational therapy services. *American Journal of Occupational Therapy, 63,* 797–803.

Authors

Debbie Amini, EdD, OTR/L, CHT, *Chairperson, Commission on Practice*
Jyothi Gupta, PhD, OTR/L, OT, *Chairperson, Commission on Education*

for

The Commission on Practice
Debbie Amini, EdD, OTR/L, CHT, *Chairperson*

and

The Commission on Education
Jyothi Gupta, PhD, OTR/L, OT, *Chairperson*

Adopted by the Representative Assembly Coordinating Council (RACC) for the Representative Assembly, 2012, in response to RA Charge # 2011AprC26

Note. This document is based on a 2010 Practice Advisory, "Services Provided by Students in Fieldwork Level II Settings." Prepared by a Commission on Practice and Commission on Education Joint Task Force:
Debbie Amini, EdD, OTR/L, CHT
Janet V. DeLany, DEd, OTR/L, FAOTA
Debra J. Hanson, PhD, OTR
Susan M. Higgins, MA, OTR/L
Jeanette M. Justice, COTA/L
Linda Orr, MPA, OTR/L

Obesity and Occupational Therapy

Obesity is a significant and wide-ranging health and social problem in the United States. Occupational therapy is a health care profession that is qualified to provide interventions with individuals, groups, and society to effect change to promote optimum health. Occupational therapy services often are used directly and indirectly to influence weight management and related health concerns through attention to healthy lifestyle choices and engagement in fulfilling occupations. The purpose of this paper is to explain the position of the American Occupational Therapy Association (AOTA) to persons within and outside the profession on the role of occupational therapists and occupational therapy assistants[1] in addressing the impact of obesity on people's ability to engage in daily activities.

Overview of Occupational Therapy's Domain and Process

Since its founding, occupational therapy has been a healing profession of practitioners who "assist clients (people, organizations, and populations) to engage in everyday activities or occupations that they want and need to do in a manner that supports health and participation" (AOTA, 2008, p. 626). Occupational therapy practitioners[2] apply their knowledge about engagement in occupation—that is, "everyday activity" (AOTA, 2008, p. 628)—to help clients who may be experiencing disease, impairment, disability, dissatisfaction, or adverse circumstances participate in their daily life in a manner that supports their health and well-being. By working with clients from this perspective, occupational therapy practitioners use everyday activities therapeutically to improve the health and quality of life of consumers and to prevent future disease or disability.

AOTA and its members are committed to improving individual quality of life; promoting community health; and supporting primary, secondary, and tertiary care for the management of obesity (AOTA, 2012). This position paper explores the growing dangers of the obesity epidemic for health and describes specific and effective services provided by occupational therapy practitioners in a variety of practice settings for clients at risk for or experiencing the negative health effects of obesity throughout the life course. It also explains how the occupational therapy profession provides expertise and leadership in working with the problem of obesity in U.S. society as it affects individuals, families, groups, and populations across the life course.

Obesity in the United States

Definitions and Prevalence

Being *overweight* (defined as having a body mass index [BMI] of 25 to 29.9) or *obese* (defined as having a BMI of 30 or greater; Centers for Disease Control and Prevention [CDC], 2012b) reduces the likelihood

---

[1]*Occupational therapists* are responsible for all aspects of occupational therapy service delivery and are accountable for the safety and effectiveness of the occupational therapy service delivery process. *Occupational therapy assistants* deliver occupational therapy services under the supervision of and in collaboration with an occupational therapist (AOTA, 2009).

[2]When the term *occupational therapy practitioner* is used in this document, it refers to both occupational therapists and occupational therapy assistants (AOTA, 2006).

of a person's participation in physical activity, including leisure activity (Trost, Owen, Bauman, Sallis, & Brown, 2002). Although only 9% of Americans believe that they have a weight problem (Lee & Oliver, 2002) and fewer than 45% of overweight and obese patients receive weight counseling from their physicians (Rose, Frank, & Carrera, 2011), an all-time high 35.5% of adult American men and 35.8% of adult American women are considered obese (Flegal, Carroll, Kit, & Ogden, 2012). The prevalence of *Grade 3 obesity,* also commonly referred to as *severe* or *morbid obesity* (defined as having a BMI over 40; Flegal et al., 2012; National Center for Health Statistics, 2007) is rising substantially faster than obesity (Sturm, 2003); the current prevalence of Grade 3 obesity is 6.3% for the population (Flegal et al., 2012).

These figures translate to more than 72 million Americans considered obese (CDC, 2011). Although statistics show that the prevalence of obesity among adults, adolescents, and children plateaued in 2009–2010 compared with 2007–2008 (Flegal et al., 2012; Ogden, Carroll, Kit, & Flegal, 2012), rates are not yet declining.

Risk for obesity is elevated for individuals who have physical disabilities such as spinal cord injuries (Krause & Broderick, 2004); persons diagnosed with schizophrenia and other forms of mental illness (Bacon, Farnworth, & Boyd, 2012; Chwastiak et al., 2009; Northey & Barnett, 2012); persons with fewer years of education or poorer economic or job status; and Latino and African American individuals (Blanchard, 2009; CDC, 2006, 2011; Cousins et al., 1992; Flegal et al., 2012; Friedman & Brownell, 1996; Institute of Medicine [IOM], 2012; Wardle, Waller, & Jarvis, 2002). As a result of increased need across all populations, the field of *bariatrics* (defined as the medical investigation, prevention, and treatment of obesity with interventions including diet and nutrition, exercise, behavior modification, lifestyle changes, surgical alternatives, and appropriate medications) is continuing to expand (Foti, 2004, 2005).

Risks and Costs

Several studies have demonstrated that obesity appears to be correlated with increased risk of both acute and chronic diseases, including Type 2 diabetes, sleep apnea, chronic low back pain, hypertension, hyperlipidemia, multiple forms of cancer, cardiovascular disease, stroke, liver and gall bladder disease, osteoarthritis, activity limitations, reproductive health complications including infertility, psychological distress, discrimination, and an increased mortality rate that is responsible for a remarkable 95.7 million years of life lost across the overweight and obese population (CDC, 2011; Expert Panel on the Identification, Evaluation, and Treatment of Overweight in Adults, 1998; Finkelstein, Brown, Wrage, Allaire, & Hoerger, 2010; Forhan, Law, Vrkljan, & Taylor, 2011; Hemminki, Li, Sundquist, & Sundquist, 2011).

The related medical costs are estimated at $147 billion annually, representing nearly 10% of all medical spending in the United States (Finkelstein, Trogdon, Cohen, & Dietz, 2009). About half of the total is paid by Medicare and Medicaid, creating a significant financial burden for taxpayers (Finkelstein & Strombotne, 2010). Job absenteeism due directly or indirectly to obesity-related illness results in costs of $12.8 billion per year and an additional $30.3 billion in medical costs for employers (Finkelstein, DiBonaventura, Burgess, & Hale, 2010; McKinnon et al., 2009). In addition, reduced productivity by obese workers while on the job, referred to as *presenteeism,* results in another $30.0 billion in losses to businesses annually (Finkelstein, DiBonaventura, et al., 2010).

Studies show that more than one-third of children aged 6 to 19 years are considered at risk for overweight or are overweight, defined as being at or above the 85th percentile of the sex-specific BMI-for-age growth chart (CDC, 2012a; Center for Health and Health Care in Schools [CHHCS], 2005; Janicke, Harman, Kelleher, & Zhang, 2009); the current prevalence of obesity among children and adolescents is 16.9% (Ogden et al., 2012). These young people are at risk for a variety of health-related concerns, including a trajectory toward obesity as an adult and the health risks associated with it (CHHCS, 2005; Nonnemaker, Morgan-Lopez, Pais, & Finkelstein, 2009; Waters et al., 2011). In addition, a bidirectional relationship between obesity and psychiatric diagnoses has been observed among children (Janicke et al., 2009).

Societal issues—such as easy access to inexpensive junk food and overexposure to junk food marketing; steadily increasing food portion sizes; decreased provision of healthy food choices and physical education in schools; lack of safety for outdoor activities in lower income areas; and the growing popularity of sedentary activities, including viewing television, playing seated video games, and using the computer—have contributed to the rapid rise of overweight and obesity in childhood (Finkelstein & Strombotne, 2010; IOM, 2012; McKinnon et al., 2009; Miller, Rosenbloom, & Silverstein, 2004). As a result, today's children are the first American generation in modern times who will not have as long a life expectancy as their parents (Nonnemaker et al., 2009).

On a societal level, obesity has been called the "last acceptable form of prejudice" (Chambliss, Finley, & Blair, 2004), one that often results in reduced education, housing, and employment opportunities (Puhl & Brownell, 2001); decreased access to and use of health care and wellness services (Wallis, 2004); exposure to stigmatization, discrimination, and bullying (IOM, 2012); and restricted social participation as a result of negative portrayals in popular media (Greenberg, Eastin, Hofschire, Lachlan, & Brownell, 2003; Moloney, 2000). Such negative consequences can have a devastating impact on individuals throughout their life, limiting their opportunities for or access to participation in their desired occupations.

Positive Results of Weight Loss

Weight loss of as little as 5% to 10% of initial body weight can result in significant improvements in measures of blood pressure, cholesterol levels, and glycemic control as well as other improved health outcomes (Expert Panel, 1998; Fabricatore & Wadden, 2003; Manson, Skerrett, Greenland, & VanItallie, 2004; Trogdon, Finkelstein, Reyes, & Dietz, 2009). Conversely, while long-term and appropriate weight loss has been shown to improve health conditions, short-term loss and rebounding with increased weight gain, inappropriate dieting methods, or extreme weight loss may have damaging effects. Typical methods used by consumers who wish to lose weight consist of adhering to a short-term calorie-restricted diet; engaging in a regular, not intense, or irregularly active exercise program; and/or a quick fix of fad diets or weight-loss drugs followed by a return to unhealthy eating habits and a sedentary lifestyle (Andrus, 2011; Heshka et al., 2003: Lowe, Miller-Kovach, Frye, & Phelan, 1999; Manson et al., 2004; Mokdad et al., 2001; Moloney, 2000; Smith & Fremouw, 1987; Willet, 2001). With millions of Americans of all ages struggling—and failing—to achieve and maintain a healthy lifestyle using current methods for weight management, it is clear that health care consumers need to implement successful approaches to attaining effective and sustainable changes in lifestyle that influence weight and, more important, produce related improvements in overall health.

Occupational Therapy's Role in Lifestyle Change

Through a knowledge of psychosocial, physical, environmental, and spiritual factors, as well as of cultural traditions and perspectives that influence performance (AOTA, 2008), occupational therapy practitioners are uniquely qualified to help consumers develop and implement an individualized, structured approach to lifestyle change. A randomized trial published in *JAMA* (Heshka et al., 2003) indicated that weight loss is more effectively achieved when a health care consumer is assisted through a structured program than when a client relies on self-help methods. Using analysis and understanding of performance patterns related to daily life activities (AOTA, 2008; Clark, 2000; Quiroga, 1995; Wilcock, 1998; Yerxa, 2002), occupational therapy practitioners provide meaningful and effective interventions that facilitate participation by the client in modifying daily life habits, roles, and patterns that contribute to chronic conditions, including obesity (Forhan et al., 2011).

For example, occupational therapy interventions are effective in fostering use of virtual reality technology to increase physical activity for patients living in a mental health residential facility (Bacon et al., 2012), engaging adolescents in increased physical activity (Ketteridge & Boshoff, 2008), adapting physical activity for children who are obese (Gill, 2011), and educating children about optimal nutritional choices (Munguba, Valdés, & da Silva, 2008).

When assessing needs, setting goals, and developing and implementing interventions to assist clients who are overweight or obese, the occupational therapy practitioner works closely with the client to design specific plans or programs to meet individual goals and desires in whatever areas of occupation are affected. Occupational therapy intervention may focus on prevention, remediation/restoration, adaptation/compensation, and maintenance programs in either long-term or short-term settings (AOTA, 2008).

Occupational therapy programs incorporate the client's personal preferences, circumstances, context, and needs into a customized healthy living regimen that takes into account any preexisting medical conditions (AOTA, 2008). Through education, strategies, and intervention planning, occupational therapy practitioners can help clients build habits, including engagement in health-promoting activities, that allow them to maintain targeted changes that influence their weight within the complex dynamic of their everyday lives. Occupational therapists provide interventions for people of diverse populations across the life course, in settings ranging from clinical to community environments.

Occupational therapy interventions in the area of weight management may include community programs of health promotion through lifestyle change; education programs; facilitation of the development of new habits and routines; Lifestyle Redesign® programs; recommendation of home modifications; adaptations/equipment; use of assistive and/or virtual technologies; compensatory training in activities of daily living and instrumental activities of daily living; wellness programs for children, teens, and adults; play and physical education in the schools; safe patient-handling programs in hospitals and skilled nursing facilities; and bariatric and postsurgical acute care interventions (Foti, 2004, 2005). Other relevant resources that can be provided by occupational therapy practitioners include adaptive equipment evaluation, home modification planning, task modification solutions, durable medical equipment considerations, compensatory strategies, caregiver training, and client resource development and advocacy (AOTA, 2008).

These and other occupational therapy services addressing obesity and related conditions may be covered by major health care payers, including Medicare, Medicaid, and private health insurance (Finkelstein & Strombotne, 2010). With the high expenses generated by obesity-related health conditions (Finkelstein et al., 2009; Finkelstein, DiBonaventura, et al., 2010; McKinnon et al., 2009), the need to reduce spending is an economic necessity. Preventing illness is consistently more cost-effective than treating it, and occupational therapy has demonstrated in past research both cost-effectiveness and success in preventing declines in health, for example, among community-dwelling older adults and other populations (Clark et al., 1997, 2012).

A study by Trogdon et al. (2009) using a return-on-investment model found that, in workplaces, a weight loss of 5% among all overweight and obese employees would result in an annual savings in medical and absenteeism costs of $90 per person. Low-cost interventions, such as a group led by an occupational therapist, could reduce costs for businesses, with even more savings realized if substantial weight loss is achieved. Thus, occupational therapy is positioned to become an ever more valuable component of the growing public health imperative to reverse obesity trends in a cost-effective manner.

Conclusion

Occupational therapy addresses the prevention and concerns of obesity through a holistic and client-centered approach to lifestyle through participation in activities that promote health. Occupational therapy interventions can facilitate weight loss and enable clients to make healthy changes in daily life, including incorporating productive and social activity as well as informed choices about eating habits and physical activity, to address obesity, thus improving health outcomes and maintaining long-term wellness.

References

American Occupational Therapy Association. (2006). Policy 1.44: Categories of occupational therapy personnel. In *Policy manual* (2011 ed., pp. 33–34). Bethesda, MD: Author.

American Occupational Therapy Association. (2008). Occupational therapy practice framework: Domain and process (2nd ed.). *American Journal of Occupational Therapy, 62,* 625–683. http://dx.doi.org/ 10.5014/ ajot.62.6.625

American Occupational Therapy Association. (2009). Guidelines for supervision, roles, and responsibilities during the delivery of occupational therapy services. *American Journal of Occupational Therapy, 63,* 797–803. http://dx.doi.org/10.5014/ajot.63.6.797

American Occupational Therapy Association. (2012). AOTA's societal statement on obesity. *American Journal of Occupational Therapy, 66*(6, Suppl.), S81–S82. http://dx.doi.org/10.5014/ajot.2012.66S81

Andrus, J. (2011). Helping patients with weight loss. *American Journal of Nursing, 111,* e1–e3. Retrieved February 12, 2012, from http://journals.lww.com/ajnonline/Fulltext/2011/07000/Helping_ Patients_ with_Weight_Loss.28.aspx

Bacon, N., Farnworth, L., & Boyd, R. (2012). The use of the Wii Fit in forensic mental health: Exercise for people at risk of obesity. *British Journal of Occupational Therapy, 75,* 61–68. http://dx.doi.org/ 10.4276/03 0802212X13286281650992

Blanchard, S. A. (2009). Variables associated with obesity among African-American women in Omaha. *American Journal of Occupational Therapy, 63,* 58–68. http://dx.doi.org/10.5014/ajot.63.1.58

Center for Health and Health Care in Schools. (2005, March). *Childhood overweight: What the research tells us.* Retrieved August 4, 2006, from www.healthinschools.org/sh/obesityfacts.asp

Centers for Disease Control and Prevention. (2006, September 12). *People with disabilities are less healthy than those without disabilities.* Retrieved October 19, 2006, from www.cdc.gov/Media/pressrel/ r060912.htm

Centers for Disease Control and Prevention. (2011, May 26). *Obesity: Halting the epidemic by making health easier—At a glance 2011.* Retrieved February 13, 2012, from www.cdc.gov/chronicdisease/resources/ publications/aag/pdf/2011/Obesity_AAG_WEB_508.pdf

Centers for Disease Control and Prevention. (2012a, April 27). *Basics about childhood obesity.* Retrieved September 6, 2012, from www.cdc.gov/obesity/childhood/basics.html

Centers for Disease Control and Prevention. (2012b, April 27). *Defining overweight and obesity.* Retrieved September 6, 2012, from www.cdc.gov/obesity/adult/defining.html

Chambliss, H. O., Finley, C. E., & Blair, S. N. (2004). Attitudes toward obese individuals among exercise science students. *Medicine and Science in Sports and Exercise, 36,* 468–474. http://dx.doi.org/10.1249/ 01.MSS.0000117115.94062.E4

Chwastiak, L. A., Rosenheck, R. A., McEvoy, J. P., Stroup, T. S., Swartz, M. S., Davis, S. M., & Lieberman, J. A. (2009). The impact of obesity on health care costs among persons with schizophrenia. *General Hospital Psychiatry, 31,* 1–7. http://dx.doi.org/10.1016/j.genhosppsych.2008.09.012

Clark, F. A. (2000). The concepts of habit and routine: A preliminary theoretical synthesis. *OTJR: Occupation, Participation and Health, 20*(Suppl. 1), 123–137.

Clark, F., Azen, S. P., Zemke, R., Jackson, J., Carlson, M., Mandel, D., . . . Lipson, L. (1997). Occupational therapy for independent-living older adults: A randomized controlled trial. *JAMA, 278,* 1321–1326. http://dx.doi.org/10.1001/jama.1997.03550160041036

Clark, F., Jackson, J., Carlson, M., Chou, C.-P., Cherry, B. J., Jordan-Marsh, M., . . . Azen, S. P. (2012). Effectiveness of a lifestyle intervention in promoting the well-being of independently living older people: Results of the Well Elderly 2 Randomised Controlled Trial. *Journal of Epidemiology and Community Health, 66,* 782–790. Retrieved February 14, 2012, from http://jech.bmj.com/content/early/2011/06/01/ jech.2009.099754.full.pdf+html

Cousins, J. H., Rubovits, D. S., Dunn, J. K., Reeves, R. S., Ramirez, A. G., & Foreyt, J. P. (1992). Family versus individually oriented intervention for weight loss in Mexican American women. *Public Health Reports, 107*, 549–555.

Expert Panel on the Identification, Evaluation, and Treatment of Overweight in Adults. (1998). Clinical guidelines on the identification, evaluation, and treatment of overweight and obesity in adults. *American Journal of Clinical Nutrition, 68*, 899–917.

Fabricatore, A. N., & Wadden, T. A. (2003). Treatment of obesity: An overview. *Clinical Diabetes, 21*, 67–72. http://dx.doi.org/10.2337/diaclin.21.2.67

Finkelstein, E. A., Brown, D. S., Wrage, L. A., Allaire, B. T., & Hoerger, T. J. (2010). Individual and aggregate years-of-life-lost associated with overweight and obesity. *Obesity, 18*, 333–339. http://dx.doi.org/10.1038/oby.2009.253

Finkelstein, E. A., DiBonaventura, M., Burgess, S. M., & Hale, B. C. (2010). The costs of obesity in the workplace. *Journal of Occupational and Environmental Medicine, 52*, 971–976. http://dx.doi.org/10.1097/JOM.0b013e3181f274d2

Finkelstein, E. A., & Strombotne, K. L. (2010). The economics of obesity. *American Journal of Clinical Nutrition, 91*(5, Suppl.), 1520S–1524S. http://dx.doi.org/10.3945/ajcn.2010.28701E

Finkelstein, E. A., Trogdon, J. G., Cohen, J. W., & Dietz, W. (2009). Annual medical spending attributable to obesity: Payer-and service-specific estimates. *Health Affairs, 28*, w822–w831. http://dx.doi.org/10.1377/hlthaff.28.5.w822

Flegal, K. M., Carroll, M. D., Kit, B. K., & Ogden, C. L. (2012). Prevalence of obesity and trends in the distribution of body mass index among US adults, 1999–2010. *JAMA, 307*, 491–497. http://dx.doi.org/10.1001/jama.2012.39

Forhan, M., Law, M., Vrkljan, B. H., & Taylor, V. H. (2011). Participation profile of adults with class III obesity. *OTJR: Occupation, Participation and Health, 31*, 135–142. http://dx.doi.org/10.3928/15394492-20101025-02

Foti, D. (2004). Bariatric care: Practical problem solving and interventions. *Physical Disabilities Special Interest Section Quarterly, 27*(4), 1–3.

Foti, D. (2005, February 7). Caring for the person of size. *OT Practice, 10*, 9–14.

Friedman, M. A., & Brownell, K. D. (1996). A comprehensive treatment manual for the management of obesity. In V. Van Hasselt & M. Hersen (Eds.), *Sourcebook of psychological treatment manuals for adult disorders* (pp. 375–422). New York: Plenum Press.

Gill, S. V. (2011). Optimising motor adaptation in childhood obesity. *Australian Occupational Therapy Journal, 58*, 386–389. http://dx.doi.org/10.1111/j.1440-1630.2011.00957.x

Greenberg, B. S., Eastin, M., Hofschire, L., Lachlan, K., & Brownell, K. D. (2003). Portrayals of overweight and obese individuals on commercial television. *American Journal of Public Health, 93*, 1342–1348. http://dx.doi.org/10.2105/AJPH.93.8.1342

Hemminki, K., Li, X., Sundquist, J., & Sundquist, K. (2011). Obesity and familial obesity and risk of cancer. *European Journal of Cancer Prevention, 20*, 438–443. http://dx.doi.org/10.1097/CEJ.0b013e32834761c0

Heshka, S., Anderson, J. W., Atkinson, R. L., Greenway, F. L., Hill, J. O., Phinney, S. D., . . . Pi-Sunyer, F. X. (2003). Weight loss with self-help compared with a structured commercial program: A randomized trial. *JAMA, 289*, 1792–1798. http://dx.doi.org/10.1001/jama.289.14.1792

Institute of Medicine. (2012). *Measuring progress in obesity prevention: Workshop report.* Washington, DC: National Academies Press.

Janicke, D. M., Harman, J. S., Kelleher, K. J., & Zhang, J. (2009). The association of psychiatric diagnoses, health service use, and expenditures in children with obesity-related health conditions. *Journal of Pediatric Psychology, 34,* 79–88. http://dx.doi.org/10.1093/jpepsy/jsn051

Ketteridge, A., & Boshoff, K. (2008). Exploring the reasons why adolescents participate in physical activity and identifying strategies that facilitate their involvement in such activity. *Australian Occupational Therapy Journal, 55,* 273–282. http://dx.doi.org/10.1111/j.1440-1630.2007.00704.x

Krause, J. S., & Broderick, L. (2004). Patterns of recurrent pressure ulcers after spinal cord injury: Identification of risk and protective factors 5 or more years after onset. *Archives of Physical Medicine and Rehabilitation, 85,* 1257–1264. http://dx.doi.org/10.1016/j.apmr.2003.08.108

Lee, T., & Oliver, J. E. (2002). *Public opinion and the politics of America's obesity epidemic* (KSG Working Paper No. RWP02-017). Boston: John F. Kennedy School of Government, Harvard University.

Lowe, M. R., Miller-Kovach, K., Frye, N., & Phelan, S. (1999). An initial evaluation of a commercial weight loss program: Short-term effects on weight, eating behavior, and mood. *Obesity Research, 7,* 51–59.

Manson, J. E., Skerrett, P. J., Greenland, P., & VanItallie, T. B. (2004). The escalating pandemics of obesity and sedentary lifestyle. A call to action for clinicians. *Archives of Internal Medicine, 164,* 249–258. http://dx.doi.org/10.1001/archinte.164.3.249

McKinnon, R. A., Orleans, C. T., Kumanyika, S. K., Haire-Joshu, D., Krebs-Smith, S. M., Finkelstein, E. A., . . . Ballard-Barbash, R. (2009). Considerations for an obesity policy research agenda. *American Journal of Preventive Medicine, 36,* 351–357. http://dx.doi.org/10.1016/j.amepre.2008.11.017

Miller, J., Rosenbloom, A., & Silverstein, J. (2004). Childhood obesity. *Journal of Clinical Endocrinology and Metabolism, 89,* 4211–4218. http://dx.doi.org/10.1210/jc.2004-0284

Mokdad, A. H., Bowman, B. A., Ford, E. S., Vinicor, F., Marks, J. S., & Koplan, J. P. (2001). The continuing epidemics of obesity and diabetes in the United States. *JAMA, 286,* 1195–1200. http://dx.doi.org/10.1001/jama.286.10.1195

Moloney, M. (2000). Dietary treatments of obesity. *Proceedings of the Nutrition Society, 59,* 601–608. http://dx.doi.org/10.1017/S0029665100000859

Munguba, M. C., Valdés, M. T. M., & da Silva, C. A. B. (2008). The application of an occupational therapy nutrition education programme for children who are obese. *Occupational Therapy International, 15,* 56–70. http://dx.doi.org/10.1002/oti.244

National Center for Health Statistics (2007, June 13). *Morbid obesity.* Retrieved September 6, 2012, from http://nchspressroom.wordpress.com/2007/06/13/morbid-obesity/

Nonnemaker, J. M., Morgan-Lopez, A. A., Pais, J. M., & Finkelstein, E. A. (2009). Youth BMI trajectories: Evidence from the NLSY97. *Obesity, 17,* 1274–1280.

Northey, A., & Barnett, F. (2012). Physical health parameters: Comparison of people with severe mental illness with the general population. *British Journal of Occupational Therapy, 75,* 100–105. http://dx.doi.org/10.4276/030802212X13286281651199

Ogden, C. L., Carroll, M. D., Kit, B. K., & Flegal, K. M. (2012). Prevalence of obesity and trends in body mass index among U.S. children and adolescents, 1999–2010. *JAMA, 307,* 483–490. http://dx.doi.org/10.1001/jama.2012.40

Puhl, R., & Brownell, K. D. (2001). Bias, discrimination, and obesity. *Obesity Research, 9,* 788–805. http://dx.doi.org/10.1038/oby.2001.108

Quiroga, V. (1995). *Occupational therapy: The first 30 years 1900–1930.* Bethesda, MD: AOTA Press.

Rose, A. E., Frank, E., & Carrera, J. S. (2011). Factors affecting weight counseling attitudes and behaviors among U.S. medical students. *Academic Medicine, 86,* 1463–1472. http://dx.doi.org/10.1097/ACM.0b013e3182312471

Smith, M. E., & Fremouw, W. J. (1987). A realistic approach to treating obesity. *Clinical Psychology Review, 7,* 449–465. http://dx.doi.org/10.1016/0272-7358(87)90022-5

Sturm, R. (2003). Increases in clinically severe obesity in the United States, 1986–2000. *Archives of Internal Medicine, 163,* 2146–2148. http://dx.doi.org/10.1001/archinte.163.18.2146

Trogdon, J., Finkelstein, E. A., Reyes, M., & Dietz, W. H. (2009). A return-on-investment simulation model of workplace obesity interventions. *Journal of Occupational and Environmental Medicine, 51,* 751–758. http://dx.doi.org/10.1097/JOM.0b013e3181a86656

Trost, S. G., Owen, N., Bauman, A. E., Sallis, J. F., & Brown, W. (2002). Correlates of adults' participation in physical activity: Review and update. *Medicine and Science in Sports and Exercise, 34,* 1996–2001. http://dx.doi.org/10.1097/00005768-200202000-00025

Wallis, L. (2004). Overweight patients face prejudice in health care. *Nursing Standard, 18,* 6.

Wardle, J., Waller, J., & Jarvis, M. J. (2002). Sex differences in the association of socioeconomic status with obesity. *American Journal of Public Health, 92,* 1299–1304. http://dx.doi.org/10.2105/AJPH.92.8.1299

Waters, E., de Silva-Sanigorski, A., Hall, B. J., Brown, T., Campbell, K. J., Gao, Y., . . . Summerbell, C. D. (2011). Interventions for preventing obesity in children. *Cochrane Database of Systematic Reviews, 2011*(12), Art. No.: CD001871. http://dx.doi.org/10.1002/14651858.CD001871.pub3

Wilcock, A. A. (1998). *An occupational perspective on health.* Thorofare, NJ: Slack.

Willet, W. C. (2001). *Eat, drink, and be healthy.* New York: Free Press.

Yerxa, E. J. (2002). Habits in context: A synthesis, with implications for research in occupational science. *OTJR: Occupation, Participation and Health, 22,* 104–110.

Authors
Faryl Saliman Reingold, OTD, OTR/L
Katie Jordan, OTD, OTR/L

for

The Commission on Practice
Debbie Amini, EdD, OTR/L, CHT, *Chairperson*

Adopted by the Representative Assembly Coordinating Council (RACC) for the Representative Assembly, 2012

Note. This revision replaces the 2007 document *Obesity and Occupational Therapy,* previously published and copyrighted in 2007 by the American Occupational Therapy Association in the *American Journal of Occupational Therapy, 61,* 701–703.

Occupational Therapy's Commitment to Nondiscrimination and Inclusion

The occupational therapy profession affirms the right of every individual to access and fully participate in society. This paper states the profession's stance on nondiscrimination and inclusion.

Nondiscrimination exists when we accept and treat all people equally. In doing so, we avoid differentiating between people because of biases or prejudices. We value individuals and respect their culture, ethnicity, race, age, religion, gender, sexual orientation, and capacities, consistent with the principles defined and described in the *Occupational Therapy Code of Ethics and Ethics Standards* (American Occupational Therapy Association [AOTA], 2010). Nondiscrimination is a necessary prerequisite for inclusion. Inclusion requires that we ensure not only that everyone is treated fairly and equitably but also that all individuals have the same opportunities to participate in the naturally occurring activities of society, such as attending social events, having access to public transportation, and participating in professional organizations. We also believe that when we do not discriminate against others and when we include all members of society in our daily lives, we reap the benefits of being with individuals who have different perspectives, opinions, and talents from our own.

We support nondiscrimination and inclusion throughout our profession. Our concerns are twofold—for the persons who receive occupational therapy services and for our professional colleagues. In professional practice, our evaluations and interventions are designed to facilitate our clients' engagement in occupations to support their health and participation in the various contexts and environments of their lives. Contexts and environments include, but are not limited to, individuals' cultural, personal, temporal, virtual, physical, and social contexts as described in the *Occupational Therapy Practice Framework: Domain and Process* (AOTA, 2014). As occupational therapists and occupational therapy assistants, we assume a collaborative partnership with clients and their significant others to support the individual's right to self-direction.

We believe that inclusion is achieved through the combined efforts of clients, their families, and significant others; health, education, and social services professionals; legislators; community members; and others. We support all individuals and their significant others' rights to fully participate in making decisions that concern their daily occupations: activities of daily living, instrumental activities of daily living, rest and sleep, work, education, play, leisure, and social participation.

AOTA and its members recognize the legal mandates concerning nondiscriminatory practices. However, the concept of nondiscrimination is not limited to that which is dictated by law. This professional association, through its members, boards, commissions, committees, officers, and staff, supports the belief that all members of the occupational therapy professional community are entitled to maximum opportunities to develop and use their abilities. These individuals also have the right to achieve productive and satisfying professional and personal lives.

We are committed to nondiscrimination and inclusion as an affirmation of our belief that the interests of all members of the profession are best served when the inherent worth of every individual is recognized and valued. We maintain that society has an obligation to provide the reasonable accommodations necessary to allow individuals access to social, educational, recreational, and vocational opportunities. By embracing the concepts of nondiscrimination and inclusion, we will all benefit from the opportunities afforded in a diverse society.

References

American Occupational Therapy Association. (2010). Occupational therapy code of ethics and ethics standards (2010). *American Journal of Occupational Therapy, 64*(6, Suppl.), S17–S26. http://dx.doi.org/10.5014/ajot.2010.64S17

American Occupational Therapy Association. (2014). Occupational therapy practice framework: Domain and process (3rd ed.). *American Journal of Occupational Therapy, 68*(Suppl. 1), S1–S48. http://dx.doi.org/10.5014/ajot.2014.682006

Authors
Ruth H. Hansen, PhD, FAOTA
Jim Hinojosa, PhD, OT, FAOTA

for

The Commission on Practice
Mary Jane Youngstrom, MS, OTR, *Chairperson*

Adopted by the Representative Assembly 1999M4

Reference citations reviewed and updated by the Commission on Practice, February 2014
Debbie Amini, EdD, OTR/L, CHT, FAOTA, *Chairperson*

Adopted by the Representative Assembly Coordinating Council (RACC) for the Representative Assembly, 2014

Note. This document replaces the 2009 document *Occupational Therapy's Commitment to Nondiscrimination and Inclusion,* previously published and copyrighted in 2009 by the American Occupational Therapy Association in the *American Journal of Occupational Therapy, 63,* 819–820. http://dx.doi.org/10.5014/ajot.63.6.819

To be published and copyrighted in 2014 by the American Occupational Therapy Association in the *American Journal of Occupational Therapy, 68*(Suppl. 3).

Occupational Therapy's Perspective on the Use of Environments and Contexts to Facilitate Health, Well-Being, and Participation in Occupations

Introduction

Occupational therapy practitioners[1] view human performance as a transactive relationship among the client (people, groups, or populations), the client's occupations (daily life activities), and environments and contexts. *Environments* are the external physical and social aspects that surround clients while they engage in an occupation. *Contexts* are the cultural, personal, temporal, and virtual aspects of this engagement; some contexts are external to the client (e.g., virtual), some are internal to the client (e.g., personal), and some may have both external features and internalized beliefs and values (e.g., cultural; American Occupational Therapy Association [AOTA], 2014b).

Using their expertise in analyzing these complex and reciprocal relationships, occupational therapy practitioners make recommendations to structure, modify, or adapt the environment and context to enhance and support performance. Both environment and context influence clients' success in desired occupations and are therefore critical aspects of any occupational therapy assessment, intervention, and outcome. This assumption is consistent with current education and health care laws and policies, which stipulate that assessment and intervention by providers take place in the natural and least restrictive environments (LREs) that support the client's successful participation. Table 1 reviews key legislation and court cases related to occupational therapy intervention and how they apply to practice.

Purpose

The purpose of this document is to articulate AOTA's position regarding how, across all areas of practice, occupational therapy practitioners select, create, and use environments and contexts to support clients as they achieve health, well-being, and participation in desired occupations.

Occupational Therapy Process

Occupational therapy practitioners collaborate with clients to identify both strengths and barriers to health, well-being, and participation. As part of this process, practitioners consider a variety of environmental and contextual factors to inform the clinical reasoning process that guides client evaluation, intervention, and targeting of outcomes.

Occupational therapy practitioners analyze the environment and context to understand how these elements can best support learning and performance. Solutions are then generated to reduce identified barriers or build on supports through modifications and adaptations.

---

[1]When the term *occupational therapy practitioner* is used in this document, it refers to both occupational therapists and occupational therapy assistants (AOTA, 2006). *Occupational therapists* are responsible for all aspects of occupational therapy service delivery and are accountable for the safety and effectiveness of the occupational therapy service delivery process. *Occupational therapy assistants* deliver occupational therapy services under the supervision of and in partnership with an occupational therapist (AOTA, 2014a).

Table 1. Legislation and Court Cases Related to Occupational Therapy Practice

Federal Law, Court Case, or Movement	Key Constructs	Application to Occupational Therapy Practice
Section 504 of the Rehabilitation Act of 1973 (Pub. L. 93–112)	• The Rehabilitation Act of 1973 is a civil rights law that states that no person may, on the basis of his or her disability, be "excluded from the participation in, or denied the benefits of . . . any program or activity receiving Federal financial assistance" (29 U.S.C. § 794(a). • In educational settings, this law requires that schools ensure equal educational opportunities for students with a qualifying disability through the provision of special education services, related services, modifications, or accommodations.	• Occupational therapy services can be used in any program funded with federal funds to ensure equal access for people with disabilities. • In educational settings, occupational therapy practitioners can participate in developing a student plan under Section 504, help suggest and implement needed modifications and accommodations, and provide related services.
No Child Left Behind Act of 2001 (NCLB; Pub. L. 107–110)	• NCLB is the most recent reauthorization of the Elementary and Secondary Education Act of 1965 (Pub. L. 89–313). • It expands accountability standards for schools receiving federal funding. • It includes children with disabilities in the accountability models developed to gauge student and school success.	• NCLB created increased motivation for schools to use all existing resources to improve the achievement of all students. • It created broader opportunities for occupational therapy to be used by schools to benefit students with and without disabilities.
Individuals With Disabilities Education Improvement Act of 2004 (IDEA; Pub. L. 108–446)	• IDEA is the law governing how early intervention services for children ages birth–3 years are provided; it addresses the provision of special education and related services to students ages 3–21. • The purpose of IDEA Part B for students ages 3–21 is "to ensure that all children with disabilities have available to them a free appropriate public education that emphasizes special education and related services designed to meet their unique needs and prepare them for further education, employment, and independent living" (34 C.F.R. 300.1[a]). • The purpose of IDEA Part C for children ages birth–3 years and their families is to enhance and expand states' capacity to provide early intervention services and to help maintain, implement, and coordinate interagency services for early intervention with children ages 0–3 years. • Of note, IDEA requires that "removal of children with disabilities from the regular educational environment occurs only if the nature or severity of the disability is such that education in regular classes cannot be achieved satisfactorily" (34 C.F.R. 300.114[a][ii]).	• IDEA identified occupational therapy as a related service for eligible children under Part B for school-age children. • It established occupational therapy as a primary service provider for children age birth–3 years under Part C. • Under both programs, occupational therapy practitioners participate in evaluation and implementation, including analyzing and adjusting the context of and environment for learning and participation in school.

(Continued)

Table 1. Legislation and Court Cases Related to Occupational Therapy Practice *(cont.)*

Federal Law, Court Case, or Movement	Key Constructs	Application to Occupational Therapy Practice
Social Security Amendments of 1965 (Medicare and Medicaid; Pub. L. 89–97)	• These amendments established a national public health care program, Medicare, to meet the needs of older Americans and people with disabilities (Social Security Disability Insurance) who qualify for services on the basis of disability status and a sufficient work history. • They established an optional state–federal program to provide health and rehabilitation services for low-income people and certain people with disabilities.	• The amendments created a system of health care financing and insurance for older Americans and for people who would otherwise not have health and other services. • It created a steady funding stream for health care, including occupational therapy. • Social, community, and individual supports can in some circumstances be paid for by Medicare. • Medicaid has many options for coverage of occupational therapy, including programs that provide community and home-based supports for long-term care.
Older Americans Act of 1965 (OAA; Pub. L. 89–73)	• The OAA created a network of local and state entities, many called Area Agencies on Aging (AAAs), that are funded through OAA resources. • Programs and services are focused on older people to plan and care for their lifelong needs. • The goal of these programs is to keep older adults living independently in their own homes. • A broad range of services are covered, based on local needs, and may address nutrition, caregiver support, community safety, and fall prevention.	• The OAA provides flexible funding options that support community health and social services programs for older adults, which may include occupational therapy. • It increased focus and emphasis on community-based living resources and the promotion of aging in place.
Omnibus Budget Reconciliation Act of 1987 (Federal Nursing Home Reform Act; Pub. L. 100–203)	• This act created a set of national minimum standards of care and a bill of rights for people living in certified nursing facilities. • It requires nursing homes to develop individualized care plans for residents that focus on maintaining or improving the ability to walk, bathe, and complete other ADLs to the maximum extent possible. • The act requires nursing homes to develop individualized care plans for residents and training of paraprofessional staff. • It protects residents' right to be free of unnecessary and inappropriate physical and chemical restraints.	• This act created requirements as well as opportunities for occupational therapy practitioners to facilitate optimum function, attention to mental health, and maximum participation. Occupational therapy practitioners' care plans and interventions in nursing facilities, whether funded through Medicare or Medicaid, should be targeted to these goals. • Occupational therapy practitioners may address environmental modifications and adaptations needed for maximum performance and safety, both in personal environments (e.g., wheelchairs, beds) as well as bedrooms, bathrooms, and common areas.
Americans With Disabilities Act of 1990 (ADA; Pub. L. 101–336)	• The ADA built on previous civil rights legislation targeted at protecting the rights and enhancing participation of other minorities. • It provides a clear mandate to end discrimination against people with disabilities in all areas of life. • The ADA includes 5 titles that address employment, state and local government services, transportation, public accommodations (i.e., public places and services), and telecommunications.	• The ADA supports initiatives and interventions, including occupational therapy expertise, that promote function and participation for people with disabilities across the lifespan. • Occupational therapy practitioners can support the end of discrimination through their knowledge of independent living, accessibility, environmental modifications, supported employment, competence-based evaluation for employment, and implementation of reasonable accommodations in all settings.

(Continued)

Table 1. Legislation and Court Cases Related to Occupational Therapy Practice *(cont.)*

Federal Law, Court Case, or Movement	Key Constructs	Application to Occupational Therapy Practice
Rehabilitation, Comprehensive Services, and Developmental Disabilities Amendments of 1978 (Pub. L. 95–602)	• These amendments provide federal funding in cooperation with states to establish a national network of consumer-run community facilities and services. • Independent living centers now exist across the country. • The amendments advocate for the removal of architectural and transportation barriers that prevent people with disabilities from sharing fully in all aspects of society.	• The amendments support provision of occupational therapy evaluation and intervention in the natural environments in which people live, work, and play to help people adapt to the realities of their physical, social, attitudinal, and political contexts. • Intervention includes consultation, program development, and advocacy with teachers in schools, supervisors in jobs, citizens' organizations, local governments, businesses, local media, and advocacy organizations.
Olmstead v. L.C. (1999)	• In a 6–3 ruling by the U.S. Supreme Court against the state of Georgia, this case affirmed the right of people with disabilities whose living situation is supported by state or federal funds to live in their community. • The ruling requires states to place people with mental disabilities in community settings rather than in institutions if at all possible. • It dictates that community placement must be appropriate; that the transfer from institutional care to a less restrictive setting is not opposed by the affected person; and that the placement can be reasonably accommodated, taking into account the resources available to the state and the needs of others with mental disabilities.	• *Olmstead v. L.C.* established the precedent for the enforcement of a federal mandate for services to be provided in the LRE and in settings of choice for people with disabilities. • The case created opportunities for occupational therapy practitioners to design accommodations, interventions, and related services to support community living for people with disabilities.

Note. ADLs = activities of daily living; LRE = least restrictive environment.

Practitioners can recommend environmental and contextual modifications and adaptations such as those in the following examples:

- *Physical environment:* Improving accessibility of kitchens (lowering counter height and creating open floor plan) for clients using wheelchairs who want to engage in the occupation of cooking. Adding visual cues in the home environment to structure homemaking tasks to increase safety and organization for people with cognitive limitations.

- *Social environment:* Encouraging a student on the autism spectrum to connect with a peer mentor to attend various activities on campus, including sporting events.

- *Personal context:* Educating older adults on community mobility options.

- *Temporal context:* Consulting with a newly retired business executive about volunteer options involving financial planning and entrepreneurship.

- *Virtual context:* Collaborating with classroom teachers to provide appropriate technology.

Occupational therapy practitioners also recognize that specific interventions may need to begin outside the natural setting in which performance takes place and be completed in a setting in which components of occupations or underlying factors and skills can be targeted. For example, during inpatient rehabilitation, an adult with a spinal cord injury would practice community mobility in a simulated community environment in the rehabilitation facility to enable independent shopping on discharge to home.

Ultimately, interventions occurring in natural or modified environments support clients where they live, work, or play and wherever occupations take place (e.g., homes, classrooms, playgrounds, work, recreation or community centers). Providing appropriate intervention in the most appropriate environment is consistent with the values and purpose of occupational therapy. Practitioners also realize that many additional factors, such as limited financial, organizational, and personnel resources and the complexity of the client's condition, may inform various service delivery options. For example, although the most natural environment in which to address cooking difficulties for a client who is experiencing poststroke weakness in one arm may be the home, the client's medical status may dictate that training occur in a subacute rehabilitation facility.

Providing opportunities for all members of society to engage in health-promoting occupations through flexibility in the analysis of the environment and context in which clients thrive is essential. Table 2 provides additional examples of how occupational therapy practitioners use and modify the context and the environment to support health and participation in occupations.

Table 2. Case Studies

Case Description	Contextual and Environmental Focus of Occupational Therapy Service Delivery	Examples of Occupational Therapy Interventions Addressing Specific Environments and Contexts	Research Evidence and Related Resources Guiding Practice
A **15-month-old boy** was born at 29 weeks' gestation. He has had difficulty sitting up, particularly during feeding, and achieving other developmental milestones. He is living at home with his family.	The focus of intervention is to support the entire family in sustaining their family life while addressing the child's developmental needs. Intervention is provided in the home with an emphasis on how to adapt the natural environment to support the child's occupational performance and development.	• After discharge from the NICU, provide direct intervention in the child's home to promote safety and establish the child's developmental skills. • Collaborate with the family to structure and modify the physical and social environments in the home to support occupational performance. • Educate the caregiver in developmental principles, positioning, and activities to facilitate feeding and development. • Consult with family and other members of the transdisciplinary team to support family goals.	• Performing everyday activities in the natural setting provides reinforcement and support to achieve and enhance performance and competence (Dunst et al., 2001; Dunst, Trivette, Hamby, & Bruder, 2006). • Helping families accommodate to the demands of daily life with a child with developmental delays helps them develop appropriate and sustainable routines congruent with the family's values and the child's developmental needs (Keogh, Bernheimer, Gallimore, & Weisner, 1998). *Additional Resources* Frolek Clark & Kingsley (2013) Kingsley & Mailloux (2013)
A **3-year-old girl** with social and emotional regulation challenges attends a center-based preschool program.	The focus of intervention is to provide early childhood services in an inclusive classroom to enhance the child's opportunities for play with peers in naturally occurring situations that arise in the classroom. Occupational therapy intervention is integrated into the classroom activities.	• Structure play groups to promote peer social interaction skills. • Direct intervention with the child and parents to promote self-regulation and establish routines to facilitate the child's transitions throughout the day. • Consult with the early childhood team to analyze the demands of the preschool class and make recommendations for adaptations to support performance.	• Center-based early intervention services have a positive effect on children's social functioning (Blok, Fukkink, Gebhardt, & Leseman, 2005). • Preschoolers with disabilities perform as well, if not better, when placed in quality inclusive classroom settings and play groups (Bailey, Aytch, Odom, Symons, & Wolery, 1999; Odom, 2000). • Parents of children with disabilities commonly report that they perceive inclusive classroom practices as contributing to their child's

(Continued)

Table 2. Case Studies *(cont.)*

Case Description	Contextual and Environmental Focus of Occupational Therapy Service Delivery	Examples of Occupational Therapy Interventions Addressing Specific Environments and Contexts	Research Evidence and Related Resources Guiding Practice
			self-esteem, confidence, and happiness as well as reshaping their own expectations of their child's ability to develop and learn with others (Buysse, Skinner, & Grant, 2001). *Additional Resources* Case-Smith (2013) Frolek Clark & Kingsley (2013) Kingsley & Mailloux (2013)
A **7-year-old student** with cognitive, motor, and speech delays participates in a special day class in a public school. He has difficulty processing sensory information, interacting with peers, focusing on academic tasks, using his hands for tasks, and maneuvering on equipment on the playground.	Guided by the child's needs, the IEP team, which includes the occupational therapist and the parents, determines that the child is having difficulty participating with typically developing peers and would benefit from a special day class for students with behavioral challenges. Although such placements are viewed as more restrictive, the regular classroom environment is currently overwhelming for the child. The goal of the tailored environment is to provide the structure necessary for the child to learn specific skills for participation in a less restrictive environment in the future.	• Educate the IEP team about the effect of the environment on sensory processing and the relationship to behavior in a school setting. • Consult with the IEP team and teachers to structure, adapt, and modify the classroom and playground environments so that the child has opportunities to meet sensory needs by participating in vestibular, tactile, and proprioceptive activities throughout the school day. • Collaborate with the student to help him establish strategies and routines for sensory regulation, emotional and behavioral deescalation, and appropriate coping skills. • Develop a peer buddy system to promote appropriate social interactions with modeling and role-play during social group. • Provide direct intervention to facilitate integration of sensory systems in an environment rich in sensory experiences and equipment.	• The student may attend to classroom instruction for longer periods of time when sensory needs are addressed (Schilling, Washington, Billingsley, & Deitz, 2003). • Teaching children self-regulation strategies (a cognitive approach to manage sensory needs) helps them manage their behavior (Barnes, Vogel, Beck, Schoenfeld, & Owen, 2008; Vaughn et al., 2003). • Supporting a school-age child's occupational performance and behavior improves participation in school (Schaaf & Nightlinger, 2007). • Suspended equipment and opportunities to carefully monitor various and safe sensory experiences is a hallmark of sensory integration intervention. These opportunities may only be available in a carefully designed environment (Parham et al., 2007). *Additional Resource* Watling, Koenig, Davies, & Schaaf (2011)
A **28-year-old man** with schizoaffective disorder lives alone. He has difficulty organizing his daily routines to manage his medications. He was recently admitted to the hospital because of an acute exacerbation of his illness. He wants to be discharged home.	The intervention focuses on developing medication routines to help the client return to his apartment. If he is unable to manage his medications, he might need to move to a group home with more structured supervision. By analyzing the social and physical environment in the client's home and community, the occupational therapy practitioner can identify external cues and resources to optimize the client's occupational performance.	• Educate the medical team and case manager about performance deficits that affect medication routines. • Request that a pharmacist or nurse teach the client how to read labels and practice filling his medication box correctly. • Advocate for reminder calls for refills from the pharmacy or another entity. • Teach the client skills to establish habits and routines that support medication management, such as regular	Environmental supports are more likely to improve functional behavior for people with schizoaffective disorder when the supports are customized for the person and situated in the person's home (Velligan et al., 2000, 2006). *Additional Resources* Arbesman & Logsdon (2011) Brown (2012) Siebert, Smallfield, & Stark (2014)

(Continued)

Table 2. Case Studies *(cont.)*

Case Description	Contextual and Environmental Focus of Occupational Therapy Service Delivery	Examples of Occupational Therapy Interventions Addressing Specific Environments and Contexts	Research Evidence and Related Resources Guiding Practice
		sleep–wake times, use of an alarm clock and calendar to track when to take and refill medication, and storage of medication in a consistent location (e.g., on a nightstand). • Provide visual cues such as a list of medications with pictures and their purpose or reminder signs. • Establish a connection with mental health support groups.	
Clients living in a shelter for homeless people want to meet basic needs, remain safe, and reduce the potential for harm.	Using a consultative model, the intervention focuses on modifying the physical and social environments to promote safety and meet the clients' basic needs.	• Establish defined areas and organize schedules within the shelter to enable clients to engage in self-care, education, work preparation, and play and leisure activities. • Design physically accessible spaces and equipment to enable clients to complete basic ADLs. • Educate clients in life skills interventions to address the environmental demands of homelessness. • Establish a self-governance and grievance committee to address safety in the shelter. • Post emergency procedures and community resources.	Life skills interventions have the potential to support the complex needs of people situated in the homeless context (Helfrich, Aviles, Badiani, Walens, & Sabol, 2006).
A 52-year-old successful businessman had a right middle cerebral artery stroke 1 year ago, resulting in left-sided weakness and decreased balance. He lives at home and has tried to return to his job as a financial consultant but has struggled to maintain his productivity at work.	Because this client may not regain all performance skills, intervention focuses on designing environmental modifications in the home, work, and community settings that will support his heath and participation in occupations.	• Adapt activity demands for participation in necessary and desired occupations. • Modify the home environment to optimize safety and reduce the impact of weakness and fatigue (Fänge & Iwarsson, 2005; Stark, 2004; Stearns et al., 2000). • Consult with the employer to modify the work environment by using assistive technology to change the task demands. • Set up an ergonomically advantageous setting by adjusting work routines and schedule to support work performance (Whiteneck, Gerhardt, & Cusick, 2004). • Consult with community agencies regarding access (e.g., transportation, public bathrooms, timing of crosswalk lights, safe railings).	• Specific strategies are effective in improving performance skills and participation in roles and routines after stroke (Ma & Trombly, 2002; Trombly & Ma, 2002). • Occupational therapists evaluate contextual factors of the work environment (e.g., work tasks, routines, tools, equipment) and use this information to plan interventions that facilitate work performance (AOTA, 2011). • Occupational therapy practitioners consult with community agencies, business owners, and building contractors, among others, to create environments that promote occupational performance for all (AOTA, 2000). *Additional Resources* Wolf, Chuh, Floyd, McInnes, & Williams (2015) Wolf, Chuh, McInnes, & Williams (2013)

(Continued)

Table 2. Case Studies *(cont.)*

Case Description	Contextual and Environmental Focus of Occupational Therapy Service Delivery	Examples of Occupational Therapy Interventions Addressing Specific Environments and Contexts	Research Evidence and Related Resources Guiding Practice
Older adults residing in an assisted-living facility are at high risk for loss of balance and falls.	The focus of intervention is to maintain the clients' occupational engagement through a multifactorial approach that includes elements such as strength and balance training; education; modifying activity demands; and creating a safe and supportive environment, including falls prevention.	• Consult with facility administrators, architects, and facility staff to design an environment that • Reflects a noninstitutional character, • Eliminates barriers to physical mobility, • Provides lighting without glare, and • Clusters small activity areas together.	• The design of the social and physical environment influences the function and well-being of older adults (Day, Carreon, & Stump, 2000). • Occupational therapy practitioners advocate for and contribute to the creation of an environment in which the demands do not exceed the client's capabilities (Cooper & Day, 2003). • Occupational therapy practitioners identify and modify environmental barriers (Davison, Bond, Dawson, Steen, & Kenny, 2005). *Additional Resource* Siebert et al. (2014)
A **74-year-old woman** with Alzheimer's disease lives in an apartment in the inner city with her husband of 45 years. She has become lethargic and no longer initiates activities. Her husband now does all the shopping, cooking, and cleaning. He is overwhelmed with the demands of caregiving.	The intervention focuses on supporting the caregiver's and the care recipient's health and participation in desired occupations and activities and enabling them to remain in their home as they age.	• Educate the caregiver about the disease process and the impact of the environment on the care recipient's occupational performance. • Recommend modifications to the home environment to manage daily care activities. • Provide emotional support and information on coping strategies and stress management to caregivers. • Facilitate use of community and family support. • Provide support and education on the uses of adaptive equipment in the home.	• People with dementia or Alzheimer's disease can live at home, remaining in their roles and contexts for a longer period of time, if given enough support from caregivers (Haley & Bailey, 1999). • An in-home skills training and environmental adaptation program (Gitlin et al., 2003) improves the quality of life for both the caregiver and the care recipient with fewer declines in the care recipient's occupational performance and less need for caregiving (Gitlin, Hauck, Dennis, & Winter, 2005). • Home-based occupational therapy is effective and cost-efficient for community-dwelling older adults and their caregivers (Graff et al., 2008). • People with Alzheimer's disease perform better at home than in unfamiliar environments; it is harder for them to adapt to new environments (Hoppes, Davis, & Thompson, 2003). *Additional Resources* Padilla (2011) Schaber (2010)

Note. ADLs = activities of daily living; AOTA = American Occupational Therapy Association; IEP = individualized education program; NICU = neonatal intensive care unit.

Summary

Occupational therapy practitioners work with a wide variety of clients across the lifespan. The goal of occupational therapy is to facilitate achievement of health, well-being, and participation in life through engagement in occupation (AOTA, 2014b). Practitioners consider current educational and health care laws and policies as they make recommendations to modify, adapt, or change environments and contexts to support or improve occupational performance. On the basis of theory, evidence, knowledge, client preferences and values, and occupational performance, they assess the intervention settings and the environmental and contextual factors influencing clients' occupational performance. In their interventions and recommendations, practitioners focus on selecting and using environments and contexts that are congruent with clients' needs and maximize participation in daily life occupations. Practitioners' expertise is essential to support clients' health and participation in meaningful occupations.

References

American Occupational Therapy Association. (2000). Occupational therapy and the Americans With Disabilities Act (ADA). *American Journal of Occupational Therapy, 54,* 622–625. http://dx.doi.org/10.5014/ajot.54.6.622

American Occupational Therapy Association. (2006). Policy 1.44: Categories of occupational therapy personnel. In *Policy manual* (2013 ed., pp. 32–33). Bethesda, MD: Author.

American Occupational Therapy Association. (2011). Occupational therapy services in facilitating work performance. *American Journal of Occupational Therapy, 65*(Suppl.), S55–S64. http://dx.doi.org/10.5014/ajot.2011.65S55

American Occupational Therapy Association. (2014a). Guidelines for supervision, roles, and responsibilities during the delivery of occupational therapy services. *American Journal of Occupational Therapy, 68*(Suppl. 3), S16–S22. http://dx.doi.org/10.5014/ajot.2014.686S03

American Occupational Therapy Association. (2014b). Occupational therapy practice framework: Domain and process (3rd ed.). *American Journal of Occupational Therapy, 68*(Suppl. 1), S1–S48. http://dx.doi.org/10.5014/ajot.2014.682006

Americans With Disabilities Act of 1990, Pub. L. 101–336, 42 U.S.C. §§ 12101–12213 (2000).

Arbesman, M., & Logsdon, D. W. (2011). Occupational therapy interventions for employment and education for adults with serious mental illness: A systematic review. *American Journal of Occupational Therapy, 65,* 238–246. http://dx.doi.org/10.5014/ajot.2011.001289

Bailey, D. B., Jr., Aytch, L. S., Odom, S. L., Symons, F., & Wolery, M. (1999). Early intervention as we know it. *Mental Retardation and Developmental Disabilities Research Reviews, 5,* 11–20. http://dx.doi.org/10.1002/(SICI)1098-2779(1999)5:1<11::AID-MRDD2>3.0.CO;2-U

Barnes, K. J., Vogel, K. A., Beck, A. J., Schoenfeld, H. B., & Owen, S. V. (2008). Self-regulation strategies of children with emotional disturbance. *Physical and Occupational Therapy in Pediatrics, 28,* 369–387. http://dx.doi.org/10.1080/01942630802307127

Blok, H., Fukkink, R., Gebhardt, E., & Leseman, P. (2005). The relevance of delivery mode and other programme characteristics for the effectiveness of early childhood intervention. *International Journal of Behavioral Development, 29,* 35–47. http://dx.doi.org/10.1080/01650250444000315

Brown, C. (2012). *Occupational therapy practice guidelines for adults with serious mental illness.* Bethesda, MD: AOTA Press.

Buysse, V., Skinner, D., & Grant, S. (2001). Toward a definition of quality inclusion: Perspectives of parents and practitioners. *Topics in Early Childhood Special Education, 24,* 146–161. http://dx.doi.org/10.1177/105381510102400208

Case-Smith, J. (2013). Systematic review of interventions to promote social–emotional development in young children with or at risk for disability. *American Journal of Occupational Therapy, 67,* 395–404. http://dx.doi.org/10.5014/ajot.2013.004713

Cooper, B. A., & Day, K. (2003). Therapeutic design of environments for people with dementia. In L. Letts, P. Rigby, & D. Stewart (Eds.), *Using environments to enable occupational performance* (pp. 253–268). Thorofare, NJ: Slack.

Davison, J., Bond, J., Dawson, P., Steen, I. N., & Kenny, R. A. (2005). Patients with recurrent falls attending accident and emergency benefit from multifactorial intervention—A randomised controlled trial. *Age and Ageing, 34,* 162–168. http://dx.doi.org/10.1093/ageing/afi053

Day, K., Carreon, D., & Stump, C. (2000). The therapeutic design of environments for people with dementia: A review of the empirical research. *Gerontologist, 40,* 397–416. http://dx.doi.org/10.1093/geront/40.4.397

Dunst, C., Bruder, M., Trivette, C., Hamby, D., Raab, M., & McLean, M. (2001). Characteristics and consequences of everyday natural learning opportunities. *Topics in Early Childhood Special Education, 21,* 68–92. http://dx.doi.org/10.1177/027112140102100202

Dunst, C. J., Trivette, C. M., Hamby, D. W., & Bruder, M. B. (2006). Influences of contrasting natural learning environment experiences on child, parent, and family well-being. *Journal of Developmental and Physical Disabilities, 18,* 235–250. http://dx.doi.org/10.1007/s10882-006-9013-9

Elementary and Secondary Education Act of 1965, Pub. L. 89–313, 20 U.S.C. §§ 2701–3386.

Fänge, A., & Iwarsson, S. (2005). Changes in ADL dependence and aspects of usability following housing adaptation—A longitudinal perspective. *American Journal of Occupational Therapy, 59,* 296–304. http://dx.doi.org/10.5014/ajot.59.3.296

Frolek Clark, G., & Kingsley, K. (2013). *Occupational therapy practice guidelines for early childhood: Birth through 5 years.* Bethesda, MD: AOTA Press.

Gitlin, L. N., Hauck, W. W., Dennis, M. P., & Winter, L. (2005). Maintenance of effects of the Home Environmental Skill-Building Program for family caregivers and individuals with Alzheimer's disease and related disorders. *Journals of Gerontology, Series A: Biological Sciences and Medical Sciences, 60,* 368–374. http://dx.doi.org/10.1093/gerona/60.3.368

Gitlin, L. N., Winter, L., Corcoran, M., Dennis, M. P., Schinfeld, S., & Hauck, W. W. (2003). Effects of the home Environmental Skill-Building Program on the caregiver–care recipient dyad: 6-month outcomes from the Philadelphia REACH Initiative. *Gerontologist, 43,* 532–546. http://dx.doi.org/10.1093/geront/43.4.532

Graff, M. J. L., Adang, E. M. M., Vernooij-Dassen, M. J. M., Dekker, J., Jönsson, L., Thijssen, M., . . . Rikkert, M. G. (2008). Community occupational therapy for older patients with dementia and their care givers: Cost effectiveness study. *BMJ, 336,* 134–138. http://dx.doi.org/10.1136/bmj.39408.481898.BE

Haley, W., & Bailey, S. (1999). Research on family caregiving in Alzheimer's disease: Implications for practice and policy. In B. Vellas & J. Fitten (Eds.), *Research and practice in Alzheimer's disease* (Vol. 2, pp. 321–332). Paris: Serdi.

Helfrich, C., Aviles, A., Badiani, C., Walens, D., & Sabol, P. (2006). Life skills interventions with homeless youth, domestic violence victims, and adults with mental illness. In K. S. Miller, G. L. Herzberg, & S. A. Ray (Eds.), *Homeless in America* (pp. 189–207). New York: Haworth Press.

Hoppes, S., Davis, L. A., & Thompson, D. (2003). Environmental effects on the assessment of people with dementia: A pilot study. *American Journal of Occupational Therapy, 57,* 396–402. http://dx.doi.org/10.5014/ajot.57.4.396

Individuals With Disabilities Education Improvement Act of 2004, Pub. L. 108–446, 20 U.S.C. §§ 1400–1482.

Keogh, B. K., Bernheimer, L. P., Gallimore, R., & Weisner, T. S. (1998). Child and family outcomes over time: A longitudinal perspective on developmental delays. In M. Lewis & C. Feiring (Eds.), *Families, risk, and competence* (pp. 269–287). Mahwah, NJ: Erlbaum.

Kingsley, K., & Mailloux, Z. (2013). Evidence for the effectiveness of different service delivery models in early intervention services. *American Journal of Occupational Therapy, 67,* 431–436. http://dx.doi.org/10.5014/ajot.2013.006171

Ma, H. I., & Trombly, C. A. (2002). A synthesis of the effects of occupational therapy for persons with stroke, Part II: Remediation of impairments. *American Journal of Occupational Therapy, 56,* 260–274. http://dx.doi.org/10.5014/ajot.56.3.260

No Child Left Behind Act of 2001, Pub. L. 107–110, 20 U.S.C. §§ 6301–8962.

Odom, A. L. (2000). Preschool inclusion: What we know and where we go from here. *Topics in Early Childhood Special Education, 20,* 20–27. http://dx.doi.org/10.1177/027112140002000104

Older Americans Act of 1965, Pub. L. 89–73, 79 Stat. 218, 42 U.S.C. §§ 3001 and 3058ff.

Olmstead v. L.C., 527 U.S. 581 (1999).

Omnibus Budget Reconciliation Act of 1987, Pub. L. 100–203, 101 Stat. 1330.

Padilla, R. (2011). Effectiveness of environment-based interventions for people with Alzheimer's disease and related dementias. *American Journal of Occupational Therapy, 65,* 514–522. http://dx.doi.org/10.5014/ajot.2011.002600

Parham, L. D., Cohn, E. S., Spitzer, S., Koomar, J. A., Miller, L. J., Burke, J. P., . . . Summers, C. A. (2007). Fidelity in sensory integration intervention research. *American Journal of Occupational Therapy, 61,* 216–227. http://dx.doi.org/10.5014/ajot.61.2.216

Rehabilitation Act of 1973, Pub. L. 93–112, 29 USC §§ 701–7961.

Rehabilitation, Comprehensive Services, and Developmental Disabilities Amendments of 1978, Pub. L. 95–602.

Schaaf, R. C., & Nightlinger, K. M. (2007). Occupational therapy using a sensory integrative approach: A case study of effectiveness. *American Journal of Occupational Therapy, 61,* 239–246. http://dx.doi.org/10.5014/ajot.61.2.239

Schaber, P. (2010). *Occupational therapy practice guidelines for adults with Alzheimer's disease and related disorders.* Bethesda, MD: AOTA Press.

Schilling, D. L., Washington, K., Billingsley, F. F., & Deitz, J. (2003). Classroom seating for children with attention deficit hyperactivity disorder: Therapy balls versus chairs. *American Journal of Occupational Therapy, 57,* 534–541. http://dx.doi.org/10.5014/ajot.57.5.534

Siebert, C., Smallfield, S., & Stark, S. (2014). *Occupational therapy practice guidelines for home modifications.* Bethesda, MD: AOTA Press.

Social Security Amendments of 1965, Pub. L. 89–97, 42 U.S.C. §§ 1395 et seq. (Medicare) and 42 U.S.C. §§ 1396 et seq. (Medicaid).

Stark, S. (2004). Removing environmental barriers in the homes of older adults with disabilities improves occupational performance. *OTJR: Occupation, Participation and Health, 24,* 32–40. http://dx.doi.org/10.1177/153944920402400105

Stearns, S. C., Bernard, S. L., Fasick, S. B., Schwartz, R., Konrad, T. R., Ory, M. G., & DeFriese, G. H. (2000). The economic implications of self-care: The effect of lifestyle, functional adaptations, and medical self-care among a national sample of Medicare beneficiaries. *American Journal of Public Health, 90,* 1608–1612. http://dx.doi.org/10.2105/AJPH.90.10.1608

Trombly, C. A., & Ma, H. I. (2002). A synthesis of the effects of occupational therapy for persons with stroke, Part I: Restoration of roles, tasks, and activities. *American Journal of Occupational Therapy, 56,* 250–259. http://dx.doi.org/10.5014/ajot.56.3.250

Vaughn, S., Kim, A.-H., Sloan, C. V. M., Hughes, M. T., Elbaum, B., & Sridhar, D. (2003). Social skills interventions for young children with disabilities: A synthesis of group design studies. *Remedial and Special Education, 24,* 2–15. http://dx.doi.org/10.1177/074193250302400101

Velligan, D. I., Bow-Thomas, C. C., Huntzinger, C., Ritch, J., Ledbetter, N., Prihoda, T. J., & Miller, A. L. (2000). Randomized controlled trial of the use of compensatory strategies to enhance adaptive functioning in outpatients with schizophrenia. *American Journal of Psychiatry, 157,* 1317–1323. http://dx.doi.org/10.1176/appi.ajp.157.8.1317

Velligan, D. I., Mueller, J., Wang, M., Dicocco, M., Diamond, P. M., Maples, N. J., & Davis, B. (2006). Use of environmental supports among patients with schizophrenia. *Psychiatric Services, 57,* 219–224. http://dx.doi.org/10.1176/appi.ps.57.2.219

Watling, T., Koenig, K., Davies, P., & Schaaf, R. (2011). *Occupational therapy practice guidelines for children and adolescents with challenges in sensory processing and sensory integration.* Bethesda, MD: AOTA Press.

Whiteneck, G. G., Gerhart, K. A., & Cusick, C. P. (2004). Identifying environmental factors that influence the outcomes of people with traumatic brain injury. *Journal of Head Trauma Rehabilitation, 19,* 191–204. http://dx.doi.org/10.1097/00001199-200405000-00001

Wolf, T. J., Chuh, A., Floyd, T., McInnis, K., & Williams, E. (2015). Effectiveness of occupation-based interventions to improve areas of occupation and social participation after stroke: An evidence-based review. *American Journal of Occupational Therapy, 69,* 6901180060. http://dx.doi.org/10.5014/ajot.2015.012195

Wolf, T. J., Chuh, A., McInnes, K., & Williams, E. (2013). *Adults with stroke: What is the evidence for the effectiveness of activity-/occupation-based interventions to improve areas of occupation and social participation after stroke?* (AOTA Critically Appraised Topics and Papers). Retrieved from http://www.aota.org/practice/productive-aging/evidence-based/cats-caps/stroke.aspx

Authors
Ellen S. Cohn, ScD, OTR/L, FAOTA
Cherylin Lew, OTD, OTR/L

With contributions from
Kate Hanauer, OTS
DeLana Honaker, PhD, OTR/L, BCP
Susanne Smith Roley, MS, OTR/L, FAOTA

for
The Commission on Education
Janet V. DeLany, DEd, OTR/L, FAOTA

Adopted by the Representative Assembly 2009CONov149
Revised by the Commission on Practice, 2014
Debbie Amini, EdD, OTR/L, CHT, FAOTA, *Chairperson*

Adopted by the Representative Assembly Coordinating Council (RACC) for the Representative Assembly, 2015

Note. This revision replaces the 2010 document *Occupational Therapy's Perspective on the Use of Environments and Contexts to Support Health and Participation in Occupations,* previously published and copyrighted in 2010 by the American Occupational Therapy Association in the *American Journal of Occupational Therapy,* 64(6, Suppl.), S57–S69. http://dx.doi.org/10.5014/ajot.2010.64S57

Citation. American Occupational Therapy Association. (2015). Occupational therapy's perspective on the use of environments and contexts to facilitate health, well-being, and participation in occupations. *American Journal of Occupational Therapy, 69*(Suppl. 3), 6913410050. http://dx.doi.org/10.5014/ajot.2015.696S05

Physical Agent Modalities

The American Occupational Therapy Association (AOTA) asserts that physical agent modalities (PAMs) may be used by occupational therapists and occupational therapy assistants in preparation for or concurrently with purposeful and occupation-based activities or interventions that ultimately enhance engagement in occupation (AOTA, 2008a, 2008b). AOTA further stipulates that PAMs may be applied only by occupational therapists and occupational therapy assistants who have documented evidence of possessing the theoretical background and technical skills for safe and competent integration of the modality into an occupational therapy intervention plan (AOTA, 2008b). The purpose of this paper is to clarify the appropriate context for use of PAMs in occupational therapy. It is the professional and ethical responsibility of occupational therapy practitioners to be knowledgeable of and adhere to applicable state laws.

Physical agent modalities are those procedures and interventions that are systematically applied to modify specific client factors when neurological, musculoskeletal, or skin conditions are present that may be limiting occupational performance. PAMs use various forms of energy to modulate pain, modify tissue healing, increase tissue extensibility, modify skin and scar tissue, and decrease edema or inflammation. PAMs are used in preparation for or concurrently with purposeful and occupation-based activities (Bracciano, 2008).

Categories of physical agents include superficial thermal agents, deep thermal agents, and electrotherapeutic agents and mechanical devices.

- *Superficial thermal agents* include but are not limited to hydrotherapy/whirlpool, cryotherapy (cold packs, ice), Fluidotherapy™, hot packs, paraffin, water, infrared, and other commercially available superficial heating and cooling technologies.

- *Deep thermal agents* include but are not limited to therapeutic ultrasound, phonophoresis, short-wave diathermy, and other commercially available technologies.

- *Electrotherapeutic agents* use electricity and the electromagnetic spectrum to facilitate tissue healing, improve muscle strength and endurance, decrease edema, modulate pain, decrease the inflammatory process, and modify the healing process. Electrotherapeutic agents include but are not limited to neuro-muscular electrical stimulation (NMES), functional electrical stimulation (FES), transcutaneous electrical nerve stimulation (TENS), high-voltage galvanic stimulation for tissue and wound repair (ESTR), high-voltage pulsed current (HVPC), direct current (DC), iontophoresis, and other commercially available technologies (Bracciano, 2008).

- *Mechanical devices* include but are not limited to vasopneumatic devices and continuous passive motion (CPM).

PAMs are categorized as preparatory methods (AOTA, 2008a) that also can be used concurrently with purposeful activity or during occupational engagement. Preparatory methods support and promote the acquisition of the performance skills necessary to enable an individual to resume or assume habits, routines, and roles for engagement in occupation.

The exclusive use of PAMs as a therapeutic intervention without direct application to occupational performance is not considered occupational therapy. When used, *PAMs are always integrated into a broader occupational therapy program* as a preparatory method for the therapeutic use of occupations or purposeful activities (AOTA, 2008a).

Occupational therapists and occupational therapy assistants must have demonstrated and verifiable competence in order to use PAMs in occupational therapy practice. The foundational knowledge necessary for proper use of these modalities requires appropriate, documented professional education, which includes continuing education courses, institutes at conferences, and accredited higher education courses or programs. Integration of PAMs in occupational therapy practice must include foundational education and training in biological and physical sciences. Modality-specific education consists of biophysiological, neurophysiological, and electrophysiological changes that occur as a result of the application of the selected modality. Education in the application of PAMs also must include indications, contraindications, and precautions; safe and efficacious administration of the modalities; and patient preparation, including the process and outcomes of treatment (i.e., risks and benefits). Education should include essential elements related to documentation, including parameters of intervention, subjective and objective criteria, efficacy, and the relationship between the physical agent and occupational performance.

Supervised use of the PAM should continue until service competency and professional judgment in selection, modification, and integration into an occupational therapy intervention plan is demonstrated and documented (AOTA, 2009).

The occupational therapist makes decisions and assumes responsibility for use of PAMs as part of the intervention plan. The occupational therapy assistant delivers occupational therapy services under the supervision of the occupational therapist. Services delivered by the occupational therapy assistant are selected and delegated by the occupational therapist (AOTA, 2009). When an occupational therapist delegates the use of a PAM to an occupational therapy assistant, both must comply with appropriate supervision and state regulatory requirements and ensure that preparation, application, and documentation are based on service competency and institutional rules. Only occupational therapists with service competency in this area may supervise the use of PAMs by occupational therapy assistants. Occupational therapy assistants may gain competency only in those modalities allowed by state and laws and regulations.

The *Occupational Therapy Code of Ethics and Ethics Standards (2010)* (AOTA, 2010) provides principles that guide safe and competent professional practice and that must be applied to the use of PAMs. The following principles from the *Code and Ethics Standards* are relevant to the use of PAMs:

Occupational therapy personnel shall:

- *Principle 1E:* provide occupational therapy services that are within each practitioner's level of competence and scope of practice (e.g., qualifications, experience, and the law).

- *Principle 1F:* use, to the extent possible, evaluation, planning, intervention techniques, and therapeutic equipment that are evidence-based and within the recognized scope of occupational therapy practice.

- *Principle 1G:* take responsible steps (e.g., continuing education, research, supervision, and training) and use careful judgment to ensure their own competence and weigh potential for client harm when generally recognized standards do not exist in emerging technology or areas of practice.

- *Principle 5F:* take responsibility for maintaining high standards and continuing competence in practice, education, and research by participating in professional development and educational activities to improve and update knowledge and skills.

- *Principle 5G:* ensure that all duties assumed by or assigned to other occupational therapy personnel match credentials, qualifications, experience, and scope of practice.

- *Principle 5H:* provide appropriate supervision to individuals for whom they have supervisory responsibility in accordance with AOTA official documents and local, state, and federal or national laws, rules, regulations, policies, procedures, standards, and guidelines. (AOTA, 2010)

References

American Occupational Therapy Association. (2008a). Occupational therapy practice framework: Domain and process (2nd ed.). *American Journal of Occupational Therapy, 62*, 625–683. http://dx.doi.org/10.5014/ajot.62.6.625

American Occupational Therapy Association. (2008b). Physical agent modalities: A position paper. *American Journal of Occupational Therapy, 62*, 691–693. http://dx.doi.org/10.5014/ajot.62.6.691

American Occupational Therapy Association. (2009). Guidelines for supervision, roles, and responsibilities during the delivery of occupational therapy services. *American Journal of Occupational Therapy, 63*, 797–803. http://dx.doi.org/10.5014/ajot.63.6.797

American Occupational Therapy Association. (2010). Occupational therapy code of ethics and ethics standards (2010). *American Journal of Occupational Therapy, 64*, S17–S26. http://dx.doi.org/10.5014/ajot.2010.64S17

Bracciano, A. G. (2008). *Physical agent modalities: Theory and application for the occupational therapist* (2nd ed.). Thorofare, NJ: Slack.

Authors

Alfred G. Bracciano, EdD, OTR, FAOTA
Scott D. McPhee, DrPH, OT, FAOTA
Barbara Winthrop Rose, MA, OTR, CVE, CHT, FAOTA

for

The Commission on Practice
Sara Jane Brayman, PhD, OTR/L, FAOTA, *Chairperson*

Adopted by the Representative Assembly 2003M37

Edited by the Commission on Practice, 2007

Revised by the Commission on Practice, 2012
Debbie Amini, EdD, OTR/L, CHT, C/NDT, *Chairperson*

Adopted by the Representative Assembly Coordinating Council (RACC) for the Representative Assembly, 2012

Note. This revision replaces the 2008 document *Physical Agent Modalities*, previously published and copyrighted in 2008 by the American Occupational Therapy Association in the *American Journal of Occupational Therapy, 62*, 691–693.

The Role of Occupational Therapy in Primary Care

The American Occupational Therapy Association (AOTA) asserts that occupational therapy practitioners are well prepared to contribute to interprofessional care teams addressing the primary care needs of individuals across the life span, particularly those with, or at risk for, one or more chronic conditions. Occupational therapy practitioners' distinct knowledge of the significant impact that habits and routines have on individuals' health and wellness will make their contribution to primary care distinct. The purposes of this position paper are to define primary care, describe the environment leading to reforms in the delivery of primary care, and establish occupational therapy's role in primary care.

Definition

Primary care is the provision of integrated, accessible health care services by clinicians who are accountable for addressing a large majority of personal health care needs, developing a sustained partnership with patients, and practicing in the context of family and community (Institute of Medicine [IOM], 1994; Patient Protection and Affordable Care Act [ACA], 2010). Evolving standards for care indicate that comprehensive primary care requires a coordinated team-based approach that promotes collaborative care, shared decision making, sustained relationships with patients and families, and quality improvement activities. New primary care delivery models have increased the emphasis on management of chronic conditions to reduce costs and improve population health (IOM, 2010; Interprofessional Education Collaborative Expert Panel, 2011; National Committee for Quality Assurance, 2011; National Quality Forum, 2012). In addition to the traditional method of delivering care, telehealth is increasingly recognized as a means to provide primary care to improve care coordination and access to services (AOTA, 2013b; Cason, 2012).

Importance of Primary Care

A combination of factors necessitates reforms to the health care delivery system. These factors include unsustainable public and private health care spending growth, an increased prevalence of chronic health conditions, and rising demand for health care services because of the aging of the population and the expected growth in the number of people with health insurance. The goals of reform are aptly summarized by the "Triple Aim": (1) improving the individual experience of care, (2) improving the health of populations, and (3) reducing the per capita cost of care (Berwick, Nolan, & Whittington, 2008). The ACA and other health care reform initiatives have incentivized increased integration and coordination of care delivery. A fundamental component of these reforms is an enhanced focus on primary care and the utilization of interprofessional teams of providers to achieve the goals of the Triple Aim (AOTA, 2013a). New models of primary care delivery are expected to be the best way to address the needs of the more than 133 million Americans with one or more chronic conditions that account for more than 75% of health care costs, as well as enhance the health and wellness of the population as a whole (Centers for Disease Control and Prevention [CDC], 2009; Grundy, Hagan, Hansen, & Grumbach, 2010).

Occupational Therapy's Role in and Preparation for Primary Care

Occupations are all activities that people engage in throughout everyday life that have meaning and value (AOTA, 2014). Successful participation in occupations can contribute to effective management of chronic conditions and improvements in health and wellness, helping to achieve fundamental goals of new primary care delivery models (Metzler, Hartmann, & Lowenthal, 2012). Occupational therapy practitioners identify those factors that support a person's ability to participate in daily life, as well as barriers (both internal and external to a person). Practitioners then provide interventions and offer strategies that capitalize on a person's strengths and address barriers to allow successful participation in occupations. As members of interprofessional primary care teams, occupational therapy practitioners are distinctly qualified to address the needs of individuals with chronic conditions with regard to limitations in daily activities. According to the CDC (2009), approximately one-fourth of people diagnosed with a chronic condition experience significant limitations in daily activities. In addition, occupational therapy practitioners can make a distinct contribution in primary care by recognizing and addressing the impact of habits and routines on the management of chronic conditions and the development of healthy lifestyles (AOTA, 2014).

Evidence shows the efficacy and cost-effectiveness of occupational therapy interventions that may be utilized in primary care settings (Borg & Davidson, 2008; Chang, Park, & Kim, 2009; Clark et al., 1997; Eklund, Sjöstrand, & Dahlin-Ivanoff, 2008; Graff et al., 2007; Gutman, Kerner, Zombek, Dulek, & Ramsey, 2009; Nagle, Valiant Cook, & Polatajko, 2002; Rexe, Lammi, & von Zweck, 2013). Research supports the use of interactions and interventions developed in accordance with client preferences, as well as culturally relevant self-management programs to enhance health behaviors, reduce disability, and improve health status and self-efficacy, while decreasing health care utilization (Arbesman & Mosley, 2012; Lorig, Ritter, & Gonzalez, 2003). These approaches serve as the hallmark of occupational therapy's client-centered occupation-based practice. Examples of specific interventions include but are not limited to

- Self-management of chronic conditions and prevention of secondary complications such as diabetes,

- Health promotion and lifestyle modification to prevent chronic conditions such as chronic obstructive pulmonary disease,

- Self-management of psychiatric conditions and promotion of mental health,

- Management of musculoskeletal conditions including pain management,

- Safety and falls prevention within the home and community environments,

- Promoting and ensuring access to community resources for social participation and community integration,

- Palliative and end-of-life care to allow for quality of life,

- Driving and community mobility resources for older adults,

- Redesign of physical environments to support participation in valued activities, and

- Family and caregiver assistance and support (Canadian Association of Occupational Therapists, 2013; Metzler et al., 2012).

Table 1 provides specific case examples of occupational therapy practitioners' contributions to primary care.

Occupational therapy practitioners are well suited to the dynamic nature of contemporary health care delivery systems by virtue of their broad educational background in the liberal arts as well as biological, physical, social, and behavioral sciences that supports an understanding of clients and the importance of occupational engagement across the life span (Accreditation Council for Occupational Therapy Education,

2012). Practitioners are prepared to be direct care providers, consultants, educators, case managers, and advocates for patients and their families.

Ethical Considerations

It is the professional and ethical responsibility of occupational therapy practitioners to provide services only within each practitioner's level of competence and scope of practice. The *Occupational Therapy Code of Ethics and Ethics Standards (2010)* (AOTA, 2010) establishes principles that guide safe and competent professional practice and that must be applied when providing primary care. Practitioners should refer to the relevant principles from these standards and comply with state and federal regulatory requirements.

References

Accreditation Council for Occupational Therapy Education. (2012). 2011 Accreditation Council for Occupational Therapy Education (ACOTE®) standards. *American Journal of Occupational Therapy, 66*(6, Suppl.), S6–S74. http://dx.doi.org/10.5014/ajot.2012.66S6

American Occupational Therapy Association. (2010). Occupational therapy code of ethics and ethics standards (2010). *American Journal of Occupational Therapy, 64*(6, Suppl.), S17– S26. http://dx.doi.org/10.5014/ajot.2010.64S17

American Occupational Therapy Association. (2013a). *Review of new models of primary care delivery.* Available online at http://www.aota.org/-/media/Corporate/files/Secure/Advocacy/Health-Care-Reform/commissioned-report.pdf

American Occupational Therapy Association. (2013b). Telehealth. *American Journal of Occupational Therapy, 67*(6, Suppl.), S69–S90. http://dx.doi.org/10.5014/ajot.2013.67S69

American Occupational Therapy Association. (2014). Occupational therapy practice framework: Domain and process (3rd ed.). *American Journal of Occupational Therapy, 68*(Suppl. 1), S1–S48. http://dx.doi.org/10.5014/ajot.2014.682006

Arbesman, M., Bazyk, S., & Nochajski, S. M. (2013). Systematic review of occupational therapy and mental health promotion, prevention, and intervention for children and youth. *American Journal of Occupational Therapy, 67*, e120–e130. http://dx.doi.org/10.5014/ajot.2013.008359

Arbesman, M., & Mosley, L. J. (2012). Systematic review of occupation- and activity-based health management and maintenance interventions for community-dwelling older adults. *American Journal of Occupational Therapy, 66*, 277–283. http://dx.doi.org/10.5014/ajot.2012.003327

Berwick, D., Nolan T., & Whittington, J. (2008). The Triple Aim: Care, health, and cost. *Health Affairs, 27*, 759–769. http://dx.doi.org/10.1377/hlthaff.27.3.759

Borg, M., & Davidson, L. (2008). The nature of recovery as lived in everyday experience. *Journal of Mental Health, 17*, 129–140. http://dx.doi.org/10.1080/09638230701498382

Canadian Association of Occupational Therapists. (2013). *CAOT position statement: Occupational therapy in primary care.* Ottawa: Author.

Case-Smith, J. (2013). Systematic review of interventions to promote social–emotional development in young children with or at risk for disability. *American Journal of Occupational Therapy, 67*, 395–404. http://dx.doi.org/10.5014/ajot.2013.004713

Cason, J. (2012). Health Policy Perspectives—Telehealth opportunities in occupational therapy through the Affordable Care Act. *American Journal of Occupational Therapy, 66*, 131–136. http://dx.doi.org/10.5014/ajot.2012.662001

Centers for Disease Control and Prevention. (2009). *Chronic diseases: The power to prevent, the call to control.* Atlanta: Author.

Chang, M., Park, B., & Kim, S. (2009). Parenting classes, parenting behavior, and child cognitive development in early Head Start: A longitudinal model. *School Community Journal, 19*(1), 155–174.

Clark, F., Azen, S. P., Carlson, M., Mandel, D., LaBree, L., Hay, J., . . . Lipson, L. (2001). Embedding health-promoting changes into the daily lives of independent-living older adults: Long-term follow-up of occupational therapy intervention. *Journals of Gerontology, Series B: Psychological Sciences and Social Sciences, 56,* 60–63. http://dx.doi.org/10.1093/geronb/56.1.P60

Clark, F., Azen, S. P., Zemke, R., Jackson, J., Carlson, M., Mandel, D., . . . Lipson L. (1997). Occupational therapy for independent-living older adults: A randomized controlled trial. *JAMA, 278,* 1321–1326. http://dx.doi.org/10.1001/jama.1997.03550160041036

Clark, G. J. F., & Schlabach, T. L. (2013). Systematic review of occupational therapy interventions to improve cognitive development in children ages birth–5 years. *American Journal of Occupational Therapy, 67,* 425–430. http://dx.doi.org/10.5014/ajot.2013.006163

Clarke, S., Oades, G. L., & Crowe, T. P. (2012). Recovery in mental health: A movement towards well-being and meaning in contrast to avoidance of symptoms. *Psychiatric Rehabilitation Journal, 25,* 297–304.

Eklund, K., Sjöstrand, J., & Dahlin-Ivanoff, S. (2008). A randomized controlled trial of a health promotion programme and its effect on ADL dependence and self-reported health problems for the elderly visually impaired. *Scandinavian Journal of Occupational Therapy, 15,* 68–74.

Fritz, H. (2014). The influence of daily routines on engaging in diabetes self-management. *Scandinavian Journal of Occupational Therapy, 21,* 232–240. http://dx.doi.org/10.3109/11038128.2013.868033

Gibson, R. W., D'Amico, M., Jaffe, L., & Arbesman, M. (2011). Occupational therapy interventions for recovery in the areas of community integration and normative life roles for adults with serious mental illness: A systematic review. *American Journal of Occupational Therapy, 65,* 247–256. http://dx.doi.org/10.5014/ajot2011.001297

Graff, M., Vernooij-Dassen, M., Thijssen, M., Deller, J., Hoefnagels, W., & Rikkert, M. G. (2007). Effects of community occupational therapy on quality of life, mood, and health status in dementia patients and their caregivers: A randomized controlled trial. *Journals of Gerontology, Series A: Biological Sciences and Medical Sciences, 62A,* 1002–1009.

Grundy, P., Hagan, K., Hansen, J., & Grumbach, K. (2010). The multi-stakeholder movement for primary care renewal and reform. *Health Affairs, 29,* 791–798. http://dx.doi.org/10.1377/hlthaff.2010.0084

Gutman, S. A., Kerner, R., Zombek, I., Dulek, J., & Ramsey, C. A. (2009). Supported education for adults with psychiatric disabilities: Effectiveness of an occupational therapy program. *American Journal of Occupational Therapy, 63,* 245–254. http://dx.doi.org/10.5014/ajot.63.3.245

Haracz, K., Ryan, S., Hazelton, M., & James, C. (2013). Occupational therapy and obesity: An integrative literature review. *Australian Occupational Therapy Journal, 60,* 356–365. http://dx.doi.org/10.1111/1440-1630.12063

Howe, T.-H., & Wang, T.-N. (2013). Systematic review of interventions used in or relevant to occupational therapy for children with feeding difficulties ages birth–5 years. *American Journal of Occupational Therapy, 67,* 405–412. http://dx.doi.org/10.5014/ajot.2013.004564

Institute of Medicine. (1994). *Defining primary care: An interim report.* Washington, DC: National Academies Press.

Institute of Medicine. (2010). *Roundtable on value and science-driven health care: The healthcare imperative: Lowering costs and improving outcomes* [Workshop Series Summary]. Washington, DC: National Academies Press.

Interprofessional Education Collaborative Expert Panel. (2011). *Core competencies for interprofessional collaborative practice: Report of an expert panel.* Washington, DC: Author.

Kingsley, K., & Mailloux, Z. (2013). Evidence for the effectiveness of different service delivery models in early intervention services. *American Journal of Occupational Therapy, 67,* 431–436. http://dx.doi.org/10.5014/ajot.2013.006171

Koome, K., Hocking, C., & Sutton, D. (2012). Why routines matter: The nature and meaning of family routines in the context of adolescent mental illness. *Journal of Occupational Science, 19,* 312–325. http://dx.doi.org/10.1080/14427591.2012.718245

Kroenke, K., Spitzer, R. L., & Williams, J. B. (2001). The PHQ–9: Validity of a brief depression severity measure. *Journal of General Internal Medicine, 16,* 606–613.

Lorig, K. R., Ritter, P. L., & Gonzalez, V. M. (2003). Hispanic chronic disease self-management: A randomized community-based outcome trial. *Nursing Research, 52,* 361–369.

Metzler, C., Hartmann, K., & Lowenthal, L. (2012). Health Policy Perspectives—Defining primary care: Envisioning the roles of occupational therapy. *American Journal of Occupational Therapy, 66,* 266–270. http://dx.doi.org/10.5014/ajot.2010.663001

Nagle, S., Valiant Cook, J., & Polatajko, H. (2002). I'm doing as much as I can: Occupational choices of persons with severe and persistent mental illness. *Journal of Occupational Science, 9,* 72–81.

National Committee for Quality Assurance. (2011). *Standards and guidelines for NCQA's patient-centered medical home (PCMH).* Washington, DC: Author.

National Quality Forum. (2012). *Multiple chronic conditions measurement framework.* Washington, DC: Author.

Orellano, E., Colón, W. I., & Arbesman, M. (2012). Effect of occupation- and activity-based interventions on instrumental activities of daily living performance among community-dwelling older adults: A systematic review. *American Journal of Occupational Therapy, 66,* 292–300. http://dx.doi.org/10.5014/ajot.2012.003053

Patient Protection and Affordable Care Act of 2010, 42 U.S.C. § 256A-1(f) (2010).

Pyatak, E. (2011). The role of occupational therapy in diabetes self-management interventions. *OTJR: Occupation, Participation and Health, 31,* 89–96.

Rexe, K., Lammi, B., & von Zweck, C. (2013). Occupational therapy: Cost-effective solutions for changing health system needs. *Healthcare Quarterly, 16,* 69–75.

Swarbrick, P., Hutchinson, D. S., & Gill, K. (2008). The quest for optimal health: Can education and training cure what ails us? *International Journal of Mental Health, 37,* 69–88.

Veseth, M., Binder, P. E., Borg, M., & Davidson, L. (2012). Toward caring for oneself in a life of ups and downs: A reflexive–collaborative exploration of recovery in bipolar disorder. *Qualitative Health Research, 22,* 119–133. http://dx.doi.org/10.1177/1049732311411487

Table 1. Case Examples Highlighting Occupational Therapy Practitioners' Contributions to Primary Care

Case Description	Considerations for Primary Care Service Delivery	Selected Examples of Occupational Therapy Interventions (all to be completed in collaboration with the patient, family, and other care team members)	Research Evidence and Related Resources Guiding Practice
A **26-year-old woman** with obesity and dyslipidemia has received regular medical care for a skin rash all over her body. After a series of misdiagnoses, it has been determined that the rash is likely a physical, acute reaction to stress. The woman is a mother and primary caretaker of a 4-year-old girl with delayed development. She reports an inability to address her own ADLs and health needs because of her daughter's hyperactive and impulsive behavior and inability to follow directions. The woman is also experiencing serious symptoms of depression, as evidenced by scores on the PHQ–9.	The intervention focuses on educating the mother about child development, effective parenting strategies, and lifestyle modifications to manage her depression and decrease her stress related to caring for a child with special needs.	• Educate the mother on the behavioral and developmental needs of the child, including establishing appropriate expectations of the child's skills. • Provide lifestyle modification interventions to facilitate development of independent problem-solving skills to manage home and community occupations and integrate sustainable health-promoting daily routines, including ADL completion and sleep hygiene. • Provide weekly goal setting and review, including self-identifying barriers and supports. • Give referrals to additional intervention services for the child.	Arbesman, Bazyk, & Nochajski (2013); Case-Smith (2013); Clark et al. (2001); Clark & Schlabach (2013); Haracz, Ryan, Hazelton, & James (2013); Kroenke, Spitzer, & Williams (2001)
A **5-month-old infant** presents with a history of repeated hospitalizations for pneumonia. The focus of the primary care visits has been on medical management of the infections causing the pneumonia. The occupational therapy screening identifies moderately increased tone on the left side, limiting participation in occupational roles.	The intervention focuses on education and support of the family members to promote successful participation by the infant in activities of play, social participation, and ADLs.	• Complete an occupational history and profile to identify barriers to participation in play, social participation, and ADLs. • Educate caregivers on strategies to prevent development of contractures and other limitations to participation in occupations. • Identify strategies for family members to facilitate participation in play, social participation, and ADLs. • Identify community resources for family support and education.	Case-Smith (2013); Chang, Park, & Kim (2009); Clark & Schlabach (2013); Howe & Wang (2013); Kingsley & Mailloux (2013)

(Continued)

Table 1. Case Examples Highlighting Occupational Therapy Practitioners' Contributions to Primary Care *(cont.)*

Case Description	Considerations for Primary Care Service Delivery	Selected Examples of Occupational Therapy Interventions *(all to be completed in collaboration with the patient, family, and other care team members)*	Research Evidence and Related Resources Guiding Practice
A **60-year-old woman** reports to her primary care physician that she has "too much going on" to improve the management of her poorly controlled hypertension and Type 2 diabetes mellitus. Secondary complications of peripheral neuropathies in both lower extremities and intermittent double vision interfere with her ability to perform ADLs, resulting in fall and safety risks. She lives with her husband and works an inconsistent schedule in a fast-food restaurant.	The intervention focuses on making lifestyle modifications to incorporate medication management, blood sugar checks, healthy eating routines, adaptations, and environmental changes into her daily life.	• Complete an occupational history and profile to identify daily routines and the presence of health-promoting and health-depleting habits. • Increase patient activation by making lifestyle modifications to incorporate medication management, blood sugar checks, healthy eating routines, adaptations, and environmental changes into her daily life. • Perform functional task analysis and activity modification to develop achievable strategies to produce quick, nutritious, and satisfying meals. • Identify ways to integrate physical activity into daily routines. • Identify adaptations and environmental changes needed to address fall risk, vision difficulties, and home safety. • Identify self-management tools, ways to monitor own progress, and barriers and supports to reaching self-identified goals.	Arbesman & Mosley (2012); Clark et al. (2001); Fritz (2014); Orellano, Colón, & Arbesman (2012); Pyatak (2011)

(Continued)

Table 1. Case Examples Highlighting Occupational Therapy Practitioners' Contributions to Primary Care *(cont.)*

Case Description	Considerations for Primary Care Service Delivery	Selected Examples of Occupational Therapy Interventions *(all to be completed in collaboration with the patient, family, and other care team members)*	Research Evidence and Related Resources Guiding Practice
A **49-year-old woman** reports to her primary care physician with lab values indicating prediabetes, hypertension, and a high lipid profile. The woman reports a history of treatment for bipolar disorder, which has been managed for 12 years with mood-stabilizing medication. She reports that side effects of the meds have included unacceptable weight gain and that lately she is experiencing increased stress leading to major changes in her mood. She is recently divorced and is maintaining primary custody of two active teenagers, one diagnosed with bipolar disorder. She expresses a need for managing her multiple medical issues as well as her family and personal challenges.	The intervention focuses on identifying barriers to incorporating the woman's medical interventions and lifestyle changes that she identifies as important into her daily schedule to improve her health.	• Complete an occupational profile to identify her valued roles, interests, typical routines, and the barriers she identifies as affecting her ability to complete day-to-day tasks. • Support her ability to identify potential solutions and problem-solving barriers. • Work with her to identify methods for self-care that include rest and leisure activities, dietary changes, exercise, and productive activities. • Establish a daily routine that includes the lifestyle changes she identifies that support improved mood and medication management as well as completing the parenting and day-to-day living tasks she values. • Connect her with resources that help her build a support network that covers emotional and parenting support, as well as valued personal relationships.	Clarke, Oades, & Crowe (2012); Gibson, D'Amico, Jaffe, & Arbesman (2011); Koome, Hocking, & Sutton (2012); Swarbrick, Hutchinson, & Gill (2008); Veseth, Binder, Borg, & Davidson (2012)

Note. ADLs = activities of daily living; PHQ–9 = Patient Health Questionnaire–9 (Kroenke et al., 2001).

Authors

Pamela Roberts, PhD, OTR/L, SCFES, CPHQ, FAOTA

Michelle E. Farmer, OTD, OTR/L

Amy Jo Lamb, OTD, OTR/L, FAOTA

Sherry Muir, MOT, OTR/L

Carol Siebert, MS, OTR/L, FAOTA

Contributors

Brian Prestwich, MD

for

The Commission on Practice

Debbie Amini, EdD, OTR/L, CHT, FAOTA, *Chairperson*

Adopted by the Representative Assembly 2014MarchCO28

Copyright © 2014 by the American Occupational Therapy Association. Previously published in the *American Journal of Occupational Therapy, 68*(Suppl. 3), S25–S33. http://dx.doi.org/10.5014/ajot.2014.686S06

The Role of Occupational Therapy in Wound Management

The American Occupational Therapy Association (AOTA) asserts that the prevention and amelioration of wounds and their impact on daily life occupations are within the scope of occupational therapy practice. Occupational therapists and occupational therapy assistants[1] routinely work with individuals and populations who are at risk for or have sustained wounds.

In the *Healthy People 2020* initiative, the U.S. Department of Health and Human Services (DHHS) called for a 10% reduction in pressure ulcer–related hospitalizations in persons age 65 or older by 2020 (DHHS, 2010), identifying this area as one of significant concern for individuals and society. This position paper serves to inform internal and external audiences, including employers and payer sources, about the role of occupational therapy related to prevention and amelioration of wounds to preserve and restore the ability of the individual to participate in meaningful, desired, and necessary daily life occupations.

Types, Incidence, and Prevalence of Wounds

Wounds, or impaired skin integrities, include abrasions, punctures, bites, surgical wounds, diabetic ulcers, pressure ulcers, traumatic wounds, venous stasis ulcers, and arterial ulcers. Certain populations either exhibit or are at risk for wounds and related complications. These populations include people with spinal cord injuries, cerebral palsy, hand injuries, diabetes, cancer, and burns and those with sensory or mobility impairments, including older adults. For example, the Centers for Disease Control and Prevention (CDC) has reported that in 2006, about 65,700 nontraumatic lower-limb amputations were performed in people with diabetes, representing approximately 60% of all nontraumatic lower-limb amputations (CDC, 2011).

Wounds and related conditions can affect a person's ability to participate fully in all daily life activities. Limitations can occur in performing self-care, work, educational activities, leisure activities, social participation, and rest and sleep. Wounds affect both the physical and the psychological well-being of individuals and can adversely affect quality of life. Pain, depression, social isolation, and anxiety can result from the existence of wounds, particularly those that are chronic in nature (Nogueira, Zanin, Miyazaki, & Godoy, 2009).

In addition, and depending on the location and severity of the wound, a person may also have difficulties with any of the following:

- Management of the wound site, including applying wound care treatments and products to promote healing as well as manage drainage or odor

- Management of clothing and footwear that may no longer fit correctly or that may worsen the wound condition

- Care, use, and application of pressure garments for scar management

---

[1]*Occupational therapists* are responsible for all aspects of occupational therapy service delivery and are accountable for the safety and effectiveness of the occupational therapy service delivery process. *Occupational therapy assistants* deliver occupational therapy services under the supervision of and in partnership with an occupational therapist (AOTA, 2009).

- Engaging in restful sleep due to the presence of pain

- Functional mobility related to the wound site or associated pain

- Engaging in physical activity necessary to prevent impairments in endurance, overall strength, cardiovascular status, pulmonary status, and cognition

- Social participation, self-efficacy, and reported quality of life resulting from discoloration of the skin, visible scars, contracting or hypertrophic scars, and conspicuous use of compression garments

- Financial stability due to an inability to work

- Maintaining role identity in all aspects of life.

Occupational Therapy's Role in Wound Management

Occupational therapy's perspective on working in this area combines an understanding of the mechanism and progression of acute and chronic wound healing and management, related body functions and structures, positive mental health, and the benefits of participation in everyday activities. Occupational therapy interventions focus on supporting health and participation through engagement in daily life activities and occupations.

The profession of occupational therapy is grounded in the principle that participation in meaningful and relevant life activities leads to life satisfaction, longevity, health, and wellness (AOTA, 2008; Christiansen, 2011). The ability to actively pursue and participate in desired life tasks and activities can be altered temporarily or for sustained periods of time due to the presence of a significant or chronic wound. In addition, diminished engagement in activity and mobility are considered risk factors for pressure ulcer–type wounds, according to the Braden Scale wound risk assessment tool (Bergstrom, Braden, Kemp, Champagne, & Ruby, 1998).

Occupational therapy practitioners[2] understand and appreciate the transactional relationship between client factors, including body functions and structures, and performance skills and performance patterns that are fundamental to participation (AOTA, 2008). When a wound is sustained, such as a severe finger laceration, direct attention to the wound itself as part of the overall occupational therapy intervention may be required to prevent or reduce occupational dysfunction that may occur secondary to this breach in the integumentary system (AOTA, 2010b).

With established service competency, following a plan of care established by an occupational therapist and as allowed by federal and state regulations and third-party payer requirements, the occupational therapy practitioner can utilize preparatory techniques such as the following:

- Application of clean dressings using the principles of moist wound care with both exudating and non-exudating wounds

- Application of wound closure strips

- Removal of sutures and wound closure strips

- Monitoring of wound status

- Mechanical debridement using forceps, cotton-tipped applicators, and wet-to-dry dressings and pulsed lavage

---

[2]When the term *occupational therapy practitioner* is used in this document, it refers to both occupational therapists and occupational therapy assistants (AOTA, 2006).

- Sharp debridement using scalpel or scissors to remove denatured tissue

- Application of appropriate topical agents to facilitate wound healing and debridement

- Application of silver nitrate for reduction of hypertrophic granulation tissue

- Application of enzymatic agents (e.g., collagenase) for debridement

- Application of negative pressure wound therapy

- Application of physical agent modalities such as whirlpool, electrical stimulation, and ultrasound.

This care may be offered as part of a team approach to intervention or in collaboration with the referring physician. In addition, occupational therapy practitioners may provide accommodations while the wound is healing. For example, education and adaptive equipment can allow a client to assist with or perform dressing changes, basic activities of daily living (ADLs), instrumental activities of daily living (IADLs), and tasks within all other areas of occupation.

Occupational therapy practitioners also are skilled in the prevention of wounds for people with various acute and chronic conditions such as spinal cord injuries, burns, lymphedema, cancer, diabetes, hand injuries, and other sensory and mobility impairments. In these cases, individual attention is given to the client's health status, environmental and contextual status, patterns of activity, and lifestyle choices as part of an overall plan to maintain skin integrity. Some interventions focus on the client (persons, organizations, and populations), others address the way activities are performed, and still others seek to change the context or environment that surrounds the client and influences performance. Interventions may focus on treatment of the actual wound, treatment of the resulting dysfunction, or prevention of the wound from occurring.

The following are examples of types of interventions and intervention approaches used in the delivery of occupational therapy services:

- Position the body to alleviate points of pressure including positioning techniques to ensure postural alignment, distribution of weight, balance, and stability.

- Fabricate and provide splints and orthotic devices to protect healing structures, prevent deformity, and secure dressings.

- Recommend support surfaces such as specialized beds and customized wheelchairs, cushions, and seating systems.

- Educate client and caregivers in skin care techniques, including moisture control and dry skin prevention.

- Educate clients and caregivers in precautions and safety techniques for all areas of occupation.

- Modify and adapt the environment for safe functional performance.

- Educate in transfer techniques to minimize risk of skin tears.

- Work with clients to identify ways to incorporate recommended prevention measures into their ongoing daily routines. These measures include pressure-relief activities (techniques and frequency) and pressure reduction equipment such as tilt-in-space wheelchairs and seat cushions.

- Educate clients and caregivers in techniques for donning and doffing pressure garments to manage swelling.

- Utilize specialized techniques for the management of upper-extremity lymphedema.

In addition, occupation-based and purposeful activities are provided and designed to engage the client in tasks that are meaningful and relevant and that support the mind, body, and spirit. Skilled selection of appropriate activities will minimize the detrimental effects of physical inactivity; loss of habits, roles, and routines; and the social isolation that may result from the presence of wounds (AOTA, 2008).

Occupational therapy practitioners recognize that, in addition to neuromusculoskeletal concerns, clients experiencing wounds also may exhibit diminished sense of self and self-efficacy, anxiety, and depression that interfere with their ability to manage currently existing wounds or participate in relevant daily occupations. Individuals who currently do not present with a wound may be at risk due to various lifestyle choices or environmental situations. Occupational therapy practitioners engage the qualities of their personality; verbal and nonverbal communication; listening skills; and empathy to encourage, facilitate, and motivate clients as they seek and achieve personal health, wellness, and occupational participation (AOTA, 2008). Practitioners consider the contextual issues that affect availability and choice with regard to wound care methods and access to tools. Advocacy efforts are initiated by practitioners as appropriate to prevent and treat wounds when individuals are faced with these concerns.

Cultural issues are also considered in the course of occupational therapy intervention. The impact of beliefs and choices is considered and integrated as part of the holistic approach to treatment. For example, parents may prefer that only organic debridement agents be used on their child's wound. An occupational therapy practitioner who is aware of this decision may advocate for the family through a team conference in which a discussion about the use of autolytic debrident versus pharmaceutical agents can take place.

Education

Occupational therapy practitioners are knowledgeable in the areas of human biology and physiology and treatment methods and interventions used as part of wound management. According to the *Accreditation Council on Occupational Therapy Education Standards* (ACOTE, 2012), occupational therapists and occupational therapy assistants must demonstrate knowledge and understanding of the structure and function of the human body to include the biological and physical sciences (B.1.1). They select and provide interventions and procedures to enhance safety, health and wellness, and performance in all areas of occupation (i. e., ADLs, IADLs, work, play, leisure, social participation, education, rest and sleep; B.5.2). In addition, occupational therapy practitioners provide development, remediation, and compensation for physical, mental, cognitive, perceptual, sensory function, neuromuscular, and behavioral skills (B.5.6) and are able to design, fabricate, apply, fit, and train in assistive technologies and devices (e.g., electronic aids to daily living, seating and positioning systems) used to enhance occupational performance and foster participation (B.5.10). Occupational therapy practitioners are able to demonstrate safe and effective application of superficial thermal and mechanical modalities as a preparatory measure to manage pain and improve occupational performance (B.5.15).

Ethical Considerations

The *Occupational Therapy Code of Ethics and Ethics Standards (2010)* (AOTA, 2010a) provides principles that guide safe and competent professional practice in all areas, including wound management. Several principles from the Code and Ethics Standards are particularly relevant to the use of wound management interventions and state that occupational therapy personnel shall

- "Provide occupational therapy services that are within each practitioner's level of competence and scope of practice (e.g., qualifications, experience, the law)" (AOTA, 2010a, p. S19, Principle 1E).

- "Use, to the extent possible, evaluation, planning, intervention techniques, and therapeutic equipment that are evidence-based and within the recognized scope of occupational therapy practice" (AOTA, 2010a, p. S19, Principle 1F).

- "Take responsible steps (e.g., continuing education, research, supervision, training) and use careful judgment to ensure competence and weigh potential for client harm when generally recognized standards do not exist in emerging technology or areas of practice" (AOTA, 2010a, p. S19, Principle 1G).

- "Take responsibility for maintaining high standards and continuing competence in practice, education, and research by participating in professional development and educational activities to improve and update knowledge and skills" (AOTA, 2010a, p. S23, Principle 5F).

- "Ensure that all duties assumed by or assigned to other occupational therapy personnel match credentials, qualifications, experience, and scope of practice" (AOTA, 2010a, p. S23, Principle 5G).

- "Provide appropriate supervision to individuals for whom they have supervisory responsibility in accordance with AOTA official documents and local, state, and federal or national laws, rules, regulations, policies, procedures, standards, and guidelines" (AOTA, 2010a, p. S23, Principle 5H).

All state laws and regulations related to wound management have precedence over AOTA policies and positions.

Table 1 presents case examples of occupational therapy's role in wound management.

Table 1. Case Examples of Occupational Therapy's Role in Wound Management

CLIENT AND BACKGROUND	ASSESSMENT AND FINDINGS	INTERVENTIONS
Geneva, age 68, was referred to an occupational therapist specializing in hand rehabilitation following an extensive palmar fasciotomy resulting from progressive Dupuytren's contracture. A full-thickness skin graft harvested from her volar wrist/forearm was used to close a full-thickness wound on the volar surface of the small finger proximal phalanx and palm that sustained extensive loss of tissue due to long-standing MP and PIP contracture. At the time of the initial occupational therapy evaluation, about 4 days postsurgery, it was noted that the donor site (about 2 cm by 5 cm) was left to heal by secondary intention. Physician orders called for the initiation of a moist wound care regimen following removal of the postsurgical dressing.	Following a saline rinse, the occupational therapy practitioner visually inspected the wound site and measured it using a disposable tape measure. Possible undermining and tunneling were assessed using a sterile cotton swab; no undermining or tunneling were found. The depth of the wound (2 mm) was measured with a tongue depressor and tape measure overlay. Observation of wound color and exudate indicated a clean red wound with early granulation tissue. Exudate was minimal/moderate and clear, as would be expected for this type of donor site. No signs of infection were present. Circumferential measurements were taken of the arm just distal and proximal to the wound; when compared with the noninvolved side, no significant differences were noted. The measurements served as a baseline for levels of edema. An analog pain scale revealed that Geneva had very minimal pain, with a score of 2 on a scale of 1–10. The occupational profile included client-centered assessment tools and outlined areas of occupation of concern to Geneva.	The occupational therapy practitioner initiated moist wound care using hydrogel to maintain an appropriately moist environment for granulation tissue growth. She covered the wound and hydrogel with semipermeable film dressing to ensure adequate oxygenation and minimize the potential for anaerobic bacterial proliferation. A secondary dry gauze dressing was applied to protect the film dressing during splint wear and functional tasks. Geneva was instructed to keep the dressing in place until her next occupational therapy visit, at which time the wound was reassessed and re-dressed as appropriate. Geneva was instructed in modification and adaptation strategies to maintain involvement in areas of occupation such as cooking and gardening, from which she derived significant personal satisfaction. This wound care regimen was administered by the occupational therapy practitioner for 2 weeks until granulation tissue bed was established. Geneva was then instructed to continue with program at home. About 2 weeks later, moist wound care was discontinued, as the wound had epithelialized fully.

(Continued)

Table 1. Case Examples of Occupational Therapy's Role in Wound Management *(cont.)*

CLIENT AND BACKGROUND	ASSESSMENT AND FINDINGS	INTERVENTIONS
Mr. Adams, age 71, was referred to home health care services following a recent fall, resulting in a pelvic fracture; increased BP; and chronic Parkinson's disease. He was discharged home from the ER with no inpatient hospitalization. Upon admission to home care, a Stage II ischial tuberosity ulcer was discovered. According to Mr. Adams, he preferred to stay in a recliner during the day and occasionally sleeps there at night if he doesn't "feel strong." Mr. Adams lives with his daughter and son-in-law, both of whom work during the day. Mr. Adams reported decreased appetite and that family are available to help with bathing if needed. He prefers to wear adult diapers, as he occasionally "cannot get to the toilet in time."	During a visit to the home, the occupational therapist visually assessed the covered wound (a nurse provided documentation of measurements and granulation tissue, and occupational therapy documentation described the type of wound and dressing present). The nurse and occupational therapist collaborated to determine whether the wound dressing was appropriate for Mr. Adams to shower. A hydrocolloid dressing was recommended to the doctor to allow a moist healing environment but provide a waterproof seal to allow bathing and prevent contamination.

Upon further visual assessment of skin integrity and evaluation of clinical factors (i.e., decreased mobility with prolonged sitting, occasional incontinence with moistness leading to potential maceration, and decreased nutrition due to poor meal planning), the occupational therapists noted 2 additional reddened areas over bony prominences on the coccyx. In addition, Mr. Adams presented with decreased pain awareness and fragile skin due to decreased weight, which contributed to pressure ulcer formation. The occupational therapist consulted with the nurse case manager to discuss a recommendation for a nutritionist consult, which the nurse followed up on and received from the doctor. | Although the home care nurse initially provided the direct application of the hydrocolloid dressing to the Stage II ulcer and monitored the wound status with photographs and diagrams, the occupational therapist was imperative in the wound care. As the wound began epithelialization, the dressing changes were reduced to every 4 days, and the nurse instructed the family in proper application, which the occupational therapist was able to reinforce during the performance of bathing. The therapist instructed Mr. Adams and his caregivers on the effects of prolonged pressure, shear forces, friction, and incontinence on the development of future ulcers and prevention of healing in the current ulcer. Bathing and toileting were addressed for thoroughness of drying skin as well as techniques for self-inspection. A toileting routine was established.

Pressure relief was addressed (Mr. Adams and his caregivers were instructed on changing position every hour, and a chair cushion was introduced for the recliner). Adequate nutrition needs (to assist with healing) were met after meal preparation alternatives were addressed with Mr. Adams, his caregivers, and a nutritionist. The wound was considered healed after full epithelialization, and as the last health care professional involved, the occupational therapist completed proper Medicare documentation and staging of the healed wound. |
| **Tanner, age 10,** qualifies for special education services at school due to multiple impairments (e.g., orthopedic, cognitive, visual). As a result of a disability, Tanner is not able to independently change his position to relieve pressure points created by the gravitational pull on his body in any position. Tanner is supported with a customized wheelchair for mobility, adapted stander, and adaptive seating in the school setting to facilitate his highest level of participation in instructional activities. Tanner is recovering from a medical intervention to address a pressure area. | Occupational therapy services evaluated Tanner's participation at school using observation, parent and teacher interviews, and the School Function Assessment (Coster, Deeney, Haltiwanger, & Haley, 1998). From the evaluation process, it was identified that Tanner required alternative positioning options at school to facilitate his highest level of functional participation in the instructional activities presented in this setting. Additionally, the classroom personnel required training on the necessity to provide Tanner with a daily schedule for change in position to facilitate healing of the pressure area. | The occupational therapist provided training for the classroom personnel on how to transfer and position Tanner in the various positioning options provided in the classroom and the functional performance they should expect from Tanner in each option. The therapist also collaborated with the classroom teacher to develop a daily positioning schedule for Tanner while at school that not only facilitated function in the setting but also provided Tanner with a change in position at least every hour. The frequency of positional changes at school was determined in consultation with Tanner's orthopedic surgeon, who is medically managing the pressure area healing process. |

(Continued)

410

Table 1. Case Examples of Occupational Therapy's Role in Wound Management *(cont.)*

CLIENT AND BACKGROUND	ASSESSMENT AND FINDINGS	INTERVENTIONS
Brian,[a] **age 36,** had a complete SCI at the T-8 level 2 years ago as a result of motor vehicle crash. He lives alone and uses a manual wheelchair for mobility. He drives a vehicle adapted with hand controls. He has been employed as a computer programmer and has had a history of pressure ulcers for the past year. Currently, he is admitted to the hospital for a UTI and a Stage 3 pressure ulcer on his left ischial tuberosity.	The rehabilitation team worked with the hospital urologist to determine the cause of Brian's recurrent UTIs. Brian uses intermittent catheterization and may not have always used the safest techniques. The team also reviewed Brian's pressure ulcer history. The pressure ulcer was cultured and treated according to the hospital's protocol, which may include dressings, whirlpool, vacuum-assisted closure, or surgery. Brian remains prone as much as possible while in the hospital. The occupational therapist evaluated Brian's ability to participate in bladder management and work. All equipment pertaining to seating (e.g., wheelchair, cushion) was evaluated for appropriateness, condition, and effectiveness. Pressure mapping may be necessary to find a wheelchair pressure reduction cushion that helps reduce the risk of pressure ulcers.	The occupational therapy practitioner reviewed with Brian strategies for reducing infection during intermittent catheterization. She discussed strategies for continued engagement in work and leisure tasks while he is hospitalized in the prone position. If necessary, Brian's wheelchair will be modified or replaced (if finances are available). Brian will participate in group and individual pressure ulcer prevention and management education sessions and will be provided with a home program to follow. Brian will be instructed on managing the ulcer (surgical site if he had surgery) with dressings and pressure redistribution (weight shifts if he is allowed to sit) during sitting or lying in bed, on nutrition, on transfers, and on sitting tolerance. Home and work site visits are recommended to help Brian identify situations that may be contributing to his recurrent pressure ulcers. He may be referred for home health services while the ulcer heals.

Note. BP = blood pressure; ER = emergency room; MP = metacarpophalangeal; PIP = proximal interphalangeal; SCI = spinal cord injury; UTI = urinary tract infection.

[a]The case study on Brian was contributed by Susan L. Garber, MA, OTR, FAOTA, FACRM.

References

Accreditation Council for Occupational Therapy Education. (2012). Accreditation Council for Occupational Therapy Education (ACOTE™) standards. *American Journal of Occupational Therapy, 66*(Suppl.), S6–S74. http://dx.doi.org/10.5014/ajot.2012.66S6

American Occupational Therapy Association. (2006). Policy 1.44: Categories of occupational therapy personnel. In *Policy manual* (2011 ed., pp. 33–34). Bethesda, MD: Author.

American Occupational Therapy Association. (2008). Occupational therapy practice framework: Domain and process (2nd ed.). *American Journal of Occupational Therapy, 62,* 525–683. http://dx.doi.org/10.5014/ajot.62.6.625

American Occupational Therapy Association. (2009). Guidelines for supervision, roles, and responsibilities during the delivery of occupational therapy services. *American Journal of Occupational Therapy, 63,* 797–803. http://dx.doi.org/10.5014/ajot.63.6.819

American Occupational Therapy Association. (2010a). Occupational therapy code of ethics and ethics standards (2010). *American Journal of Occupational Therapy, 64*(Suppl.), S17–S26. http://dx.doi.org/10.5014/ajot.2010.64S17

American Occupational Therapy Association. (2010b). Scope of practice. *American Journal of Occupational Therapy, 64*(Suppl.), S70–S77. http://dx.doi.org/10.5014/ajot.2010.64S70

Bergstrom, N., Braden, B. J., Kemp, M., Champagne, M., & Ruby, E. (1998). Reliability and validity of the Braden Scale: A multi-site study. *Nursing Research, 47,* 261–269.

Centers for Disease Control and Prevention. (2011). *National estimates and general information on diabetes and prediabetes in the United States, 2011* (National Diabetes Fact Sheet). Atlanta: Author.

Christiansen, C. (2011). The importance of participation in everyday activities. In C. H. Christiansen & K. M. Matuska (Eds.), *Ways of living: Intervention strategies to enable participation* (4th ed., pp. 1–26). Bethesda, MD: AOTA Press.

Coster, W. J., Deeney, T., Haltiwanger, J., & Haley, S. M. (1998). *School Function Assessment.* San Antonio, TX: Psychological Corporation.

Nogueira, G., Zanin, C., Miyazaki, M., & Godoy, J. (2009). Venous leg ulcers and emotional consequences. *International Journal of Lower Extremity Wounds, 8,* 194–196.

U.S. Department of Health and Human Services. (2010, December). OA-10. Reduce the rate of pressure ulcer–related hospitalizations among older adults. In *Healthy People 2020: Summary of objectives.* Retrieved December 29, 2011, from www.healthypeople.gov/2020/topicsobjectives2020/pdfs/OlderAdults.pdf

Additional Resources

Baker, T., Boyce, J., Gairy, P., & Mighty, G. (2011). Interprofessional management of a complex continuing care patient admitted with 18 pressure ulcers: A case report. *Ostomy Wound Management, 57*(2), 38–47.

Blanche, E. I., Fogelberg, D., Diaz, J., Carlson, M., & Clark, F. (2011). Manualization of occupational therapy interventions: Illustrations from the Pressure Ulcer Research Program. *American Journal of Occupational Therapy, 65,* 711–719. http://dx.doi.org/10.5014/ajot.2011.001172

Braden, B., & Bergstrom, N. (1988).*The Braden Scale.* Retrieved June 13, 2013, from http://www.in.gov/isdh/files/Braden_Scale.pdf

Author

Debbie Amini, EdD, OTR/L, CHT

for

The Commission on Practice
Debbie Amini, EdD, OTR/L, CHT, *Chairperson*

Adopted by the Representative Assembly 2012CO19

Note. This document replaces the 2009 Wound Management White Paper.

Scope of Practice

Statement of Purpose

The purpose of this document is to

A. Define the scope of practice in occupational therapy by

1. Delineating the domain of occupational therapy practice and services provided by occupational therapists and occupational therapy assistants;

2. Delineating the dynamic process of occupational therapy evaluation and intervention services used to achieve outcomes that support the participation of clients in everyday life activities (occupations); and

3. Describing the education and certification requirements needed to practice as an occupational therapist and occupational therapy assistant;

B. Inform consumers, health care providers, educators, the community, funding agencies, payers, referral sources, and policymakers regarding the scope of occupational therapy.

Introduction

The occupational therapy scope of practice is based on the American Occupational Therapy Association (AOTA) documents *Occupational Therapy Practice Framework: Domain and Process* (AOTA, 2014b) and *The Philosophical Base of Occupational Therapy* (AOTA, 2011b), which states that "the use of occupation to promote individual, community, and population health is the core of occupational therapy practice, education, research, and advocacy" (p. S65). Occupational therapy is a dynamic and evolving profession that is responsive to consumer and societal needs, to system changes, and to emerging knowledge and research.

This document is designed to support and be used in conjunction with the *Definition of Occupational Therapy Practice for the AOTA Model Practice Act* (AOTA, 2011a). Although this document may be a resource to augment state statutes and regulations that govern the practice of occupational therapy, it does not supersede existing laws and other regulatory requirements. Occupational therapists and occupational therapy assistants are required to abide by relevant statutes and regulations when providing occupational therapy services. State statutes and other regulatory requirements typically include statements about educational requirements to practice occupational therapy, procedures to practice occupational therapy legally within the defined area of jurisdiction, the definition and scope of occupational therapy practice, and supervision requirements for occupational therapy assistants.

It is the position of AOTA that a referral is not required for the provision of occupational therapy services, but referrals for such services are generally affected by laws and payment policy. AOTA's position is also that "an occupational therapist accepts and responds to referrals in compliance with state or federal laws, other regulatory and payer requirements, and AOTA documents" (AOTA 2010b, Standard II.2, p. S108). State laws and other regulatory requirements should be viewed as minimum criteria to practice occupational therapy. Ethical guidelines that ensure safe and effective delivery of occupational therapy services to clients always guide occupational therapy practice (AOTA, 2010a). Policies of payers such as insurance companies also must be followed.

Occupational therapy services may be provided by two levels of practitioners: (1) the occupational therapist and (2) the occupational therapy assistant, as well as by occupational therapy students under appropriate supervision (AOTA, 2012). Occupational therapists function as autonomous practitioners, are responsible for all aspects of occupational therapy service delivery, and are accountable for the safety and effectiveness of the occupational therapy service delivery process.

The occupational therapy assistant delivers occupational therapy services only under the supervision of and in partnership with the occupational therapist (AOTA, 2014a). When the term *occupational therapy practitioner* is used in this document, it refers to both occupational therapists and occupational therapy assistants (AOTA, 2011c).

Definition of Occupational Therapy

The *Occupational Therapy Practice Framework* (AOTA, 2014b) defines *occupational therapy* as

> the therapeutic use of everyday life activities (occupations) with individuals or groups for the purpose of enhancing or enabling participation in roles, habits, and routines in home, school, workplace, community, and other settings. Occupational therapy practitioners use their knowledge of the transactional relationship among the person, his or her engagement in valuable occupations, and the context to design occupation-based intervention plans that facilitate change or growth in client factors (body functions, body structures, values, beliefs, and spirituality) and skills (motor, process, and social interaction) needed for successful participation. Occupational therapy practitioners are concerned with the end result of participation and thus enable engagement through adaptations and modifications to the environment or objects within the environment when needed. Occupational therapy services are provided for habilitation, rehabilitation, and promotion of health and wellness for clients with disability- and non–disability-related needs. These services include acquisition and preservation of occupational identity for those who have or are at risk for developing an illness, injury, disease, disorder, condition, impairment, disability, activity limitation, or participation restriction. (p. S1)

Occupational Therapy Practice

Occupational therapists and occupational therapy assistants are experts at analyzing the client factors, performance skills, performance patterns, and contexts and environments necessary for people to engage in their everyday activities and occupations. The practice of occupational therapy includes

A. Evaluation of factors affecting activities of daily living (ADLs), instrumental activities of daily living (IADLs), rest and sleep, education, work, play, leisure, and social participation, including

   1. Client factors, including body functions (e.g., neuromuscular, sensory, visual, perceptual, cognitive) and body structures (e.g., cardiovascular, digestive, integumentary, genitourinary systems)

   2. Habits, routines, roles, and rituals

   3. Physical and social environments and cultural, personal, temporal, and virtual contexts and activity demands that affect performance

   4. Performance skills, including motor, process, and social interaction skills.

B. Approaches to identify and select interventions, such as

   1. Establishment, remediation, or restoration of a skill or ability that has not yet developed or is impaired

2. Compensation, modification, or adaptation of activity or environment to enhance performance

3. Maintenance and enhancement of capabilities without which performance in everyday life activities would decline

4. Health promotion and wellness to enable or enhance performance in everyday life activities

5. Prevention of barriers to performance.

C. Interventions and procedures to promote or enhance safety and performance in ADLs, IADLs, rest and sleep, education, work, play, leisure, and social participation, for example,

1. Occupations and activities

   a. Completing morning dressing and hygiene routine using adaptive devices

   b. Playing on a playground with children and adults

   c. Engaging in a driver rehabilitation and community mobility program

   d. Managing feeding, eating, and swallowing to enable eating and feeding performance.

2. Preparatory methods and tasks

   a. Exercises, including tasks and methods to increase motion, strength, and endurance for occupational participation

   b. Assessment, design, fabrication, application, fitting, and training in assistive technology and adaptive devices

   c. Design and fabrication of splints and orthotic devices and training in the use of prosthetic devices

   d. Modification of environments (e.g., home, work, school, community) and adaptation of processes, including the application of ergonomic principles

   e. Application of physical agent modalities and use of a range of specific therapeutic procedures (e.g., wound care management; techniques to enhance sensory, perceptual, and cognitive processing; manual therapy techniques) to enhance performance skills

   f. Assessment, recommendation, and training in techniques to enhance functional mobility, including wheelchair management

   g. Explore and identify effective tools for regulating nervous system arousal levels in order to participate in therapy and/or in valued daily activities.

3. Education and training

   a. Training in self-care, self-management, home management, and community or work reintegration

   b. Education and training of individuals, including family members, caregivers, and others.

4. Advocacy

   a. Efforts directed toward promoting occupational justice and empowering clients to seek and obtain resources to fully participate in their daily life occupations.

5. Group interventions

   a. Facilitate learning and skill acquisition through the dynamics of group or social interaction across the life span.

6. Care coordination, case management, and transition services

7. Consultative services to groups, programs, organizations, or communities.

Scope of Practice: Domain and Process

The scope of practice includes the domain and process of occupational therapy services. These two concepts are intertwined, with the *domain* defining the focus of occupational therapy and the *process* defining the delivery of occupational therapy.

The *domain* of occupational therapy is the everyday life activities (occupations) that people find meaningful and purposeful. Within this domain, occupational therapy services enable clients to participate in their everyday life activities in their desired roles, contexts and environments, and life situations.

Clients may be individuals or persons, groups, or populations. The occupations in which clients engage occur throughout the life span and include

- ADLs (self-care activities);

- IADLs (activities to support daily life within the home and community that often require complex interactions, e.g., household management, financial management, child care);

- Rest and sleep (activities relating to obtaining rest and sleep, including identifying the need for rest and sleep, preparing for sleep, and participating in rest and sleep);

- Education (activities to participate as a learner in a learning environment);

- Work (activities for engaging in remunerative employment or volunteer activities);

- Play (activities pursued for enjoyment and diversion);

- Leisure (nonobligatory, discretionary, and intrinsically rewarding activities); and

- Social participation (the ability to exhibit behaviors and characteristics expected during interaction with others within a social system).

Within their domain of practice, occupational therapists and occupational therapy assistants consider the repertoire of occupations in which the client engages, the performance skills and patterns the client uses, the contexts and environments influencing engagement, the features and demands of the activity, and the client's body functions and structures. Occupational therapists and occupational therapy assistants use their knowledge and skills to help clients conduct or resume daily life activities that support function and health throughout the life span. Participation in activities and occupations that are meaningful to the client involves emotional, psychosocial, cognitive, and physical aspects of performance. Participation in meaningful activities and occupations enhances health, well-being, and life satisfaction.

The domain of occupational therapy practice complements the World Health Organization's (WHO's) conceptualization of *participation* and *health* articulated in the *International Classification of Functioning, Disability and Health* (*ICF*; WHO, 2001). Occupational therapy incorporates the basic constructs of *ICF*, including environment, participation, activities, and body structures and functions, when providing interventions to enable full participation in occupations and maximize occupational engagement.

The *process* of occupational therapy refers to the delivery of services and includes evaluating, intervening, and targeting of outcomes. Occupation remains central to the occupational therapy process, which is client centered, involving collaboration with the client throughout each aspect of service delivery. During the evaluation, the therapist develops an occupational profile; analyzes the client's ability to carry out everyday life activities; and determines the client's occupational needs, strengths, barriers to participation, and priorities for intervention.

OCCUPATIONS	CLIENT FACTORS	PERFORMANCE SKILLS	PERFORMANCE PATTERNS	CONTEXTS AND ENVIRONMENTS
Activities of daily living (ADLs)*	Values, beliefs, and spirituality	Motor skills	Habits	Cultural
Instrumental activities of daily living (IADLs)	Body functions	Process skills	Routines	Personal
Rest and sleep	Body structures	Social interaction skills	Rituals	Physical
Education			Roles	Social
Work				Temporal
Play				Virtual
Leisure				
Social participation				

*Also referred to as *basic activities of daily living (BADLs)* or *personal activities of daily living (PADLs)*.

Exhibit 1. Aspects of the domain of occupational therapy.
All aspects of the domain transact to support engagement, participation, and health. This exhibit does not imply a hierarchy.

Source. From "Occupational Therapy Practice Framework: Domain and Process" (3rd ed., p. S4), by American Occupational Therapy Association, 2014, *American Journal of Occupational Therapy, 68*(Suppl. 1), S1–S48. http://dx.doi.org/10.5014/ajot.2014.682006. Copyright © 2014 by the American Occupational Therapy Association. Used with permission.

Evaluation and intervention may address one or more aspects of the domain (Exhibit 1) that influence occupational performance. Intervention includes planning and implementing occupational therapy services and involves activities and occupations, preparatory methods and tasks, education and training, and advocacy. The occupational therapist and occupational therapy assistant in partnership with the occupational therapist utilize occupation-based theories, frames of reference, evidence, and clinical reasoning to guide the intervention (AOTA, 2014b).

The outcome of occupational therapy intervention is directed toward "achieving health, well-being, and participation in life through engagement in occupations" (AOTA, 2014b, p. S4). Outcomes of the intervention determine future actions with the client and include occupational performance, prevention (of risk factors, disease, and disability), health and wellness, quality of life, participation, role competence, well-being, and occupational justice (AOTA, 2014b).

Sites of Intervention and Areas of Focus

Occupational therapy services are provided to persons, groups, and populations. People served come from all age groups. Practitioners work with individuals one to one, in groups, or at the population level to address occupational needs and issues, for example, in mental health; work and industry; rehabilitation, disability, and participation; productive aging; and health and wellness.

Along the continuum of service, occupational therapy services may be provided to clients throughout the life span in a variety of settings. The settings may include, but are not limited to, the following:

- Institutional settings (inpatient; e.g., acute care, rehabilitation facilities, psychiatric hospitals, community and specialty-focused hospitals, nursing facilities, prisons),

- Outpatient settings (e.g., hospitals, clinics, medical and therapy offices),

- Home and community settings (e.g., residences, group homes, assisted living, schools, early intervention centers, day care centers, industry and business, hospice, sheltered workshops, transitional-living facilities, wellness and fitness centers, community mental health facilities), and

- Research facilities.

Education and Certification Requirements

To practice as an occupational therapist, the individual trained in the United States

- Has graduated from an occupational therapy program accredited by the Accreditation Council for Occupational Therapy Education (ACOTE®; 2012) or predecessor organizations;

- Has successfully completed a period of supervised fieldwork experience required by the recognized educational institution where the applicant met the academic requirements of an educational program for occupational therapists that is accredited by ACOTE or predecessor organizations;

- Has passed a nationally recognized entry-level examination for occupational therapists; and

- Fulfills state requirements for licensure, certification, or registration.

To practice as an occupational therapy assistant, the individual trained in the United States

- Has graduated from an occupational therapy assistant program accredited by ACOTE or predecessor organizations;

- Has successfully completed a period of supervised fieldwork experience required by the recognized educational institution where the applicant met the academic requirements of an educational program for occupational therapy assistants that is accredited by ACOTE or predecessor organizations;

- Has passed a nationally recognized entry-level examination for occupational therapy assistants; and

- Fulfills state requirements for licensure, certification, or registration.

AOTA supports licensure of qualified occupational therapists and occupational therapy assistants (AOTA, 2009). State and other legislative or regulatory agencies may impose additional requirements to practice as occupational therapists and occupational therapy assistants in their area of jurisdiction.

References

American Council for Occupational Therapy Education. (2012). 2011 Accreditation Council for Occupational Therapy Education (ACOTE®) standards. *American Journal of Occupational Therapy, 66,* S6–S74. http://dx.doi.org/10.5014/ajot.2012.66S6

American Occupational Therapy Association. (2009). Policy 5.3: Licensure. In *Policy manual* (2013 ed., pp. 60–61). Bethesda, MD: Author.

American Occupational Therapy Association. (2010a). Occupational therapy code of ethics and ethics standards (2010). *American Journal of Occupational Therapy, 64*(Suppl.), S17–S26. http://dx.doi.org/10.5014/ajot.2010.64S17

American Occupational Therapy Association. (2010b). Standards of practice for occupational therapy. *American Journal of Occupational Therapy, 64*(Suppl.), S106–S111. http://dx.doi.org/10.5014/ajot.2010.64S106

American Occupational Therapy Association. (2011a). *Definition of occupational therapy practice for the AOTA Model Practice Act.* Retrieved from http://www.aota.org/-/media/Corporate/Files/Advocacy/State/Resources/PracticeAct/Model%20Definition%20of%20OT%20Practice%20%20Adopted%2041411.ashx

American Occupational Therapy Association. (2011b). The philosophical base of occupational therapy. *American Journal of Occupational Therapy, 65*(Suppl.), S65. http://dx.doi.org/10.5014/ajot.2011.65S65

American Occupational Therapy Association. (2011c). Policy 1.44: Categories of occupational therapy personnel. In *Policy manual* (2013 ed., pp. 32–33). Bethesda, MD: Author.

American Occupational Therapy Association. (2012). Fieldwork Level II and occupational therapy students: A position paper. *American Journal of Occupational Therapy, 66*(6, Suppl.), S75–S77. http://dx.doi.org/10.5014/ajot.2012.66S75

American Occupational Therapy Association. (2014a). Guidelines for supervision, roles, and responsibilities during the delivery of occupational therapy services. *American Journal of Occupational Therapy, 68*(Suppl. 1), S16–S22. http://dx.doi.org/ajot.2014.686S03

American Occupational Therapy Association. (2014b). Occupational therapy practice framework: Domain and process (3rd ed.). *American Journal of Occupational Therapy, 68*(Suppl. 1), S1–S48. http://dx.doi.org/10.5014/ajot.2014.682006

World Health Organization. (2001). *International classification of functioning, disability and health.* Geneva: Author.

Authors
The Commission on Practice:
Sara Jane Brayman, PhD, OTR/L, FAOTA, *Chairperson*
Gloria Frolek Clark, MS, OTR/L, FAOTA
Janet V. DeLany, DEd, OTR/L
Eileen R. Garza, PhD, OTR, ATP
Mary V. Radomski, MA, OTR/L, FAOTA
Ruth Ramsey, MS, OTR/L
Carol Siebert, MS, OTR/L
Kristi Voelkerding, BS, COTA/L
Patricia D. LaVesser, PhD, OTR/L, *SIS Liaison*
Lenna Aird, *ASD Liaison*
Deborah Lieberman, MHSA, OTR/L, FAOTA, *AOTA Headquarters Liaison*

for

The Commission on Practice
Sara Jane Brayman, PhD, OTR/L, FAOTA, *Chairperson*, 2002–2005

Adopted by the Representative Assembly 2004C23

Edited by the Commission on Practice 2014
Debbie Amini, EdD, OTR/L, CHT, FAOTA, *Chairperson*

Adopted by the Representative Assembly Coordinating Council (RACC) for the Representative Assembly, 2014

Note. This document replaces the 2010 document *Scope of Practice,* previously published and copyrighted in 2010 by the American Occupational Therapy Association in the *American Journal of Occupational Therapy, 64*(6, Suppl.), S70–S77. http://dx.doi.org/10.5014/ajot.2010.64S70

Telehealth

The purpose of this paper is to provide the current position of the American Occupational Therapy Association (AOTA) regarding the use of telehealth by occupational therapists and occupational therapy assistants[1] to provide occupational therapy services. This document describes the use of telehealth within occupational therapy practice areas, as described in the existing research. Additionally, occupational therapy practitioner[2] qualifications, ethics, and regulatory issues related to the use of telehealth as a service delivery model within occupational therapy are outlined. Occupational therapy practitioners are the intended audience for this document, although others involved in supervising, planning, delivering, regulating, and paying for occupational therapy services also may find it helpful.

Telecommunication and information technologies have prompted the development of an emerging model of health care delivery called *telehealth,* which involves health care services, health information, and health education. AOTA defines *telehealth* as the application of evaluative, consultative, preventative, and therapeutic services delivered through telecommunication and information technologies. Occupational therapy services provided by means of a telehealth service delivery model can be *synchronous,* that is, delivered through interactive technologies in real time, or *asynchronous,* using store-and-forward technologies. Occupational therapy practitioners can use telehealth as a mechanism to provide services at a location that is physically distant from the client, thereby allowing for services to occur where the client lives, works, and plays, if that is needed or desired (AOTA, 2010d). An overview of telehealth technologies is included in Appendix A. *Telerehabilitation* within the larger realm of telehealth is the application of telecommunication and information technologies for the delivery of rehabilitation services. Key terms related to telehealth and telehealth technologies are defined in Appendix B.

Use of Telehealth Within Occupational Therapy

Occupational therapy practitioners use telehealth as a service delivery model to help clients develop skills; incorporate assistive technology and adaptive techniques; modify work, home, or school environments; and create health-promoting habits and routines. Benefits of a telehealth service delivery model include increased accessibility of services to clients who live in remote or underserved areas, improved access to providers and specialists otherwise unavailable to clients, prevention of unnecessary delays in receiving care, and workforce enhancement through consultation and research among others (Cason, 2012a, 2012b). By removing barriers to accessing care, including social stigma, travel, and socioeconomic and cultural barriers, the use of telehealth as a service delivery model within occupational therapy leads to improved access to care and ameliorates the impact of personnel shortages in underserved areas. Occupational therapy outcomes aligned with telehealth include the facilitation of occupational performance, adaptation, health and wellness, prevention, and quality of life.

---

[1]The *occupational therapist* is responsible for all aspects of occupational therapy service delivery and is accountable for the safety and effectiveness of the occupational therapy service delivery process. The *occupational therapy assistant* delivers occupational therapy services under the supervision of and in partnership with the occupational therapist (AOTA, 2009).

[2]When the term *occupational therapy practitioner* is used in this document, it refers to both occupational therapists and occupational therapy assistants (AOTA, 2006).

Telehealth has potential as a service delivery model in each major practice area within occupational therapy. Note that given the variability of client factors, activity demands, performance skills, performance patterns, and contexts and environments, the candidacy and appropriateness of a telehealth service delivery model "should be determined on a case-by-case basis with selections firmly based on clinical judgment, client's informed choice, and professional standards of care" (Brennan et al., 2010, p. 33). See Appendix C for applications and evidence supporting the use of telehealth within occupational therapy practice areas.

Evaluation Using Telehealth Technologies: Tele-Evaluation

The traditional telephone system continues to be a low-cost alternative for effectively conducting interview assessments by various health care professionals (Cooper et al., 2002; Dreyer, Dreyer, Shaw, & Wittman, 2001; Winters, 2002), and advanced communication technologies have broadened the possibilities for conducting evaluations. Studies have described the use of telehealth in areas that are of concern to occupational therapy, such as evaluation and consultative services for wheelchair prescription (Barlow, Liu, & Sekulic, 2009; Schein, Schmeler, Brienza, Saptono, & Parmanto, 2008; Schein, Schmeler, Holm, Saptono, & Brienza, 2010; Schein et al., 2011), neurological assessment (Savard, Borstad, Tkachuck, Lauderdale, & Conroy, 2003), adaptive equipment prescription and home modification (Sanford et al., 2007), and ergonomic assessment (Baker & Jacobs, 2013).

Clinical reasoning guides the selection and application of appropriate telehealth technologies necessary to evaluate client needs and environmental factors. Therapists should consider the reliability and validity of specific assessment tools when administered remotely. Researchers have investigated the reliability of assessments such as the Functional Reach Test and European Stroke Scale (Palsbo, Dawson, Savard, Goldstein, & Heuser, 2007); the Kohlman Evaluation of Living Skills and the Canadian Occupational Performance Measure (Dreyer et al., 2001); and the FIM™, the Jamar Dynamometer, the Preston Pinch Gauge, the Nine-Hole Peg Test, and the Unified Parkinson's Disease Rating Scale (Hoffman, Russell, Thompson, Vincent, & Nelson, 2008) and found these tools to be reliable when administered remotely through telehealth technologies. In some cases, an in-person assistant, such as a paraprofessional or other support person, may be used to relay assessment tool measurements or other measures (e.g., environmental, wheelchair and seating) to the remote therapist during the evaluation process.

When choosing a telehealth model for conducting an evaluation, occupational therapists need to consider the client's diagnosis, client's preference, access to technology, and ability to measure outcomes when using that model. The occupational therapist may determine that an in-person evaluation is required for some clients. Because of the evolving knowledge and technology related to telehealth, occupational therapists should review the latest research to remain current about the appropriate use of telehealth technologies for conducting evaluations.

Intervention Using Telehealth Technologies: Teleintervention and Telerehabilitation

A telehealth model of service delivery may be used for providing interventions that are preventative, habilitative, or rehabilitative in nature. When planning and providing interventions delivered with telehealth technologies, Scheideman-Miller et al. (2003) reported that the appropriateness and maintenance of the technology and the sustainability of participation by the client are important factors to consider. As related to occupational therapy interventions, some factors to consider include technology availability and options for the occupational therapy practitioner and the client; the safety, effectiveness, sustainability, and quality of interventions provided exclusively through telehealth or in combination with in-person interventions; the client's choice about receiving interventions by means of telehealth technologies; the client's outcomes, including the client's perception of services provided; reimbursement; and compliance with federal and state laws, regulation, and policy, including licensure requirements (Cason & Brannon, 2011).

Consultation Using Telehealth Technologies: Teleconsultation

Teleconsultation is a virtual consultation that includes the

- Expert provider and client,

- Expert provider and local provider with the client present, or

- Expert provider and local provider without the client present.

Teleconsultation uses telecommunication and information technologies for the purpose of obtaining health and medical information or advice.

Teleconsultation has been used to overcome the shortage of various rehabilitation professionals across the United States. For example, an occupational therapist or prosthetist can remotely evaluate and adjust a client's prosthetic device using computer software with videoconferencing capability and remote access to a local clinician's computer screen despite the physical distance between the expert and client (Whelan & Wagner, 2011). Similarly, Schein et al. (2008) demonstrated positive outcomes associated with teleconsultation between a remote seating specialist and a local therapist for evaluating wheelchair prescriptions. The Veterans Health Administration is using teleconsultation for veterans with traumatic brain injuries in a process that involves interactive videoconferencing technology and Web-based management systems (Girard, 2007). In the practice area of pediatrics, Wakeford (2002) used videoconferencing technologies to consult on play performance in children with special needs.

Practitioners should contact state professional licensure boards in their state as well as in the state where the client is located for further clarification on policies related to teleconsultation before rendering services. Some states do have consultation and licensure exemption provisions, although application of the consultation and licensure exemption provisions to facilitate temporary (i.e., consultative) interstate occupational therapy practice using telehealth technologies has not been established (Cason & Brannon, 2011).

Monitoring Using Telehealth Technologies: Telemonitoring

Occupational therapy practitioners can use telehealth technologies to monitor a client's adherence to an intervention program, assist a client in progressing toward achieving desired outcomes, and track and respond to follow-up issues and concerns within a client's natural environments. For example, the Gator Tech Smart House (Mann & Milton, 2005) developed at the University of Florida provides an array of *self-m*onitoring *a*nalysis and *r*eporting *t*echnology (SMART) technologies that monitor and cue clients remotely. Examples include the SmartShoe (Naditz, 2009), which determines fall risk by analyzing walking behavior patterns in a client's own environment and sends the information to a remote site. Similarly, home exercise programs can be monitored remotely using a *haptic* (touch-sensitive) control interface to track a client's hand position while providing resistive forces remotely (Popescu, Burdea, Bouzit, & Hentz, 2000).

Tang and Venables (2000) used smartphones to deliver rehabilitation interventions remotely by using wireless Internet or Intranet access and by providing frequent prompts and cues regarding when and how to complete daily living occupations. Wireless technologies such as these are expanding opportunities for occupational therapy practitioners to implement interventions using telehealth technologies where clients live, work, and play and to provide services throughout the day rather than only within the occupational therapy clinic.

Appendix D provides case examples of how occupational therapy practitioners use telehealth technologies to support health and participation in occupations.

Practitioner Qualifications and Ethical Considerations

AOTA asserts that the same ethical and professional standards that apply to in-person delivery of occupational therapy services also apply to the delivery of services by means of telehealth technologies. Occupational therapy practitioners should refer to the *Occupational Therapy Code of Ethics and Ethics Standards (2010)* (AOTA, 2010a). As stated in this document, occupational therapy practitioners are responsible for ensuring their individual competence in the areas in which they provide services. In addition, Principle 1B of the *Code and Ethics Standards* states that "occupational therapy personnel shall provide appropriate evaluation and a plan of intervention for all recipients of occupational therapy services specific to their needs" (AOTA, 2010a, p. S19). This requirement reinforces the importance of careful consideration about whether evaluation or intervention through a telehealth service delivery model will best meet the client's needs and is the most appropriate method of providing services given the client's situation.

Clinical and ethical reasoning guides the selection and application of appropriate telehealth technology necessary to evaluate and meet client needs. Occupational therapy practitioners should consider whether the use of technology and service provision through telehealth will ensure the safe, effective, appropriate delivery of services. To determine whether providing occupational therapy by means of telehealth is in the best interest of the client, the occupational therapist must consider the following:

- Complexity of the client's condition

- Knowledge, skill, and competence of the occupational therapy practitioner

- Nature and complexity of the intervention

- Requirements of the practice setting

- Client's context and environment.

Additionally, the American Telemedicine Association's "A Blueprint for Telerehabilitation Guidelines" outlines important administrative, clinical, technical, and ethical principles associated with the use of telehealth (Brennan et al., 2010). Occupational therapy practitioners may use various educational approaches to gain competency in using telehealth technologies. They may gain an understanding about basic telehealth service delivery model and telehealth technologies as a part of entry-level education (Standard B.1.8; Accreditation Council for Occupational Therapy Education, 2012) or may participate in continuing education opportunities as clinicians to acquire expertise in this area (Theodorus & Russell, 2008). Examples of ethical considerations related to telehealth are outlined in Table 1.

The *Specialized Knowledge and Skills in Technology and Environmental Interventions for Occupational Therapy Practice* document (AOTA, 2010b) describes the knowledge and skills necessary for entry- and advanced-level practice in technology. Practitioners should have a working knowledge of the hardware, software, and other elements of the technology they are using and have technical support personnel available should problems arise (Schopp, Hales, Brown, & Quetsch, 2003). They should use evidence, mentoring, and continuing education to maintain and enhance their competency related to the use of a telehealth service delivery model within occupational therapy.

Supervision Using Telehealth Technologies

State licensure laws, institution-specific guidelines regarding supervision of occupational therapy students and personnel, the AOTA *Guidelines for Supervision, Roles, and Responsibilities During the Delivery of Occupational Therapy Services* (AOTA, 2009), and the *Occupational Therapy Code of Ethics and Ethics Standards (2010)* (AOTA, 2010a) must be followed, regardless of the method of supervision. Telehealth technologies may be used within those guidelines to the extent that they take into account the unique characteristics of telehealth supervision, to support students and practitioners working in isolated or rural areas (Miller, Miller,

Table 1. Ethical Considerations and Strategies for Practice Using Telehealth Technologies

ETHICAL CONSIDERATIONS	STRATEGIES FOR ETHICAL PRACTICE
Fully inform the client regarding the implications of a telehealth service delivery model versus an in-person service delivery model.	Occupational therapy personnel shall . . .
	"Establish a collaborative relationship with recipients of service including families, significant others, and caregivers in setting goals and priorities throughout the intervention process. This includes full disclosure of the benefits, risks, and potential outcomes of any intervention; the personnel who will be providing the intervention(s); and/or any reasonable alternatives to the proposed intervention." (Principle 3A)
	"Obtain consent before administering any occupational therapy service, including evaluation, and ensure that recipients of service (or their legal representatives) are kept informed of the progress in meeting goals specified in the plan of intervention/care." (Principle 3B)
Abide by laws and scope of practice related to licensure and provision of occupational therapy services using telehealth technologies.	"Occupational therapy personnel shall comply with institutional rules, local, state, federal, and international laws and AOTA documents applicable to the profession of occupational therapy." (Principle 5)
Adhere to professional standards.	Occupational therapy personnel shall . . .
	"Provide occupational therapy services that are within each practitioner's level of competence and scope of practice (e.g., qualification, experience, the law)." (Principle 1E)
	"Take responsible steps (e.g., continuing education, research, supervision, training) and use careful judgment to ensure their own competence and weigh potential for client harm when generally recognized standards do not exist in emerging technology or areas of practice." (Principle 1G)
	"Take responsibility for maintaining high standards and continuing competence in practice, education, and research by participating in professional development and educational activities to improve and update knowledge and skills." (Principle 5F)
	"Occupational therapy personnel shall comply with institutional rules, local, state, federal, and international laws and AOTA documents applicable to the profession of occupational therapy." (Principle 5)
Understand and abide by approaches that ensure that privacy, security, and confidentiality are not compromised as a result of using telehealth technologies.	Occupational therapy personnel shall . . .
	"Ensure that confidentiality and the right to privacy are respected and maintained regarding all information obtained about recipients of service, students, research participants, colleagues, or employees. The only exceptions are when a practitioner or staff member believes that an individual is in serious foreseeable or imminent harm. Laws and regulations may require disclosure to appropriate authorities without consent." (Principle 3G)
	"Maintain the confidentiality of all verbal, written, electronic, augmentative, and nonverbal communications, including compliance with HIPAA regulations." (Principle 3H)
Understand and adhere to procedures if there is any compromise of security related to health information.	Report any breach of security to an appropriate health privacy officer, or seek guidance of an independent legal counsel.

(Continued)

Table 1. Ethical Considerations and Strategies for Practice Using Telehealth Technologies *(cont.)*

ETHICAL CONSIDERATIONS	STRATEGIES FOR ETHICAL PRACTICE
Assess the effectiveness of interventions provided through telehealth technologies by consulting current research and conducting ongoing monitoring of client response.	Occupational therapy personnel shall . . . "Refer to other health care specialists solely on the basis of the needs of the client." (Principle 1I) "Reevaluate and reassess recipients of service in a timely manner to determine if goals are being achieved and whether intervention plans should be revised." (Principle 1C) "Use, to the extent possible, evaluation, planning, intervention techniques, and therapeutic equipment that are evidence-based and within the recognized scope of occupational therapy practice." (Principle 1F)
Recognize the need to be culturally competent in the provision of services via telehealth, including language, ethnicity, socioeconomic and educational background that could affect the quality and outcomes of services provided.	Occupational therapy personnel shall . . . "Provide services that reflect an understanding of how occupational therapy service delivery can be affected by factors such as economic status, age, ethnicity, race, geography, disability, marital status, sexual orientation, gender, gender identity, religion, culture, and political affiliation." (Principle 4F) "Make every effort to facilitate open and collaborative dialogue with clients and/or responsible parties to facilitate comprehension of services and their potential risks/benefits." (Principle 3J)

Note. HIPAA = Health Insurance Portability and Accountability Act of 1996 (Pub. L. 104–191). Ethical principles are from AOTA's (2010a) *Occupational Therapy Code of Ethics and Ethics Standards (2010).*

Burton, Sprang, & Adams, 2003; Hubbard, 2000). However, practitioners engaged in telehealth supervision should be cautious when relying on legal or other standards that were not necessarily established with telehealth supervision in mind. Factors that may affect the model of supervision and frequency of supervision include the complexity of client needs, number and diversity of clients, skills of the occupational therapist and the occupational therapy assistant, type of practice setting, requirements of the practice setting, and other regulatory requirements (AOTA, 2009). Supervision must comply with applicable state and federal practice regulations, state and federal insurance programs, relevant workplace policies, and the *Occupational Therapy Code of Ethics and Ethics Standards (2010)* (AOTA, 2010a).

Legal and Regulatory Considerations

Occupational therapy practitioners are to abide by state licensure laws and related occupational therapy regulations regarding the use of a telehealth service delivery model within occupational therapy (Cwiek, Rafiq, Qamar, Tobey, & Merrell, 2007). Given the inconsistent adoption and nonuniformity of language regarding the use of telehealth within occupational therapy, it is incumbent upon the practitioner to check a state's statutes, regulations, and policies before beginning to practice using a telehealth service delivery model. Typically, information may be found on state licensure boards' Web sites. The absence of statutes, regulations, or policies that guide the practice of occupational therapy by means of telehealth delivery should not be viewed as authorization to do so. State regulatory boards should be contacted directly in the absence of written guidance to determine the appropriateness of using telehealth technologies for the delivery of occupational therapy services within their jurisdictions. In addition, the policies and guidelines of payers should be consulted. At this time, occupational therapy practitioners are to comply with the licensure and regulatory requirements in the state where they are located and the state where the client is located (Cason & Brannon, 2011).

Occupational therapy practitioners are to abide by Health Insurance Portability and Accountability Act (HIPAA, 1996; Pub. L. 104–191) regulations to maintain security, privacy, and confidentiality of all records and interactions. Additional safeguards inherent in the use of technology to deliver occupational therapy services must be considered to ensure privacy and security of confidential information (Watzlaf, Moeini, & Firouzan, 2010; Watzlaf, Moeini, Matusow, & Firouzan, 2011). Occupational therapy practitioners are to consult with their practice setting's privacy officer or legal counsel or to consult with independent legal counsel if they are in independent or other practice outside of an institutional setting to ensure that the services they provide through telehealth are consistent with protocol and HIPAA regulations.

Funding and Reimbursement

It is the position of AOTA that occupational therapy services provided with telehealth technologies should be valued, recognized, and reimbursed the same as occupational therapy services provided in person. At this writing, Medicare does not list occupational therapy practitioners as eligible providers of services delivered through telehealth technologies. However, AOTA supports the inclusion of occupational therapy practitioners on Medicare's approved list of telehealth providers. The U.S. Department of Defense and Veteran's Health Administration use occupational therapy practitioners for select telehealth programming.

Opportunities for reimbursement exist through some state Medicaid programs; insurance companies; and private pay with individuals, school districts, agencies, and organizations. Medicaid reimbursement is available at the discretion of each state, because it is subject to specific requirements or restrictions within a state. It is recommended that occupational therapy practitioners contact their state Medicaid or other third-party payers to determine the guidelines for reimbursement of services provided through telehealth technologies.

When billing occupational therapy services provided by means of telehealth technologies, practitioners must distinguish the service delivery model, often designated with a *modifier* (Cason & Brannon, 2011). However, regardless of whether the services are reimbursed or the practitioner is responsible for completing paperwork related to billing, the nature of the service delivery as being performed through telehealth should be thoroughly documented.

Summary

Telehealth is a service delivery model that uses telecommunication technologies to deliver health-related services at a distance. Occupational therapy practitioners are using synchronous or asynchronous telehealth technologies to provide evaluative, consultative, preventative, and therapeutic services to clients who are physically distant from the practitioner. Occupational therapy practitioners using telehealth as a service delivery model must adhere to the *Occupational Therapy Code of Ethics and Ethics Standards (2010)* (AOTA, 2010a), maintain the *Standards of Practice for Occupational Therapy* (AOTA, 2010c), and comply with federal and state regulations to ensure their competencies as practitioners and the well-being of their clients.

Occupational therapy practitioners must give careful consideration as to whether evaluation or intervention through a telehealth service delivery model will best meet the client's needs and provide the most appropriate method of providing services given the individual's situation. Clinical and ethical reasoning guides the selection and application of appropriate telehealth technology necessary to evaluate and meet client needs.

References

Accreditation Council for Occupational Therapy Education. (2012). 2011 Accreditation Council for Occupational Therapy Education (ACOTE®) standards. *American Journal of Occupational Therapy, 66*(6, Suppl.), S6–S74. http://dx.doi.org/10.5014/ajot.2012.66S6

American Medical Association. (2011). *CPT 2012*. Chicago: Author.

American Occupational Therapy Association. (2006). Policy 1.44: Categories of occupational therapy personnel. In *Policy manual* (2009 ed., pp. 33–34). Bethesda, MD: Author.

American Occupational Therapy Association. (2009). Guidelines for supervision, roles, and responsibilities during the delivery of occupational therapy services. *American Journal of Occupational Therapy, 63,* 797–803. http://dx.doi.org/10.5014/ajot.63.6.797

American Occupational Therapy Association. (2010a). Occupational therapy code of ethics and ethics standards (2010). *American Journal of Occupational Therapy, 64*(6, Suppl.), S17–S26. http://dx.doi.org/ 10.5014/ ajot.2010.64S17

American Occupational Therapy Association. (2010b). Specialized knowledge and skills in technology and environmental interventions for occupational therapy practice. *American Journal of Occupational Therapy, 64*(6, Suppl.), S44–S56. http://dx.doi.org/10.5014/ajot.2010.64S44

American Occupational Therapy Association. (2010c). Standards of practice for occupational therapy. *American Journal of Occupational Therapy, 64*(6, Suppl.), S106–S111. http://dx.doi.org/10.5014/ajot.2010.64S106

American Occupational Therapy Association. (2010d). Telerehabilitation. *American Journal of Occupational Therapy, 64*(6, Suppl.), S92–S102. http://dx.doi.org/10.5014/ajot.2010.64S92

Backman, C. L., Village, J., & Lacaille, D. (2008). The Ergonomic Assessment Tool for arthritis: Development and pilot testing. *Arthritis and Rheumatism, 59,* 1495–1503. http://dx.doi.org/10.1002/art.24116

Baker, N., & Jacobs, K. (2010). Tele-ergonomics: A novel approach to computer workstation ergonomic assessment and modification. In *Proceedings of the Human Factors and Ergonomics Society 54th Annual Meeting (2010)* (p. 36). Santa Monica, CA: Human Factors and Ergonomics Society.

Baker, N., & Jacobs, K. (2013). Tele-ergonomics. In S. Kumar & E. Cohn (Eds.), *Telerehabilitation* (pp. 163–174). London: Springer.

Barlow, I. G., Liu, L., & Sekulic, A. (2009). Wheelchair seating assessment and intervention: A comparison between telerehabilitation and face-to-face service. *International Journal of Telerehabilitation, 1,* 17–28. http://dx.doi.org/10.5195/ijt.2009.868

Bendixen, R., Horn, K., & Levy, C. (2007). Using telerehabilitation to support elders with chronic illness in their homes. *Topics in Geriatric Rehabilitation, 23,* 47–51.

Bendixen, R., Levy, C., Lutz, B. J., Horn, K. R., Chronister, K., & Mann, W. C. (2008). A telerehabilitation model for victims of polytrauma. *Rehabilitation Nursing, 33,* 215–220. http://dx.doi.org/10.1002/j.2048-7940.2008.tb00230.x

Bendixen, R., Levy, C., Olive, E., Kobb, R., & Mann, W. (2009). Cost-effectiveness of a telerehabilitation program to support chronically ill and disabled elders in their homes. *Telemedicine and e-Health, 15,* 31–38. http://dx.doi.org/10.1089/tmj.2008.0046

Brennan, D., Tindall, L., Theodoros, D., Brown, J., Campbell, M., Christiana, D., . . . Lee, A. (2010). A blueprint for telerehabilitation guidelines. *International Journal of Telerehabilitation, 2,* 31–34. http://dx.doi.org/10.5195/ijt.2010.6063

Brewer, B. R., Fagan, M., Klatzky, R. L., & Matsuoka, Y. (2005). Perceptual limits for a robotic rehabilitation environment using visual feedback distortion. *IEEE Transactions on Neural Systems and Rehabilitation Engineering, 13,* 1–11. http://dx.doi.org/10.1109/TNSRE.2005.843443

Bruce, C., & Sanford, J. A. (2006). Development of an evidence-based conceptual framework for workplace assessment. *Work, 27,* 381–389.

Cason, J. (2009). A pilot telerehabilitation program: Delivering early intervention services to rural families. *International Journal of Telerehabilitation, 1,* 29–38. http://dx.doi.org/10.5195/ijt.2009.6007

Cason, J. (2011). Telerehabilitation: An adjunct service delivery model for early intervention services. *International Journal of Telerehabilitation, 3,* 19–28. http://dx.doi.org/10.5195/ijt.2011.6071

Cason, J. (2012a). An introduction to telehealth as a service delivery model within occupational therapy. *OT Practice, 17*(7), CE1–CE8.

Cason, J. (2012b). Telehealth opportunities in occupational therapy through the Affordable Care Act. *American Journal of Occupational Therapy, 66,* 131–136. http://dx.doi.org/10.5014/ajot.2012.662001

Cason, J., & Brannon, J. A. (2011). Telehealth regulatory and legal considerations: Frequently asked questions. *International Journal of Telerehabilitation, 3,* 15–18. http://dx.doi.org/10.5195/ijt.2011.6077

Chumbler, N., Quigley, P., Sanford, J., Griffiths, P., Rose, D., Morey, M., . . . Hoenig, H. (2010). Implementing telerehabilitation research for stroke rehabilitation with community dwelling veterans: Lessons learned. *International Journal of Telerehabilitation, 2,* 15–21. http://dx.doi.org/10.5195/ijt.2010.6047

Cooper, R., Fitzgerald, S., Boninger, M. L., Cooper, R. A., Shapcott, N., & Cohen, L. (2002). Using telerehabilitation to aid in selecting a wheelchair. In R. Simpson (Ed.), *RESNA 2002 annual conference proceedings* (pp. 245–247). Minneapolis, MN: RESNA Press.

Cwiek, M. A., Rafiq, A., Qamar, A., Tobey, C., & Merrell, R. C. (2007). Telemedicine licensure in the United States: The need for a cooperative regional approach. *Telemedicine and e-Health, 13,* 141–147. http://dx.doi.org/10.1089/tmj.2006.0029

Darkins, A., Ryan, P., Kobb, R., Forster, L., Edmonson, E., Wakefield, B., & Lancaster, A. E. (2008). Care coordination/home telehealth: The systematic implementation of health informatics, home telehealth, and disease management to support the care of veteran patients with chronic conditions. *Telemedicine and e-Health, 14,* 1118–1126. http://dx.doi.org/10.1089/tmj.2008.0021

Diamond, B. J., Shreve, G. M., Bonilla, J. M., Johnston, M. V., Morodan, J., & Branneck, R. (2003). Telerehabilitation, cognition and user accessibility. *NeuroRehabilitation, 18,* 171–177.

Dreyer, N. C., Dreyer, K. A., Shaw, D. K., & Wittman, P. P. (2001). Efficacy of telemedicine in occupational therapy: A pilot study. *Journal of Allied Health, 30,* 39–42.

Federal Communications Commission. (2010). *Voice-over-Internet protocol.* Retrieved from www.fcc.gov/voip/

Forducey, P. G., Ruwe, W. D., Dawson, S. J., Scheideman-Miller, C., McDonald, N. B., & Hantla, M. R. (2003). Using telerehabilitation to promote TBI recovery and transfer of knowledge. *NeuroRehabilitation, 18,* 103–111.

Gallagher, T. E. (2004). Augmentation of special-needs services and information to students and teachers "ASSIST"—A telehealth innovation providing school-based medical interventions. *Hawaii Medical Journal, 63,* 300–309.

Germain, V., Marchand, A., Bouchard, S., Drouin, M. S., & Guay, S. (2009). Effectiveness of cognitive behavioural therapy administered by videoconference for posttraumatic stress disorder. *Cognitive Behaviour Therapy, 38,* 42–53. http://dx.doi.org/10.1080/16506070802473494

Girard, P. (2007). Military and VA telemedicine systems for patients with traumatic brain injury. *Journal of Rehabilitation Research and Development, 44,* 1017–1026. http://dx.doi.org/10.1682/JRRD.2006.12.0174

Gros, D. F., Yoder, M., Tuerk, P. W., Lozano, B. E., & Acierno, R. (2011). Exposure therapy for PTSD delivered to veterans via telehealth: Predictors of treatment completion and outcome and comparison to treatment delivered in person. *Behavior Therapy, 42,* 276–283. http://dx.doi.org/10.1016/j.beth.2010.07.005

Harada, N. D., Dhanani, S., Elrod, M., Hahn, T., Kleinman, L., & Fang, M. (2010). Feasibility study of home telerehabilitation for physically inactive veterans. *Journal of Rehabilitation Research and Development, 47,* 465–475. http://dx.doi.org/10.1682/JRRD.2009.09.0149

Harrison, A., Derwent, G., Enticknap, A., Rose, F. D., & Attree, E. A. (2002). The role of virtual reality technology in the assessment and training of inexperienced powered wheelchair users. *Disability and Rehabilitation, 24,* 599–606. http://dx.doi.org/10.1080/09638280110111360

Health Insurance Portability and Accountability Act, Pub. L. 104–191, 101 Stat. 1936 (1996).

Hegel, M. T., Lyons, K. D., Hull, J. G., Kaufman, P., Urguhart, L., Li, Z., & Ahles, T. A. (2011). Feasibility study of a randomized controlled trial of a telephone-delivered problem solving occupational therapy intervention to reduce participation restrictions in rural breast cancer survivors undergoing chemotherapy. *Psycho-Oncology, 20,* 1092–1101. http://dx.doi.org/10.1002/pon.1830

Heimerl, S., & Rasch, N. (2009). Delivering developmental occupational therapy consultation services through telehealth. *Developmental Disabilities Special Interest Section Quarterly, 32*(3), 1–4.

Hermann, V. H., Herzog, M., Jordan, R., Hofherr, M., Levine, P., & Page, S. J. (2010). Telerehabilitation and electrical stimulation: An occupation-based, client-centered stroke intervention. *American Journal of Occupational Therapy, 64,* 73–81. http://dx.doi.org/10.5014/ajot.64.1.73

Hoffman, H. G., Patterson, D. R., & Carrougher, G. J. (2000). Use of virtual reality for adjunctive treatment of adult burn pain during physical therapy: A controlled study. *Clinical Journal of Pain, 16,* 244–250. http://dx.doi.org/10.1097/00002508-200009000-00010

Hoffmann, T., Russell, T., Thompson, L., Vincent, A., & Nelson, M. (2008). Using the Internet to assess activities of daily living and hand function in people with Parkinson's disease. *NeuroRehabilitation, 23,* 253–261.

Hori, M., Kubota, M., Kihara, T., Takahashi, R., & Kinoshita, A. (2009). The effect of videophone communication (with Skype and webcam) for elderly patients with dementia and their caregivers. *Gan To Kagaku Ryoho, 36S,* 36–38. Retrieved from www.ncbi.nlm.nih.gov/pubmed/20443395

Hubbard, S. (2000, December 4 & 18). A case example of remote supervision. *OT Practice, 5,* 16–18.

Individuals With Disabilities Education Act Amendments of 1997, Pub. L. 105–117, 20 U.S.C. § 1400 *et seq.*

Kairy, D., Lehoux, P., Vincent, C., & Visintin, M. (2009). A systematic review of clinical outcomes, clinical process, healthcare utilization and costs associated with telerehabilitation. *Disability and Rehabilitation, 31,* 427–47. http://dx.doi.org/10.1080/09638280802062553

Kelso, G., Fiechtl, B., Olsen, S., & Rule, S. (2009). The feasibility of virtual home visits to provide early intervention: A pilot study. *Infants and Young Children, 22,* 332–340. http://dx.doi.org/10.1097/IYC.0b013e3181b9873c

Kim, J. B., & Brienza, D. M. (2006). Development of a remote accessibility assessment system through three-dimensional reconstruction technology. *Journal of Rehabilitation Research and Development, 43,* 257–272. http://dx.doi.org/10.1682/JRRD.2004.12.0163

Kim, J. B., Brienza, D. M., Lynch, R. D., Cooper, R. A., & Boninger, M. L. (2008). Effectiveness evaluation of a remote accessibility assessment system for wheelchair users using virtualized reality. *Archives of Physical Medicine and Rehabilitation, 89,* 470–479. http://dx.doi.org/10.1016/j.apmr.2007.08.158

Lewis, J. A., Boian, R. F., Burdea, G., & Deutsch, J. E. (2005). Remote console for virtual telerehabilitation. *Studies in Health Technology and Informatics, 111,* 294–300.

Lewis, J. A., Deutsch, J. E., & Burdea, G. (2006). Usability of the remote console for virtual reality telerehabilitation: Formative evaluation. *Cyberpsychology and Behavior, 9,* 142–147. http://dx.doi.org/10.1089/cpb.2006.9.142

Mann, W. C., & Milton, B. R. (2005). Home automation and SMART homes to support independence. In W. C. Mann (Ed.), *Smart technology for aging, disability, and independence* (pp. 33–66). Hoboken, NJ: Wiley.

Merians, A. S., Jack, D., Boian, R., Tremaine, M., Burdea, G. C., Adamovich, S. V., . . . Poizner, H. (2002). Virtual reality–augmented rehabilitation for patients following stroke. *Physical Therapy, 82,* 898–915.

Miller, T. W., Miller, J. M., Burton, D., Sprang, R., & Adams, J. (2003). Telehealth: A model for clinical supervision in allied health. *Internet Journal of Allied Health Sciences and Practice, 1*(2), 1–8.

Naditz, A. (2009). Still standing: Telemedicine devices and fall prevention. *Telemedicine and e-Health, 15,* 137–141. http://dx.doi.org/10.1089/tmj.2009.9989

Neubeck, L., Redfern, J., Fernandez, R., Briffad, T., Bauman, A., & Freedman, S. B. (2009). Telehealth interventions for the secondary prevention of coronary heart disease: A systematic review. *European Journal of Preventive Cardiology, 16,* 281–289. http://dx.doi.org/0.1097/HJR.0b013e32832a4e7a

Palsbo, S. E., Dawson, S. J., Savard, L., Goldstein, M., & Heuser, A. (2007). Televideo assessment using Functional Reach Test and European Stroke Scale. *Journal of Rehabilitation Research and Development, 44,* 659–664. http://dx.doi.org/10.1682/JRRD.2006.11.0144

Popescu, V. G., Burdea, G. C., Bouzit, M., & Hentz, V. R. (2000). A virtual-reality-based telerehabilitation system with force feedback. *IEEE Transactions on Information Technology in Biomedicine, 4,* 45–51. http://dx.doi.org/10.1109/4233.826858

Rand, D., Katz, N., & Weiss, P. L. (2009). Intervention using the VMall for improving motor and functional ability of the upper extremity in poststroke participants. *European Journal of Physical and Rehabilitation Medicine, 45,* 113–121.

Rand, D., Kizony, R., & Weiss, P. T. (2008). The Sony PlayStation II EyeToy: Low-cost virtual reality for use in rehabilitation. *Journal of Neurologic Physical Therapy, 32,* 155–163. http://dx.doi.org/10.1097/NPT.0b013e31818ee779

Rand, D., Weiss, P. L., & Katz, N. (2009). Training multitasking in a virtual supermarket: A novel intervention after stroke. *American Journal of Occupational Therapy, 63,* 535–542. http://dx.doi.org/10.5014/ajot.63.5.535

Sanford, J., Hoenig, H., Griffiths, P., Butterfield, T., Richardson, P., & Hargraves, K. (2007). A comparison of televideo and traditional in-home rehabilitation in mobility impaired older adults. *Physical and Occupational Therapy in Geriatrics, 25,* 1–18. http://dx.doi.org/10.1080/J148v25n03_01

Savard, L., Borstad, A., Tkachuck, J., Lauderdale, D., & Conroy, B. (2003). Telerehabilitation consultations for clients with neurologic diagnoses: Cases from rural Minnesota and American Samoa. *NeuroRehabilitation, 18,* 93–102.

Scheideman-Miller, C., Clark, P. G., Moorad, A., Post, M. L., Hodge, B. G., & Smeltzer, S. (2003, January). Efficacy and sustainability of a telerehabilitation program. In *Proceedings of the 36th Annual Hawaii International Conference on System Sciences* (pp. 11–21). Washington, DC: IEEE Computer Society.

Schein, R. M., Schmeler, M. R., Brienza, D., Saptono, A., & Parmanto, B. (2008). Development of a service delivery protocol used for remote wheelchair consultation via telerehabilitation. *Telemedicine and e-Health, 14,* 932–938.

Schein, R. M., Schmeler, M. R., Holm, M. B., Pramuka, M., Saptono, A., & Brienza, D. M. (2011). Telerehabilitation assessment using the Functioning Everyday with a Wheelchair-Capacity instrument. *Journal of Rehabilitation Research and Development, 48,* 115–124. http://dx.doi.org/10.1682/JRRD.2010.03.0039

Schein, R. M., Schmeler, M. R., Holm, M. B., Saptono, A., & Brienza, D. M. (2010). Telerehabilitation wheeled mobility and seating assessments compared with in person. *Archives of Physical Medicine and Rehabilitation, 91,* 874–878. http://dx.doi.org/10.1016/j.apmr.2010.01.017

Schmeler, M. R., Schein, R. M., McCue, M., & Betz, K. (2009). Telerehabilitation and clinical applications: Research, opportunities, and challenges. *International Journal of Telerehabilitation, 1,* 59–72. http://dx.doi.org/10.5195/ijt.2009.6014

Schopp, L. H., Hales, J. W., Brown, G. D., & Quetsch, J. L. (2003). A rationale and training agenda for rehabilitation informatics: Roadmap for an emerging discipline. *NeuroRehabilitation, 18,* 159–170.

Sheridan, T. B. (1992). Musings on telepresence and virtual presence. *Presence, 1,* 120–125.

Steel, K., Cox, D., & Garry, H. (2011). Therapeutic videoconferencing interventions for the treatment of long-term conditions. *Journal of Telemedicine and Telecare, 17,* 109–117. http://dx.doi.org/ 10.1258/ jtt.2010.100318

Tang, P., & Venables, T. (2000). "Smart" homes and telecare for independent living. *Journal of Telemedicine and Telecare, 6,* 8–14. http://dx.doi.org/10.1258/1357633001933871

Theodorus, D., & Russell, T. (2008). Telerehabilitation: Current perspectives. *Current Principles and Practices of Telemedicine and e-Health, 131,* 191–209.

Verburg, G., Borthwick, B., Bennett, B., & Rumney, P. (2003). Online support to facilitate the reintegration of students with brain injury: Trials and errors. *NeuroRehabilitation, 18,* 113–123.

Wakeford, L. (2002, November 25). Telehealth technology for children with special needs. *OT Practice, 7,* 12–16.

Watzlaf, V., Moeini, S., & Firouzan, P. (2010). VoIP for telerehabilitation: A risk analysis for privacy, security, and HIPAA compliance, Part I. *International Journal of Telerehabilitation, 2,* 3–14. http://dx.doi.org/ 10.5195/ijt.2010.6056

Watzlaf, V., Moeini, S., Matusow, L., & Firouzan, P. (2011). VoIP for telerehabilitation: A risk analysis for privacy, security, and HIPAA compliance, Part II. *International Journal of Telerehabilitation, 3,* 3–10. http:// dx.doi.org/10.5195/ijt.2011.6070

Weiss, P. L., & Jessel, A. S. (1998). Virtual reality applications to work. *Work, 11,* 277–293.

Whelan, L., & Wagner, N. (2011). Technology that touches lives: Teleconsultation to benefit persons with upper limb loss. *International Journal of Telerehabilitation, 3,* 19–22. http://dx.doi.org/10.5195/ijt.2011.6080

Winters, J. M. (2002). Telerehabilitation research: Emerging opportunities. *Annual Review of Biomedical Engineering, 4,* 287–320. http://dx.doi.org/10.1146/annurev.bioeng.4.112801.121923

Additional Resources

American Telemedicine Association's Telerehabilitation Special Interest Group/Resources, www.americantelemed.org/i4a/pages/index.cfm?pageid=3328

Center for Telehealth and e-Health Law (CTel), http://ctel.org/

International Journal of Telerehabilitation, http://telerehab.pitt.edu/ojs/index.php/telerehab

Journal of Telemedicine and Telecare, http://jtt.rsmjournals.com/

Rehabilitation Engineering Research Center for Telerehabilitation, www.rerctr.pitt.edu

Telehealth Resource Centers, www.telehealthresourcecenter.org/

Telemedicine and e-Health, www.liebertpub.com/TMJ

Authors

Jana Cason, DHS, OTR/L, FAOTA
Kim Hartmann, PhD, OTR/L, FAOTA
Karen Jacobs, EdD, CPE, OTR/L, FAOTA
Tammy Richmond, MS, OTR/L, FAOTA

for

The Commission on Practice
Debbie Amini, EdD, OTR/L, CHT, *Chairperson*

The COP would like to acknowledge the contributions of the authors of the 2010 Telerehabilitation
Position Paper:
Mark R. Schmeler, PhD, OTR/L, ATP
Richard M. Schein, PhD
Andrea Fairman, MOT, OTR/L, CPRP
Amanda Brickner, MOT, OTR/L
William C. Mann, PhD, OTR

Adopted by the Representative Assembly Coordinating Council (RACC) for the Representative Assembly, 2012

Revised by the Commission on Practice 2012

Appendix A. Overview of Telehealth Technologies

Synchronous Technologies: Videoconferencing

Synchronous technologies enable the exchange of health information in *real time* (i.e., live) by interactive audio and video between the patient or client and a health care provider located at a distant site. Several options for videoconferencing are available; they include voice over the Internet protocol (VoIP) services, mobile videoconferencing systems, "plain old telephone service" (POTS), videoconferencing, and high-definition television (HDTV) technologies (see Table A1).

VoIP services use a computer, special VoIP phone, or traditional phone with adapter to convert voice into a digital signal that travels over the Internet (Federal Communications Commission, 2010). Integrated with video software, VoIP provides a mechanism for Internet-based videoconferencing. Similarly, mobile video-conferencing uses a mobile device (e.g., smartphone, electronic tablet) with videoconferencing capabilities to transmit audio and video over a wireless or cellular network. POTS videoconferencing primarily uses an analog telephone line or landline to support audio and video transmission through a videophone or specialized equipment connected to a television. HDTV videoconferencing requires an HD television, console, HD camera, remote control, and high-speed broadband connection at both locations. Unlike the technologies described above and marketed for consumer use, telehealth networks use high-end videoconferencing technologies (e.g., Polycom, Tandberg) and fiber-optic telephone lines (e.g., T1 lines) or high-speed Internet to connect sites.

Advantages of VoIP, mobile, POTS, and consumer HDTV technologies include service provision within the context where occupations naturally occur (e.g., home, work, community), minimal infrastructure requirements, and lower costs for equipment and connectivity (e.g., residential service plan, data plan). Disadvantages may include privacy, security, and confidentiality risks; lack of infrastructure (e.g., limited access to high-speed Internet/broadband; inadequate bandwidth for connectivity); recurring expense (e.g., residential service plan, data plan); diminished sound or image quality; and technological challenges associated with end-user experience and expertise with videoconferencing technology (Cason, 2011; see Table A1).

Asynchronous Technologies

Telehealth applications that are asynchronous, commonly referred to as "store-and-forward" data transmission, may include video clips, digital photographs, virtual technologies, and other forms of electronic communications. With *asynchronous technologies,* the provider and client are not connected at the same time. Potential applications for asynchronous telehealth technologies within occupational therapy include home assessments and recommendations for home modifications that are based on recorded data of the home environment; recommendations for inclusion of ergonomic principles and workstation modifications that are based on recorded data of the work environment; and secure viewing of video segments for evaluation and intervention purposes.

Technologies That May Be Synchronous or Asynchronous

Telemonitoring Technologies

Occupational therapy practitioners providing services through telehealth technologies can take advantage of *self-m*onitoring *a*nalysis and *r*eporting *t*echnology (SMART) to monitor a client's occupational performance within the home and community. SMART technologies that are wireless allow the occupational therapy practitioner to provide services within varied environments without restricting the client's movements within those environments. These technologies provide information that allows an offsite occupational therapy practitioner to assess performance and modify services and the environment and also enable occupational therapy practitioners to understand the real-life occupations and performance challenges of the client and to plan appropriate interventions. As a result, occupational therapy practitioners can tailor environmental accommodations for clients with physical limitations or can develop individualized technology-based cueing systems for clients with cognitive disabilities so that they can live more independently.

Virtual Reality Technologies

Virtual reality (VR) typically refers to the use of interactive simulations created with computer hardware and software to present users with opportunities to engage in environments that appear and feel similar to real-world objects and events (Sheridan, 1992; Weiss & Jessel, 1998). Although typical use of VR technologies does not constitute a telehealth service delivery model, live data (synchronous) streamed to a remote occupational therapy practitioner or recorded data (asynchronous) used by an occupational therapy practitioner to monitor and adjust a client's course of treatment would constitute the use of VR technologies within a telehealth service delivery model. Occupational therapy practitioners can use a telehealth service delivery model with VR technologies when conducting evaluations and providing interventions. A remote console telerehabilitation system (ReCon, Rutgers University, New Brunswick, NJ) incorporating VR technology provides occupational therapy practitioners with three-dimensional representations of the client's movements, VR-based exercise progress, and motor performance updates (Lewis, Boian, Burdea, & Deutsch, 2005; Lewis, Deutsch, & Burdea, 2006). Telehealth combined with VR has been used to provide feedback and information remotely as part of occupational therapy intervention (Merians et al., 2002), to distract people from physical pain, and to improve their adherence to therapeutic exercises (Hoffman, Patterson, & Carrougher, 2000).

Further, VR provided through telehealth technologies is effective in enabling people to compare the difference between their desired level of occupational engagement and their current functional status after a stroke (Brewer, Fagan, Klatzky, & Matsuoka, 2005; Merians et al., 2002; Rand, Katz, & Weiss, 2009; Rand, Weiss, & Katz, 2009), using virtual environments as part of the assessment and training of users of power wheelchairs (Harrison, Derwent, Enticknap, Rose, & Attree, 2002), and evaluating and determining home accessibility using three-dimensional construction of the architectural features of the environment (Kim & Brienza, 2006; Kim, Brienza, Lynch, Cooper, & Boninger, 2008).

Low-cost video capture gaming systems (e.g., Nintendo Wii, Sony Playstation's EyeToy and MOVE, XBOX-360 Kinect) were not developed specifically for rehabilitation, but they offer an easy-to-set-up, fun, and less expensive alternative to the expensive VR systems (Rand, Kizony, & Weiss, 2008). Although typical use of gaming systems does not constitute telehealth, live data (synchronous) streamed to a remote occupational therapy practitioner or recorded data (asynchronous) used by an occupational therapy practitioner to monitor and adjust a client's course of treatment would constitute a telehealth application of the devices.

Table A1. Telehealth Technologies

TECHNOLOGY TYPE	EXAMPLES	CONSIDERATIONS
Synchronous	• Voice over Internet protocol software • Mobile videoconferencing • Consumer high-definition television videoconferencing • "Plain old telephone service" • Videoconferencing • Telehealth network with commercial videoconferencing system • Virtual reality (VR) technologies (with live-streaming data to remote practitioner)	• Confidentiality (security, privacy) • Integrity (information protected from changes by unauthorized users) • Availability (information, services) • Cost–benefit ratio • Socioeconomic considerations • Leveraging existing infrastructure (equipment and personnel) • Technology connection requirements (e.g., broadband, T1 line) • Sound and image quality
Asynchronous	• Video recording devices • Cameras (photographs) • Devices enabling electronic communication • VR technologies (with store-and-forward data to remote practitioner)	• Equipment accessibility • Provider and end-user comfort, experience, and expertise with technology

Synchronous (interactive) or asynchronous (store-and-forward data)	• Telemonitoring technologies
	  – Home monitoring systems/devices
	  – Wireless sensors
	• VR technologies
	  – Remote use of VR systems/devices	

Note. From "Telerehabilitation: An Adjunct Service Delivery Model for Early Intervention Services," by J. Cason, 2011, *International Journal of Telerehabilitation, 3*(1), p. 24. http://dx.doi.org/10.5195/ijt.2011.6071 Copyright © 2011 by Jana Cason. Adapted with permission.

Appendix B. Glossary

asynchronous—A method of exchanging health information whereby the provider and patient or client are not connected at the same time; commonly referred to as "store-and-forward" data transmission and may include video clips, digital photographs, virtual technologies, and other forms of electronic communications.

eHealth—A broad term encompassing health-related information and educational resources (e.g., health literacy Web sites and repositories, videos, blogs), commercial "products" (e.g., apps), and direct services delivered electronically (often through the Internet) by professionals, nonprofessionals, businesses, or consumers. May also be written as *e-Health* or *E-Health;* sometimes used interchangeably with *health informatics.*

haptic technology—A tactile feedback technology that takes advantage of a user's sense of touch by applying forces, vibrations, or motions upon the user.

health informatics—Use of information technologies for health care data collection, storage, and analysis to enhance health care decisions and improve quality and efficiency of health care services.

mHealth—The delivery of health-related information and services using mobile communication technology (e.g., smartphone, electronic tablet, or other mobile devices).

modifier—A modifier used in conjunction with a *Current Procedural Terminology* (American Medical Association, 2011) code to identify the type of technology used within a telehealth service delivery model. GT is the most common modifier; it indicates use of interactive audio and video telecommunications technology. The GQ modifier designates the use of asynchronous technologies; reimbursement for this modifier is limited.

privacy officer—A position or office that responds to concerns over the use of personal information, including medical data and financial information. It ensures adherence to regulations but is not limited to legislation concerning the protection of patient medical records (e.g., Health Insurance Portability and Accountability Act of 1996, Pub. L. 104–191).

protocol—A written document specifying standard operating policies and procedures for application of telehealth technologies in delivering services.

synchronous—A method of exchanging health information in real time (i.e., live) between the patient or client and a health care provider located at a distant site.

telehealth—The application of evaluative, consultative, preventative, and therapeutic services delivered through telecommunication and information technologies.

telehealth technologies—The hardware and software used in delivering services remotely by means of a telehealth service delivery model.

telemedicine—Medical services delivered through communication and information technologies.

telerehabilitation—The application of telecommunication and information technologies for the delivery of rehabilitation services.

virtual reality A computer-simulated environment of the real world; can be coupled with telehealth technologies as part of a telehealth service delivery model.

Appendix C. Applications of Telehealth Within Occupational Therapy Practice Areas

Children and Youth

Evidence supports the use of a telehealth service delivery model to deliver appropriate early intervention (EI) and school-based services effectively and efficiently. EI services, mandated by Part C of the Individuals With Disabilities Education Act Amendments of 1997 (IDEA; Pub. L. 105–117), are designed to promote development of skills and enhance the quality of life of infants and toddlers who have been identified as having a disability or developmental delay (Cason, 2011). Telehealth technology supports delivery of EI services (Cason, 2009, 2011; Heimerl & Rasch, 2009; Kelso, Fiechtl, Olsen, & Rule, 2009).

Similarly, evidence supports the use of telehealth for the delivery of occupational therapy services within the school setting for evaluation and intervention (Gallagher, 2004) as well as for reintegration of students with traumatic injury following acute rehabilitation (Verburg, Borthwick, Bennett, & Rumney, 2003). Telehealth may be used within school-based interprofessional team models for wellness programming, including efforts to combat the obesity epidemic among children and for programming targeting prevention of violence among youth (Cason, 2012b). School-based occupational therapy services focus on helping children with disabilities participate in and, thus, benefit from the instructional program.

In addition to what has been stated, telehealth technology may provide another avenue for the occupational therapy practitioner to observe the child's level of participation in a school setting without risk of altering the setting by being physically present. This unobtrusive observation strategy can allow the occupational therapy practitioner to consult with the teacher and offer strategies to alter the child's level of participation (e.g., strategies to facilitate a child's use of self-regulation skills, encourage appropriate interaction with peers, or facilitate the child's physical participation in an instructional activity).

The potential benefit of this observation strategy is to ensure the maintenance of the day-to-day integrity of the classroom while providing the practitioner with an understanding of the specific sensory, cognitive, physical, and emotional demands placed on the child in the setting. This technology may also provide the ability to record observations that contribute to the therapist's data collection during evaluation; this information can then be used as a baseline from which to support Individualized Education Program teams in developing goals and objectives and measuring progress in the child's level of participation in the setting. In rural or large urban school districts, this technology can assist the occupational therapy practitioner with more efficiently supporting multiple campuses that may be located across large distances, thereby facilitating the interprofessional team process as well as reducing costs incurred to allow a practitioner the time and transportation resources to support multiple campuses.

Productive Aging

The growing number of older adults in the United States creates opportunities for occupational therapy practitioners to use telehealth to promote health and wellness, prevention, and productive aging while reducing health care costs. The use of telerehabilitation to remotely monitor and provide self-management strategies to older adults who are chronically ill and living in their homes has been found to decrease hospitalizations and nursing home stays (Bendixen, Levy, Olive, Kobb, & Mann, 2009). Interactive videoconferencing technologies promote health and aging in place among older adults (Bendixen, Horn, & Levy, 2007; Harada et al., 2010; Hori, Kubota, Kihara, Takahashi, & Kinoshita, 2009). The use of home monitoring devices such as *self-m*onitoring *a*nalysis and *r*eporting *t*echnology (SMART) enable occupational therapy practitioners to remotely monitor clients' occupational performance and provide recommendations for environmental modifications and interventions to support occupational performance (Mann & Milton, 2005).

Health and Wellness

Telehealth also supports health and wellness and prevention programming through assessment and management of obesity (Neubeck et al., 2009) and chronic diseases such as diabetes mellitus, congestive heart failure, and hypertension (Darkins et al., 2008; Steel, Cox, & Garry, 2011).

Mental Health

Opportunities exist for occupational therapy practitioners to use telehealth to promote participation and psychological and social functioning for clients within the home, at work, and in the community through engagement in meaningful occupations. Research demonstrates efficacy of telehealth as a delivery model for psychological and behavioral interventions among individuals with posttraumatic stress disorder (PTSD) and other mental health issues (Germain, Marchand, Bouchard, Drouin, & Guay, 2009; Gros, Yoder, Tuerk, Lozano, & Acierno, 2011).

Rehabilitation, Disability, and Participation

In the practice area of rehabilitation, disability, and participation, the use of a telehealth service delivery model promotes occupational performance, adaptation, participation, and quality of life for clients with polytrauma, neurological, and orthopedic conditions. Telehealth provides remote access to occupational therapy services through assessment of physical function and goal setting, integration of individualized exercise interventions, training in adaptive strategies such as environmental modifications and energy conservation, and consultation on durable medical and adaptive equipment (Chumbler et al., 2010; Sanford et al., 2007).

Published studies support the use of telehealth in improving functional outcomes with individuals with stroke (Chumbler et al., 2010; Hermann et al., 2010), survivors of breast cancer (Hegel et al., 2011), veterans with polytrauma (Bendixen et al., 2008), and individuals with traumatic brain injury (Diamond et al., 2003; Forducey et al., 2003; Girard, 2007; Verburg et al., 2003). Additional studies have used a telehealth service delivery model to evaluate activities of daily living and hand function in individuals with Parkinson's disease (Hoffman, Russell, Thompson, Vincent, & Nelson, 2008) and other neurological impairments (Savard, Borstad, Tkachuck, Lauderdale, & Conroy, 2003). Seating experts used telehealth to provide remote wheelchair prescription and consultation to individuals with neurological and orthopedic conditions (Barlow, Liu, & Sekulic, 2009; Schein, Schmeler, Holm, Saptono, & Brienza, 2010; Schein et al., 2011). In addition to positive clinical outcomes, evidence indicates a high level of practitioner and client satisfaction associated with a telehealth service delivery model (Kairy, Lehoux, Vincent, & Visintin, 2009; Steel et al., 2011).

Work and Industry

Schmeler, Schein, McCue, and Betz (2009) detailed the use of assistive technology via a telehealth service delivery model for clinical and vocational applications. Telehealth is also being used to support work through remote assessment and analysis of work spaces. Bruce and Sanford (2006) described using teleconferencing to complete remote assessments and discussed the need for a highly structured and comprehensive assessment tool to be able to complete remote assessments.

Backman, Village, and Lacaille (2008) developed the Ergonomic Assessment Tool for Arthritis (EATA) to evaluate the workplace for people with arthritis. The EATA was designed so that the worker could gather the data for the assessment without an expert visiting the workplace. Pilot testing of the method indicated that workers could successfully gather the necessary information for appropriate intervention identification (Baker & Jacobs, 2013). Baker and Jacobs (2010) developed a systematic two-step program, the Telerehabilitation Computer Ergonomics System *(tele-CES)*. This systematic program will allow ergonomically trained health professionals to (1) remotely assess the computer workstation and (2) on basis of the assessment, generate explicit, participant-specific workstation modification recommendations. The recommendations will be easily implemented; reduce pain, discomfort, and fatigue; and eliminate barriers to productivity.

Appendix D. Telehealth Case Examples

CASE DESCRIPTION	USE OF TELEHEALTH	OUTCOME
Lisa is a 70-year-old woman who has difficulty performing her daily occupations because of a stroke resulting in right-sided weakness. Although she had learned compensatory techniques for completing activities of daily living (ADLs), instrumental ADLs, and work, she still wants to increase the use of her right hand, particularly for tasks related to managing her farm. Lisa learned of a program in a nearby community using new technology that might be beneficial for people with hemiparesis; however, the clinic is 2 hours from her home.	Lisa meets with her occupational therapist in a clinic for the initial evaluation. During the evaluation, Lisa learns additional strategies for incorporating the use of her right hand to perform her farm work. She is fitted for a functional electrical stimulation orthosis that she can use at home once it is programmed in the clinic. Twice each week, Lisa meets with her occupational therapist by computer, using a Web camera and online video software. As Lisa continues to make progress, the occupational therapist instructs her in how to more effectively use her right hand for completion of ADLs and farm chores.	Lisa is able to make functional gains in using her right hand for everyday occupations. She reports that she is able to rely less on compensatory strategies and use her right hand more easily, especially while completing ADLs. Lisa achieved these outcomes with only two trips to the clinic and without therapist travel.
José is a 35-year-old administrative assistant working at an urban university. He has been employed in this position for 5 years. Recently, he began experiencing discomfort in his neck, shoulder, and back areas. He reported this discomfort, which he associated with computer work, to his immediate supervisor.	Josh scheduled an appointment with an occupational therapist who had expertise in ergonomic workstation evaluation. During his initial contact with the occupational therapist, he requested that because of his busy schedule, he would prefer to have his evaluation conducted through telehealth technology. The occupational therapist asked Josh to have photographs taken of him while working at his office computer workstation. The occupational therapist requested that the photographs be from multiple angles and then e-mailed to a secure platform, where the therapist would be able to review them. In addition, Josh was asked to keep a time log for a week into which he would input information on his activities along with when he experienced discomfort. A telephone consultation was arranged, during which the occupational therapist reviewed findings from the photographs along with the time log. Josh reported on the time log that he sat at his computer workstation 100% of the time during the work day. During this time, he multitasked by using a hand-held telephone while keying. It was observed from the photographs that Josh was using a notebook computer, which placed him in an awkward posture for computing.	Explicit workstation modification recommendations were provided by the occupational therapist by means of a telephone consultation with Josh. The recommendations included raising the notebook computer so that his head was not positioned in flexion or extension and that the monitor was about arm's length away (closed fist) and using a keyboard and mouse as input devices. An adjustable keyboard tray was recommended for the keyboard and mouse. On the basis of data from the time log, the occupational therapist encouraged Josh to change his work behaviors by taking regular stretch breaks every 20 minutes. A second telephone consultation occurred within 2 weeks. Josh reported that his supervisor ordered the external notebook computer accessories and that this new workstation arrangement had reduced his discomfort.

(Continued)

Appendix D. Telehealth Case Examples *(cont.)*

CASE DESCRIPTION	USE OF TELEHEALTH	OUTCOME
Angela is a 10-year-old girl with a complicated medical history that includes spina bifida. She is significantly limited in her ability to be mobile in the home and community. Although she uses a basic power wheelchair to drive around town and attend her family activities, it is in poor condition and too small for her. Angela cannot adequately reposition herself or properly perform a weight shift because of decreased upper-extremity strength and range of motion.	Angela has trouble traveling and sitting for long distances. She and her mother meet with an occupational therapy generalist in person at a nearby clinic. Concurrently, an occupational therapist who has expertise in wheeled mobility participates in an occupational therapy session remotely using a videoconferencing system. The remote occupational therapist provides consultation to the local occupational therapist, Angela, and her mother about seating system frames, bases, and accessories; policy implications and funding mechanisms; and wheeled mobility and seating options.	After interviewing Angela and her mother and observing Angela navigate in her current chair, the remote occupational therapist recommends the appropriate power wheelchair and power seat functions. Upon approval from the insurance company, the remote occupational therapist uses the videoconferencing system to monitor the delivery, evaluate the fitting, and provide feedback and advice to Angela about use of the wheelchair within the community and home. Angela has benefited from services without the need to travel a long distance. The local practitioner gained additional knowledge about wheeled mobility and seating options.
Ethan is a 55-year-old self-employed entrepreneur who has severe depression, anxiety, and isolation after head and neck cancer resection surgery. The surgery left one side of his face disfigured. He plans to have reconstructive surgery in the future. Meanwhile, Ethan has difficulties with eating, fatigue, facial–body image, depression, and pain. He lives alone and over 50 minutes away from the hospital/outpatient therapy clinic. Ethan was seen by an occupational therapist in the hospital and prescribed outpatient occupational therapy for his physical and mental impairments. Due to travel distance to the outpatient therapy clinic and anxiety associated with being seen in public, Ethan is interested in the option to continue his therapy at home through secure videoconferencing technology.	Ethan completed a telehealth participation screening and initial occupational therapy evaluation during his hospital stay. It was determined that he would continue with occupational therapy twice a week via telehealth using secure videoconferencing software and a Web camera within his home environment. During the biweekly occupational therapy sessions delivered via telehealth technologies, focus is on establishing a therapeutic wellness plan and implementing compensatory eating techniques, pain management and relaxation techniques, stress management, and engagement in progressive physical activities. Ethan completes a home program and a daily journal sent to him by his occupational therapist through electronic communications technology.	Ethan is able to manage his physical and mental impairments and is able to leave his house to purchase groceries and complete other errands in his community. His pain is tolerable, and breathing and stamina have improved to allow 20–30 minutes of physical activity after 6 weeks of occupational therapy delivered through telehealth technologies. Ethan continues his daily journaling. The occupational therapist will follow up with Ethan via telehealth technologies weekly until reconstruction surgery and again after surgery to make sure Ethan continues his wellness plan.

Value of Occupational Therapy Assistant Education to the Profession

The American Occupational Therapy Association (AOTA) recognizes the value, necessity, and viability of occupational therapy assistant education. Occupational therapy assistant educational programs meet standards of performance established by the Accreditation Council for Occupational Therapy Education (ACOTE®) to produce competent entry-level occupational therapy assistants who are eligible for national certification and state licensure. Occupational therapy assistants work collaboratively with occupational therapists in contributing to the profession's pursuit of providing high-quality, cost-effective services to promote health and wellness by meeting society's occupational needs. Occupational therapy assistant education provides a sound foundation for practice with the development of competent skill sets to fulfill various professional roles within contemporary practice. These roles include direct care provider, educator, and advocate for the profession and the consumer (ACOTE, 2012).

The collaboration of occupational therapy assistants with occupational therapists in service delivery ensures greater affordability and accessibility of occupational therapy services for all populations so that more of society's occupational needs can be effectively met. The rising costs of higher education can impose limits on one's pursuit of a career in occupational therapy. Affordability, accessibility, and reduced time commitment are key components of an occupational therapy assistant education that enable timely entry of skilled occupational therapy practitioners into the workforce to meet the growing demand for services within the expanding health care environment. Occupational therapy assistants are equipped to promote the value and role of occupational therapy services with persons across the lifespan in rehabilitation, habilitation, prevention, wellness, chronic disease management, and other critical areas while providing skilled occupational therapy services to improve client outcomes at lower costs (AOTA, 2014a). In this way, occupational therapy assistant education produces highly skilled practitioners who, in partnership with occupational therapists, help to achieve the triple aim of health care reform to improve the individual experience of care, improve the health of populations, and reduce the cost of care (AOTA, 2014b).

Ensuring a diverse workforce is a priority within health care. Occupational therapy assistant educational programs are housed in academic institutions that are designed to meet the needs of a diverse student body that is representative of the surrounding communities in which graduates ultimately become employed and serve. Many students within occupational therapy assistant educational programs bring a variety of life experiences and commitment to their local communities that enrich the teaching–learning process and community engagement. These factors, in combination with an education based on rigorous accreditation standards that develop knowledge in the domain and process of occupational therapy; competencies in the application of culturally relevant, client-centered, evidence-based, and occupation-based interventions; and skills in the areas of written and verbal communication, leadership and management, scholarship, advocacy, and professional values, ethics, and responsibilities, result in the occupational therapy assistant becoming a vital partner with the occupational therapist and a valued member of the interprofessional team.

The Commission on Education (COE) recognizes that occupational therapy assistant education adds an important and valued dimension to the provision of occupational therapy services. The COE is committed to the support of occupational therapy assistant education by seeking role clarification, promoting collaboration among educational programs for occupational therapy assistants and occupational therapists, and advocating for the qualifications of occupational therapy assistants within all contexts of service delivery.

References

Accreditation Council for Occupational Therapy Education. (2012). 2011 Accreditation Council for Occupational Therapy Education (ACOTE®) standards. *American Journal of Occupational Therapy, 66*(Suppl.), S6–S74. http://dx.doi.org/10.5014/ajot.2012.66S6

American Occupational Therapy Association. (2014a). *Health care reform and the occupational therapy assistant.* Retrieved from http://www.aota.org/-/media/Corporate/Files/Advocacy/Health-Care-Reform/Overview/HCR_OTA.pdf

American Occupational Therapy Association. (2014b). The role of occupational therapy in primary care. *American Journal of Occupational Therapy, 68*(Suppl. 3), S25–S33. http://dx.doi.org/10.5014/ajot.2014.686S06

Authors
Claudia Miller, OTD, OTR/L
Matthew Mekkes, MS, OTR/L
Maureen Nardella, MS, OTR/L
Renee Ortega, MA, COTA
Kim Qualls, MS, OTR/L

for

The Commission on Education
Andrea Bilics, PhD, OTR/L, FAOTA, *Chairperson*
Tina DeAngelis, EdD, OTR/L
Jamie Geraci, MS, OTR/L
Julie McLaughlin Gray, PhD, OTR/L
Michael Iwama, PhD, OT(C)
Julie Kugel, OTD, MOT, OTR/L
Kate McWilliams
Maureen Nardella, MS, OTR/L
Renee Ortega, MA, COTA
Kim Qualls, MS, OTR/L
Tamra Trenary, OTD, OTR/L, BCPR
Neil Harvison, PhD, OTR/L, FAOTA, *AOTA Headquarters Liaison*

Adopted by the Representative Assembly 2015AprC10

Standards

Standards for Continuing Competence

Continuing competence is a process involving the examination of current competence and the development of capacity for the future. It is a component of ongoing professional development and lifelong learning. Continuing competence is a dynamic and multidimensional process in which the occupational therapist and occupational therapy assistant develop and maintain the knowledge, performance skills, interpersonal abilities, critical reasoning, and ethical reasoning skills necessary to perform current and future roles and responsibilities within the profession. The pursuit of continuing competence advances the occupational therapy practitioner and the profession. Continuing competence is maintained through self-assessment of the practitioner's capacities in the core of occupational therapy, which reflects knowledge of the domain of the profession and the process used in service delivery.

Occupational therapists and occupational therapy assistants use the following standards to assess, maintain, and document continuing competence. Basic to these standards is the belief that all occupational therapists and occupational therapy assistants share core values and knowledge, guiding actions within their roles and responsibilities. The core of occupational therapy involves "the therapeutic use of everyday activities (occupations) with individuals or groups for the purpose of enhancing or enabling participation in roles, habits, and routines in home, school, workplace, community, and other settings" (American Occupational Therapy Association [AOTA], 2014, p. S1).

Standard 1. Knowledge

Occupational therapists and occupational therapy assistants shall demonstrate understanding and integration of the information required for the multiple roles and responsibilities they assume. The individual must demonstrate

- Mastery of the core of the practice and profession of occupational therapy as it is applied in the multiple responsibilities assumed;

- Expertise in client-centered occupational therapy practice and related primary responsibilities;

- Integration of relevant evidence, literature, and epidemiological data related to primary responsibilities and to the consumer population(s) served by occupational therapy;

- Integration of current AOTA documents and legislative, legal, and regulatory requirements into occupation- and evidence-based practice; and

- The ability to seek new knowledge to meet client needs as well as the demands of a dynamic profession.

Standard 2. Critical Reasoning

Occupational therapists and occupational therapy assistants shall use reasoning processes to make sound judgments and decisions. The individual must demonstrate

- Deductive and inductive reasoning in making decisions specific to roles and responsibilities;

- Problem-solving skills necessary to carry out responsibilities;

- The ability to analyze occupational performance as influenced by client and environmental factors;

- The ability to reflect on one's own practice of occupational therapy;

- Management and synthesis of information from a variety of sources in support of making decisions;

- Application of evidence, research findings, and outcome data in making decisions; and

- The ability to assess previous assumptions against new evidence and revise decision-making processes.

Standard 3. Interpersonal Skills

Occupational therapists and occupational therapy assistants shall develop and maintain their professional relationships with others within the context of their roles and responsibilities. The individual must demonstrate

- Use of effective communication methods that match the abilities, personal factors, learning styles, and therapeutic needs of consumers and others;

- Cultural competence through effective interaction with people from diverse backgrounds;

- Integration of feedback from clients, supervisors, and colleagues to modify one's professional behavior and therapeutic use of self;

- Collaboration with clients, families, significant others, and professionals to attain optimal consumer outcomes; and

- The ability to develop, sustain, and refine interprofessional and team relationships to meet identified outcomes.

Standard 4. Performance Skills

Occupational therapists and occupational therapy assistants shall demonstrate the expertise, proficiencies, and abilities to competently fulfill their roles and responsibilities by employing the art and science of occupational therapy in the delivery of services. The individual must demonstrate expertise in

- Practice grounded in the core of occupational therapy;

- The therapeutic use of self, the therapeutic use of client-centered occupations and activities, the consultation process, and the education process to bring about change (AOTA, 2014);

- Integrating current evidence-based practice techniques and technologies;

- Updating performance based on current evidence-based literature with consideration given to client interest and practitioner judgment; and

- Using quality improvement processes that prevent practice error and optimize client outcomes.

Standard 5. Ethical Practice

Occupational therapists and occupational therapy assistants shall identify, analyze, and clarify ethical issues or dilemmas to make responsible decisions within the changing context of their roles and responsibilities. The individual must demonstrate in practice

- Understanding and adherence to the *Occupational Therapy Code of Ethics (2015)* (AOTA, 2015), other relevant codes of ethics, and applicable laws and regulations;

- The use of ethical principles and the profession's core values to understand complex situations;

- The integrity to make and defend decisions based on ethical reasoning; and

- Integration of varying perspectives in the ethics of clinical practice.

References

American Occupational Therapy Association. (2014). Occupational therapy practice framework: Domain and process (3rd ed.). *American Journal of Occupational Therapy, 68*(Suppl. 1), S1–S48. http://dx.doi. org/10.5014/ajot.2014.682006

American Occupational Therapy Association. (2015). Occupational therapy code of ethics (2015). *American Journal of Occupational Therapy, 69*(Suppl. 3), 6913410030. http://dx.doi.org/10.5014/ajot.2015.696S03

Authors

The Commission on Continuing Competence and Professional Development

Clare Giuffrida, MS, PhD, OTR/L, FAOTA

Leslie Jackson, MEd, OT, FAOTA

Anne B. James, PhD, OTR/L

Christy Nelson, PhD, OTR/L, FAOTA

Marla Robinson MSc, OTR/L, BCPR, *Chairperson, Board for Advanced and Specialty Certifications*

Winifred Shultz-Krohn, PhD, OTR/L, BCP, FAOTA, *Chairperson*

Maria Elena E. Louch, OT, *AOTA Staff Liaison for the Commission on Continuing Competence and Professional Development*

Adopted by the Representative Assembly 1999

Revisions adopted 2005C243

Edited 2006

Revisions adopted 2010CApr12

Revisions adopted 2015CApr16

Note. This document replaces the 2010 document *Standards for Continuing Competence*, previously published and copyrighted in 2010 by the American Occupational Therapy Association in the *American Journal of Occupational Therapy, 64*(6, Suppl.), S103–S105. http://dx.doi.org/10.5014/ajot.2010.64S103

Citation. American Occupational Therapy Association. (2015). Standards for continuing competence. *American Journal of Occupational Therapy, 69*(Suppl. 3), 6913410055. http://dx.doi.org/10.5014/ajot.2015.696S16

Standards of Practice for Occupational Therapy

This document defines minimum standards for the practice of occupational therapy. The *practice of occupational therapy* means the therapeutic use of occupations (everyday life activities) with persons, groups, and populations for the purpose of participation in roles and situations in the home, school, workplace, community, or other settings.

Occupational therapy services are provided for habilitation, rehabilitation, and the promotion of health and wellness to those who have or are at risk for developing an illness, injury, disease, disorder, condition, impairment, disability, activity limitation, or participation restriction. Occupational therapy addresses the physical, cognitive, psychosocial, sensory–perceptual, and other aspects of performance in a variety of contexts and environments to support engagement in occupations that affect physical and mental health, well-being, and quality of life (American Occupational Therapy Association [AOTA], 2011). The overarching goal of occupational therapy is to support people in participation in life through engagement in occupation for "habilitation, rehabilitation, and promotion of health and wellness for clients with disability- and non–disability-related needs" (AOTA, 2014b, p. S1).

The *Standards of Practice for Occupational Therapy* are requirements for occupational therapists and occupational therapy assistants for the delivery of occupational therapy services. *The Reference Manual of the Official Documents of the American Occupational Therapy Association, Inc.* (AOTA, 2015b) contains documents that clarify and support occupational therapy practice, as do various issues of the *American Journal of Occupational Therapy*. These documents are reviewed and updated on an ongoing basis for their applicability.

Education, Examination, and Licensure Requirements

All occupational therapists and occupational therapy assistants must practice under federal and state laws. To practice as an occupational therapist, the individual must

- Have graduated from an occupational therapy program accredited by the Accreditation Council for Occupational Therapy Education (ACOTE®) or predecessor organizations;

- Have successfully completed a period of supervised fieldwork experience required by the recognized educational institution where the applicant met the academic requirements of an educational program for occupational therapists that is accredited by ACOTE or predecessor organizations;

- Have passed the entry-level examination for occupational therapists approved by the state occupational therapy regulatory board or agency; and

- Fulfill state requirements for licensure, certification, or registration. Internationally educated occupational therapists must complete occupational therapy education programs (including fieldwork requirements) that are deemed comparable (by the credentialing body recognized by the state occupational therapy regulatory board or agency) to entry-level occupational therapy education programs in the United States.

To practice as an occupational therapy assistant, the individual must

- Have graduated from an occupational therapy assistant program accredited by ACOTE or prede-cessor organizations;

- Have successfully completed a period of supervised fieldwork experience required by the recognized educational institution where the applicant met the academic requirements of an educational pro-gram for occupational therapy assistants that is accredited by ACOTE or predecessor organizations;

- Have passed the entry-level examination for occupational therapy assistants approved by the state occupational therapy regulatory board or agency; and

- Fulfill state requirements for licensure, certification, or registration.

Definitions

The following definitions are used in this document. All definitions are retrieved from the *Occupational Therapy Practice Framework: Domain and Process* (AOTA, 2014b) unless noted otherwise:

- *Activities:* Actions designed and selected to support the development of performance skills and performance patterns to enhance occupational engagement (AOTA, 2014b, p. S41).

- *Assessments:* "Specific tools or instruments that are used during the evaluation process" (AOTA, 2010, p. S107).

- *Client:* Person or persons (including those involved in the care of a client), group (collective of individuals, e.g., families, workers, students, or community members), or population (collective of groups or individuals living in a similar locale—e.g., city, state, or country—or sharing the same or like concerns) (AOTA, 2014b, p. S41).

- *Evaluation:* "Process of obtaining and interpreting data necessary for intervention. This includes planning for and documenting the evaluation process and results" (AOTA, 2010, p. S107).

- *Intervention:* "Process and skilled actions taken by occupational therapy practitioners in collabo-ration with the client to facilitate engagement in occupation related to health and participation. The intervention process includes the plan, implementation, and review" (AOTA, 2010, p. S107; see Table 6).

- *Occupation*: Daily life activities in which people engage. Occupations occur in context and are influenced by the interplay among client factors, performance skills, and performance patterns. Occupations occur over time; have purpose, meaning, and perceived utility to the client; and can be observed by others (e.g., preparing a meal) or be known only to the person involved (e.g., learning through reading a textbook). Occupations can involve the execution of multiple activi-ties for completion and can result in various outcomes. The *Framework* identifies a broad range of occupations categorized as activities of daily living, instrumental activities of daily living, rest and sleep, education, work, play, leisure, and social participation (AOTA, 2014b, p. S43).

- *Outcome:* End result of the occupational therapy process; what clients can achieve through occu-pational therapy intervention (AOTA, 2014b, p. S44).

- *Reevaluation*: Reappraisal of the client's performance and goals to determine the type and amount of change that has taken place (AOTA, 2014b, p. S45).

- *Screening:* Obtaining and reviewing data relevant to a potential client to determine the need for further evaluation and intervention.

- *Transitions*: Actions coordinated to prepare for or facilitate a change, such as from one functional level to another, from one life [change] to another, from one program to another, or from one environment to another.

Standard I. Professional Standing and Responsibility

1. An occupational therapy practitioner (occupational therapist or occupational therapy assistant) delivers occupational therapy services that reflect the philosophical base of occupational therapy and are consistent with the established principles and concepts of theory and practice.

2. An occupational therapy practitioner is knowledgeable about and delivers occupational therapy services in accordance with AOTA standards, policies, and guidelines and state, federal, and other regulatory and payer requirements relevant to practice and service delivery.

3. An occupational therapy practitioner maintains current licensure, registration, or certification as required by law or regulation.

4. An occupational therapy practitioner abides by the *Occupational Therapy Code of Ethics (2015)* (AOTA, 2015a).

5. An occupational therapy practitioner abides by the *Standards for Continuing Competence* (AOTA, 2015c) by establishing, maintaining, and updating professional performance, knowledge, and skills.

6. An occupational therapist is responsible for all aspects of occupational therapy service delivery and is accountable for the safety and effectiveness of the occupational therapy service delivery process (AOTA, 2014a).

7. An occupational therapy assistant is responsible for providing safe and effective occupational therapy services under the "direct and indirect" supervision of and in partnership with the occupational therapist and in accordance with laws or regulations and AOTA documents (AOTA, 2014a).

8. An occupational therapy practitioner maintains current knowledge of legislative, political, social, cultural, societal, and reimbursement issues that affect clients and the practice of occupational therapy.

9. An occupational therapy practitioner is knowledgeable about evidence-based practice and applies it ethically and appropriately to provide occupational therapy services consistent with best practice approaches.

10. An occupational therapy practitioner obtains the client's consent throughout the occupational therapy process.

11. An occupational therapy practitioner is an effective advocate for the client's intervention and/or accommodation needs.

12. An occupational therapy practitioner is an integral member of the interdisciplinary collaborative health care team. He or she consults with team and family members to ensure the client-centeredness of evaluation and intervention practices.

13. An occupational therapy practitioner respects the client's sociocultural background and provides client-centered and family-centered occupational therapy services.

Standard II. Screening, Evaluation, and Reevaluation

1. An occupational therapist is responsible for all aspects of the screening, evaluation, and reevaluation process.

2. An occupational therapist accepts and responds to referrals in compliance with state or federal laws, other regulatory and payer requirements, and AOTA documents.

3. An occupational therapist, in collaboration with the client, evaluates the client's ability to participate in daily life tasks, roles, and responsibilities by considering the client's history, goals, capacities, and needs; analysis of task components; the activities and occupations the client wants and needs to perform; and the environments and context in which these activities and occupations occur.

4. An occupational therapist initiates and directs the screening, evaluation, and reevaluation process and analyzes and interprets the data in accordance with federal and state laws, other regulatory and payer requirements, and AOTA documents.

5. An occupational therapy assistant contributes to the screening, evaluation, and reevaluation process by administering delegated assessments and by providing verbal and written reports of observations and client capacities to the occupational therapist in accordance with federal and state laws, other regulatory and payer requirements, and AOTA documents.

6. An occupational therapy practitioner uses current assessments and assessment procedures and follows defined protocols of standardized assessments and needs assessment methods during the screening, evaluation, and reevaluation process.

7. An occupational therapist completes and documents the results of the occupational therapy evaluation. An occupational therapy assistant may contribute to the documentation of evaluation results. An occupational therapy practitioner abides by the time frames, formats, and standards established by practice settings, federal and state laws, other regulatory and payer requirements, external accreditation programs, and AOTA documents.

8. An occupational therapy practitioner communicates screening, evaluation, and reevaluation results within the boundaries of client confidentiality and privacy regulations to the appropriate person, group, or population.

9. An occupational therapist recommends additional consultations or refers clients to appropriate resources when the needs of the client can best be served by the expertise of other professionals or services.

10. An occupational therapy practitioner educates current and potential referral sources about the scope of occupational therapy services and the process of initiating occupational therapy services.

Standard III: Intervention Process

1. An occupational therapist has overall responsibility for the development, documentation, and implementation of the occupational therapy intervention plan based on the evaluation, client goals, best available evidence, and professional and clinical reasoning. When delegating aspects of the occupational therapy intervention to the occupational therapy assistant, the occupational therapist is responsible for providing appropriate supervision.

2. An occupational therapist ensures that the intervention plan is documented within the time frames, formats, and standards established by the practice settings, agencies, external accreditation programs, state and federal laws, and other regulatory and payer requirements.

3. An occupational therapy practitioner collaborates with the client to develop and implement the intervention plan, on the basis of the client's needs and priorities, safety issues, and relative benefits and risks of the interventions and service delivery.

4. An occupational therapy practitioner coordinates the development and implementation of the occupational therapy intervention with the intervention provided by other professionals, when appropriate.

5. An occupational therapy practitioner uses professional and clinical reasoning, available evidence-based practice, and therapeutic use of self to select and implement the most appropriate types of interventions. Preparatory methods and tasks, education and training, advocacy, and group interventions are used, with meaningful occupations as the primary treatment modality, both as an ends and a means.

6. An occupational therapy assistant selects, implements, and makes modifications to therapeutic interventions that are consistent with the occupational therapy assistant's demonstrated competency and delegated responsibilities, the intervention plan, and requirements of the practice setting.

7. An occupational therapist modifies the intervention plan throughout the intervention process and documents changes in the client's needs, goals, and performance.

8. An occupational therapy assistant contributes to the modification of the intervention plan by exchanging information with and providing documentation to the occupational therapist about the client's responses to and communications throughout the intervention.

9. An occupational therapy practitioner documents the occupational therapy services provided within the time frames, formats, and standards established by the practice settings, agencies, external accreditation programs, federal and state laws, other regulatory and payer requirements, and AOTA documents.

Standard IV. Transition, Discharge, and Outcome Measurement

1. An occupational therapist is responsible for selecting, measuring, documenting, and interpreting expected and achieved outcomes that are related to the client's ability to engage in occupations.

2. An occupational therapist is responsible for documenting changes in the client's performance and capacities and for transitioning the client to other types or intensity of service or discontinuing services when the client has achieved identified goals, reached maximum benefit, or does not desire to continue services.

3. An occupational therapist prepares and implements a transition or discontinuation plan based on the client's needs, goals, performance, and appropriate follow-up resources.

4. An occupational therapy assistant contributes to the transition or discontinuation plan by providing information and documentation to the supervising occupational therapist related to the client's needs, goals, performance, and appropriate follow-up resources.

5. An occupational therapy practitioner facilitates the transition or discharge process in collaboration with the client, family members, significant others, other professionals (e.g., medical, educational, social services), and community resources, when appropriate.

6. An occupational therapist is responsible for evaluating the safety and effectiveness of the occupational therapy processes and interventions within the practice setting.

7. An occupational therapy assistant contributes to evaluating the safety and effectiveness of the occupational therapy processes and interventions within the practice setting.

8. The occupational therapy practitioner responsibly reports outcomes to payers and referring entities as well as to relevant local, regional, and national databases and registries, when appropriate.

References

American Occupational Therapy Association. (2010). Standards of practice for occupational therapy. *American Journal of Occupational Therapy, 64*(6, Suppl.), S106–S111. http://dx.doi.org/10.5014/ajot.2010.64S106

American Occupational Therapy Association. (2011). *Definition of occupational therapy practice for the AOTA Model Practice Act.* Retrieved from http://www.aota.org/-/media/Corporate/Files/Advocacy/State/Resources/PracticeAct/Model%20Definition%20of%20OT%20Practice%20%20Adopted%2041411.ashx

American Occupational Therapy Association. (2014a). Guidelines for supervision, roles, and responsibilities during the delivery of occupational therapy services. *American Journal of Occupational Therapy, 68*(Suppl. 3), S16–S22. http://dx.doi.org/10.5014/ajot.2014.686S03

American Occupational Therapy Association. (2014b). Occupational therapy practice framework: Domain and process (3rd ed.). *American Journal of Occupational Therapy, 68*(Suppl. 1), S1–S48. http://dx.doi.org/10.5014/ajot.2014.682006

American Occupational Therapy Association. (2015a). Occupational therapy code of ethics (2015). *American Journal of Occupational Therapy, 69*(Suppl. 3), 6913410030. http://dx.doi.org/10.5014/ajot.2015.696S03

American Occupational Therapy Association. (2015b). *The reference manual of the official documents of the American Occupational Therapy Association, Inc.* (20th ed.). Bethesda, MD: AOTA Press.

American Occupational Therapy Association. (2015c). Standards for continuing competence. *American Journal of Occupational Therapy, 69*(Suppl. 3), 6913410055. http://dx.doi.org/10.5014/ajot.2015.696S16

Authors

Revised by the Commission on Practice, 2015:

Kathleen Kannenberg, MA, OTR/L, CCM, *Chairperson*

Salvador Bondoc, OTD, OTR/L, FAOTA

Cheryl Boop, MS, OTR/L

Meredith P. Gronski, OTD, OTR/L

Kimberly Kearney, COTA/L

Marsha Neville, PhD, OT

Janet M. Powell, PhD, OTR/L, FAOTA

Jerilyn (Gigi) Smith, PhD, OTR/L

Julie Dorsey, OTD, OTR/L, CEAS, *SIS Liaison*

Dottie Handley-More, MS, OTR/L, *Immediate-Past SIS Liaison*

Shannon Kelly, OT, *ASD Liaison*

Kiel Cooluris, MOT, OTR/L, *Immediate-Past ASD Liaison*

Deborah Lieberman, MHSA, OTR/L, FAOTA, *AOTA Headquarters Liaison*

For

The Commission on Practice
Kathleen Kannenberg, MA, OTR/L, CCM, *Chairperson*

The COP wishes to acknowledge the authors of the 2010 edition of this document: Janet V. DeLany, DEd, OTR/L, FAOTA, *Chairperson;* Debbie Amini, MEd, OTR/L, CHT; Ellen Cohn, ScD, OTR/L, FAOTA; Jennifer Cruz, MAT, MOTS, *ASD Liaison;* Kimberly Hartmann, PhD, OTR/L, FAOTA, *SISC Liaison;* Jeanette Justice, COTA/L; Kathleen Kannenberg, MA, OTR/L, CCM; Cherylin Lew, OTD, OTR/L; James Marc-Aurele, MBA, OTR/L; Mary Jane Youngstrom, MS, OTR, FAOTA; Deborah Lieberman, MHSA, OTR/L, FAOTA, *AOTA Headquarters Liaison*.

Adopted by the Representative Assembly, 2015NovCO14

Note. These standards are intended as recommended guidelines to assist occupational therapy practitioners in the provision of occupational therapy services. These standards serve as a minimum standard for occupational therapy practice and are applicable to all individual populations and the programs in which these individuals are served.

This revision replaces the 2010 document *Standards of Practice for Occupational Therapy* (previously published and copyrighted in 2010 by the American Occupational Therapy Association in the *American Journal of Occupational Therapy, 64*(Suppl.), S106–S111. http://dx.doi.org/10.5014/ajot.2010.64S106

Citation. American Occupational Therapy Association. (2015). Standards of practice for occupational therapy. *American Journal of Occupational Therapy, 69*(Suppl. 3), 6913410057. http://dx.doi.org/10.5014/ajot.2015.696S06

Statements

Academic Terminal Degree

Although there are doctoral-degree programs in occupational therapy and occupational science, currently it is customary for occupational therapy faculty to have a doctorate in related areas of science or social science, including but not limited to education, neuroscience, public health, psychology, policy, law, or sociology. Thus, a degree in any of these areas would be considered a terminal degree for occupational therapists in academia.

Author

René Padilla, PhD, OTR/L, FAOTA

for

The Commission on Education
René Padilla, PhD, OTR/L, FAOTA, *Chairperson (2007–2010)*

Adopted by the Representative Assembly 2008C4

Reviewed by the Commission on Education, 2013, with no changes
Andrea Bilics PhD, OTR, *Chairperson (2013–2016)*

Adopted by the Representative Assembly Coordinating Council for the Representative Assembly (2013)

Note. This revision replaces the 2008 document *Academic Terminal Degree*, previously published and copyrighted in 2008 by the American Occupational Therapy Association in the *American Journal of Occupational Therapy, 62,* 704. http://dx.doi.org/10.5014/ajot.62.6.704

Citation. American Occupational Therapy Association. (2015). Academic terminal degree. *American Journal of Occupational Therapy, 69,* 6913410007. http://dx.doi.org/10.5014/ajot.2015.696S20

Assistive Technology and Occupational Performance

Purpose

The purpose of this statement is to clarify the role and describe the distinct perspective of occupational therapy practitioners (occupational therapists and occupational therapy assistants)[1] in providing ethical, competent occupational therapy services using assistive technology (AT) as an intervention to improve clients' performance, enable participation, or maintain their meaningful engagement in occupation. This document also may be used to inform recipients of occupational therapy services, the public, and other health and education professionals about the process, expertise, and professional reasoning used by occupational therapy practitioners related to the application of AT.

Background

Occupational therapy practitioners have a long-standing, documented expertise in providing client services that incorporate technology, even before the U.S. government provided a legal definition of *assistive technology*.[2] In the early 1900s, technology was embedded in occupational therapy practice. Floor looms, human-powered saws, and jigs to hold therapy projects were used extensively and managed expertly by practitioners. After World War II, adaptive technologies appeared prolifically in the occupational therapy literature. In her Eleanor Clarke Slagle Lecture, Muriel Zimmerman (1960) articulated a "basic philosophy and technical approach [to the] selection, design . . . and methods of fabrication" of AT to enable occupational performance by occupational therapy practitioners (p. 17). Since the passing of the Technology-Related Assistance Act of 1988 and its subsequent reauthorizations, the literature has actively described AT use by occupational therapy practitioners (American Occupational Therapy Association [AOTA], 2010; Angelo & Smith, 1993; Gitlow, Dininno, Choate, Luce, & Flecky, 2011; Gitlow & Sanford, 2003; Goodrich, 2003, 2004, 2005; Goodrich, Gitlow, & Schoonover, 2009; Hammel & Angelo, 1996; Hammel & Smith, 1993; Kanny, Anson, & Smith, 1991) and provided references to the evolution of occupational therapy knowledge and skills with regard to AT (Goodman, Tiene, & Luft, 2002; Goodman et al., 2012; Lenker, 2005; Lenker, Scherer, Fuhrer, Jutai, & Deruyter, 2005; Rust & Smith, 2005; Watson, Ito, Smith, & Andersen, 2010).

Educational standards for entry-level occupational therapy practice now mandate training in the use of AT to enhance occupational performance (Accreditation Council for Occupational Therapy Education® [ACOTE®], 2012). Furthermore, ACOTE (2012) mandates that entry-level occupational therapists should be able to evaluate, design, fit, and fabricate ATs.

Definitions

Occupations are "daily life activities" (AOTA, 2014b, p. S4) in which individuals engage for their purpose, meaning, and perceived utility. The profession asserts that engagement in occupation facilitates health, participation, and well-being (AOTA, 2014b). Successful engagement in occupation involves the interplay of performance skills, performance patterns, and context and environment. As such, occupational therapy

---

[1] *Occupational therapists* are responsible for all aspects of occupational therapy service delivery and are accountable for the safety and effectiveness of the occupational therapy service delivery process. *Occupational therapy assistants* deliver occupational therapy services under the supervision of and in partnership with an occupational therapist (AOTA, 2014a).

[2] The first legal reference to assistive technology was the Technology-Related Assistance Act of 1988 (Pub. L. 100–407), which was later repealed in 1998 and replaced with the Assistive Technology Act of 1998 (Pub. L. 105–394).

practitioners consider this dynamic interplay in applying AT adaptation or modification to create access and promote independent performance of a given task.

Technology, in its broadest sense, is ubiquitous and used daily. As defined by Merriam-Webster (2016), *technology* does not always connote complexity but is simply a tool developed or used to make things happen. The Assistive Technology Act of 2004 (Pub. L. 108–364) defines *assistive technology* as "any item, piece of equipment, or product system, whether acquired commercially off the shelf, modified, or customized, that is used to increase, maintain, or improve functional capabilities of individuals with disabilities" (29 U.S.C. § 2202(2)). When everyday technology ranging from simple (e.g., hook-and-loop fasteners, reachers, built-up eating utensils, nonslip grip mats) to complex (e.g., tablets, smart phones, computer software, game consoles) is adapted, modified, or applied by a skilled professional to improve the capabilities of individuals with disabilities, the technology becomes *assistive* in nature. As technology evolves and becomes more integrated into individuals' daily lives, the distinction between what is *assistive* and what is *enabling* becomes blurred.

Although all occupational therapy practitioners use some form of tool or technology in everyday practice (e.g., simple switch computer access, magnifier, pencil grip, tablet or smartphone app, static display or limited message communication device), other rehabilitation technologies require more in-depth levels of training. These include robotics, complex computer access configurations (e.g., access through eye gaze), complex augmentative communication systems (e.g., multifunction integrated devices with dynamic display), powered mobility, complex seating and positioning systems, and complex home modification systems (e.g., smart home technology). Information on AT resources is available at Disability.gov's (n.d.). *Guide to Assistive and Accessible Technologies.*

Occupation as a Foundation in AT Interventions

The provision of AT interventions is a client-centered process and often involves a team of professionals. Occupational therapy practitioners who participate in a professional care team may encounter overlap in skills among the other team members. Although occupational therapy practitioners may share similar competencies with other professionals in the provision of AT, they possess a professional reasoning and theoretical foundation that is uniquely grounded in occupation.

Theoretical models that inform occupational therapy practice delineate the dynamic interplay and transactional relationship among the client, the client's occupation, and the environment and contexts within which the occupation is performed (Dunn, Brown, McClain, & Westman, 1994; Kielhofner & Burke, 1980; Law et al., 1996; Schkade & Schultz, 1992). These theoretical models have strong parallels with (and some have provided foundation for) many frameworks used in the decision-making processes to effectively provide AT. These frameworks, which include the Human Activity Assistive Technology Model (Cook & Polgar, 2015), the Student, Environments, Tasks, and Tools Framework (Zabala, 2005), the Matching Persons and Technology Assessment Process (Institute for Matching Person and Technology, 2015; Scherer, Jutai, Fuhrer, Demers, & Deruyter, 2007), and the Integrated Multi-Intervention Paradigm for Assessment and Application of Concurrent Treatments (IMPACT2; Smith, 2005), share common constructs of client, activity or task, environment, and technology (see Appendix A for additional information).

More specifically, when applying these frameworks in the occupational therapy process, practitioners consider the

1. Needs, capabilities, goal orientation, values, and beliefs of the *client;*

2. Client's *occupation* and tasks involved;

3. *Contexts and environment* that support or present barriers to performance; and

4. *Intervention*s that match the person, occupation, and environment with interventions (inclusive of AT) to enable performance expectations of the desired occupation.

Thus, at the most fundamental level, occupational therapy practitioners, who are guided by evidence and a theoretical framework, perform an AT decision-making process when conducting evaluations and providing interventions, as reflected in the *Occupational Therapy Practice Framework: Domain and Process* (AOTA, 2014b). Furthermore, these frameworks can help drive research in occupational therapy.

Occupational Therapy Process With AT

The process by which occupational therapy practitioners apply AT to enhance or enable client engagement in occupation is client centered and evidence based. Because of the varying complexity of technology-based interventions, the occupational therapy process may require varying levels of proficiency (i.e., entry level, advanced level, specialized skill sets) from occupational therapy practitioners (Hammel & Angelo, 1996).

The occupational therapy process begins with the evaluation performed by the occupational therapist. The therapist possesses a unique approach of identifying the "just-right" fit and clarifying the interplay of client, occupation, and performance to then incorporate interventions that may include AT. Through the evaluation process, the therapist analyzes the client's contexts and goals (what the client wants and needs to do) in relation to the client's performance skills and motivation (what the client is capable of doing) and the factors that limit or facilitate successful engagement in occupation, including the environment and the availability of technology.

On the basis of the evaluation results, the occupational therapist, in collaboration with the client, designs an intervention plan that bridges the gap between what the client wants and needs to do and what the client is capable of doing. The therapist considers AT as one option among many. As such, the therapist designs, fabricates, applies, modifies, and provides training with various forms of assistive technologies and tools as part of the intervention process to promote participation in occupation and enable access. The occupational therapy assistant, under the supervision of the occupational therapist, may also play a role in identification and provision of AT training.

The AT may be a "means" or an aid to an occupational performance (e.g., adaptive equipment, switches, mobility aids) but could also be part of the "end," as AT opens alternative media for occupational engagement. Examples of the latter include using social media for participation in the virtual context or engaging in leisure pursuits using virtual gaming platforms.

The success of the AT intervention lies not in the technology itself but in occupational therapy practitioners' competence in analyzing, problem solving, and creating a shared understanding of the client–occupation–intervention interplay among those who are supporting a client's participation and engagement in occupations. See Table 1 for case examples of the occupational therapy process using AT interventions.

Technology Interventions as Evidence-Based Practice

Evidence-based practice (EBP) is the integration of the best available evidence, including current research, client evaluation data, and the availability of AT interventions with the occupational therapy practitioner's professional judgment, informed by the client's perspective, to address that client's occupational needs. Because AT is highly individualized to each client in the client's specific context, the focus of EBP is not in the technology itself but the use of AT devices and services as part of a dynamic system of occupational therapy–related interventions.

This context makes the traditional evidence from an EBP paradigm (i.e., evidence drawn from randomized controlled trials with client populations and subsequent meta-analyses) difficult to obtain, as the provision of and training in the use of AT are highly individualized (Clayback et al., 2015). Moreover, AT continues to rapidly advance in its development, often forging ahead of evidence-based research with human participants. Thus, occupational therapy practitioners must stay informed of current and emerging technological advancements and consider the best evidence available while continuing to hone their skills in functional performance, task and activity, and environmental analysis and adaptations to enhance performance outcomes.

Several AT tools have evolved over time and are supported by literature to address various barriers to participation related to a disabling condition that can interfere with an individual's occupational performance. For example, the use of text-to-speech software has been identified to address barriers to accessing printed texts for those who have visual impairments or those who have a learning difference that impedes the processing of language in text form. The technology has become more functional and reliable through a feedback loop between users and developers. Similarly, complex wheelchair mobility and seating systems continue to evolve through advances in engineering.

Despite technological advancements, to attain a client's desired occupational performance outcome requires occupational therapy practitioners to match the available technology with a client's individualized occupational needs. Practitioners draw evidence from their own professional reasoning in evaluating the interaction among client–occupation–intervention to determine the effectiveness of the AT in supporting client-centered outcomes. Therapists develop an intervention plan involving AT using their understanding of the relationship between client (client factors, performance skills, and performance patterns) and occupation (the meaningful and purposeful daily life activities defined by the client) in the natural context or environment. Occupational therapy assistants collaborate in the process of planning the AT intervention, implementing the plan, and evaluating the plan's effectiveness.

Funding decisions are made frequently on the basis of available evidence that supports practice (Clayback et al., 2015). Thus, it is important for occupational therapy practitioners to use evidence-based, occupation-focused, and psychometrically sound tools to regularly and reliably document the effects of AT devices and services on participation and occupational performance and to work with researchers to help generate this evidence.

Ethics in Occupational Therapy Practice Using Technology

It is the professional and ethical responsibility of occupational therapy practitioners to provide services only within their own level of competence and scope of practice. The *Occupational Therapy Code of Ethics (2015)* (AOTA, 2015) establishes principles that guide safe and competent professional practice, and these must be applied when developing a plan of care and implementing the intervention. Practitioners should refer to the relevant principles from the Code of Ethics as well as comply with state and federal regulatory requirements. Occupational therapy practitioners must ensure that they possess the necessary knowledge and skills related to technology and environmental interventions to effectively support their clients in the evaluation, intervention, and outcomes measurement processes. A full range of AT is available to accomplish meaningful interventions to support efficient participation in daily occupations. Because these technologies continue to rapidly advance, practitioners have a responsibility to actively engage in professional development opportunities to keep informed of these advances and to maintain current skills to support practice.

Occupational Therapy Practitioner Qualifications for Using Technology in Practice

Due to the wide range of options and the constant evolution of AT devices, occupational therapy practitioners may vary in their expertise on the basis of the type of technology; for example, practitioners who have specialized skills in developing and applying mobile apps may not be as skilled in other AT and would require the expertise of other practitioners who have specialized skills in, say, complex wheeled mobility and seating systems to fully address the needs of a particular client. Fundamental to occupational therapy practice are skills in the analyses of client factors (body structures and functions), performance skills, demands of a task or activity, performance of that task or activity, and environmental and contextual barriers and supports to performance—all of which are basic prerequisites to designing effective interventions incorporating AT.

Occupational therapy practice with AT encompasses a broad range of knowledge and skills including, but not limited to,

- Evaluating AT needs;

- Developing and implementing an intervention plan that supports occupational or task performance with AT;

- Training client, caregivers, and team members on appropriate and effective use of AT;

- Coordinating services and resources with an interprofessional team;

- Advocating for reimbursement or funding for AT devices and services; and

- Engaging in outcomes measurement and in scholarly endeavors to build evidence to support occupational therapy practice with AT.

These competencies are considered minimum requirements for entry into occupational therapy practice (ACOTE, 2012). More specifically, Standards B.5.8–B.5.11, B.5.19, and B.5.20 clearly articulate the important functions of occupational therapy practitioners as they relate to AT.

Beyond these entry-level competencies are avenues to pursue advanced competencies through ongoing professional development and continuing competence both within and outside of the occupational therapy profession. Two certifications given by the Rehabilitation Engineering and Assistive Technology Society of North America (RESNA) that signify specialized AT skills are the Assistive Technology Professional (ATP) and the Seating and Mobility Specialist (SMS) certifications (RESNA, 2015). However, these credentials are not a prerequisite to demonstrating specialized skills and knowledge in AT.

Because technological developments are rapid and continuous, ongoing professional development and continuing competency are key to effective practice of AT. Furthermore, as AT devices diversify into various models or platforms, it is necessary to engage in interprofessional and intraprofessional collaboration with colleagues who may have unique expertise.

Summary

Use of AT as a means of intervention to support a client to participate in a desired occupation has always been an integral component of occupational therapy practice. Occupational therapy practitioners collaborate with the client and other professionals and use their understanding of a client's functioning, the task or occupation, and the environment or context to apply AT of varying complexity to support the client's occupational performance. As technology continues to evolve, becoming even more ubiquitous in modern society, it will remain commonplace and intertwined in everyday living. Not only have technological innovations changed ways of living, they also have been harnessed to improve health and reduce the effects of disability.

Amid continuous technological evolution, the client-centered focus of occupational therapy practice remains. It is still important to focus on the client, the occupation, and the environment and context when designing interventions that use technology. All occupational therapy practitioners are skilled in analyzing client needs, the tasks, the demands of an occupation, and the environment but may partner with a multidisciplinary team to relate more complex aspects of technology and person–environment factors in the decision-making process. Practitioners must know when the occupational therapy process requires the additional input of more advanced or specialized personnel. As evidence that supports the use of AT to achieve specific outcomes continues to emerge, practitioners must stay abreast of the developments in technology so that they may be incorporated into the occupational therapy process.

References

Accreditation Council for Occupational Therapy Education. (2012). 2011 Accreditation Council for Occupational Therapy Education (ACOTE®) standards. *American Journal of Occupational Therapy, 66*(6, Suppl.), S6–S74. http://dx.doi.org/10.5014/ajot.2012.66S6

American Occupational Therapy Association. (2010). Specialized knowledge and skills in technology and environmental interventions for occupational therapy practice. *American Journal of Occupational Therapy, 64*(6, Suppl.), S44–S56. http://dx.doi.org/10.5014/ajot.2010.64S44

American Occupational Therapy Association. (2014a). Guidelines for supervision, roles, and responsibilities during the delivery of occupational therapy services. *American Journal of Occupational Therapy, 68*(Suppl. 3), S16–S22. http://dx.doi.org/10.5014/ajot.2014.686S03

American Occupational Therapy Association. (2014b). Occupational therapy practice framework: Domain and process (3rd ed.). *American Journal of Occupational Therapy, 68*(Suppl. 1), S1–S48. http://dx.doi.org/10.5014/ajot.2014.682006

American Occupational Therapy Association. (2015). Occupational therapy code of ethics (2015). *American Journal of Occupational Therapy, 69*(Suppl. 3), 6913410030. http://dx.doi.org/10.5014/ajot.2015.696S03

Angelo, J., & Smith, R. O. (1993). An analysis of computer-related articles in occupational therapy periodicals. *American Journal of Occupational Therapy, 47,* 25–29. http://dx.doi.org/10.5014/ajot.47.1.25

Assistive Technology Act of 1998, Pub. L. 105–394, 34 CFR §300.5, 92 NAC 51-003.04.

Assistive Technology Act of 2004, Pub. L. 108–364, 29 U.S.C. 3001 et seq.

Cannella, H. I., O'Reilly, M. F., & Lancioni, G. E. (2005). Choice and preference assessment research with people with severe to profound developmental disabilities: A review of the literature. *Research in Developmental Disabilities, 26,* 1–15. http://dx.doi.org/10.1016/j.ridd.2004.01.006

Charters, E., Gillett, L., & Simpson, G. K. (2015). Efficacy of electronic portable assistive devices for people with acquired brain injury: A systematic review. *Neuropsychological Rehabilitation, 25,* 82–121. http://dx.doi.org/10.1080/09602011.2014.942672

Clayback, D., Hostak, R., Leahy, J. A., Minkel, J., Piper, M., Smith, R. O., & Vaarwerk, T. (2015). Standards for assistive technology funding: What are the right criteria? *Assistive Technology Outcomes and Benefits, 9*(1), 38–53. https://www.atia.org/wp-content/uploads/2015/10/ATOBV9N1.pdf

Cook, A. M., & Polgar, J. M. (Eds.). (2015). *Assistive technologies: Principles and practice* (4th ed.). St. Louis, MO: Mosby.

Disability.gov. (n.d.). *Guide to assistive and accessible technologies.* Retrieved June 23, 2016, from https://www.disability.gov/resource/disability-govs-guide-assistive-technology/

Dunn, W., Brown, C., McClain, L., & Westman, K. (1994). The Ecology of Human Performance: A contextual perspective on human occupation. In C. B. Royeen (Ed.), *The practice of the future: Putting occupation back into therapy* (AOTA Self-Study Series). Rockville, MD: American Occupational Therapy Association.

Gitlow, L., Dininno, D., Choate, L., Luce, R., & Flecky, K. (2011). The provision of assistive technology by occupational therapists who practice in mental health. *Occupational Therapy in Mental Health, 27,* 178–190. http://dx.doi.org/10.1080/0164212X.2011.567352

Gitlow, L., & Sanford, T. (2003). Assistive technology education needs of allied health professionals in a rural state. *Journal of Allied Health, 32,* 46–51.

Goodman, G., Kovach, L., Fisher, A., Elsesser, E., Bobinski, D., & Hansen, J. (2012). Effective interventions for cumulative trauma disorders of the upper extremity in computer users: Practice models based on systematic review. *Work (Reading, Mass.), 42,* 153–172. http://dx.doi.org/10.3233/WOR-2012-1341

Goodman, G., Tiene, D., & Luft, P. (2002). Adoption of assistive technology for computer access among college students with disabilities. *Disability and Rehabilitation, 24,* 80–92. http://dx.doi.org/10.1080/09638280110066307

Goodrich, B. (2003, September). AT in schools. *Technology Special Interest Section Quarterly, 13,* 2–3.

Goodrich, B. (2004, March). Universal design for learning and occupational therapy. *School System Special Interest Section Quarterly, 11,* 1–4.

Goodrich, B. (2005, May). S.W.I.T.C.H.: A process for integrating assistive technology into the user's occupation. *OT Practice, 10,* CE1–CE7.

Goodrich, B., Gitlow, L., & Schoonover, J. (2009). *Understanding the assistive technology process to promote school-based occupation outcomes* (AOTA Online Course). Bethesda, MD: American Occupational Therapy Association.

Hammel, J., & Angelo, J. (1996). Technology competencies for occupational therapy practitioners. *Assistive Technology, 8,* 34–42. http://dx.doi.org/10.1080/10400435.1996.10132271

Hammel, J. M., & Smith, R. O. (1993). The development of technology competencies and training guidelines for occupational therapists. *American Journal of Occupational Therapy, 47,* 970–979. http://dx.doi.org/10.5014/ajot.47.11.970

Horn, E. M., & Kang, J. (2012). Supporting young children with multiple disabilities: What do we know and what do we still need to learn. *Topics in Early Childhood Special Education, 31,* 241–248. http://dx.doi.org/10.1177/0271121411426487

Institute for Matching Person and Technology. (2015). *Matching Person and Technology (MPT) Assessment Process.* Retrieved from http://www.matchingpersonandtechnology.com/mptdesc.html

Joe, J., & Demiris, G. (2013). Older adults and mobile phones for health: A review. *Journal of Biomedical Informatics, 46,* 947–954. http://dx.doi.org/10.1016/j.jbi.2013.06.008

Kanny, E., Anson, D., & Smith, R. O. (1991). Technology training for occupational therapists: A survey of entry-level curricula. *OTJR: Occupation, Participation and Health, 11,* 311–319.

Kielhofner, G., & Burke, J. P. (1980). A model of human occupation, Part 1. Conceptual framework and content. *American Journal of Occupational Therapy, 34,* 572–581. http://dx.doi.org/10.5014/ajot.34.9.572

Law, M., Cooper, B., Strong, S., Stewart, D., Rigby, P., & Letts, L. (1996). The Person–Environment–Occupation Model: A transactive approach to occupational perfection. *Canadian Journal of Occupational Therapy, 63,* 9–23. http://dx.doi.org/10.1177/000841749606300103

Lenker, J. A. (2005). AT outcomes research: Important considerations for conducting clinically relevant studies. *Occupational Therapy Now, 7,* 15–18.

Lenker, J. A., Scherer, M. J., Fuhrer, M. J., Jutai, J. W., & Deruyter, F. (2005). Psychometric and administrative properties of measures used in assistive technology device outcomes research. *Assistive Technology, 17,* 7–22. http://dx.doi.org/10.1080/10400435.2005.10132092

Mendiola, M. F., Kalnicki, M., & Lindenauer, S. (2015). Valuable features in mobile health apps for patients and consumers: Content analysis of apps and user ratings. *JMIR mHealth and uHealth, 3,* e40. http://dx.doi.org/10.2196/mhealth.4283

Merriam-Webster. (2016). *Technology.* Retrieved from http://www.merriam-webster.com/dictionary/technology

Rehabilitation Engineering and Assistive Technology Society of North America. (2015). *Get certified.* Retrieved from http://www.resna.org/certification

Rust, K. L., & Smith, R. O. (2005). Assistive technology in the measurement of rehabilitation and health outcomes: A review and analysis of instruments. *American Journal of Physical Medicine and Rehabilitation, 84,* 780–793, quiz 794–796. http://dx.doi.org/10.1097/01.phm.0000179520.34844.0e

Saunders, M. D., Saunders, R. R., Mulugeta, A., Henderson, K., Kedziorski, T., Hekker, B., & Wilson, S. (2005). A novel method for testing learning and preferences in people with minimal motor movement. *Research in Developmental Disabilities, 26,* 255–266. http://dx.doi.org/10.1016/j.ridd.2004.03.002

Scherer, M., Jutai, J., Fuhrer, M., Demers, L., & Deruyter, F. (2007). A framework for modelling the selection of assistive technology devices (ATDs). *Disability and Rehabilitation: Assistive Technology, 2,* 1–8. http://dx.doi.org/10.1080/17483100600845414

Schkade, J. K., & Schultz, S. (1992). Occupational adaptation: Toward a holistic approach for contemporary practice, Part 1. *American Journal of Occupational Therapy, 46,* 829–837. http://dx.doi.org/10.5014/ajot.46.9.829

Smith, R. O. (2005). *IMPACT2 Model.* Retrieved from http://www.r2d2.uwm.edu/archive/impact2model.html

Technology-Related Assistance Act of 1988, Pub. L. 100-407, 102 Stat. 1045.

Udvari-Solner, A., Causton-Theoharis, J., & York-Barr, J. (2004). Developing adaptations to promote participation in inclusive environments. In F. P. Orelove, D. Sobsey, & R. K. Silberman (Eds.), *Educating children with multiple disabilities: A collaborative approach* (pp. 151–192). Baltimore: Brookes.

Watson, A. H., Ito, M., Smith, R. O., & Andersen, L. T. (2010). Effect of assistive technology in a public school setting. *American Journal of Occupational Therapy, 64,* 18–29. http://dx.doi.org/10.5014/ajot.64.1.18

Xie, B., Watkins, I., Golbeck, J., & Huang, M. (2012). Understanding and changing older adults' perceptions and learning of social media. *Educational Gerontology, 38,* 282–296. http://dx.doi.org/10.1080/03601277.2010.544580

Zabala, J. S. (2005). *Using the SETT Framework to level the learning field for students with disabilities.* Retrieved from http://www.joyzabala.com/uploads/Zabala_SETT_Leveling_the_Learning_Field.pdf

Zimmerman, M. E. (1960). Devices: Development and direction (Eleanor Slagle Lecture). *Proceedings of the 1960 Annual Conference.* New York: American Occupational Therapy Association.

Authors

Beth Goodrich, OTR, ATP, PhD, FAOTA
Lynn Gitlow, PhD, OTR/L, ATP, FAOTA
Roger O. Smith, PhD, OT, FAOTA, RESNA Fellow

for

The Commission on Practice
Kathleen Kannenberg, MA, OTR/L, CCM, *Chairperson*

Adopted by the Representative Assembly 2016AprilC3

Citation. American Occupational Therapy Association. (2016). Assistive technology and occupational performance. *American Journal of Occupational Therapy, 70,* 7012410030. http://dx.doi.org/10.5014/ajot.2016.706S02

Table 1. Case Examples of Occupational Therapy Using AT

Case Description (Setting, Client Profile)	Considerations for Technology Interventions (Clinical Reasoning)	Examples of Occupational Therapy Interventions and Role of Occupational Therapy Practitioners	Evidence and Related Resources Guiding Occupational Therapy Practice
Older adult as primary caretaker for spouse with Alzheimer's disease	*Occupational Goals:* The client's desired occupation is to enable her spouse to age in place with her as his primary caretaker. *Occupational Analysis:* The client factors and performance skills providing strengths on which an intervention plan is designed are her intact cognitive processes and emotional stability, allowing her to be highly organized in the care of her husband. Barriers to successful participation in her desired occupation are her physical stamina, strength, and musculoskeletal changes causing pain. *AT Consideration:* A tablet may provide ease of use and reliable functionality that does not overly challenge the client's confidence for success or skill development.	Although the client's emotional stability is a strength, the nature of the occupation limits the client's ability to maintain social contact with family and friends. Thus, the OT will train and support the client in accessing social media using a tablet to maintain contact with family and friends. Because of the client's limited comfort with technology, this requires ongoing training and monitoring to facilitate the client's success. The client finds great satisfaction in preparing meals for her husband, but sometimes her reduced stamina for the day's work limits her ability to complete the day with a prepared meal. The OT completes an activity analysis in collaboration with the client to consider her options for conserving energy and to allow for the unexpected challenges that may occur in a day. Building on the client's strength in organizing her day, the OT supports the client in mapping out the day's schedule for a 2-week time span using the calendar function built into the tablet. A list of common tasks in each day supports the client to accomplish this with ease and efficiency.	Research on the use of social media by older adults is still emerging as this population continues to adopt social media and tablets. One qualitative study offers guidance to occupational therapy practitioners in using social media with older adults: (1) introducing the concepts first before introducing the features, (2) addressing concerns about privacy, and (3) making social media more personally relevant and meaningful (Xie, Watkins, Golbeck, & Huang, 2012). The evidence for using health-focused mobile apps for older adults is also emerging but promising, particularly in terms of health monitoring and managing chronic symptoms such as pain and fatigue. In their review of literature on the use of mobile apps for older adults, Joe and Demiris (2013) suggested that health care providers should consider age-related decline, fine motor abilities, and visual and somatosensory acuity when presenting mobile devices and apps. Therefore, the OT should explore accessibility features of the tablet device (e.g., large letters, icons). Regardless of client age, the use of health-focused apps is most successful when the apps are gamified, provide reminders, have tracking functions, and have the perception of usability by the client (Mendiola, Kalnicki, & Lindenauer, 2015).
Child with cognitive, physical, and communication impairments at school.	*Occupational Goal:* The client's desired occupation is to participate in the learning activities presented in his classroom at school.	To align the design of learning activities with state-mandated educational standards, the OT partners with the classroom teacher to identified academic learning goals to focus on with the switch-activated learning activities. Once learning goals are clarified, the OT works with the classroom teacher to design activity sequences to support the child's skill development toward the learning goals.	A collaborative approach to address educational standards and achieve optimal outcomes through the use AT and related adaptations is viewed as best practice (Horn & Kang, 2012; Udvari-Solner, Causton-Theoharis, & York-Barr, 2004). The collaborative partnership among team members including the teacher and OT with expertise in AT services and AT devices should take place from the initial provision of the AT, through how the AT is implemented to support learning, and the ongoing assessment of the AT's utility and effectiveness.

(Continued)

Table 1. Case Examples of Occupational Therapy Using AT *(cont.)*

Case Description (Setting, Client Profile)	Considerations for Technology Interventions (Clinical Reasoning)	Examples of Occupational Therapy Interventions and Role of Occupational Therapy Practitioners	Evidence and Related Resources Guiding Occupational Therapy Practice
	Occupational Analysis: In evaluating factors that facilitate successful implementation of the intervention, the OT identified the following: (1) the willingness of the teacher to invest in the work and collaborate with the OT to successfully engage the child in meaningful learning experiences and (2) the availability of two consistent and reliable switch access sites, using the client's head for one switch activation site and using the ulnar side of the child's right hand as a second site. Concurrently, the OT must consider the teacher's lack of experience with switch-controlled learning activities, the child's physical growth and development in relation to his existing and future needs for seating and positioning, and the child's limited motor skills to activate the switches and limited understanding of cause-and-effect in switch-activated learning activities. *AT Consideration:* Switch activation of learning activities may include numerical, alphabetical, and pictorial options. A potential modification to the head array and the right armrest of the seating system may be configured to accommodate the proper placement of the switches.	The teacher and the OT collaborate to design 3 consistent two-choice sequences that will initiate the child's training in two-switch activation while engaged in learning activities. The OT sets up the two-switch access to the classroom computer and trains the teacher how to support the child in using the switches with the choice sequences and how to use the choice sequences to facilitate the child's participation in learning activities. The OT provides this support across multiple sessions with the teacher and the child, modeling with the child while the teacher observes, coaching the teacher's implementation of the switch activation with the child, and monitoring the data the teacher collects while implementing the AT with the child when the OT is not present. The OT also participates in a full team review of the child's progress with developing switch activation skills every 2 weeks so that the multidisciplinary team is providing a consistent continuity of care across the multiple services the child receives at school. The OT keeps in mind the need to collaborate in the future with a seating and mobility specialist as the child outgrows his current seating and mobility system.	Specific to switch adaptations, an empirical review of studies on AT for children with multiple and profound impairments indicates that choice interventions can lead to a decrease in inappropriate behaviors and an increase in appropriate behaviors (Cannella, O' Reilly, & Lancioni, 2005). Furthermore, Saunders and colleagues (2005) suggested that two-choice conditions using AT switches produce convincing indicators of learning.
Young adult survivor of TBI from a car accident 2 years ago	*Occupational Goal:* The client's desired goal is to finish her college degree, which was interrupted by the injury. *Occupational Analysis:* The client has achieved a level of modified independence in self-care activities and mobility with the use of a 4-point cane at home and a power chair in the community, which support her decreased balance and low endurance. Because of the client's physical limitations, the OT suggested pursuing degree completion through online learning. Initial evaluation	The OT collaborated with the client to explore strategies to enhance her occupational performance related to online learning. The OT provided remedial interventions to improve the client's ocular motility and strength while teaching her how to adjust the visual contrast and resolution of the computer screen.	In a systematic review of the efficacy of EPADs for people with TBI (Charters, Gillett, & Simpson, 2015), the authors found sufficient evidence to recommend the use of EPAD reminder systems to support everyday functioning. Mobile devices such as iPhones and Androids are a suitable substitute for EPADs. With the multitude of available apps in the marketplace, the therapist and the client have many options to choose from, but selecting the appropriate app may be a daunting task. AOTA's website (http://www.aota.org/Practice/Rehabilitation–Disability/RDP-apps.aspx) has resources for app recommendations.

(Continued)

Table 1. Case Examples of Occupational Therapy Using AT *(cont.)*

Case Description (Setting, Client Profile)	Considerations for Technology Interventions (Clinical Reasoning)	Examples of Occupational Therapy Interventions and Role of Occupational Therapy Practitioners	Evidence and Related Resources Guiding Occupational Therapy Practice
	indicates that the client is proficient in operating a desktop computer with a large screen and a mobile tablet/digital reader. However, her main complaints include headaches, blurry vision, and photosensitivity after an hour of use. Her mental endurance is also limited; when mentally fatigued, her memory, attention, and executive functioning declines. *AT Consideration:* The adaptability features of a desktop or laptop computer may be useful. In addition, use of a portable electronic device such as a tablet, larger smartphone, or reader can be explored.	In addition, the OT suggested using the alarm functions of the client's mobile device and installed a task reminder app (e.g., Any.do) not only to cue her to take visual and mental breaks but also to provide external strategies to assist with memory and executive tasks (e.g., sequencing, organization).	

Note. AOTA = American Occupational Therapy Association; AT = assistive technology; EPAD = electronic portable assistive device; OT = occupational therapist; TBI = traumatic brain injury.

Appendix A. Assistive Technology Frameworks

Matching Person and Technology (MPT) Assessment Process (Scherer, Jutai, Fuhrer, Demers, & Deruyter, 2007)

The MPT Model, developed by Dr. Marcia Scherer, consists of three constructs—the person, the technology and the milieu—that interact together to guide the process of matching a person with assistive technology (AT). More information may be found at http://www.matchingpersonandtechnology.com/mptdesc.html.

Student, Environments, Tasks, and Tools (SETT) Framework (Zabala, 2005)

The SETT framework was developed by Joy Zabala and is widely used in school-based settings. The framework considers the student, the environment, the task, and the tool to systematically guide AT evaluation and intervention. More information about the SETT framework may be found at http://www.joyzabala.com/uploads/CA_Kananaskis__SETT_Horses_Mouth.pdf.

Human Activity Assistive Technology (HAAT) Model (Cook & Polgar, 2015)

The HAAT model developed by Cook and Hussey considers 4 constructs in guiding a systematic process of matching a person with AT. These include the human, the activity, the AT, and the context. An in-depth description and application of the model is found in Cook and Polgar (2015).

Integrated Multi-Intervention Paradigm for Assessment and Application of Concurrent Treatments (IMPACT2) Model (Smith, 2005)

The IMPACT2 Model presents a 6-stage decision-making process for evaluating the need for and designing intervention using AT. The model also delineates variables that must be assessed or measured to determine the effectiveness of AT interventions. The model and its 6 stages—Preintervention, Context, Baseline, Intervention Approaches, Outcome Covariates, and Outcomes—are described online at http://www.r2d2.uwm.edu/archive/impact2model.html.

Cognition, Cognitive Rehabilitation, and Occupational Performance

The American Occupational Therapy Association (AOTA) asserts that occupational therapists and occupational therapy assistants, through the use of occupations and activities, facilitate individuals' cognitive functioning to enhance occupational performance, self-efficacy, participation, and perceived quality of life. Cognition is integral to effective performance across the broad range of daily occupations such as work, educational pursuits, home management, and play and leisure. Cognition also plays an integral role in human development and in the ability to learn, retain, and use new information in response to changes in everyday life.

The purpose of this statement is to clarify the role of occupational therapy in evaluating and addressing cognitive functioning and the provision of cognitive rehabilitation to maintain and improve occupational performance. The intended primary audience for this statement is practitioners within the profession of occupational therapy. The statement also may be used to inform recipients of occupational therapy services, practitioners in other disciplines, and the wider community regarding occupational therapy theory and methods and to articulate the expertise of occupational therapy practitioners in addressing cognition and cognitive dysfunction.

Occupational therapy theory and research support the principle that cognition is essential to the performance of everyday tasks (Toglia & Kirk, 2000). Occupational therapy practitioners'[1] educational preparation and focus on occupational performance are grounded in an understanding of the relationship between cognitive processes and performance of daily life occupations. This understanding is in keeping with the disciplinary perspective of occupational therapy that emphasizes engagement in the client's desired occupations as a means of promoting cognitive functioning and occupational performance (Baum & Katz, 2010; Giles, 2010). Occupation is understood as both the means and the end of occupational therapy intervention. Participation in occupations enhances client functioning in areas such as cognition, the improvement in which leads to enhanced participation in desired daily activities.

Occupational therapy practitioners administer assessments and interventions that focus on cognition as it relates to participation and occupational performance. Furthermore, occupational therapy practitioners believe that cognitive functioning can only be understood and facilitated fully within the context of occupational performance. This understanding of the relationship among the client, his or her roles, daily occupations, and context make occupational therapy a profession that is uniquely qualified to address cognitive deficits that negatively affect the daily life experience of the individual.

Occupational therapy practitioners may choose from a range of interventions that use engagement in the client's desired occupations and activities with a focus on function-based outcomes. Considerable progress has been made over the past decade in advancing the knowledge of cognition and in identifying effective rehabilitative strategies.

---

[1]When the term *occupational therapy practitioner* is used in this document, it refers to both occupational therapists and occupational therapy assistants (AOTA, 2006). *Occupational therapists* are responsible for all aspects of occupational therapy service delivery and are accountable for the safety and effectiveness of the occupational therapy service delivery process. *Occupational therapy assistants* deliver occupational therapy services under the supervision of and in partnership with an occupational therapist (AOTA, 2009).

Definitions

In this document, *cognition* refers to information-processing functions carried out by the brain (Diller & Weinberg, 1993) that include attention, memory, executive functions (i.e., planning, problem solving, self-monitoring, self-awareness), comprehension and formation of speech (Sohlberg & Mateer, 1989), calculation ability (Roux, Boetto, Sacko, Chollet, & Trémoulet, 2003), visual perception (Warren, 1993), and praxis skills (Donkervoort, Dekker, Stehmann-Saris, & Deelman, 2001). Cognitive processes can be conscious or unconscious (Eysenck & Keane, 1990) and often are divided into basic-level skills (e.g., attention and memory processes) and executive functions (Schutz & Wanlass, 2009).

Cognitive dysfunction (or cognitive impairment) can be defined as functioning below expected normative levels or loss of ability in any area of cognitive functioning. The term *cognitive rehabilitation* has been widely discussed and used in a variety of contexts. However, there is no singular, consensus-based definition. In general, it refers to a broad category of "therapeutic interventions designed to improve cognitive functioning and participation in activities that may be affected by difficulties in one or more cognitive domains" (Brain Injury Association of America, 2011, p. 1). When occupational therapy practitioners provide intervention to improve cognitive functioning (i.e., cognitive rehabilitation), the therapeutic goal is always to enhance some aspect of occupational performance.

Occupations refer to "everyday activities" that are important to the individual and that help define the individual to himself or herself and others and that serve an individual's life roles (AOTA, 2008; Baum & Christiansen, 2005). Occupations help structure everyday life and contribute to health and well-being. Engagement in occupation as the focus of occupational therapy intervention involves addressing both the neurologically mediated occupational performance deficits and the individual's psychological responses to those deficits.

Cognitive Dysfunction

Cognitive dysfunction may occur across the lifespan and may be associated with a wide range of clinical conditions. Cognitive dysfunction can be transient or permanent, progressive or static, general or specific, and of different levels of severity affecting individuals in different domains of their lives. Even subtle cognitive impairments consistently influence social participation, subjective well-being, academics, employment, and functional performance across different ages and populations (Foster et al., 2011; Frittelli et al., 2009; Wadley, Okonkwo, Crowe, & Ross-Meadows, 2008). Most often, cognitive impairments are categorized by severity (mild or major neurocognitive disorder; American Psychiatric Association, 2000) or the clinical condition that causes the dysfunction (i.e., by diagnostic group).

Cognitive rehabilitation interventions for persons with stroke, traumatic brain injury (TBI), and dementias have the most robust empirical support (Cicerone et al., 2011; Golisz, 2009; Rohling, Faust, Beverley, & Demakis, 2009), and persons with these conditions are among the most frequently seen by occupational therapy practitioners. Additionally, occupational therapy practitioners address cognitive barriers to functioning resulting from developmental disorders, environmental factors, or disease. Specifically, these populations include those experiencing cognitive dysfunction related to

- Human genetics and/or development (e.g., environmental deprivation, fetal alcohol syndrome, learning disabilities, pervasive developmental disorders);
- Neurologic disease, events, injuries, and disorders (e.g., stroke, TBI, Parkinson's and Huntington's diseases, HIV/AIDS, Alzheimer's disease and related dementias, rheumatoid arthritis, diabetes, lupus, Lyme disease, multiple sclerosis, chronic fatigue syndrome, chronic obstructive pulmonary disease, cardiac and circulatory conditions);
- Mental illness (e.g., schizophrenia, major depressive disorder, bipolar disorder, substance use disorders); or

- Transient or continuing life stresses or changes (e.g., stress-related disorders, pain syndromes, anxiety disorders, grief and loss).

In addition to rehabilitative approaches, occupational therapy practitioners recognize that there are many circumstances in which interventions to support cognitive functions can optimize occupational performance and quality of life. Habilitative approaches to cognitive functioning can be appropriate for populations with normative neurological development (e.g., interventions to enhance executive functions in the school-age population; see Case 1 in Appendix C) and the well elderly (in an attempt to prevent cognitive disability and occupational performance problems). Occupational therapy practitioners are at the forefront of using novel approaches to assess and enhance function among these diverse populations (Rand, Basha-Abu Rukan, Weiss, & Katz, 2009).

Occupational Therapy Service Delivery

The occupational therapy service delivery process is broadly composed of evaluation and intervention leading to the outcome of participation in areas of occupation. Occupational therapists are often a valuable part of an interdisciplinary team in which practitioner knowledge of cognition, participation, and context complements the interventions of other clinicians on the team, including, but not limited to, neuropsychologists and speech–language pathologists.

Evaluation of Occupational Performance

Occupational therapy evaluation focuses on determining what the client most needs and wants to be able to do and identifying the factors that either support or hinder the desired performance (AOTA, 2008). The *Occupational Therapy Practice Framework: Domain and Process* (2nd ed., AOTA, 2008) identifies the underlying factors and areas of occupation that occupational therapy practitioners consider during the evaluation and intervention process (i.e., client factors, performance skills, performance patterns, context and environment, activity demands). The interaction between a person's cognitive functioning and each factor is transactional in nature and, as such, cognitive functioning is always embedded in occupational performance and cannot be accurately understood in isolation.

In addition, the relationship of cognitive dysfunction to occupational performance is complex. Therefore, a thorough understanding of the contributions of various client factors and the current level of client participation must be sought (Giles, 2011; Lowenstein & Acevedo, 2010).

Occupational therapists examine cognition and performance from multiple perspectives and use multiple methods during the evaluation process, including interviewing the client and others (e.g., parent, teacher, caregiver), cognitive screening, performance-based assessments, environmental assessment, and specific cognitive measures.

The Cognitive Functional Evaluation (CFE) process is an example of a multifaceted approach used by occupational therapists for individuals with suspected cognitive disabilities (Baum & Katz, 2010; Hartman-Maeir, Katz, & Baum, 2009). The CFE process is intended to be customized to each person's needs and can include up to six types of assessments, as outlined in Appendix A.

Models for Intervention and Cognitive Rehabilitation

Occupational therapy scholars have developed several theoretical models that explain and guide intervention. These models, and the specific approaches and methods that they espouse, are used by occupational therapy practitioners to address cognition and to provide evidence-based cognitive rehabilitation as it affects occupational performance. These models include, but are not limited to, the

- Dynamic Interactional Model (Toglia, 2011),
- Cognitive Rehabilitation Model (Averbach & Katz, 2011),

- Cognitive Disabilities Model (Allen, Earhart, & Blue, 1992),

- Cognitive Orientation to Daily Occupational Performance model (CO–OP; Polatajko, Mandich, & McEwen, 2011), and the

- Neurofunctional Approach (NFA; Giles, 2010, 2011; Giles & Clark-Wilson, 1993; Parish & Oddy, 2007; Vanderploeg et al., 2008).

The development of occupational therapy theoretical models is ongoing, as is the refinement of their applicability to particular client populations, severity of deficits, and environmental contexts. Additional information about these theoretical models is included in Appendix B.

Key Features of Interventions

Many occupational therapy intervention models are multimodal and include a range of strategies adapted to an individual client's needs. Occupational therapists may select different approaches to address different types of occupational performance deficits in the same client. The following key features are found within various models and can assist practitioners in choosing an approach or approaches that are best suited to the client.

Global Strategy Learning and Awareness Approaches

Global strategy learning focuses on improving awareness of cognitive processes and assisting clients to develop higher order compensatory approaches (e.g., internal problem solving and reasoning strategies) versus attempting to remediate basic cognitive deficits. This type of intervention relies on the holistic analysis skills of the occupational therapist in understanding the whole person and helping the client deconstruct his or her own performance. This approach enables clients to be able to generalize the application of these compensatory strategies to novel circumstances (Dawson et al., 2009; Polatajko et al., 2011). Case studies illustrating these approaches can be found in Appendix C (see Cases 1–3).

Domain-Specific Strategy Training

Domain-specific strategy training focuses on teaching clients particular strategies to manage specific perceptual or cognitive deficits versus being taught the task itself. For example, the client may learn an internal routine to scan the whole environment to assist with left-sided neglect, may learn a social skills strategy to manage interpersonal interactions, or may learn to use a mental checklist to identify things to be recorded in a personal digital assistant. Case studies illustrating these approaches can be found in Appendix C (see Cases 3 and 4).

Cognitive Retraining Embedded in Functional Activity

In cognitive retraining, cognitive processes are addressed within the context of the activity (e.g., attention retraining during driving reeducation); the retraining is "context specific." The transfer-appropriate processing hypothesis of Park, Moscovitch, and Robertson (1999) suggests that performance on a particular task after training will improve to the extent that processing operations required to carry out that task overlap with the processes engaged during training. For example, problem-solving strategies developed in the context of a simple front-closing shirt-donning activity will carry over to a front-closing jacket-donning activity when that process is engaged.

Specific-Task Training

Specific-task training assists clients to perform a specific functional behavior (Mastos, Miller, Eliasson, & Imms, 2007; Parish & Oddy, 2007). In specific-task training, the therapist attempts to circumvent the cognitive deficit that hampers performance by teaching an actual functional task. The intervention is designed to help the individual achieve the occupational performance goal by learning a routine so that the cognitive deficits no longer interfere with occupational performance (Giles, 2010; Giles & Clark-Wilson, 1993).

"Errorless" learning is often used in preference to trial-and-error learning. By addressing basic-skills training, clients may be able to improve self-awareness, mental efficiency, and organization, resulting in continued cognitive improvements (Parish & Oddy, 2007). Case studies illustrating these approaches can be found in Appendix C (see Cases 3–6).

Environmental Modifications and Use of Assistive Technology

Environmental modifications and simplifications are a component of most of the approaches described. Part of the process of occupational therapy intervention involves addressing the complexity of activity demands and altering environmental contexts to enhance the match between the client's abilities and the environmental demands (Evans et al., 2000; Wilson, Baddeley, Evans, & Shiel, 1994). Several technology-based cognitive prosthetics have been developed as a scheduling assistant (to assist with memory impairment) and for task initiation and task guidance (to cue persons with cognitive impairment to undertake and complete functional routines; Bergman, 2003; Gorman, Dayle, Hood, & Rumrell, 2003; Wilson, Scott, Evans, & Emslie, 2003).

The cueing systems may be used as an ongoing prosthetic or as a way to "extend" therapy and to become second nature as the client internalizes the routine. When occupational therapists think about the environment, they do not limit themselves to consideration of the physical environment (Giles, Wager, Fong, & Waraich, 2005). In addition to physical objects, Barris, Kielhofner, Levine, and Neville (1985) conceptualized other aspects of the environment that influence behavior, including the structure and sequence of tasks, the content of the social network, and values and beliefs embedded in culture (Giles, 2011). Case studies illustrating these approaches can be found in Appendix C (see Cases 2, 6, and 7).

Contributions to the Interdisciplinary Team

Occupational therapy practitioners are important members of interdisciplinary rehabilitation teams. As part of these teams, practitioners bring a unique focus on occupational performance as both an intervention and an outcome (AOTA, 2008; Baum & Katz, 2010; Giles, 2010). Interdisciplinary programs that address cognition are variously described as *comprehensive outpatient programs, postacute rehabilitation,* and *holistic neurologic rehabilitation* (Geurtsen, van Heugten, Martina, & Geurts, 2010; Turner-Stokes, 2008; Turner-Stokes, Nair, Sedki, Disler, & Wade, 2005) and often emphasize the integration of cognitive, interpersonal, and functional interventions within a therapeutic milieu.

Occupational therapy practitioners bring an understanding of the interrelatedness of the mind, body, and spirit and the transactional relationship of client factors, the environment, and occupational performance to the rehabilitation team (AOTA, 2008). Clients in these programs have been found to show increased self-awareness, increased self-efficacy for symptom management, increased perceived quality of life, and increased community integration (Cicerone et al., 2008, 2011).

Advancing Future Research

Considerable progress has been made over the past decade in advancing knowledge and rehabilitative strategies that improve the clients' occupational performance, self-efficacy, and perceived quality of life. Occupational therapy practitioners use existing and emerging evidence as summarized in systematic reviews (such as Cicerone et al., 2000, 2005, 2011) and the *Occupational Therapy Practice Guidelines for Adults With Traumatic Brain Injury* (Golisz, 2009) to guide their approach to evaluation and intervention. All of the occupational therapy approaches described in this statement have (at minimum) case-series and proof-of-concept designs showing effectiveness, and some have been found effective in large-scale, multi- center, randomized controlled trials (Giles, 2010; Vanderploeg et al., 2008).

There is now a general consensus among several payers (including insurance companies and Medicare contractor policy statements) that sufficient information is available to support evidence-based protocols and implement empirically supported treatments for disability caused by cognitive impairment after TBI and stroke (Rohling et al., 2009). However, although there is some support from systematic reviews of cognitive interventions for persons with Alzheimer's disease, multiple sclerosis, and schizophrenia, no consensus as yet exists for these and other diagnostic groupings in regard to cognitive rehabilitation (McGurk, Twamley, Sitzer, McHugo, & Mueser, 2007; Sitzer, Twamley, & Jeste, 2006; Wykes, Huddy, Cellard, McGurk, & Czobor, 2011; Zarit & Femia, 2008). Occupational therapy practitioners continue to work to advance the evidence base in these areas.

Qualifications of Occupational Therapy Practitioners

Occupational therapy practitioners are well qualified to assess and address cognitive performance issues affecting daily activity performance because of their education and training in cognitive functioning, task analysis, learning, diagnostic conditions, and a holistic understanding of the wide range of factors and contexts that affect performance (Accreditation Council for Occupational Therapy Education [ACOTE], 2012). The occupational therapist is responsible for the overall evaluation process, interpretation of the results, development, and management of the intervention plan. The occupational therapy assistant can perform those portions of the assessment as delegated by the occupational therapist, in which service competency has been established and in keeping with state laws and other regulations. All occupational therapy practitioners assume ethical responsibility for maintaining competence and determining whether they are qualified for independent or supervised practice (ACOTE, 2012).

AOTA asserts the importance of cognition to human performance and to the superordinate goals of occupational therapy. On the basis of theoretical models and evidence-supported methods and approaches, occupational therapy practitioners assess and address cognition so that clients may optimally perform the roles and activities that advance their productivity, wellness, and life satisfaction.

References

Accreditation Council for Occupational Therapy Education. (2012). 2011 Accreditation Council for Occupational Therapy Education (ACOTE®) standards. *American Journal of Occupational Therapy, 66*(6, Suppl.), S6–S74. http://dx.doi.org/10.5014/ajot.2012.66S6

Allen, C. K., Earhart, C., & Blue, T. (1992). *Occupational therapy treatment goals for the physically and cognitively disabled.* Rockville, MD: American Occupational Therapy Association.

American Occupational Therapy Association. (2006). Policy 1.44: Categories of occupational therapy personnel. In *Policy manual* (2011 ed., pp. 33–34). Bethesda, MD: Author.

American Occupational Therapy Association. (2008). Occupational therapy practice framework: Domain and process (2nd ed.). *American Journal of Occupational Therapy, 62,* 625–683. http://dx.doi.org/ 10.5014/ ajot.62.6.625

American Occupational Therapy Association. (2009). Guidelines for supervision, roles, and responsibilities during the delivery of occupational therapy services. *American Journal of Occupational Therapy, 63,* 797–803. http://dx.doi.org/10.5014/ajot.63.6.797

American Psychiatric Association. (2000). *Diagnostic and statistical manual of mental disorders* (4th ed., text rev.). Washington, DC: Author.

Amundson, S. J. (1995). *Evaluation Tool of Children's Handwriting.* Homer, AK: OT Kids.

Arnadottir, G. (1990). *Brain and behavior: Assessing cortical dysfunction through activities of daily living (ADL)*. St. Louis, MO: Mosby.

Arnadottir, G. (2011). Impact of neurobehavioral deficits on activities of daily living. In G. Gillen (Ed.), *Stroke rehabilitation: A function-based approach* (3rd ed., pp. 456–500). St. Louis, MO: Elsevier/Mosby.

Averbach, S., & Katz, N. (2011). Cognitive rehabilitation: A retraining model for clients with neurological disabilities. In N. Katz (Ed.), *Cognition, occupation, and participation across the life span: Neuroscience, neurorehabilitation, and models of intervention in occupational therapy* (3rd ed., pp. 277–298). Bethesda, MD: AOTA Press.

Barris, R., Kielhofner, G., Levine, R. E., & Neville, A. (1985). Occupation as interaction with the environment. In G. Kielhofner (Ed.), *A model for human occupation* (pp. 42–62). Baltimore: Williams & Wilkins.

Baum, C. M., & Christiansen, C. H. (2005). Person–environment–occupation–performance: An occupation-based framework for practice. In C. Christiansen, C. M. Baum, & J. Bass-Haugen (Eds.), *Occupational therapy: Performance, participation, and well-being* (pp. 242–267). Thorofare, NJ: Slack.

Baum, C. M., Connor, L. T., Morrison, T., Hahn, M., Dromerick, A. W., & Edwards, D. F. (2008). Reliability, validity, and clinical utility of the Executive Function Performance Test: A measure of executive function in a sample of people with stroke. *American Journal of Occupational Therapy, 62,* 446–455. http://dx.doi.org/10.5014/ajot.62.4.446

Baum, C. M., & Edwards, D. (2008). *Activity Card Sort* (2nd ed.). Bethesda, MD: AOTA Press.

Baum, C. M., & Katz, N. (2010). Occupational therapy approach to assessing the relationship between cognition and function. In T. D. Marcotte & I. Grant (Eds.), *Neuropsychology of everyday functioning* (pp. 63–90). New York: Guilford Press.

Baum, C. M., Morrison, T., Hahn, M., & Edwards, D. F. (2003). *Executive Function Performance Test: Test protocol booklet*. St. Louis, MO: Washington University School of Medicine, Program in Occupational Therapy.

Bergman, M. M. (2003). The essential steps cognitive orthotic. *NeuroRehabilitation, 18,* 31–46.

Brain Injury Association of America. (2011). *Cognitive rehabilitation evidence*. Retrieved July 5, 2011, from www.BIAUSA.org

Brown, C. E., & Dunn, W. (2002). *Adolescent/Adult Sensory Profile: User's manual*. San Antonio, TX: Psychological Corporation.

Brown, L., & Alexander, J. (1991). *Self-Esteem Index*. Austin, TX: Pro-Ed.

Burns, T. (1991). *Cognitive Performance Test: A measure of cognitive capacity for the performance of routine tasks*. Minneapolis: Minneapolis Veterans Administration Medical Center, GRECC Center.

Cermak, S. A., & Maeir, A. (2011). Cognitive rehabilitation of children and adults with attention-deficit/hyperactivity disorder. In N. Katz (Ed.), *Cognition, occupation, and participation across the life span: Neuroscience, neurorehabilitation, and models of intervention in occupational therapy* (3rd ed., pp. 249–276). Bethesda, MD: AOTA Press.

Chui, T., Oliver, R., Ascott, P., Choo, L. C., Davis, T., Gaya, A., . . . Letts, L. (2006). *Safety Assessment of Function and the Environment for Rehabilitation–Health Outcome Measurement and Evaluation (SAFER–Home), Version 3 manual*. Toronto: COTA Health.

Cicerone, K. D., Dahlberg, C., Kalmar, K., Langenbahn, D. M., Malec, J. F., Bergquist, T. F., . . . Morse, P. A. (2000). Evidence-based cognitive rehabilitation: Recommendations for clinical practice. *Archives of Physical Medicine and Rehabilitation, 81,* 1596–1615. http://dx.doi.org/10.1053/apmr.2000.19240

Cicerone, K. D., Dahlberg, C., Malec, J. F., Langenbahn, D. M., Felicetti, T., Kneipp, S., . . . Catanese, J. (2005). Evidence-based cognitive rehabilitation: Updated review of the literature from 1998 through 2002. *Archives of Physical Medicine and Rehabilitation, 86,* 1681–1692. http://dx.doi.org/10.1016/j.apmr.2005.03.024

Cicerone, K. D., Langenbahn, D. M., Braden, C., Malec, J. F., Kalmar, K., Fraas, M., . . . Ashman, T. (2011). Evidence-based cognitive rehabilitation: Updated review of the literature from 2003 through 2008. *Archives of Physical Medicine and Rehabilitation, 92,* 519–530. http://dx.doi.org/10.1016/j.apmr.2010.11.015

Cicerone, K. D., Mott, T., Azulay, J., Sharlow-Galella, M. A., Ellmo, W. J., Paradise, S., & Friel, J. C. (2008). A randomized controlled trial of holistic neuropsychologic rehabilitation after traumatic brain injury. *Archives of Physical Medicine and Rehabilitation, 89,* 2239–2249. http://dx.doi.org/10.1016/j.apmr.2008.06.017

Corcoran, M. (Ed.). (2006). *Neurorehabilitation for dementia-related diseases* (AOTA Self-Paced Clinical Course). Bethesda, MD: American Occupational Therapy Association.

Dawson, D. R., Gaya, A., Hunt, A., Levine, B., Lemsky, C., & Polatajko, H. J. (2009). Using the Cognitive Orientation to Occupational Performance (CO–OP) with adults with executive dysfunction following traumatic brain injury. *Canadian Journal of Occupational Therapy, 76,* 115–127. http://dx.doi.org/10.1177/000841740907600209

Diller, L., & Weinberg, J. (1993). Response styles in perceptual retraining. In W. A. Gordon (Ed.), *Advances in stroke rehabilitation* (pp. 162–182). Boston: Andover Medical.

Donkervoort, M., Dekker, J., Stehmann-Saris, F. C., & Deelman, B. G. (2001). Efficacy of strategy training in left-hemisphere stroke patients with apraxia: A randomized clinical trial. *Neuropsychological Rehabilitation, 11,* 549–566. http://dx.doi.org/10.1080/09602010143000093

Evans, J. J., Wilson, B. A., Schuri, U., Andrade, J., Baddeley, A., Bruna, O., . . . Taussik, I. (2000). A comparison of "errorless" and "trial-and-error" learning methods for teaching individuals with acquired memory deficits. *Neuropsychological Rehabilitation, 10,* 67–101. http://dx.doi.org/10.1080/096020100389309

Eysenck, M. W., & Keane, M. T. (1990). *Cognitive psychology: A student's handbook.* East Sussex, England: Erlbaum.

Fisher, A. G., & Bray Jones, K. (2010a). *Assessment of Motor and Process Skills: Vol. 1. Development, standardization, and administration manual* (7th ed.). Fort Collins, CO: Three Star Press.

Fisher, A. G., & Bray Jones, K. (2010b). *Assessment of Motor and Process Skills: Vol. 2. User manual* (7th ed.). Fort Collins, CO: Three Star Press.

Folstein, M. F., Folstein, S. E., & McHugh, P. R. (1975). "Mini-Mental State." A practical method for grading the cognitive state of patients for the clinician. *Journal of Psychiatric Research, 12,* 189–198. http://dx.doi.org/10.1016/0022-3956(75)90026-6

Foster, E. R., Cunnane, K. B., Edwards, D. F., Morrison, M. T., Ewald, G. A., Geltman, E. M., & Zazulia, A. R. (2011). Executive dysfunction and depressive symptoms associated with reduced participation of people with severe congestive heart failure. *American Journal of Occupational Therapy, 65,* 306–313. http://dx.doi.org/10.5014/ajot.2011.000588

Frittelli, C., Borghetti, D., Iudice, G., Bonanni, E., Maestri, M., Tognoni, G., . . . Iudice, A. (2009). Effects of Alzheimer's disease and mild cognitive impairment on driving ability: A controlled clinical study by simulated driving test. *International Journal of Geriatric Psychiatry, 24,* 232–238. http://dx.doi.org/10.1002/gps.2095

Gentry, T., Wallace, J., Kvarfordt, C., & Lynch, K. B. (2008). Personal digital assistants as cognitive aids for individuals with severe traumatic brain injury: A community-based trial. *Brain Injury, 22,* 19–24. http://dx.doi/org/10.1080/02699050701810688

Geurtsen, G. J., van Heugten, C. M., Martina, J. D., & Geurts, A. C. H. (2010). Comprehensive rehabilitation programmes in the chronic phase after severe brain injury: A systematic review. *Journal of Rehabilitation Medicine, 42,* 97–110. http://dx.doi.org/10.2340/16501977-0508

Giles, G. M. (2010). Cognitive versus functional approaches to rehabilitation after traumatic brain injury: Commentary on a randomized controlled trial. *American Journal of Occupational Therapy, 64,* 182–185. http://dx.doi.org/10.5014/ajot.64.1.182

Giles, G. M. (2011). A neurofunctional approach to rehabilitation after brain injury. In N. Katz (Ed.), *Cognition, occupation, and participation across the life span: Neuroscience, neurorehabilitation, and models of intervention in occupational therapy* (3rd ed., pp. 351–381). Bethesda, MD: AOTA Press.

Giles, G. M., & Clark-Wilson, J. (Eds.). (1993). *Brain injury rehabilitation: A neurofunctional approach.* San Diego, CA: Singular.

Giles, G. M., Wager, J., Fong, L., & Waraich, B. S. (2005). Twenty-month effectiveness of a non-aversive, long-term, low-cost programme for persons with persisting neurobehavioural disability. *Brain Injury, 19,* 753–764. http://dx.doi.org/10.1080/02699050500110108

Gillen, G. (2009). *Cognitive and perceptual rehabilitation: Optimizing function.* St. Louis, MO: Mosby.

Gillespie, L. D., Robertson, M. C., Gillespie, W. J., Lamb, S. E., Gates, S., Cumming, R. G., & Rowe, B. H. (2009). Interventions for preventing falls in older people living in the community. *Cochrane Database of Systematic Reviews, 2012*(9), Art. No. CD007146. http://dx.doi.org/10.1002/14651858.CD007146.pub2

Gioia, G. A., Isquith, P. K., Guy, S. C., & Kenworthy, L. (2000). *Behavior Rating Inventory of Executive Function.* Lutz, FL: Psychological Assessment Resources.

Gitlin, L. N. (2003). Conducting research on home environments: Lessons learned and new directions. *Gerontologist, 43,* 628–637. http://dx.doi.org/10.1093/geront/43.5.628

Gitlin, L. N., & Corcoran, M. (Eds.). (2005). *An occupational therapy guide to helping caregivers of persons with dementia: The Home Environment Skill-Building Program.* Bethesda, MD: AOTA Press.

Gitlin, L. N., Schinfeld, S., Winter, L., Corcoran, M., Boyce, A. A., & Hauck, W. W. (2002). Evaluating home environments of persons with dementia: Interrater reliability and validity of the Home Environmental Assessment Protocol (HEAP). *Disability and Rehabilitation, 24,* 59–71. http://dx.doi.org/10.1080/09638280110066325

Goldenberg, G., Daumuller, M., & Hagmann, S. (2001). Assessment and therapy of complex activities of daily living in apraxia. *Neuropsychological Rehabilitation, 11,* 549–566. http://dx.doi.org/10.1080/09602010042000204

Goldenberg, G., & Hagman, S. (1998). Therapy of activities of daily living in patients with apraxia. *Neuropsychological Rehabilitation, 8,* 123–141. http://dx.doi.org/10.1080/713755559

Golisz, K. (2009). *Occupational therapy practice guidelines for adults with traumatic brain injury.* Bethesda, MD: AOTA Press.

Gorman, P., Dayle, R., Hood, C.-A., & Rumrell, L. (2003). Effectiveness of the ISAAC cognitive prosthetic system for improving rehabilitation outcomes with neurofunctional impairment. *NeuroRehabilitation, 18,* 57–67.

Guy, S. C., Isquith, P. K., & Gioia, G. A. (2004). *Behavior Rating Inventory of Executive Function—Self-Report Version*. Lutz, FL: Psychological Assessment Resources.

Hartman-Maeir, A., Katz, N., & Baum, C. M. (2009). Cognitive Functional Evaluation (CFE) process for individuals with suspected cognitive disabilities. *Occupational Therapy in Health Care, 23,* 1–23.

Izal, M., Montorio, I., Márquez, M., & Losada, A. (2005). Caregivers' expectations and care receivers' competence: Lawton's ecological model of adaptation and aging revisited. *Archives of Gerontology and Geriatrics, 41,* 129–140. http://dx.doi.org/10.1016/j.archger.2005.01.001

Josman, N. (2011). The Dynamic Interactional Model in schizophrenia. In N. Katz (Ed.), *Cognition, occupation, and participation across the lifespan: Neuroscience, neurorehabilitation, and models of intervention in occupational therapy* (3rd ed., pp. 203–221). Bethesda, MD: AOTA Press.

Katz, N. (2006). *Routine Task Inventory–Expanded manual*. Retrieved from www.allen-cognitive-network. org

Katz, N., Itzkovich, M., Averbuch, S., & Elazar, B. (1989). Loewenstein Occupational Therapy Cognitive Assessment (LOTCA) battery for brain-injured patients: Reliability and validity. *American Journal of Occupational Therapy, 43,* 184–192. http://dx.doi.org/10.5014/ajot.43.3.184

Katzman, R., Brown, T., Fuld, P., Peck, A., Schechter, R., & Schimmel, H. (1983). Validation of a short Orientation–Memory–Concentration Test of cognitive impairment. *American Journal of Psychiatry, 140,* 734–739.

Kielhofner, G. (2009). *Conceptual foundations of occupational therapy* (3rd ed.). Philadelphia: F. A. Davis.

Law, M., Baptiste, S., Carswell, A., McColl, M. A., Polatajko, H., & Pollock, N. (1998). *Canadian Occupational Performance Measure* (2nd rev. ed.). Ottawa, ON: CAOT Publications.

Law, M., Baptiste, S., Carswell, A., McColl, M. A., Polatajko, H., & Pollock, N. (2005). *Canadian Occupational Performance Measure* (4th ed.). Ottawa, ON: CAOT Publications.

Law, M., Cooper, B., Strong, S., Stewart, D., Rigby, P., & Letts, L. (1996). The Person–Environment–Occupation Model: A transactive approach to occupational performance. *Canadian Journal of Occupational Therapy, 63,* 10–23.

Lawton, M. P., & Nahemow, L. (1973). Ecology and the aging process. In C. Eisdorfer & M. P. Lawton (Eds.), *Psychology of adult development and aging* (pp. 619–674). Washington, DC: American Psychological Association.

Lowenstein, D., & Acevedo, A. (2010). The relationship between activities of daily living and neuropsychological performance. In T. D. Marcotte & I. Grant (Eds.), *Neuropsychology of everyday functioning* (pp. 93–112). New York: Guilford Press.

Mastos, M., Miller, K., Eliasson, A. C., & Imms, C. (2007). Goal-directed training: Linking theories of treatment to clinical practice for improved functional activities in daily life. *Clinical Rehabilitation, 21,* 47–55. http://dx.doi.org/10.1177/0269215506073494

McGurk, S. R., Twamley, E. W., Sitzer, D. I., McHugo, G. J., & Mueser, K. T. (2007). A meta-analysis of cognitive remediation in schizophrenia. *American Journal of Psychiatry, 164,* 1791–1802. http://dx.doi.org/10.1176/appi.ajp.2007.07060906

Nasreddine, Z. S., Phillips, N. A., Bédirian, V., Charbonneau, S., Whitehead, V., Collin, I., . . . Chertkow, H. (2005). The Montreal Cognitive Assessment, MoCA: A brief screening tool for mild cognitive impairment. *Journal of the American Geriatrics Society, 53,* 695–699. http://dx.doi.org/10.1111/j.1532-5415.2005.53221.x

Neistadt, M. E. (1992). The Rabideau Kitchen Evaluation–Revised: An assessment of meal preparation skill. *OTJR: Occupation, Participation and Health, 12,* 242–253.

Parish, L., & Oddy, M. (2007). Efficacy of rehabilitation for functional skills more than 10 years after extremely severe brain injury. *Neuropsychological Rehabilitation, 17,* 230–243. http://dx.doi.org/10.1080/09602010600750675

Park, N. W., Moscovitch, M., & Robertson, I. H. (1999). Divided attention impairments after traumatic brain injury. *Neuropsychologia, 37,* 1119–1133. http://dx.doi.org/10.1016/S0028-3932(99)00034-2

Polatajko, H. J., & Mandich, A. (2004). *Enabling occupation in children: The Cognitive Orientation to Daily Occupational Performance.* Ottawa, ON: CAOT Publications.

Polatajko, H. J., Mandich, A., & McEwen, S. E. (2011). Cognitive Orientation to Daily Occupational Performance (CO–OP): A cognitive-based intervention for children and adults. In N. Katz (Ed.), *Cognition, occupation, and participation across the life span: Neuroscience, neurorehabilitation, and models of intervention in occupational therapy* (3rd ed., pp. 299–321). Bethesda, MD: AOTA Press.

Rand, D., Basha-Abu Rukan, S., Weiss, P. L., & Katz, N. (2009). Validation of the Virtual MET as an assessment tool for executive functions. *Neuropsychological Rehabilitation, 19,* 583–602. http://dx.doi.org/10.1080/09602010802469074

Riska-Williams, L., Allen, C. A., Austin, S., David, S., Earhart, C., & McCraith, D. B. (2007). *Manual for the ACLS–5 and LACLS–5.* Camarillo, CA: ACLS & LACLS Committee.

Robertson, I. H., Ward, T., Ridgeway, V., & Nimmo-Smith, I. (1994). *The Test of Everyday Attention.* Bury St. Edmunds, England: Thames Valley Test Company.

Rocke, K., Hays, P., Edwards, D., & Berg, C. (2008). Development of a performance assessment of executive function: The Children's Kitchen Task Assessment. *American Journal of Occupational Therapy, 62,* 528–537. http://dx.doi.org/10.5014/ajot.62.5.528

Rohling, M. L., Faust, M. E., Beverly, B., & Demakis, G. (2009). Effectiveness of cognitive rehabilitation following acquired brain injury: A meta-analytic re-examination of Cicerone et al.'s (2000, 2005) systematic reviews. *Neuropsychology, 23,* 20–39. http://dx.doi.org/10.1037/a0013659

Roux, F. E., Boetto, S., Sacko, O., Chollet, F., & Trémoulet, M. (2003). Writing, calculating, and finger recognition in the region of the angular gyrus: A cortical stimulation study of Gerstmann syndrome. *Journal of Neurosurgery, 99,* 716–727. http://dx.doi.org/10.3171/jns.2003.99.4.0716

Schutz, L. E., & Wanlass, R. L. (2009). Interdisciplinary assessment strategies for capturing the elusive executive. *American Journal of Physical Medicine and Rehabilitation, 88,* 419–422. http://dx.doi.org/10.1097/PHM.0b013e3181a0e2d3

Shallice, T., & Burgess, P. W. (1991). Deficits in strategy application following frontal lobe damage in man. *Brain, 114,* 727–741. http://dx.doi.org/10.1093/brain/114.2.727

Sheikh, J. L., & Yesavage, J. A. (1986). Geriatric Depression Scale (GDS): Recent evidence and development of a shorter version. *Clinical Gerontologist, 5,* 165–173.

Sitzer, D. I., Twamley, E. W., & Jeste, D. V. (2006). Cognitive training in Alzheimer's disease: A meta-analysis of the literature. *Acta Psychiatrica Scandinavica, 114,* 75–90. http://dx.doi.org/10.1111/j.1600-0447.2006.00789.x

Sohlberg, M. M., & Mateer, C. A. (1989). *Introduction to cognitive rehabilitation.* New York: Guilford Press.

Tariq, S. H, Tumosa, N., Chibnall, J. T., Perry, M. H., III, & Morley, J. E. (2006). Comparison of the Saint Louis University Mental Status Examination and the Mini-Mental State Examination for detecting dementia and mild neurocognitive disorder: A pilot study. *American Journal of Geriatric Psychiatry, 14,* 900–910. http://dx.doi.org/10.1097/01.JGP.0000221510.33817.86

Toglia, J. P. (1993). *The Contextual Memory Test.* Tucson, AZ: Therapy Skill Builders.

Toglia, J. P. (2011). The Dynamic Interactional Model of Cognition in cognitive rehabilitation. In N. Katz (Ed.), *Cognition, occupation, and participation across the life span: Neuroscience, neurorehabilitation, and models of intervention in occupational therapy* (3rd ed., pp. 161–201). Bethesda, MD: AOTA Press.

Toglia, J. P., Johnston, M. V., Goverover, Y., & Dain, B. (2010). A multicontext approach to promoting transfer of strategy use and self regulation after brain injury: An exploratory study. *Brain Injury, 24,* 664–677. http://dx.doi.org/10.3109/02699051003610474

Toglia, J. P., & Kirk, U. (2000). Understanding awareness deficits following brain injury. *NeuroRehabilitation, 15,* 57–70.

Turner-Stokes, L. (2008). Evidence for the effectiveness of multi-disciplinary rehabilitation following acquired brain injury: A synthesis of two systematic approaches. *Journal of Rehabilitation Medicine, 40,* 691–701. http://dx.doi.org/10.2340/16501977-0265

Turner-Stokes, L., Nair, A., Sedki, I., Disler, P. B., & Wade, D. (2005). Multi-disciplinary rehabilitation for acquired brain injury in adults of working age. *Cochrane Database of Systematic Reviews, 2005*(3), Art. No. CD004170. http://dx.doi.org/10.1002/14651858.CD004170.pub2

Vanderploeg, R. D., Schwab, K., Walker, W. C., Fraser, J. A., Sigford, B. J., Date, E. S., . . . Warden, D. L. (2008). Rehabilitation of traumatic brain injury in active duty military personnel and veterans: Defense and Veterans Brain Injury Center randomized controlled trial of two rehabilitation approaches. *Archives of Physical Medicine and Rehabilitation, 89,* 2227–2238. http://dx.doi.org/10.1016/j.apmr.2008 .06.015

van Heugten, C. M., Dekker, J., Deelman, B. G., Stehmann-Saris, J. C., & Kinebanian, A. (1999). Assessment of disabilities in stroke patients with apraxia: Internal consistency and inter-observer reliability. *OTJR: Occupation, Participation and Health, 19,* 55–73.

van Heugten, C. M., Dekker, J., Deelman, B. G., van Dijk, A., Stehmann Saris, J. C., & Kinebanian, A. (2000). Measuring disabilities in stroke patients with apraxia: A validation of an observational method. *Neuropsychological Rehabilitation, 10,* 401–414. http://dx.doi.org/10.1080/096020100411989

Wadley, V. G., Okonkwo, O., Crowe, M., & Ross-Meadows, L. A. (2008). Mild cognitive impairment and everyday function: Evidence of reduced speed in performing instrumental activities of daily living. *American Journal of Geriatric Psychiatry, 16,* 416–424. http://dx.doi.org/10.1097/01.JGP.00003107 80.04465.13

Warren, M. (1993). A hierarchical model for evaluation and treatment of visual perceptual dysfunction in adult acquired brain injury, Part 1. *American Journal of Occupational Therapy, 47,* 42–54. http://dx.doi. org/10.5014/ajot.47.1.42

Wilson, B. A., Alderman, N., Burgess, A. W., Emslie, H., & Evans, J. J. (1996). *Behavioral assessment of the dysexecutive syndrome.* Bury St. Edmunds, England: Thames Valley Test Company.

Wilson, B. A., Baddeley, A., Evans, J. J., & Shiel, A. (1994). Errorless learning in the rehabilitation of memory impaired people. *Neuropsychological Rehabilitation, 4,* 307–326. http://dx.doi.org/10.1080/ 09602019408401463

Wilson, B. A., Clare, E., Baddeley, A. D., Cockburn, J., Watson, P., & Tate, R. (1999). *The Rivermead Behavioural Memory Test–Extended Version.* London: Pearson Assessment.

Wilson, B. A., Cockburn, J., & Baddeley, A. (1991). *The Rivermead Behavioral Memory Test.* Bury St. Edmunds, England: Thames Valley Test Company.

Wilson, B. A., Cockburn, J., & Baddeley, A. D. (2003). *The Rivermead Behavioural Memory Test* (2nd ed.). London: Pearson Assessment.

Wilson, B. A., Scott, H., Evans, J., & Emslie, H. (2003). Preliminary report of a NeuroPage service within a health care system. *NeuroRehabilitation, 18,* 3–8.

Wykes, T., Huddy, V., Cellard, C., McGurk, S. R., & Czobor, P. (2011). A meta-analysis of cognitive remediation for schizophrenia: Methodology and effect sizes. *American Journal of Psychiatry, 168,* 472–485. http://dx.doi.org/10.1176/appi.ajp.2010.10060855

Zarit, S. H., & Femia, E. E. (2008). A future for family care and dementia intervention research? Challenges and strategies. *Aging and Mental Health, 12,* 5–13. http://dx.doi.org/10.1080/13607860701616317

Related Readings

Gitlin, L. N., Winter, L., Dennis, M. P., Corcoran, M., Schinfeld, S., & Hauck, W. W. (2002). Strategies used by families to simplify tasks for individuals with Alzheimer's disease and related disorders: Psychometric analysis of the Task Management Strategy Index (TMSI). *Gerontologist, 42,* 61–69. http://dx.doi.org/10.1093/geront/42.1.61 PubMed

Katz, N. (Ed.). (2011). *Cognition, occupation, and participation across the life span: Neuroscience, neurorehabilitation, and models of intervention in occupational therapy* (3rd ed.). Bethesda, MD: AOTA Press.

Authors
Gordon Muir Giles, PhD, OTR/L, FAOTA
Mary Vining Radomski, PhD, OTR/L, FAOTA
Tina Champagne, OTD, OTR/L
Mary A. Corcoran, PhD, OT/L, FAOTA
Glen Gillen, EdD, OTR/L, FAOTA
Heather Miller Kuhaneck, PhD, OTR/L, FAOTA
M. Tracy Morrison, OTD, OTR/L
Barbara Nadeau, MA, OTR/L
Izel Obermeyer, MS, OTR/L
Joan Toglia, PhD, OTR/L
Timothy J. Wolf, OTD, MSCI, OTR/L

for

The Commission on Practice
Debbie Amini, EdD, OTR/L, CHT, *Chairperson*

Adopted by the Representative Assembly 2012OctCO21

Appendix A. Types of Cognitive Evaluations in Occupational Therapy Based on Cognitive Functional Evaluation Process

EVALUATION TYPE	DESCRIPTION	EXAMPLES
Interview	Provides the occupational therapist with background information from the client or significant others and delineates the client's occupational profile (occupational history, current status, and occupational goals) as well as the client's views regarding the nature of any deficits he or she might have.	• Activity Card Sort (Baum & Edwards, 2008) • Canadian Occupational Performance Measure (Law et al., 1998)
Cognitive screening tools	Used to create a preliminary overview of the client's strengths and weaknesses using standardized assessments.	• Mini-Mental State Examination (Folstein, Folstein, & McHugh, 1975) • Short Blessed Memory Test (Katzman et al., 1983) • Montreal Cognitive Assessment (Nasreddine et al., 2005) • Allen Cognitive Level Screen–5 (Riska-Williams et al., 2007) • Loewenstein Occupational Therapy Cognitive Assessment (Katz, Itzkovich, Averbuch, & Elazar, 1989) • St. Louis University Mental Status Examination (Tariq, Tumosa, Chibnall, Perry, & Morley, 2006)
Performance-based assessments that may be used to assess cognitive- and executive function–based performance deficits once those have been established	Used to identify the occupational performance concerns to address in occupational therapy intervention. These measures themselves may or may not implicate specific cognitive or executive function deficits, and this relationship is established on the basis of the skilled observation of the occupational therapist.	• Routine Task Inventory (Katz, 2006) • Rabideau Kitchen Task Assessment–Revised (Neistadt, 1992) • Assessment of Motor and Process Skills (AMPS; Fisher & Bray Jones, 2010a, 2010b) • Executive Function Performance Test (EFPT; Baum, Morrison, Hahn, & Edwards, 2003) • Multiple Errands Test (Shallice & Burgess, 1991) • Árnadóttir OT-ADL Neurobehavioral Evaluation (Arnadottir, 1990) • Children's Kitchen Task Assessment (Rocke, Hays, Edwards, & Berg, 2008)
Measures of specific cognitive functions and client factors (e.g., memory, attention), preferably those with established ecological validity	Used to develop a detailed understanding of the client's occupational performance deficits or to inform in the design of interventions to help clients overcome occupational performance deficits.	• Contextual Memory Test (Toglia, 1993) • Rivermead Behavioral Memory Test (Wilson et al., 1999; Wilson, Cockburn, & Baddeley, 1991, 2003) • Test of Everyday Attention (Robertson, Ward, Ridgeway, & Nimmo-Smith, 1994) • Behavioral Assessment of the Dysexecutive Syndrome (Wilson, Alderman, Burgess, Emslie, & Evans, 1996)
Specific measures of cognitive performance in the context of specific occupations	Used to determine how specific cognitive deficits manifest themselves in occupational performance.	• ADL checklist for neglect • EFPT (Baum et al., 2008) • AMPS (Fisher & Bray Jones, 2010a, 2010b)
Environmental assessment	Provides the therapist with information about the environment and context in which the client needs to function in his or her daily life.	• Safety Assessment of Function and the Environment for Evaluation (Chui et al., 2006) • Home Environmental Assessment Protocol (Gitlin et al., 2002)

Appendix B. Theoretical Models Guiding Occupational Therapy Cognitive Rehabilitation

Occupational therapy scholars have developed several theoretical models that explain and guide the intervention approaches used by occupational therapy practitioners to address the impact of cognition on occupational performance.

Toglia's Dynamic Interactional Model (Toglia, 2011) was developed for persons with stroke or traumatic brain injury (TBI) but is relevant to many people with cognitive dysfunction, including children with attention deficit hyperactivity disorder and adolescents (Cermak & Maeir, 2011; Josman, 2011). The Dynamic Interactional Model utilizes multiple activities in a variety of contexts to help individuals understand performance problems and develop strategies to enhance occupational performance. The overall goal of multicontextual intervention is to help the client gain more control over symptoms by efficiently and independently using strategies for information processing (Toglia, Johnston, Goverover, & Dain, 2010).

The **Cognitive Rehabilitation Model of Katz and Averbach** (Averbach & Katz, 2011) provides a comprehensive approach to clients with neurological impairment of differing severities. The approach focuses on enhancing retained cognitive abilities, the development of self-awareness, and the use of remedial cognitive-training strategies (targeting specific areas of cognitive function such as visual perception, visual–motor organization, and thinking operations), learning strategies (interventions designed to help the client develop learning strategies), and remedial strategies (to develop basic activities of daily living [ADLs]).

Allen's Cognitive Disabilities Model (Allen, Earhart, & Blue, 1992) has been applied to persons with dementia, TBI, and severe mental health disorders. The Cognitive Disabilities Model provides a way to describe deficits arising from damage in the physical or chemical structures of the brain and producing observable limitations in "routine task behavior." The Allen battery of assessments provides tools that are used to predict what a person will be able to do (level, mode, patterns) across multiple domains of functioning; identifies the assistance that he or she will require, including safety considerations; and guides appropriate communication and teaching methods when appropriate (Allen et al., 1992; Kielhofner, 2009).

The **Cognitive Orientation to Daily Occupational Performance (CO–OP)** model was developed for children with developmental coordination disorder but has been used widely with neurological and adult populations and across different types of dysfunction (Polatajko, Mandich, & McEwen, 2011). CO–OP is a client-centered problem-solving and performance-based intervention that facilitates performance acquisition through a process of guided discovery of strategies that enable learning of skills. Strategies may be global and provide a general method of approaching any problem (i.e., goal, plan, do, check) or domain-specific (i.e., relating to one area of dysfunction only).

The **Neurofunctional Approach** was developed for persons with independent living goals after TBI but has also been applied to persons after stroke and other acquired neurological impairment (Giles, 2010, 2011; Giles & Clark-Wilson, 1993; Parish & Oddy, 2007; Vanderploeg et al., 2008). The client and therapist collaboratively select specific performance goals. A task analysis is developed, and a "constraint" model is used to establish the client's specific strengths and limitations and construct specific interventions to allow learning to take place (e.g., "cue experimentation" to determine the types of cues the client needs to be successful). Automatic behavioral routines are viewed as the foundation of effective functional and behavioral competencies for all individuals. Interventions are specifically tailored to the client's abilities and are experiential. Evidence from social psychology, learning theory, errorless learning, self-generation, and overlearning literature is used in the design of task-specific skill-retraining programs.

Several occupational therapy models focus on the influence of the environment and the modification of task demands on cognition and function. The **Cognitive Disabilities Model** is an important occupational therapy model that assists in the development of an understanding of a client's needs for environmental support (Kielhofner, 2009). Many other occupational therapy models (Baum & Christiansen, 2005; Gitlin, 2003; Law et al., 1996) trace their roots to the **Press-Competence Model** (Izal, Montorio, Márquez, & Losada, 2005; Lawton & Nahemow, 1973), which was developed to explain the transactional relationship between an individual's capacity and attributes of the environment (e.g., natural, physical, social). Gitlin and Corcoran's (2005) **Environmental Skill-Building Program** is designed to help family caregivers of persons with dementia learn specific strategies to modify their living space and develop a more supportive environment so that the person with dementia will exhibit fewer disruptive behaviors and experience a slower rate of decline and dependence in instrumental and basic ADLs.

Appendix C. Cognition Case Examples

Case 1. Students in a 5th-Grade Classroom: Improving cognitive performance using the Multicontext Approach

CLIENT DESCRIPTION	EVALUATION AND GOAL-SETTING	OCCUPATIONAL THERAPY INTERVENTION AND OUTCOME
The teachers and principal expressed concerns about the organizational skills of **5th graders,** who, in this district, are required for the first time to manage lockers and switch classes. The class included 35 students (7 with special needs) with an average age of 10 years and had 3 teacher's aides.	*Occupational Profile:* The occupational therapist interviewed the principal and teachers. The teachers indicated that more than half of the students had difficulty keeping track of class materials and homework and often lost or misplaced required materials. *Analysis of Occupational Performance:* The therapist observed the classroom and analyzed the classroom and locker routines and the school demands placed on the students' organizational skills. *Goal Setting:* Analysis of interviews and classroom observations indicated that disorganization of lockers, desks, and folders appeared to contribute to students' difficulties. The teachers agreed with this analysis. Goals were for students to be able to 1. Identify at least 2 strategies for improving locker or desk organization; 2. Recognize situations in which they need to use organizational strategies; and 3. Apply self-generated organizational strategies to other school and home activities.	*Intervention Approach:* The occupational therapist collaborated with the teacher to design a 12-session pilot program to address the identified goals and assess initial feasibility, student engagement, and response. The therapist led each weekly 42-minute session. The teacher reinforced the information between sessions. The program was based on the Multicontext Approach (Toglia, Johnston, Goverover, & Dain, 2010), which provides a framework to promote strategy use and metacognitive skills across different situations. Activities are systematically varied to help persons make connections across activities. The approach emphasizes anticipation of challenges and self-monitoring skills. During the intervention sessions, students discussed identifying "roadblocks" and challenges to staying organized in school and daily life (e.g., locker, desk, folders, backpack). Once students identified these, they generated strategies. For example, to address locker management, students were asked to develop or draw a personalized locker plan and checklist, carry it out, and then assess whether it worked for them. During the week, students made daily ratings of their locker organization. Next session they identified factors that influenced their performance and revised or generated new strategies. Students were encouraged to use organizational strategies in different activities (e.g., homework, backpack, binder, folder, or desk organization; organizing information on a page or worksheet). Every session focused on making connections to previous sessions. *Outcome:* The lead teacher indicated that 80% of the students came to class prepared, with the correct materials. The majority of students rated their lockers as more organized and reported high satisfaction with the program. Students indicated that although their lockers could still become disorganized, they knew when to stop, reorganize, or make a new plan.

Case 2. Client With Asperger's Syndrome: Addressing cognition to optimize occupational performance at school using a CO–OP and Environmental Adaptation Approach

Cody, age 12 and in 6th grade, was diagnosed with Asperger's syndrome at age 8. Cody currently lives with his mother, father, and 2 siblings. He received occupational therapy through his school system and from an occupational therapist in private practice beginning in kindergarten and	*Occupational Profile:* Cody stated that he dislikes writing by hand, cannot read his own notes, and often wastes time in school so he can do schoolwork at home on the computer. He reported having trouble concentrating and being distracted by noise and classroom activity. He described him-	*Intervention Approach:* The occupational therapy practitioner used the CO–OP approach (Polatajko & Mandich, 2004) to develop the intervention plan. In the CO–OP approach, children develop their own goals and are guided in developing and applying cognitive strategies.

(Continued)

Appendix C. Cognition Case Examples *(cont.)*

CLIENT DESCRIPTION	EVALUATION AND GOAL-SETTING	OCCUPATIONAL THERAPY INTERVENTION AND OUTCOME
continuing through 3rd grade. Following 3rd grade, his occupational therapy services were discontinued, but he continued to use assistive technology to reduce the writing demands of schoolwork. Cody's mother requested renewed occupational therapy services for him at an outpatient facility because of her concerns with his coordination and self-image and his reported concerns regarding relationships with his peers.	self as bad at sports because he doesn't have good reflexes. His interests are primarily sedentary and digital. Cody's mother reported that he needs structure and routine and becomes upset when routines are altered. A phone interview with his teacher suggested that Cody is disorganized with his work, has trouble initiating appropriate activity, does not seek assistance, and often loses track of time. *Analysis of Occupational Performance:* While completing the Evaluation Tool of Children's Handwriting (ETCH; Amundson, 1995), Cody exhibited problems with both legibility and speed. Cody's scores on the Self-Esteem Index (Brown & Alexander, 1991) indicated that he is most comfortable with himself and his family relationships and least comfortable with himself in relation to his peers. His scores on the Sensory Profile (Brown & Dunn, 2002) indicated difficulties with sensory seeking and sensitivity. Cody's score on the Behavior Rating Inventory of Executive Function (BRIEF; Gioia, Isquith, Guy, & Kenworthy, 2000) and the BRIEF Self-Report (Guy, Isquith, & Gioia, 2004) suggested problems with inhibition, behavioral shift, emotional control, planning and organizing, and task completion. Cody reported feeling comfortable and secure in his family and discussed his difficulties easily. He reported being motivated to play sports and games with his peers. *Goal Setting:* Cody, his mother, and the occupational therapist collaborated to set therapy goals. After 6 months, Cody will 1. Independently manage the homework process (knowing what homework is required and due dates, initiating its completion, and turning it in on time); 2. Complete homework while seated at the kitchen table; 3. Write legibly during note taking and homework; 4. Sit at a desk and attend during class time; and 5. Select at least 1 peer sport to try.	For the first month, Cody attended twice-weekly occupational therapy sessions. Cody was then seen monthly and provided with home practice and phone consultation for strategy implementation and modification. Therapy focused on the use of cognitive strategies to improve performance as well as environmental and task adaptations. Cognitive–behavioral interventions were taught to assist Cody with the specific social situations he identified as difficult; role-playing was completed in occupational therapy. The skills were then practiced with a peer. These included the problem-solving steps of 1. Stopping and thinking before acting, 2. Identifying the problem, 3. Thinking about 2 or 3 possible solutions, 4. Considering the consequences of each action, and 5. Deciding on and implementing a strategy. Cody was also taught skills of task analysis so he could begin to develop his own adaptations. By gaining control over his own behaviors, he hoped to improve his ability to engage with peers. *Outcome:* After 6 months, Cody participated in a reevaluation. Improvements were noted in all goal areas. Cody had begun playing soccer with neighborhood friends. His handwriting was more legible. The combination of improved legibility and the use of technology allowed him to take notes, read them, complete his written class work, and document to his teacher what he was learning. He was better able to attend to his classroom activities using the strategies he had implemented at school. He also found that by keeping data on his performance, with his mother's help, he was able to see how much better he was doing and that motivated him to continue and practice. Cody reported that his self-esteem is better now that he believes he can learn the things he wants to learn.

Case 3. Client With Mild Stroke: Addressing cognition to advance occupational performance using a combined Problem-Solving and Task-Specific Approach and Environmental Adaptation Approach

Until a month ago, **Martha, age 65,** was living independently in the community with her husband. Martha had worked as a circuit judge for the previous 10 years. She has 3 children and 3 grandchildren younger than age 5. Martha had cared for her grandchildren every Saturday while her daughter worked. Martha frequently trav-	*Occupational Profile:* The occupational therapist conducted an informal interview with Martha and her husband and concluded that Martha was aware of her deficits. Martha revealed she found situations that are out of her control to be the most difficult: "I don't like not knowing what is going to happen. I lose my cool,	*Intervention Approach:* A goal-setting/problem-solving approach aims to empower the client so that the client uses a specific problem-solving framework to develop (with the occupational therapist's guidance) his or her own self-training program, which when successful acts as reinforcement for the whole process.

Appendix C. Cognition Case Examples *(cont.)*

CLIENT DESCRIPTION	EVALUATION AND GOAL-SETTING	OCCUPATIONAL THERAPY INTERVENTION AND OUTCOME
eled for work and pleasure. One month ago, Martha fell down a flight of stairs in her home. *Symptom/Complaints:* Since the fall, Martha has felt dizzy and fatigued and reported several functional changes. For example, it takes more effort for her to smile and make facial expressions. She reports difficulty picking up items, such as her hairbrush, and holding on to them during functional tasks. Prior to her fall she enjoyed spending time with her grandchildren, but now she feels impatient and intolerant with them. During a recent work trip, Martha lost track of time while having a meal at the airport and missed her flight. *Medical Evaluation and Referral to Occupational Therapy:* Martha's physician referred her to an imaging center for a MRI scan. The physician informed Martha that she had had a stroke. Martha was referred to a neurologist, who told her she had had a mild stroke, due to a clot in her right anterior cerebral artery, damaging the middle region of her right frontal lobe. The neurologist noted that Martha had mild facial weakness and dysarthria and mild weakness in her left hand. The neurologist recommended that Martha take a couple of weeks to rest before returning to work. He also referred her to outpatient occupational therapy.	and that is when I make mistakes." According to Martha and her family, these errors are new and appear to be a consequence of her stroke. The Canadian Occupational Performance Measure (COPM; Law et al., 2005) was used to identify Martha's priorities for treatment. The Activity Card Sort (Baum & Edwards, 2008) revealed that Martha retained only 80% of her usual activities since her stroke. Among the activities she had given up were eating in restaurants, playing golf, dancing, going to parties and picnics, and doing laundry and yard work. *Analysis of Occupational Performance:* The occupational therapist used informal observation methods as Martha worked on complex everyday tasks, such as child care, to assess Martha's ability to deal with unforeseen frustrations and challenges. The Executive Function Performance Test (EFPT) helped determine the underlying factors that limited Martha's occupational performance (Baum, Morrison, Hahn, & Edwards, 2003; Baum et al., 2008). The EFPT results suggested that Martha required some support in planning and organizing complex tasks (e.g., paying bills). Additionally, results from the EFPT suggested Martha could use support in terms of her judgment during high-stress times. During the EFPT assessment, the occupational therapist noted Martha would get off task if she felt challenged on test items (e.g., bill paying). Martha accurately predicts the environmental factors that result in her performance errors. Problematic situations for Martha are dynamic and novel, such as going to a conference or going out to lunch. Additionally, Martha has motor weakness that affects her speech, facial expressions, and ability to grasp objects. On the basis of Martha's occupational therapy evaluation, the following long-term (1-month) goals were established: 1. Resume caring for her grandchildren with support from her husband 1 day a week. 2. Schedule all weekly meetings independently using an organizing system. 3. Complete desired functional activities using her upper extremity as an active assist. 4. Continue with desired leisure activities through planning and engaging in trips to novel restaurants with her husband.	Appropriate steps for problem-solving training include problem orientation, definition, and formulation; generation of alternatives; decision making; and solution verification. Task-specific training requires task analysis and a graded approach as the client accomplishes sequential tasks. Using both training methods, Martha accomplished her goal to improve child care skills by identifying specific aspects of child care that resulted in her feeling stressed and frustrated. Martha was encouraged to define the problem (e.g., "When the children yell, I feel anxious and frustrated"). She was then encouraged to formulate alternatives to reacting in a negative manner. With practice Martha improved at self-monitoring and needed her husband's assistance less and less. With the encouragement and guidance of the occupational therapy practitioner, Martha identified her organizational problems and identified the use of a day planner as a preferred solution. Martha also developed methods that worked for her in entering and checking for information. Martha developed a program to work on her upper extremity and used her day planner to arrange a novel restaurant trip for her and her husband once per week. *Outcome:* After 1 month of twice-weekly occupational therapy sessions, the COPM was readministered, and Martha reported significant improvements in both her performance and satisfaction with performance associated with tasks of importance to her. She was taking care of her grandchildren (with her husband) and routinely using a planner to organize her day and to plan restaurant trips. In addition to upper-extremity exercises, Martha continued to set and meet daily goals involving use of her left upper extremity to perform routine tasks. Martha and the occupational therapist discussed whether the therapist could be of assistance in problem solving about return to work. Martha reported that she had not yet determined if she was going to transition back to work at a reduced schedule or retire, but she felt confident that she would be able to make the right decision.

(Continued)

Appendix C. Cognition Case Examples *(cont.)*

Case 4. Client With Severe Stroke: Addressing cognition to advance occupational performance using a Task-Specific, Strategy-Training Approach

CLIENT DESCRIPTION	EVALUATION AND GOAL-SETTING	OCCUPATIONAL THERAPY INTERVENTION AND OUTCOME
Jamie, age 55, was healthy and living independently in the community with her husband Carl prior to a left middle cerebral artery occlusion and subsequent fall. Following 6 days at the acute hospital, the acute care team documented her ADL/mobility status as maximum assist and determined that Jamie was a candidate for inpatient rehabilitation.	*Occupational Profile:* On admission, Jamie presented with global aphasia, so an interview with Carl served to develop Jamie's occupational profile. Carl reported that Jamie enjoyed long walks, trying new recipes, and was planning her daughter's wedding. Carl reported that Jamie "takes pride in her appearance" and "always has a positive outlook on life." Carl saw himself as Jamie's primary support. He reported that Jamie becomes tearful when he has to assist her in feeding. *Analysis of Occupational Performance:* The occupational therapist administered the A–ONE (Arnadottir, 1990, 2011) instrument, which helped determine the underlying factors that limited occupational performance. Jamie required maximum assistance for self-care and mobility due to the presence of ideational apraxia (e.g., using a comb as a toothbrush, putting her sock on her hand), motor apraxia (e.g., inability to plan left-sided movements to propel her wheelchair, unable to generate motor plans for tooth brushing resulting in clumsy and awkward movements), impaired organization and sequencing (attempting to don socks after donning her shoes, attempting to get out of bed prior to removing the blanket), and impaired motor function (i.e., a flaccid right upper extremity preventing Jamie from washing her left arm or right axilla, weak right lower extremity making transfers unsafe). The Assessment of Disabilities in Stroke Patients With Apraxia (van Heugten et al., 1999, 2000) revealed that Jamie required physical assistance to initiate task performance, to execute the correct sequence of action, and to correct her errors. *Goal Setting:* On the basis of the evaluation, the following long-term (1-month) goals were established: 1. Jamie will complete grooming tasks with supervision and 3 demonstration cues for object use; 2. Jamie will transfer to the toilet with minimal assist for sequencing; 3. Jamie will prepare a simple sandwich with minimal assist; and 4. Jamie will eat a sandwich with supervision.	*Intervention Approach:* Following goal identification, a task-specific strategy-training approach was chosen (Donkervoort, Dekker, Stehmann-Saris, & Deelman, 2001), because it is focused on improving occupational performance and has been shown to promote generalization (Gillen, 2009). The intervention is aimed at improving the performance of those with apraxia by teaching them internal (e.g., verbalizing steps during task performance) or external (e.g., referring to a sequence of pictures) compensatory strategies that enable more independent functioning despite the persisting apraxia. Strategy training occurred in the context of ADLs. A task-specific errorless-completion approach (Goldenberg, Daumuller, & Hagmann, 2001; Goldenberg & Hagman, 1998) was used during mealtimes for achieving errorless completion of feeding. *Outcome:* Jamie spent 18 days in inpatient rehabilitation. Jamie met her grooming goal, surpassed her toileting goal, and met her feeding goal (Goals 1, 2, and 4, respectively). Although improvement was noted, Jamie did not meet her meal preparation goal (Goal 3) by discharge, as her performance still fluctuated between minimal and moderate assistance. The team and Carl decided that Jamie would be discharged home with a home health aide and occupational, speech, and physical therapy.

Case 5. Client With Severe Traumatic Brain Injury: Addressing cognition to advance occupational performance using Specific-Skill Training and an Environmental Modification Approach

Chloe, age 19, had sustained a traumatic brain injury 2 years ago when she collided with a tree while skiing. At the scene she had a Glasgow Coma Scale of 8 and was intubated. Injuries included a right basilar skull fracture, bilateral subarachnoid hemorrhage, a mandibular fracture, and a fractured right wrist. Chloe was transported via	*Occupational Profile:* The occupational therapist met with Chloe and her mother to develop the occupational profile. Chloe's daily activities consist primarily of watching TV and occasionally completing simple household chores assigned by her mother. Chloe uses her smartphone to text message her mother more than 30 times a day,	*Intervention Approach:* Occupational therapy was provided as a weekly consultative service and was a collaboration among the therapist, Chloe, and her support staff. A compensatory approach using an electronic memory aid (Gentry, Wallace, Kvarfordt, & Lynch, 2008) was chosen, as Chloe was already comfortable with the use of

Appendix C. Cognition Case Examples *(cont.)*

CLIENT DESCRIPTION	EVALUATION AND GOAL-SETTING	OCCUPATIONAL THERAPY INTERVENTION AND OUTCOME

medical helicopter to a Level 1 trauma center.

Six weeks later, Chloe was transferred to a subacute rehabilitation hospital where she received occupational therapy, physical therapy, and speech and language therapy for 1 month before being discharged home.

Two years postinjury, Chloe has been unable to hold a job and lives at home with her mother. Chloe's most recent neuropsychological evaluation indicated significant impairments in visual and verbal memory and processing speed as well as in verbal comprehension. Deficits also were noted in executive functioning, including problem solving and planning and organization.

Chloe recently was approved to receive services through her state's Brain Injury Medicaid Waiver program. This program provides support staff for individuals who meet specified financial and functional criteria so that individuals who have sustained a severe brain injury can remain in the community rather than be institutionalized. Chloe was approved to have support staff 8 hours per day while her mother was at work. An occupational therapy consult was ordered to provide input to the program.

asking repetitive questions and for reassurance. Chloe states that she feels anxious and does not know what to do. Chloe states that the memory book that she was asked to use "made her look stupid"; however, she verbalizes that she "can't remember anything."

Prior to her injury, Chloe was very active and was on the softball and volleyball teams at school. She also liked to cook but no longer does so because she "burns stuff." Chloe stated that she loves animals and wants to be a veterinarian.

Analysis of Occupational Performance: The occupational therapist administered several measures of functional cognition and observed Chloe plan, shop for, and prepare a simple meal. Chloe required moderate cueing when making the grocery list and at the grocery store to proceed to the next step of the task. She required reorientation to the task twice because she stated she could not remember what she was doing. She was able to use the list, locate needed items, and pay for items appropriately, although she reported being anxious throughout the shopping trip and rechecked the list multiple times. She was able to make the sandwich without cueing but required a verbal cue to turn off the stove.

Goal Setting: Chloe and her mother agreed that developing strategies to manage Chloe's memory deficits would have the largest impact on her functional status. A list of goals was established:

1. Chloe will refer to her smartphone to determine the next activity in her day with minimal cues from staff.
2. Chloe will refer to her smartphone to determine the next step of IADL tasks with minimal cues from staff.
3. Chloe will refer to her smartphone to determine the next steps in each task in a volunteer position at local animal shelter with minimal cues from staff.

her smartphone and regarded this device as socially acceptable. Chloe's staff were instructed to enter her daily schedule into the calendar of the smartphone each morning. Chloe was then cued at the completion of each task to check her calendar and determine what activity she should do next.

When Chloe was comfortable with using the calendar function, a task management application was added to the phone. The occupational therapist worked with staff to enter step-by-step instructions for IADLs that initially required moderate verbal cueing from staff. Staff then cued Chloe to check the next step in the phone rather than helping her with tasks.

When Chloe was comfortable with using the smartphone for familiar tasks, the therapist worked with her and her staff to program steps for tasks undertaken as part of a volunteer job at a local animal shelter.

Outcome: After 6 months the Brain Injury Medicaid Waiver program hours were decreased from 8 hours per day to 4 hours per day because Chloe was now using the smartphone to guide her through IADLs. However, through the frequent repetition of task performance the same way each day, Chloe is relying less on the phone with no increase in errors.

Text messages to her mother have decreased from 30 messages per day to 3 per day. Chloe volunteers 15 hours per week at the local animal shelter and rarely reports feeling anxious. Any new tasks need to be programmed into the smartphone and monitored for the first few weeks. Chloe has learned that for any new tasks she must rely on her smartphone.

Case 6. Client With Alzheimer's Disease: Addressing cognition to advance occupational performance using an Task/Environmental Modification Approach

Raymond, age 79, lives with his wife Dorothy in a small central Pennsylvania town. Raymond and Dorothy have lived in the same house for 42 years, where they have raised 5 children. Very few upgrades have been made to the home, so all the bedrooms and the only full bath are on the second floor (clawfoot tub only).

The event that first led to medical evaluation occurred 1 year ago, when Raymond became lost when driving to a neighboring town and ended up 150 miles beyond his intended destination. A state trooper

Occupational Profile: Dorothy responds to most of the questions at the initial interview, with Raymond responding only if specifically asked. Dorothy reports that Raymond is requiring assistance for most self-care tasks, with the exception of feeding and toileting, in which he is independent.

Raymond owned his own furniture repair business before retiring and until about 3 months ago was able to make very simple repairs around the house or in his workshop. Dorothy does not feel it is currently safe for him to work unsupervised.

Intervention Approach: The intervention approach was based on the Person–Environment–Occupation–Performance model and involved teaching Dorothy and Raymond to use environmental and verbal cuing, plus task simplification during self-care, leisure, and work activities and to provide a calming atmosphere.

The occupational therapist proposed 6 visits per month (twice weekly for 2 weeks; once weekly for 2 weeks) followed by a reevaluation. In collaboration with Dorothy, the therapist worked with Raymond to

(Continued)

Appendix C. Cognition Case Examples *(cont.)*

CLIENT DESCRIPTION	EVALUATION AND GOAL-SETTING	OCCUPATIONAL THERAPY INTERVENTION AND OUTCOME

helped him when his car ran out of gas, and Raymond was returned home to a worried Dorothy. Subsequently, Raymond was diagnosed with Alzheimer's disease, and over the following year his symptoms have progressed, triggering a referral to occupational therapy by Raymond's internist.

Raymond no longer drives or does home chores and is angry about these losses. Dorothy says he is easily angered and bored. She is concerned that he will "sit around the house all day and do nothing."

Dorothy wants to help her husband and has given up activities she enjoys to do so. The occupational therapist is concerned about role overload for Dorothy.

Analysis of Occupational Performance: Direct observation of Raymond in his workshop and the Cognitive Performance Test (Burns, 1991) provided findings for symptoms consistent with the moderate stage of Alzheimer's disease and difficulties completing detailed tasks. This score was consistent with Dorothy's report of Raymond's need for assistance with most IADLs and supervision and setup for ADLs. The occupational therapist also administered the following assessments:

1. *Geriatric Depression Scale* (Sheikh & Yesavage, 1986). Raymond's score on this measure indicated that he should visit his physician for diagnostic testing for possible major depressive disorder. Dorothy's score was within the normal range.
2. *Safety Assessment of Function and the Environment for Rehabilitation–Health Outcome Measurement and Evaluation* (SAFER–Home), Version 3 (Chui et al., 2006). Using this tool, the therapist determined that overall safety issues were moderate and were primarily isolated to lighting and bathroom issues.
3. *Task Management Strategy Index* (TMSI; Gitlin et al., 2002). This tool was administered to Dorothy to assess her use of task simplification and objects modification. Scores suggested that training was needed in environmental and verbal cueing and guidance.

Goal Setting: On the basis of Raymond's occupational profile, the analysis of occupational performance, and consultation with Dorothy, the following long-term (1-month) goals were established:

1. Through use of environmental and verbal cueing, Raymond will
   • Dress and bathe independently on 5 of 7 days,
   • Complete simple home chores with distant supervision, and
   • Assemble simple wooden kits with distant supervision.
2. Engage in desired activities, with agitated outbursts reduced to no more than 1 per week.

determine the types of cueing that work best to support his occupational performance. The overall approach was to support his retained procedural memory with cues (e.g., lists or other types of instructions, placement of objects, verbal instruction).

Interventions with empirical evidence were implemented (Corcoran, 2006; Gillespie et al., 2009; Gitlin & Corcoran, 2005) and included the folllowing approaches:

1. *Environmental Cueing*—Modifying objects so their use is unambiguous (may require use of labels), eliminating power tools or other items that could cause injury, reducing the number of items available (clutter), and improved lighting for safety. In addition, suggestions were made regarding specific adaptive equipment for bathing and a monitoring system to provide distant supervision. Raymond's favorite music was used to create a calming atmosphere.
2. *Verbal Cueing*—To avoid conflict, Dorothy was taught to use implicit guiding by setting up the environment and making appropriate activity choices. When explicit guidance is needed, Dorothy was taught to provide instructions one step at a time in a neutral voice. Dorothy also decided to make or purchase audio or video recordings with explicit instructions for wooden assembly kits. Dorothy was shown how to provide tactile guidance.
3. *Task Simplification*—Dorothy and Raymond learned to choose simple activities or to modify existing activities so they involve few steps and reduced opportunities for errors.

Outcome: At the 4-week reevaluation visit, the occupational therapist observed Raymond during a leisure activity in the workshop, interviewed the couple, and readministered the SAFER–HOME and the TMSI. Scores improved on the standardized tests, and the couple reported that all goals were met. The therapist developed a discharge plan that included identification of behaviors that should trigger a request for additional occupational therapy (e.g., reduced performance in ADLs or leisure activities, daily agitation, increased risk of or actual falls or injury).

Appendix C. Cognition Case Examples *(cont.)*

Case 7. Client With Schizophrenia: Addressing cognition to optimize occupational performance based on the Cognitive Disabilities Model

CLIENT DESCRIPTION	EVALUATION AND GOAL-SETTING	OCCUPATIONAL THERAPY INTERVENTION AND OUTCOME
George, age 62, resides in a group home that has 24-hour staff supervision. George was diagnosed with schizophrenia, paranoid type, at age 21. He works at a local furniture workshop but is having difficulty with attendance, staying on task, and some aspects of job satisfaction. George was referred to occupational therapy to evaluate his abilities, goals, and employment expectations and also the job site.	*Occupational Profile:* George described two key areas of challenge at work: (1) work performance limitations and (2) strained interactions with his supervisor. George could explain most of the steps of his upholstery job, but he had difficulties with memory and sequencing when demonstrating the tasks. Additionally he reported problems with task transitions and indicated that he is frequently expected to shift to a new task before achieving mastery of the prior task.

George reported that he likes his job but that his boss is often angry with him and he does not know why. George's boss appeared equally frustrated and confused. For example, the boss appeared puzzled by George's daily questions about familiar tasks. In private, George's boss admitted that he thought George was lazy.

Analysis of Occupational Performance: Using clinical observations within the work setting, an analysis of cognitive performance actions with the Allen level and mode correlations (Allen, Earhart, & Blue, 1992) was completed for 3 of George's job activities (e.g., measuring, cutting, and gluing fabric) on 3 different days. George's scores on the Allen Cognitive Level Battery ranged between 4.4 and 4.6, suggesting that "scaffolding" would help George optimize his work performance. At this cognitive level and mode range, assistance for setup and organization, sequencing, and cues as needed is recommended.

Goal Setting: The following long-term (3-month) goals were established:
1. George will demonstrate an increase of 25% in his productivity, with assistance for setup, the use of pictures outlining the steps of each task, and one full demonstration of each task and object use prior to the supervisor leaving George to complete the task.
2. George will increase attendance from 50% to 90% of the time.
3. George will check in at the end of each shift on a daily basis to discuss with his supervisor what works and what might be more helpful in order for George to meet his vocational goals.
4. George will report a 75% increase in job satisfaction by the end of 3 months. | *Intervention Approach:* The occupational therapist met with George's supervisor to provide education about schizophrenia to help him better understand George's experiences and needs. The supervisor was very appreciative of this information, which heightened his receptiveness to the therapist's recommendations. The therapist also met jointly with George and his boss to explain the results of the evaluation process, review George's work-related goals, and discuss recommended types and amount of assistance. Together they decided to create a weekly schedule in which George spends each day doing one specific task in the upholstery department rather than multiple tasks in the same day.

The occupational therapist developed pictorial sequencing booklets for each task that George was to complete. The supervisor agreed to provide the organizational setup for the day's tasks and one full demonstration of the directions at the start of each shift. He would then observe George fully complete what was demonstrated and provide any needed additional verbal cues. These external cues (e.g., setup, demonstration, referring to a sequence of pictures) provided the compensatory strategies necessary to enable George to function more independently and productively at work.

Outcome:
- *Goal 1:* George demonstrated an increase of 40% in his productivity rate.
- *Goal 2:* George demonstrated an increase of 95% in his attendance at work.
- *Goal 3:* George and his supervisor met at the end of each workday 100% of the time and identified and addressed all issues that came up within their sessions.
- *Goal 4:* George reported an increase in his job satisfaction by 80%. |

Note. ADLs = activities of daily living; CO–OP = Cognitive Orientation to Daily Occupational Performance; IADLs = instrumental activities of daily living.

Driving and Community Mobility

The American Occupational Therapy Association (AOTA) affirms the role of occupational therapy practitioners[1] in addressing community mobility as an instrumental activity of daily living (IADL) essential for the health and well-being of individuals and for the effective functioning of systems and organizations dedicated to keeping humans mobile within society. Furthermore, AOTA recognizes that driving in particular is a critical component of community mobility in the context of living within an industrialized nation and asserts that occupational therapy practitioners are poised to address driving at various levels to evaluate and intervene relative to individual performance as well as contribute to the overall health and safety of the public.

The purpose of this statement is to define driving and community mobility from an occupational perspective, outline the role of occupational therapy in driving and community mobility, and situate the profession of occupational therapy in collaboration with other professions and organizations working toward safe and effective community mobility. The primary audience for this paper is occupational therapy practitioners, but it may also prove useful to stakeholders outside of the profession, including service recipients, related professionals, and the general public.

Throughout the lifespan, community mobility contributes to health and quality of life by supporting independence, social connectedness, a sense of identity, and access to health services and the community (Oxley & Whelan, 2008; Satariano et al., 2012). Within the context of industrialized nations such as the United States, driving in particular is linked to personal freedom and independence, and the inability to drive as well as the loss of the driving privilege are characterized by increased risk for social isolation, depression, and loneliness (Curl, Stowe, Cooney, & Proulx, 2014; Liddle, Reaston, Pachana, Mitchell, & Gustafsson, 2014).

Driving and community mobility are included within the domain of occupational therapy (AOTA, 2014b) and in the profession's *Scope of Practice* (AOTA, 2014c) as an IADL. Subsequently, all services in the realm of driving rehabilitation and community mobility are covered under typical malpractice insurance. Occupational therapy practitioners can further reduce liability risks through implementation of best practices, clear communication, thorough documentation, and limitation of practice to tasks within one's trained skill set (Pierce, 2009). Appendix A illustrates some of the aspects of driving and community mobility within the domain of occupational therapy practice and describes the complexity and influence of this critical IADL.

Definitions

Driving and *community mobility* are defined within the *Occupational Therapy Practice Framework: Domain and Process* (3rd ed.)., which guides practice in the United States, in the following way: "planning and moving around in the community and using public or private transportation, such as driving, walking, bicycling, or accessing and riding in buses, taxi cabs, or other transportation systems" (American Occupational Therapy

---

[1]When the term *occupational therapy practitioner* is used in this document, it refers to both occupational therapists and occupational therapy assistants (AOTA, 2015b). *Occupational therapists* are responsible for all aspects of occupational therapy service delivery and are accountable for the safety and effectiveness of the occupational therapy service delivery process. *Occupational therapy assistants* deliver occupational therapy services under the supervision of and in partnership with an occupational therapist (AOTA, 2014a).

Association [AOTA], 2014b, p. S19). In other occupational therapy literature, community mobility is described as moving about in the life space outside one's home (Rantakokko, Portegijs, Viljanen, Iwarsson, & Rantanen, 2013) and is viewed as essential for social participation and access to engagement in other everyday life activities (Ravulaparthy, Youn, & Goulias, 2013; Siren, Hjorthol, & Levin, 2015). These life activities are categorized as occupations in the lexicon of occupational therapy practice, and community mobility is considered a discrete area of occupation as well as an enabler of other occupations (Stav & McGuire, 2012).

Other definitions that inform work within driving and community mobility can be found in Appendix B. These definitions are not all-inclusive of terminology used within the profession but represent the most commonly used language in this domain of practice.

Occupational Therapy Service Provision

Occupational therapy practitioners possess the foundational education and training necessary to address driving and community mobility as an IADL as identified in the *Framework*. Throughout the evaluation and intervention process, occupational therapy practitioners recognize and address factors related to diseases, health conditions, atypical development, or aging that affect performance in driving and community mobility. The goal of service provision in this area of occupation is to optimize community mobility across the lifespan and in the context of all levels of ability.

Occupational therapy practitioners address driving and community mobility in a variety of practice settings with clients along the entire continuum of service provision. Clients of all ages and conditions may present with difficulties in driving and community mobility, including those with developmental or learning challenges, orthopedic injuries, neurological conditions, mental health conditions, and age-related changes and illnesses. In addition, environmental and contextual barriers such as community design, access to transit, population density, and slope or topography of the community may limit engagement in driving and community mobility.

All occupational therapy practitioners, including generalists, use assessment and clinical reasoning skills across IADL performance areas to interpret information about the client's factors and performance skills, performance patterns, and contextual and environmental factors to deduce strengths and potential risks related to occupational performance in driving and community mobility. This comprehensive set of skills positions occupational therapy as a critical and essential health care discipline to meet the complex demands of driving and community mobility concerns.

All occupational therapy practitioners share the common goals of supporting participation in the community, optimizing independence in community mobility, and preventing and reducing crash-related injuries and fatalities. Clients may be persons, groups, or populations. The extent of that therapeutic attention in all practice areas is provided along a continuum of expertise and focus from generalists through specialists. Appendix C provides examples of clients served, their respective community mobility concerns, and examples of possible occupational therapy services.

The following general principles apply to service provision along the entire spectrum of practice:

- Evaluating the ability to safely engage in driving and community mobility and ultimately determining an individual's ability to safely and independently travel in the community should be based on performance in context, not solely on diagnosis or age.

- Complex clinical reasoning during observation of performance in multiple areas of IADL performance as well as the administration and interpretation of evidence-based assessments are necessary to effectively determine the ability to engage in driving and community mobility.

- Interventions to enhance performance and safety in driving and community mobility should consider the community context as well as the client's potential for new learning.

- All clients and caregivers can benefit from education about safety and injury prevention in driving and relevant modes of transportation.

- Early identification of impairment relative to transportation provides clients and families the opportunity to plan (e.g., therapy, vehicle choice), explore options (e.g., program costs, accessible communities), and access desired interventions.

- Transitions to driving cessation should consider the client's need for continued engagement in community-based occupation and mobility throughout the community.

Generalist Practice in Driving and Community Mobility

Occupational therapy generalist practitioners address driving and community mobility as part of a larger mission to optimize occupational engagement through inquiry about community mobility needs, assessment of performance skills related to driving and community mobility, referral to other disciplines or specialists, and recommendation of discontinued or alternative driving or community mobility. Working with individual clients whose health or functional status may interfere with safe and effective community mobility, generalists have the education and skills to identify performance deficits, assess contributing skill or capacity impairments, and provide skilled interventions aimed at remediating or adapting performance. This process includes considering the strategic, operational, and tactical factors related to driving (Dickerson & Bédard, 2014) and the client's performance in this and other IADLs.

Specific to driving, generalist practitioners have the ability to determine those clients at risk for compromised driving performance and the responsibility to be aware of state regulations regarding minimum criteria for safe driving. Generalist practitioners must also use a referral process to driving rehabilitation specialists (DRSs) for those clients who are medically or developmentally at risk for impaired driving or for clients whose performance in other IADLs indicates they would benefit from specialized driving and community mobility services.

Relevant to other forms of community mobility, all occupational therapy practitioners have the education and skills to determine individual, occupational, and environmental factors that interfere with successful performance. Standards that guide occupational therapy education ensure that basic information about community mobility modes and resources is within the scope of knowledge of all occupational therapy practitioners (Accreditation Council for Occupational Therapy Education, 2012). This knowledge combined with the core therapeutic processes used by occupational therapy practitioners ensures that determining the fit between the community mobility task demands and the abilities of an individual is within the purview of generalist practitioners.

Although no specific certification is required of practitioners engaging in system-level community mobility work such as public transportation use and paratransit eligibility, advanced knowledge and training are strongly encouraged. Examples of specific community mobility training include Child Passenger Safety Certification sponsored by Safe Kids Worldwide (2013) and travel training options offered by Easter Seals Project Action (2013b).

Specialist Practice in Driving and Community Mobility

AOTA asserts that occupational therapists and occupational therapy assistants require advanced education prior to working directly in specialized driving and community mobility services. These practitioners offer a highly skilled and focused approach specific to driving and community mobility that leads to recommendation of the safest mobility outcome, provision of interventions and training in the use of adaptive equipment, advocacy and recommendations for system modifications, and execution of in vivo assessment and intervention either directly or via a proxy provider who partners in specific client situations. Specialist occupational therapy practitioners administer evidence-based assessments, when available, specific to the demands of driving, including clinical assessments of motor and praxis skills, sensory–perceptual skills, emotional regulation skills, cognitive skills, and communication and social skills. In addition, reaction time, knowledge of traffic rules, and on-road driving skills are typically assessed.

The primary purpose of conducting or contributing to these comprehensive evaluations is to determine the client's occupational performance potential to safely engage in driving or community mobility. Occupational therapy assistants contribute to this evaluation process by administering delegated assessments and reporting results toward the comprehensive evaluation. All practitioners contribute to education and support of caregivers and significant others through community mobility evaluation, intervention, and transitions.

Occupational therapy practitioners who specialize in realms of community mobility other than driving may seek focused training in certain areas (see above), but no specific advanced credential exists that represents this work. Development of expertise in areas such as travel training, work with paratransit systems, or pedestrian safety, to offer a few examples, is often accomplished through mentored experience in the field. Advanced practice in community mobility requires an understanding of the transportation or mobility system being addressed and skilled application of occupational therapy evaluation and intervention processes within these contexts.

Specific to driving, practitioners who conduct comprehensive driving evaluations are trained as DRSs and may be credentialed through the AOTA Board and Specialty Certification program (see http://tinyurl.com/jt8vp67) or certified through the Association for Driver Rehabilitation Specialists (ADED; n.d.-a; see http://www.aded.net). Those who are credentialed through AOTA Board and Specialty Certification are approved through a peer-reviewed process in which a professional portfolio representing excellence and substantive work in this realm is required. Once approved, practitioners may use the credentials SCDCM or SCDCM–A (specialty certified in driving and community mobility as an occupational therapist or occupational therapy assistant). Occupational therapy practitioners who seek certification through ADED are eligible to obtain the CDRS (certified driver rehabilitation specialist) after presenting qualifying credentials, having a specified number of hours of direct experience, and passing a certification exam.

Practitioners who conduct on-road evaluations must comply with state-specific requirements that may include being trained as driving instructors by the state-level entity administering that credential. This is especially relevant to providing training to novice drivers or persons whose driver license has expired. These practitioners have advanced training and experience in conducting not only in-clinic but also in vivo assessment of driving performance and are recognized by other health professionals as essential providers of driving rehabilitation services.

Evaluation processes carried out by specialists in driving and community mobility are characterized by the presentation of varying challenges and complexities during the in vivo observation and assessment of performance evaluation process to replicate actual driving or traveling experiences for a valid judgment of performance and safety. Those who are occupational therapists

- Administer comprehensive driving or community mobility evaluations;
- Recommend continued, modified, or cessation of driving or community travel;
- Suggest appropriate modifications or adaptive equipment for driving or community travel; and
- Provide retraining or specialized education for safe and effective travel through the community using the appropriate mode of transportation.

Specialist occupational therapy practitioners follow the evaluation with an individualized plan to provide intervention services to individuals for whom safe driving or community mobility is a possibility or will require intervention to transition from driver to passenger (National Highway Traffic Safety Administration [NHTSA], 2009; NHTSA & American Society on Aging, 2007). Interventions for the client with potential to travel in the community may include referral to an occupational therapy generalist for remediation of performance skills, education in adaptive strategies, remediation of driving performance, and training in the use of equipment to optimize performance and safety while operating or traveling in a motor vehicle.

The AOTA *Spectrum of Driver Services: Right Services for the Right People at the Right Time* (Lane et al., 2014) was developed as a guide to distinguish programs by services, training, credentials, and expected outcome. See http://www.aota.org/-/media/Corporate/Files/Practice/Aging/Driving/Spectrum-of-Driving-Services-2014.pdf.

Roles of Occupational Therapists and Occupational Therapy Assistants

The roles of occupational therapists and occupational therapy assistants in providing community mobility services differ according to the AOTA supervision guidelines (AOTA, 2014a). Consistent with these guidelines, occupational therapists carry the overall responsibility for the evaluation and intervention process. Therapists oversee the evaluation process and may delegate specific assessments to an occupational therapy assistant if that assistant has demonstrated competency in administration of the individual assessment. Examples include clinic-based tests of vision, cognition, and motor performance or the on-road assessment.

Occupational therapists are responsible for interpreting the results of any assessments and incorporating the results into the analysis of the entire evaluation. Therapists also may delegate the responsibility of implementing the intervention to occupational therapy assistants in accordance with the therapist's plan and the client's intervention goals. The *Guidelines for Supervision, Roles, and Responsibilities During the Delivery of Occupational Therapy Services* (AOTA, 2014a) recommend that occupational therapists and occupational therapy assistants develop a collaborative plan for supervision to guide the evaluation and the intervention process. The supervision must follow occupational therapy state licensure guidelines as well as the policies of the workplace and the *Occupational Therapy Code of Ethics* (AOTA, 2015a).

External Influences on Service Delivery in Driving and Community Mobility

Federal, state, and local laws, regulations, and policies are variable throughout the United States and therefore influence the delivery of occupational therapy services related to driving and community mobility in different ways. Occupational therapy practitioners need to govern their practice in consideration of laws and guidelines related to driver licensing (NHTSA & American Association of Motor Vehicle Administrators, 2009), medical reporting, Americans With Disabilities Act of 1990 (Pub. L. 101–336) requirements, paratransit eligibility, bicycling and pedestrian travel, and child passenger safety.

Reimbursement for driving and community mobility services also varies considerably from state to state and influences payment for occupational therapy services. The existing mechanisms for reimbursement for professional services and vehicle modifications include the Veterans Affairs system, Medicare and Medicaid in some states, state vocational rehabilitation departments, state workers' compensation, auto insurance, legal settlements, and self-pay. Community mobility services are paid for by several funding sources, including paratransit budgets, transit agencies, state departments of vocational rehabilitation, offices on aging, school systems, and grant funding through a variety of sources such as the United We Ride and Safe Routes to School initiatives.

Ethical Concerns in Driving and Community Mobility

In addition to ethical responsibilities that apply to all occupational therapy practice (AOTA, 2015a), some concerns relevant to driving and community mobility require the attention of occupational therapy practitioners. Literature and legal case precedents point in particular to two areas:

1. The duty to warn of the potential danger of impaired performance

2. The enhanced need to recognize factors that compromise performance as public health safety risks, not just individual issues (Slater, 2014).

A consensus statement on ethics specific to driving provides guidance to practitioners working in this area of practice. Among the recommendations in the statement are an emphasis on the use of current and appropriate assessment tools, the duty to avoid harm as well as promote engagement in occupation, and the obligation to warn clients and relevant regulatory agencies on the basis of the foreseeable likelihood of danger from the actions of an impaired client (Slater, 2014).

The consensus statement also notes that literature highlights the need to attend to the increased risk of unsafe driving due to impaired cognition, which occupational therapists may encounter working with clients who have not only traumatic or progressive conditions but also mental health concerns (Love, Welsh, Knabb, Scott, & Brokaw, 2008). Occupational therapy practitioners have a legal and ethical responsibility to be aware of laws in their state that pertain to reporting obligations and a professional responsibility to stay informed on recommendations for ethical practice (Slater, 2014).

Approaches to Driving and Community Mobility in Occupational Therapy

In accordance with the *Occupational Therapy Practice Framework* (AOTA, 2014b), approaches to intervention include specific strategies that are implemented on the basis of the clients' desired outcomes, evaluation data, and best available evidence. Each overarching approach outlined in the *Framework* is addressed in Table 1 relative to practice in driving and community mobility, although the examples are not meant to be all inclusive.

Table 1. Occupational Therapy Intervention Approaches in Driving and Community Mobility

Intervention Approach	Driving and Community Mobility Examples
Create/Promote (health promotion)	• Advocate for transportation equity • Collaborate with public transportation systems to ensure consumer knowledge about transit options • Provide staff training to paratransit operators and schedulers • Offer CarFit™ programs, which provide driver–vehicle fit education within the community • Contribute to planning and designs for communities and roadways to optimize travel for motorists, bicyclists, and pedestrians • Consult with automobile manufacturers for continuous improvement of vehicle–driver and vehicle–passenger fit • Provide instruction to novice drivers with learning or disabling conditions.
Establish/Restore (remediation, restoration)	• Offer (or refer for) specialized driving rehabilitation services to individuals experiencing compromised driving performance, once skills and recovery are optimized • Conduct cognitive retraining related to community mobility • Deliver travel training for safe and effective use of public transportation • Provide caregiver education related to capacity for community mobility • Remediate motor skills to operate a vehicle.
Maintain	• Conduct car seat checks in the community • Promote wellness related to driving and community mobility • Offer walking wellness programs • Work with municipalities to maintain bike and walking routes.
Modify (compensation or adaptation)	• Prescribe and train in the use of adaptive driving equipment • Recommend environmental modifications for accessibility at bus stops and transit stations • Recommend vehicle modifications to enhance access for drivers and passengers • Propose bicycle modifications for optimized travel • Suggest altered driving routes or travel times • Recommend restricted driver licenses.
Prevent (disability prevention)	• Advocate and consult for safe pedestrian routes • Review proposed policies and legislation • Recommend restricted licensing • Support evidence-based policies implementing graduated licensing • Reduce risk of injury through educational programming such as CarFit™.

Summary

Driving and community mobility is a growing area of importance. The association among personal mobility, transportation, and occupational engagement is increasingly relevant to clients across the lifespan, to the community, and to other organizations across the spectrum of healthcare and human services.

The skills, knowledge base, and scope of practice of occupational therapy enhanced by advanced education in driving and community mobility place the profession in the forefront of driving and community mobility services. The focus on injury prevention, engagement in occupation, and the intervention strategies used in driving rehabilitation and community mobility services are consistent with *The Philosophical Base of Occupational Therapy* (AOTA, 2011) and, therefore, warrant attention in all areas of occupational therapy practice. Occupational therapy practitioners provide a critical and essential combination of skills and abilities to support individuals' driving and community mobility and thus to expand or maintain their engagement in community activities and their quality of life.

References

AAA, AARP, & American Occupational Therapy Association. (2015). *CarFit technician manual.* Washington, DC: American Automobile Association.

AARP. (2005). *Beyond 50.05: A report to the nation on livable communities: Creating environments for successful aging.* Washington, DC: Author. Retrieved from http://assets.aarp.org/rgcenter/il/beyond_50_communities.pdf

Abley, S. (2005). *Walkability scoping paper.* Retrieved from http://www.levelofservice.com/walkability-research.pdf

Accreditation Council for Occupational Therapy Education. (2012). 2011 Accreditation Council for Occupational Therapy Education (ACOTE®) standards. *American Journal of Occupational Therapy, 66*(6, Suppl.), S6–S74. http://dx.doi.org/10.5014/ajot.2012.66S6

ADED: The Association for Driver Rehabilitation Specialists. (n.d.-a). *Association for Driver Rehabilitation Specialists.* Retrieved from http://www.aded.net

ADED. (n.d.-b). *Learn about: CDRS.* Retrieved from http://www.aded.net/?page=210

American Academy of Pediatrics. (2011). Policy Statement—Child passenger safety. *Pediatrics, 127,* 788–793. http://dx.doi.org/10.1542/peds.2011-0213

American Geriatrics Society, & Pomidor, A. (Eds.). (2016, January). *Clinician's guide to assessing and counseling older drivers, 3rd edition* (Report No. DOT HS 812 228). Washington, DC: National Highway Traffic Safety Administration.

American Occupational Therapy Association. (2011). The philosophical base of occupational therapy. *American Journal of Occupational Therapy, 65*(6, Suppl.), S65. http://dx.doi.org/10.5014/ajot.2011.65s65

American Occupational Therapy Association. (2014a). Guidelines for supervision, roles, and responsibilities during the delivery of occupational therapy services. *American Journal of Occupational Therapy, 68*(Suppl. 3), S16–S22. http://dx.doi.org/10.5014/ajot.2014.686S03

American Occupational Therapy Association. (2014b). Occupational therapy practice framework: Domain and process (3rd ed.). *American Journal of Occupational Therapy, 68*(Suppl. 1), S1–S48. http://dx.doi.org/10.5014/ajot.2014.682006

American Occupational Therapy Association. (2014c). Scope of practice. *American Journal of Occupational Therapy, 68*(Suppl. 3), S34–S40. http://dx.doi.org/10.5014/ajot.2014.686S04

American Occupational Therapy Association. (2015a). Occupational therapy code of ethics (2015). *American Journal of Occupational Therapy, 69*(Suppl. 3), 6913410030. http://dx.doi.org/10.5014/ajot.2015.696S03

American Occupational Therapy Association. (2015b). Policy A.23: Categories of occupational therapy personnel. In *Policy manual* (pp. 25–26). Bethesda, MD: Author. Retrieved from http://www.aota.org/-/media/corporate/files/aboutaota/governance/2015-policy-manual.pdf

American Occupational Therapy Association. (2015c). Standards of practice for occupational therapy. *American Journal of Occupational Therapy, 69*(Suppl. 3), 6913410057. http://dx.doi.org/10.5014/ajot.2015.696S06

American Public Transportation Association. (1994). *Glossary of transit terminology.* Retrieved from http://www.apta.com/resources/reportsandpublications/Documents/Transit_Glossary_1994.pdf

Americans With Disabilities Act of 1990, Pub. L. 101–336, 42 U.S.C. § 12101.

Barlow, J. H., Cullen, L. A., Foster, N. E., Harrison, K., & Wade, M. (1999). Does arthritis influence perceived ability to fulfill a parenting role? Perceptions of mothers, fathers and grandparents. *Patient Education and Counseling, 37,* 141–151. http://dx.doi.org/10.1016/S0738-3991(98)00136-0

Best, K. L., Miller, W. C., Huston, G., Routhier, F., & Eng, J. J. (2016). Pilot study of a peer-led wheelchair training program to improve self-efficacy using a manual wheelchair: A randomized controlled trial. *Archives of Physical Medicine and Rehabilitation, 97,* 37–44. http://dx.doi.org/10.1016/j.apmr.2015.08.425

Beverly Foundation, & AAA Foundation for Traffic Safety. (2004). *Supplemental transportation programs for seniors: A report on STPs in America.* Pasadena, CA: Beverly Foundation.

Bicycle Safety Resource Center. (2009). *Federal Highway Administration.* Retrieved from http://www.bicyclinginfo.org/education/resource/fhwa.html?/ee/fhwa.html

Boulias, C., Meikle, B., Pauley, T., & Devlin, M. (2006). Return to driving after lower-extremity amputation. *Archives of Physical Medicine and Rehabilitation, 87,* 1183–1188. http://dx.doi.org/10.1016/j.apmr.2006.06.001

Brown, C. (2009). Functional assessment and intervention in occupational therapy. *Psychiatric Rehabilitation Journal, 32,* 162–170. http://dx.doi.org/10.2975/32.3.2009.162-170

Chee, D. Y., Lee, H. C., Falkmer, M., Barnett, T., Falkmer, O., Siljehav, J., & Falkmer, T. (2015). Viewpoints on driving of individuals with and without autism spectrum disorder. *Developmental Neurorehabilitation, 18,* 26–36. http://dx.doi.org/10.3109/17518423.2014.964377

Classen, S., Dickerson, A., & Justiss, M. D. (2012). Occupational therapy driving evaluation: Using evidence-based screening and assessment tools. In M. J. McGuire & E. Schold Davis (Eds.), *Driving and community mobility: Occupational therapy strategies across the lifespan* (pp. 221–278). Bethesda, MD: AOTA Press.

Classen, S., Levy, C., McCarthy, D., Mann, W. C., Lanford, D., & Waid-Ebbs, J. K. (2009). Traumatic brain injury and driving assessment: An evidence-based literature review. *American Journal of Occupational Therapy, 63,* 580–591. http://dx.doi.org/10.5014/ajot.63.5.580

Community Transportation Association of America. (2010). *Glossary of transportation terms.* Retrieved from http://web1.ctaa.org/webmodules/webarticles/articlefiles/GlossaryOfTransportationTerms.pdf

Crabtree, J., Troyer, J. D., & Justiss, M. D. (2009). The intersection of driving with a disability and being a public transportation passenger with a disability. *Topics in Geriatric Rehabilitation, 25,* 163–172. http://dx.doi.org/10.1097/TGR.0b013e3181a1043a

Curl, A. L., Stowe, J. D., Cooney, T. M., & Proulx, C. M. (2014). Giving up the keys: How driving cessation affects engagement in later life. *Gerontologist, 54,* 423–433. http://dx.doi.org/10.1093/geront/gnt037

Di Stefano, M., Lovell, R., Stone, K., Oh, S., & Cockfield, S. (2009). Supporting individuals to make informed personal mobility choices. *Topics in Geriatric Rehabilitation, 25,* 55–72. http://dx.doi.org/10.1097/TGR.0b013e3181914b2a

Dickerson, A. E., & Bédard, M. (2014). Decision tool for clients with medical issues: A framework for identifying driving risk and potential to return to driving. *Occupational Therapy in Health Care, 28,* 194–202. http://dx.doi.org/10.3109/07380577.2014.903357

Dickerson, A. E., & Schold Davis, E., (2012). Welcome to the team! Who are the stakeholders? In M. J. McGuire & E. Schold Davis (Eds.), *Driving and community mobility: Occupational therapy strategies across the lifespan* (pp. 49–77). Bethesda, MD: AOTA Press.

Easter Seals Project Action. (2013a). *Glossary of disability and transit terms.* Retrieved from http://www.projectaction.com/glossary-of-disability-and-transit-terms/

Easter Seals Project Action. (2013b). *Travel training resources.* Retrieved from http://www.projectaction.com/travel-training-resources/

Federal Highway Administration. (2001). *Highway design handbook: For older drivers and pedestrians* (Report No. FHWA-RD-01-103). McLean, VA: U.S. Department of Transportation.

Fisher, A. G. (2009). *Occupational Therapy Intervention Process Model: A model for planning and implementing top-down, client-centered, and occupation-based interventions.* Fort Collins, CO: Three Star Press.

Fisher, A. G., & Griswold, L. A. (2014). Performance skills: Implementing performance analyses to evaluate quality of occupational performance. In B. A. B. Schell, G. Gillen, & M. Scaffa (Eds.), *Willard and Spackman's occupational therapy* (12th ed., pp. 249–264). Philadelphia: Lippincott Williams & Wilkins.

Griffin, J., & Priddy, D. A. (2005). Assessing paratransit eligibility under the Americans With Disabilities Act in the rehabilitation setting. *Archives of Physical Medicine and Rehabilitation, 86,* 1267–1269. http://dx.doi.org/10.1016/j.apmr.2004.10.034

Hunt, L. A., Brown, A. E., & Gilman, I. P. (2010). Drivers with dementia and outcomes of becoming lost while driving. *American Journal of Occupational Therapy, 64,* 225–232. http://dx.doi.org/10.5014/ajot.64.2.225

International Transport Forum. (2009). *Cognitive impairment, mental health and transport: Design with everyone in mind.* Retrieved from http://www.internationaltransportforum.org/pub/pdf/09Cognitive.pdf

Kielhofner, G. (2008). *The Model of Human Occupation: Theory and application* (4th ed.). Philadelphia: Lippincott Williams & Wilkins.

Lane, A., Green, E., Dickerson, A. E., Schold Davis, E., Rolland, B., & Stohler, J. T. (2014). Driver rehabilitation programs: Defining program models, services and expertise. *Occupational Therapy in Health Care, 28,* 177–187.

Law, M., Cooper, B., Strong, S., Stewart, D., Rigby, P., & Letts, L. (1996). Person–Environment–Occupation Model: A transactive approach to occupational performance. *Canadian Journal of Occupational Therapy, 63,* 9–23. http://dx.doi.org/10.1177/000841749606300103

Liddle, J., Reaston, T., Pachana, N., Mitchell, G., & Gustafsson, L. (2014). Is planning for driving cessation critical for the well-being and lifestyle of older drivers? *International Psychogeriatrics, 26,* 1111–1120. http://dx.doi.org/10.1017/S104161021400060X

Lillie, S. (2006). Transportation, community mobility, and driving assessment. In H. M. Pendleton & W. Schultz-Krohn (Eds.), *Pedretti's occupational therapy: Practice skills for physical dysfunction* (6th ed., pp. 224–247). St. Louis, MO: Mosby.

Love, C. M., Welsh, R. K., Knabb, J. J., Scott, S. T., & Brokaw, D. W. (2008). Working with cognitively impaired drivers: Legal issues for mental health professionals to consider. *Journal of Safety Research, 39,* 535–545. http://dx.doi.org/10.1016/j.jsr.2008.09.001

National Center for Mobility Management. (2016). *Mobility management.* Retrieved May 31, 2016, from http://nationalcenterformobilitymanagement.org/mobility-management/#sthash.RA47d4d1.dpuf

National Center for Safe Routes to School. (n.d.). *Safe routes.* Retrieved May 31, 2016, from http://www.saferoutesinfo.org/

National Highway Traffic Safety Administration. (2009). *Driving transitions education: Tools, scripts, and practice exercises* (DOT HS 811 152). Washington, DC: Author.

National Highway Traffic Safety Administration. (2014, April). Older driver safety. In *Uniform Guidelines for state highway safety programs* (DOT HS 812 007D). Retrieved May 31, 2016, from http://www.nhtsa.gov/nhtsa/whatsup/tea21/tea21programs/pages/812007D-HSPG13-OlderDriverSafety.pdf

National Highway Traffic Safety Administration, & American Association of Motor Vehicle Administrators. (2009). *Driver fitness medical guidelines.* Washington, DC: National Highway Traffic Safety Administration.

National Highway Traffic Safety Administration, & American Society on Aging. (2007). *DriveWell: Promoting older driver safety and mobility in your community.* Washington, DC: National Highway Traffic Safety Administration.

O'Neil, J., Bull, M. J., Slaven, J. E., & Talty, J. L. (2012). Grandparents and child passenger safety. *Accident Analysis and Prevention, 49,* 354–359. http://dx.doi.org/10.1016/j.aap.2012.02.011

Oxley, J., & Whelan, M. (2008). It cannot be all about safety: The benefits of prolonged mobility. *Traffic Injury Prevention, 9,* 367–378. http://dx.doi.org/10.1080/15389580801895285

Perkinson, M. A., Berg-Weger, M. L., Carr, D. B., Meuser, T. M., Palmer, J. L., Buckles, V. D., . . . Morris, J. C. (2005). Driving and dementia of the Alzheimer type: Beliefs and cessation strategies among stakeholders. *Gerontologist, 45,* 676–685. http://dx.doi.org/10.1093/geront/45.5.676

Pierce, S. (2009, September 29). *Driving evaluation programs: Development and effective service delivery* (AOTA Webinar Series). Bethesda, MD: Retrieved from http://www.aota.org/-/media/corporate/files/practice/aging/driving/toolkit/driving/developingdrivingevaluationprogramwebinar.pdf

Rantakokko, M., Portegijs, E., Viljanen, A., Iwarsson, S., & Rantanen, T. (2013). Life-space mobility and quality of life in community-dwelling older people. *Journal of the American Geriatrics Society, 61,* 1830–1832. http://dx.doi.org/10.1111/jgs.12473

Ravulaparthy, S., Yoon, S. Y., & Goulias, K. G. (2013). Linking elderly transport mobility and subjective well-being. *Transportation Research Record, 2382,* 28–36. http://dx.doi.org/10.3141/2382-04

Safe Kids Worldwide. (2013). *National child passenger safety certification.* Retrieved from http://cert.safekids.org/

Safe Kids Worldwide. (2015). *Bike safety.* Retrieved from http://www.safekids.org/bike

Satariano, W. A., Guralnik, J. M., Jackson, R. J., Marottoli, R. A., Phelan, E. A., & Prohaska, T. R. (2012). Mobility and aging: New directions for public health action. *American Journal of Public Health, 102,* 1508–1515. http://dx.doi.org/10.2105/AJPH.2011.300631

Siren, A., Hjorthol, R., & Levin, L. (2015). Different types of out-of-home activities and well-being amongst urban residing old people with mobility impediments. *Journal of Transport and Health, 2,* 14–21. http://dx.doi.org/10.1016/j.jth.2014.11.004

Slater, D. Y.; National Highway Traffic Safety Administration, & American Occupational Therapy Association. (2014). Consensus statements on occupational therapy ethics related to driving. *Occupational Therapy in Health Care, 28,* 163–168. http://dx.doi.org/10.3109/07380577.2014.903356

Stav, W. B. (2015). *Occupational therapy practice guidelines for driving and community mobility for older adults.* Bethesda, MD: AOTA Press.

Stav, W. B., & Lieberman, D. (2008). From the desk of the editor. *American Journal of Occupational Therapy, 62,* 127–129. http://dx.doi.org/10.5014/ajot.62.2.127

Stav, W. B., & McGuire, M. J. (2012). Introduction to driving and community mobility. In M. J. McGuire & E. Schold Davis (Eds.), *Driving and community mobility: Occupational therapy strategies across the lifespan* (pp. 1–18). Bethesda, MD: AOTA Press.

Stepaniuk, J. A., Tuokko, H., McGee, P., Garrett, D. D., & Benner, E. L. (2008). Impact of transit training and free bus pass on public transportation use by older drivers. *Preventive Medicine, 47,* 335–337. http://dx.doi.org/10.1016/j.ypmed.2008.03.002

Stern, E. (2007). Driving safely at home after combat driving. *Military OneSource.* Retrieved from http://www.militaryonesource.com/portals/0/aspx/material_getpdf.ashx?MaterialID=15086

Womack, J., & Silverstein, N. (2010). The big picture: Comprehensive community mobility. In M. J. McGuire & E. Schold Davis (Eds.), *Driving and community mobility: Occupational therapy strategies across the lifespan* (pp. 19–31). Bethesda: AOTA Press.

Yonkman, J., O'Neil, J., Talty, J., & Bull, M. J. (2010). Transporting children in wheelchairs in passenger vehicles: A comparison of best practice to observed and reported practice in a pilot sample. *American Journal of Occupational Therapy, 64,* 804–808. http://dx.doi.org/10.5014/ajot.2010.09162

Authors
Elin Schold Davis, OTR/L, CDRS
Wendy B. Stav, PhD, OTR/L, SCDCM, FAOTA
Jenny Womack, MS, MA, OTR/L, C/PH, SCDCM, FAOTA

for

The Commission on Practice
Kathleen Kannenberg, MA, OTR/L, CCM, *Chairperson*

Adopted by the Representative Assembly Coordinating Council (RACC) for the Representative Assembly

Revised by the Commission on Practice 2015

Note. This revision replaces the 2010 document *Driving and Community Mobility,* previously published and copyrighted in 2010 by the American Occupational Therapy Association in the *American Journal of Occupational Therapy, 64*(6, Suppl.), S112–S124. http://dx.doi.org/10.5014/ajot.2010.64S112

Citation. American Occupational Therapy Association. (2016). Driving and community mobility. *American Journal of Occupational Therapy, 70*(Suppl. 2), 7012410050. http://dx.doi.org/10.5014/ajot.2016.706S04

Appendix A. Domain of Occupational Therapy Specific to Driving and Community Mobility

Aspects of the Domain (AOTA, 2014b)	Examples
Areas of occupation • IADLs • Driving and community mobility	"Planning and moving around in the community and using public or private transportation, such as driving, walking, bicycling, or accessing and riding taxi cabs, or other transportation systems" (AOTA, 2014b, p. S19). In addition to being an IADL, driving and community mobility is an occupation enabler, because it allows for engagement in several other areas of occupation including education, work, leisure, social participation, and other IADLs (Stav & Lieberman, 2008).
Performance skills (motor skills, process skills, social interaction skills)	• Driving and community mobility require one to possess and execute adequate performance skills. • Individuals must use motor skills to physically move in a planned, coordinated, sequenced manner to operate a motor vehicle, travel using transit services, or exert bodily control while walking or bicycling. • Driving and community mobility require process skills to use sufficient attention, sequencing, organization, and navigation skills while moving through the dynamic, unpredictable environment of the community. • Communication and social skills are used as individuals exchange information, relate, and physically communicate to move through a community in which other individuals are also mobile.
Client factors (values, beliefs, spirituality; body functions; body structures)	Persons, groups, and populations assign meaning to and derive meaning from driving and community mobility based on their own values, beliefs, and spirituality as well as the values and beliefs of society and culture. To successfully engage in driving and community mobility, clients use their body functions—mental functions, sensory functions, neuromusculoskeletal and movement-related functions, voice and speech functions, and cardiovascular and respiratory system functions, as well as related body structures—to effectively and safely move about in the community.
Performance patterns (habits, routines, roles)	Driving and community mobility involve performance patterns using habits to operate equipment and routines to travel on an established route. Individuals fulfill the duties and responsibilities of a community traveler (e.g., driver, passenger, pedestrian) as well as life roles by engaging in community mobility.
Context and environment (cultural, personal, temporal, virtual, social)	• The environment and context in which driving and community mobility take place are critical in understanding who, what, where, when, how, and why individuals move through the community. • The cultural context may dictate which driver in a family with 5 licensed individuals operates an automobile during an outing. • An individual's personal context indicates whether travel will be performed as a passenger or operator on the basis of age or socioeconomic status. • Temporal context affects community mobility on the basis of the stage of life, time of day, season of year, and duration of driving. • Virtual contexts such as driving simulators and the use of personal computers for various mobility supports are influencing engagement in and performance of community mobility. • The physical environment relates to travel in urban or rural settings; on different types of roadways; over a street, sidewalk, or path; or using underground, waterway, air, or land travel. • The social context may influence independent vs. group travel.

Note. AOTA = American Occupational Therapy Association; IADL = instrumental activity of daily living.

Appendix B. Glossary of Driving and Community Mobility Terminology for Occupational Therapy

Overarching Terminology

Instrumental activities of daily living (IADLs): Activities to support daily life within the home and community that often require more complex interactions than those used in activities of daily living (AOTA, 2014b, p. S19).

Occupation enabler: An occupation, device, or factor that supports engagement in other occupations.

Occupational performance: Act of doing and accomplishing a selected action (performance skill), activity, or occupation (Fisher, 2009; Fisher & Griswold, 2014; Kielhofner, 2008) that results from the dynamic transaction among the client, the context, and the activity; improving or enabling skills and patterns in occupational performance leads to engagement in occupations or activities (adapted in part from Law et al., 1996, p. 16).

Driving and Community Mobility Terminology

Adaptive driving equipment/adaptive driving technology: After-market modifications to vehicle controls, seating, doorways, entrance and exit, or mobility device management and storage on a vehicle to accommodate for driver or passenger impairments.

Americans With Disabilities Act of 1990 (ADA; Pub. L. 101–336): Federal law that requires public transit agencies that provide fixed-route service to provide "complementary paratransit" services to people with disabilities who cannot use the fixed-route bus or rail service because of a disability. The ADA regulations specifically define a population of customers who are entitled to this service as a civil right. The regulations also define minimum service characteristics that must be met for this service to be considered equivalent to the fixed-route service it is intended to complement. In general, ADA complementary paratransit service must be provided within 3/4 of a mile of a bus route or rail station, at the same hours and days, for no more than twice the regular fixed route fare (Community Transportation Association of America [CTAA], 2010).

Bikeability: The extent to which the built or natural environment is friendly for bicycling.

Certified driver rehabilitation specialist (CDRS): A person who meets the educational and experiential requirements and successfully completes the certification examination provided by the Association for Driver Rehabilitation Specialists (ADED, n.d.-a).

Community mobility assessment: "An assessment of a specific performance skill related to walking in the community, using transportation, negotiating travel using transit, and interacting with other travelers that is conducted in the naturalistic context of the community" (Stav, 2015, p. 118).

Community mobility evaluation: "The evaluation process measures client factors, performance skills, and contexts in which the client engages in community mobility to identify strengths and areas of need" (AOTA, 2015c, p. 2; Stav & McGuire, 2012, p. 12). The process may include identification of available, accessible, and appropriate transportation options for the client and assessment of the client's ability to use the transportation options, navigate through the community using the transportation, and interact with other users and transportation operators.

Community transportation: The family of transportation services in a community, including public and private sources, that are available to respond to the mobility needs of all community members (CTAA, 2010).

Comprehensive driving evaluation: An in-depth evaluation of driving performance skills and client factors related to driving (Pierce, 2009). The evaluation process includes self-report, clinical assessment, and behind-the-wheel assessment (Classen, Dickerson, & Justiss, 2012); interpretation of results leads to determination of fitness to drive and development of an intervention plan.

Driver rehabilitation specialist/driving rehabilitation specialist (DRS): A specialist who "plans, develops, coordinates, or implements driving rehabilitation services for individuals with disabilities" (Dickerson & Schold Davis, 2012, p. 51) and "works with people of all ages and abilities, exploring alternative transportation solutions for drivers with special needs" (ADED, n.d.-b, para. 1).

Driver–vehicle fit: The match between a driver and the vehicle to allow for proper use of vehicle safety features and vehicle operation to optimize comfort, driving performance, safety, and reduction of injuries in the event of a crash.

Driving screening: "The process of obtaining and reviewing data relevant to a potential client to determine the need for further [driving or community mobility] evaluation and intervention" (AOTA, 2015c, p. 2).

Fitness to drive: A driver's ability to operate a motor vehicle safely in the light of the driver's state of health (National Highway Traffic Safety Administration & American Association of Motor Vehicle Administrators 2009).

Fixed-route transportation: Transit services in which vehicles run on regular, scheduled routes with fixed stops and no deviation. Typically, fixed-route service is characterized by printed schedules or timetables, designated bus stops where passengers board and exit, and the use of larger transit vehicles (CTAA, 2010).

Livability: A term used to describe communities that have affordable and appropriate housing, supportive community services, and adequate mobility options that facilitate personal independence and the engagement of inhabitants in civic and social life (AARP, 2005).

Mobility manager: An individual who designs the delivery of transportation services that begins and ends with the customer. The mobility manager works to develop a community vision in which the entire transportation network—public transit, private operators, cycling and walking, volunteer drivers, and others—works together with customers, planners, and stakeholders to deliver the transportation options that best meet a community's needs (National Center for Mobility Management, 2016).

Paratransit/ADA complementary paratransit: Types of passenger transportation that are more flexible than conventional fixed-route transit but more structured than the use of private automobiles. *Paratransit* is a broad term that may be used to describe any means of shared-ride transportation other than fixed-route mass transit services. Paratransit services usually use smaller vehicles (fewer than 25 passengers) and provide advance-reservation, demand-responsive service that is either curb-to-curb or door-to-door. Paratransit services that are provided to accommodate passengers with disabilities who are unable to use fixed-route service and that meet specific service equivalency tests are called *ADA complementary paratransit services.*

Paratransit eligibility: The process of determination of a traveler's functional limitation relative to fixed-route public transportation that may then qualify him or her for ADA complementary paratransit services (see above). Some systems determine eligibility on a trip-by-trip basis, whereas others provide all-or-none eligibility (Womack & Silverstein, 2010).

Public transportation: Transportation by a means of conveyance that provides general or specialized service to the public that is regular and continuous (American Public Transportation Association, 1994). Public transportation is alternatively referred to as *mass transportation, mass transit,* or simply *transit.* Public transportation typically connotes services that are funded in whole or part by public tax revenues.

Supplemental transportation programs (STPs): Also called *STPs for seniors,* these types of transportation options are provided to supplement or complement the efforts of family members, neighbors, and friends to provide options that enable older adults to stop driving without losing their ability to go places. They also fill in the gaps where traditional transit options are unavailable or cannot accommodate the special needs of older travelers (Beverly Foundation & AAA Foundation for Traffic Safety, 2004).

Travel training/travel instruction: Short-term, intensive instruction (usually one-on-one) designed to teach people with disabilities and seniors to travel safely and independently on fixed-route public transportation in their community. Travel instruction professionals must be able to determine how different disabilities affect a person's ability to travel and develop appropriate methods to teach travel skills based on these abilities (Easter Seals Project Action, 2013a).

Walkability: The extent to which the built environment is walking friendly (Abley, 2005) for a diverse population of people with varying abilities.

Appendix C. Case Examples of Driving and Community Mobility Services

Service Recipients	Community Mobility Concerns	Occupational Therapy Services
Individuals		
Traveling in a car with a 3-year-old with CP	• Secure, safe seating for the child • Adherence to state child passenger safety laws.	• Assistance in selection of appropriate child safety seat for the child's size, weight, and age • Family education for seat installation • Family education for managing extensor tone and fastening the child • Introduction to DRS for long-term planning to inform and build awareness that includes future vehicle choices and potential resources for possible future driving • Development of a child safety seat loan closet for short-term client needs. (American Academy of Pediatrics, 2011; Yonkman, O'Neil, Talty, & Bull, 2010)
Fastening a child into a safety seat by a parent with RA	• Secure, safe seating for the child • Adherence to state child passenger safety laws • Joint protection for the parent • Energy conservation for the parent.	• Assistance in the identification of the appropriate seat for child's size, weight, and age • Assistance in the identification of child safety seats for ease of use • Parent education for seat installation • Identification of child safety seat installation stations • Client education in joint protection and energy conservation related to seat installation and child fastening • Training in the use of adaptive equipment to aide in fastening • Consideration of specialized driver rehabilitation services for exploration of equipment or vehicle modification to ease long-term caregiver burden and safety for ingress and egress. (Barlow, Cullen, Foster, Harrison, & Wade, 1999; O'Neil, Bull, Slaven, & Talty, 2012)

Bicycling by an 8-year-old with MD	• Strength and coordination to operate a bicycle
	• Balance to remain upright on the bicycle
	• Awareness of risks and rules of the road.
		• Evaluation to determine potential for independent bicycling
		• Therapeutic exercise and activity for
		  ○ Strength
		  ○ Coordination
		  ○ Balance.
		• Client and family education on environmental awareness and rules of the road.
		(Bicycle Safety Resource Center, 2009; Safe Kids Worldwide, 2015)

Learning to drive for a 16-year-old with ASD	• Interpersonal relations with other road users using nonverbal communication • Coordination to operate a motor vehicle • Awareness of the driving environment and risks • Awareness of rules of the road.	• Provision of therapeutic exercises and activities to support future readiness for driving or readiness to participate in driving rehabilitation program • Referral to an OT specialist in driving for individualized structured driver education • Evaluation to determine potential for driving • Client education for environmental awareness consistent with client's cognitive capacities and learning needs • Assistance with applying for a driver license. (Chee et al., 2015)

Appendix C. Case Examples of Driving and Community Mobility Services *(cont.)*

Service Recipients	Community Mobility Concerns	Occupational Therapy Services
Traveling in a community as a 19-year-old pedestrian with SCI	• Negotiation of intersections • Navigation across uneven terrain.	• Client education for curb cuts and safety awareness • Route planning for accessible paths • Training in advocacy strategies for promotion of accessible communities. (Best, Miller, Huston, Routhier, & Eng, 2016)

Return to driving for a 45-year-old after TBI	• Operation of the vehicle controls with impaired motor skills and abnormal muscle tone
	• Full and accurate visual access to the driving environment
	• Safe maneuvering in the driving environment using
	  ○ Attention
	  ○ Memory
	  ○ Judgment
	  ○ Planning
	  ○ Organization
	  ○ Impulse control.
	• Transfer in and out of the vehicle
	• Storage of mobility aids
	• Self-awareness of deficits and correlation to driving safety.
		• Determination of readiness for transition to specialized driving rehabilitation services
		• Evaluation to identify client-centered transportation options and potential to return to driving*
		• Client and family education related to delayed return to driving
		• Assessment to determine capability of learning how to use adaptive equipment and traffic safety rules*
		• Therapeutic exercises and activities to maximize
		  ○ Sensory–perceptual skills
		  ○ Motor and praxis skills
		  ○ Emotional regulation skills
		  ○ Cognitive skills
		  ○ Communication and social skills
		  ○ BTW training.*
		• Recommendation of and training in the use of adaptive equipment*
		• Assistance in the selection of an automobile capable of accommodating adaptive equipment*
		• Assistance with applying for a modified driver license
		• Guidance for applying to vehicle manufacturer for an adaptive equipment rebate.
		(Classen et al., 2009; Lillie, 2006).

Return to driving for a 20-year-old wounded veteran with a traumatic right lower-extremity amputation and PTSD related to combat driving	• Operation of the vehicle foot pedals with a prosthetic limb or obtaining a left-foot gas pedal modification
	• Continuation of dangerous combat driving postdeployment:
	  ○ Maneuvering around traffic
	  ○ Avoiding roadside debris
	  ○ Proceeding through traffic lights and stop signs.
	• Panic attacks when driving under bridges
	• Safety related to return to driving.
		• Evaluation to determine potential for safe return to driving*
		• Assessment to determine capability to learn how to use adaptive equipment*
		• Referral for psychological counseling to address PTSD concerns
		• BTW training*
		• Recommendation and training in the use of adaptive equipment*
		• Assistance in the selection of an automobile capable of accommodating adaptive equipment*
		• Assistance with applying for a modified driver license
		• Guidance in applying to veteran's benefits for a vehicle stipend and to vehicle manufacturer for an adaptive equipment rebate.
		(Boulias, Meikle, Pauley, & Devlin, 2006; Stern, 2007)

Driving for a 64-year-old woman with dementia	• Safe operation of an automobile in a variety of driving environments, particularly unfamiliar roads or routes, due to impairment • Memory • Judgment • Cognitive processing speed • Recognition of errors	• Comprehensive driving evaluation to determine potential for continued driving* • Identification of plan for driving restrictions, transition, and reevaluation • Analysis of a person's historical and current daily occupational patterns as part of an occupational profile to identify community mobility needs

(Continued)

Appendix C. Case Examples of Driving and Community Mobility Services *(cont.)*

Service Recipients	Community Mobility Concerns	Occupational Therapy Services

	• Potential for wandering and getting lost
	• Capacity to flexibly and effectively respond to complex or unexpected events, such as road construction and detours
	• Capacity to problem solve and seek or accept assistance.
		• Assistance in the transition to driving cessation, including
		  ○ Identification of transportation alternatives and service delivery resources in the client's area
		  ○ Training in supervised travel on existing transit systems, assistance with the application for paratransit, and family education
		  ○ Referral to counseling or support services to address feelings of loss related to driving cessation
		  ○ Provision of support for family members
		  ○ Provision of cessation strategies to counter persistent determination to drive.
		(American Geriatrics Society & Pomidor, 2016; Hunt, Brown, & Gilman, 2010; Perkinson et al., 2005)

Traveling by transit systems for an adult with schizophrenia	• Safe and timely negotiation of routes and transfers
	• Management of fare or bus pass
	• Potential for victimization.
		• Travel training in the use of the local transit system
		• Therapeutic activities for
		  ○ Money management
		  ○ Time management
		  ○ Trip planning
		  ○ Community reintegration.
		• Assistance in the application for prepaid bus passes
		• Exploration of support options, including travel escort or specialized transportation providers via guidance through mobility managers
		• Advocacy for services of mobility managers and travel trainers
		• Training in strategies to protect one's person and possessions.
		(Brown, 2009; International Transport Forum, 2009)

Groups

Service Recipients	Community Mobility Concerns	Occupational Therapy Services

Transit company seeking to increase ridership among passengers with disabilities and reduce costly paratransit services	• Consumer awareness of disability-friendly transportation services
	• Availability and accessibility of
	  ○ Vehicles
	  ○ Bus stops
	  ○ Shelters.
	• Leniency of paratransit eligibility
	• Disability awareness
	• Ability of drivers to operate lift and wheelchair tie-downs and to manage behavioral issues
	• Ability of facility schedulers to meet the needs of riders with cognitive impairments.
		• Accessibility evaluations and recommendations for vehicles, bus stops, and shelters to elevate to ADA compliance
		• Modification of paratransit eligibility evaluation
		• Equipment training for drivers
		• Advocacy for services of mobility managers and travel trainers
		• Sensitivity training of drivers and schedulers.
		(Crabtree, Troyer, & Justiss, 2009; Griffin & Priddy, 2005)

Populations

Service Recipients	Community Mobility Concerns	Occupational Therapy Services

Populations that need to safely engage in mobility within the community	• Roadway design to support older drivers
	• Bike lanes, pedestrian paths, and sidewalks to support multiple modes of transportation
	• Signage visible to road users of varying literacy and visual levels
	• Access to common areas.
		• Collaboration with municipal planning organizations to promote
		  ○ Multiuser roadway design
		  ○ Inclusion of bicycle and pedestrian paths
		  ○ Centralized common areas of equidistant travel from all residences
		  ○ Separation of locations with many high-risk drivers (e.g., high school and senior center should not be across the street from each other)
		  ○ Legible signage with large fonts and symbols (Federal Highway Administration, 2001).

Appendix C. Case Examples of Driving and Community Mobility Services *(cont.)*

Service Recipients	Community Mobility Concerns	Occupational Therapy Services
		• Travel training programs to increase acceptance and use of transit. (Di Stefano, Lovell, Stone, Oh, & Cockfield, 2009; Stepaniuk, Tuokko, McGee, Garrett, & Benner, 2008) • Participation in multidisciplinary programming, such as Safe Routes to School (National Center for Safe Routes to School, n.d.).

Population of older drivers at risk for injuries and fatalities during crashes	• Increased frailty and fragility of the aging body, which is less able to sustain energy forces of a crash
	• Knowledge about operation and use of safety features that have emerged in the past several decades
	• Poor driver–vehicle fit among older drivers.
		• Provision of education to stakeholder groups (NHTSA & American Society on Aging, 2007)
		• Participation in CarFit events to
		  ○ Measure driver–vehicle fit
		  ○ Identify areas of concern
		  ○ Offer education related to proper adjustment of vehicle safety features (e.g., air bag, seat belt, head restraint) and positioning of driver's body in the vehicle
		  ○ Educate about availability of commonly used assistive devices and specialized services (AAA, AARP, & AOTA, 2015).

Population of medically at risk drivers, placing all road users at risk with undefined medical reporting guidelines	• Drivers with medical impairments at increased risk for crashes
	• Subsequent increased risk of injury and fatality for all road users
	• Narrow or nonexistent medical reporting guidelines
	• Confidentiality of reporting
	• Legal immunity for reporting parties
	• Evidence-based guidelines supporting licensing decisions
	• Potential for overrestriction when licensing decisions are made without consideration of addressing impairments through rehabilitation
	• Potential for noncompliance (continued driving) when license is canceled without driver or family support to understand and enforce nondriving.
		• Conduct a systematic review of diagnostic groups and report to state licensing agency (NHTSA & AAMVA, 2009)
		• Advocate for the development of new and more comprehensive medical reporting laws inclusive of
		  ○ Recognition of occupational therapy as a discipline capable of reporting
		  ○ Confidentiality of reporting
		  ○ Legal immunity for reporters.
		• Serve as a member of state Medical Review Board or state constituency group
		• Advocate for the development of a state Medical Review Board offering a pathway of services that include screening, clinician assessment, and occupational therapy DRS where indicated.
		(NHTSA, 2014).

*Services performed by an occupational therapy practitioner who specializes in driving rehabilitation.

Note. AAMVA = American Association of Motor Vehicle Administrators; ADA = Americans With Disabilities Act; AOTA = American Occupational Therapy Association; ASD = autism spectrum disorder; BTW = behind the wheel; CP = cerebral palsy; DRS = driver rehabilitation specialist; MD = muscular dystrophy; NHTSA = National Highway Traffic Safety Administration; OT = occupational therapist; PTSD = posttraumatic stress disorder; RA = rheumatoid arthritis; SCI = spinal cord injury; TBI = traumatic brain injury.

Occupational Therapy Fieldwork Education: Value and Purpose

The purpose of fieldwork education is to propel each generation of occupational therapy practitioners from the role of student to that of practitioner. Through the fieldwork experience, future practitioners achieve competence in applying the occupational therapy process and using evidence-based interventions to meet the occupational needs of a diverse client population. Fieldwork experiences may occur in a variety of practice settings, including medical, educational, and community-based programs. Moreover, fieldwork placements also present the opportunity to introduce occupational therapy services to new and emerging practice environments.

Fieldwork experiences constitute an integral part of the occupational therapy and occupational therapy assistant education curricula. Through fieldwork education, students learn to apply theoretical and scientific principles learned from their academic programs, to address actual client needs within the context of authentic practice environments. During fieldwork experiences, each student develops competency to ascertain client occupational performance needs to identify supports or barriers affecting health and participation, and to document interventions provided. Fieldwork education also provides opportunities for the student to develop advocacy, leadership, and managerial skills in a variety of practice settings, while incorporating principles of evidence-based practice and client-centered care. Finally, the student develops a professional identity as an occupational therapy practitioner, aligning his or her professional judgments and decisions with the American Occupational Therapy Association (AOTA) *Standards of Practice* (AOTA, 2015b) and the *Occupational Therapy Code of Ethics* (AOTA, 2015a).

As students proceed through their fieldwork experiences, performance expectations become progressively more challenging. *Level I fieldwork* experiences occur concurrently with academic coursework, and the goal "is to introduce students to the fieldwork experience, to apply knowledge to practice, and to develop understanding of the needs of clients" (Accreditation Council for Occupational Therapy Education® [ACOTE®], 2012, p. S61). Furthermore, Level I is "designed to enrich didactic coursework through directed observation and participation in selected aspects of the occupational therapy process" (ACOTE, 2012, p. S61).

Level II fieldwork experiences occur at or near the conclusion of the didactic phase of occupational therapy curricula and are designed to "develop competent, entry-level, generalist practitioners" (ACOTE, 2012, p. S62). Level II fieldwork features "in-depth experience(s) in delivering occupational therapy services to clients, focusing on the application of purposeful and meaningful occupation" (ACOTE, 2012, p. S62). For the occupational therapist student, there is an additional exposure to "research, administration, and management of occupational therapy services" (ACOTE, 2012, p. S62). Students should be "exposed to a variety of clients across the lifespan and to a variety of settings" (ACOTE, 2012, p. S62).

The value of fieldwork transcends the obvious benefits directed toward the student. Supervising students enhances fieldwork educators' own professional development by providing exposure to current practice trends, evidence-based practice, and research. Moreover, the experience of fieldwork supervision is recognized by the National Board for Certification in Occupational Therapy and many state regulatory boards as a legitimate venue for achieving continuing competency requirements for occupational therapy practitioners.

Another benefit to the fieldwork site of sponsoring a fieldwork education program is the recruitment of qualified occupational therapy personnel. Through the responsibilities expected during Level II fieldwork, occupational therapy staff and administration are given opportunity for an in-depth view of a student's potential as a future employee. In turn, an active fieldwork program allows the student, as a potential employee, to view firsthand the agency's commitment to the professional growth of its occupational therapy personnel and to determine the fit of his or her professional goals with agency goals. The fieldwork program also creates a progressive, state-of-the-art image to the professional community, consumers, and other external audiences through its partnership with the academic programs.

In summary, fieldwork education is an essential bridge between academic education and authentic occupational therapy practice. Through the collaboration between academic faculty and fieldwork educators, students are given the opportunity to achieve the competencies necessary to meet the present and future occupational needs of individuals, groups and, indeed, society as a whole.

References

Accreditation Council for Occupational Therapy Education. (2012). 2011 Accreditation Council for Occupational Therapy Education (ACOTE®) standards. *American Journal of Occupational Therapy, 66*(6, Suppl.), S6–S74. http://dx.doi.org/10.5014/ajot.2012.66S6

American Occupational Therapy Association. (2015a). Occupational therapy code of ethics (2015). *American Journal of Occupational Therapy, 69*(Suppl. 3), 6913410030. http://dx.doi.org/10.5014/ajot.2015.696S03

American Occupational Therapy Association. (2015b). Standards of practice for occupational therapy. *American Journal of Occupational Therapy, 69*(Suppl. 3), 6913410057. http://dx.doi.org/10.5014/ajot.2015.696S06

Authors

Donna Brzykcy, MS, OTR
Jamie Geraci, MS, OTR/L
Renee Ortega, MA, COTA
Tamra Trenary, OTD, OTR/L, BCPR
Kate McWilliams, MSOT, OTR/L

for

The Commission on Education
Andrea Bilics, PhD, OTR/L, FAOTA, *Chairperson*
Tina DeAngelis, EdD, OTR/L
Jamie Geraci, MS, OTR/L
Michael Iwama, PhD, OT(C)
Julie Kugel, OTD, MOT, OTR/L
Julie McLaughlin Gray, PhD, OTR/L, FAOTA
Kate McWilliams, MSOT, OTR/L
Maureen S. Nardella, MS, OTR/L
Renee Ortega, MA, COTA
Kim Qualls, MS, OTR/L
Tamra Trenary, OTD, OTR/L, BCPR
Neil Harvison, PhD, OTR/L, FAOTA, *AOTA Headquarters Liaison*

Adopted by the Representative Assembly 2016

Citation. American Occupational Therapy Association. (2016). Occupational therapy fieldwork education: Value and purpose. *American Journal of Occupational Therapy, 70*(Suppl. 2), 7012410060. http://dx.doi.org/10.5014/ajot.2016.706S06

Occupational Therapy for Children and Youth Using Sensory Integration Theory and Methods in School-Based Practice

The American Occupational Therapy Association (AOTA) recognizes that occupational therapists and occupational therapy assistants[1] working within public school settings may provide intervention to students in general and special education programs. When the processing and integrating of sensory information interferes with a child's performance in school activities, occupational therapy practitioners[2] may use sensory-based interventions or a sensory integration (SI) approach (Ayres, 1972a) to support the child's ability to participate in his or her educational program. Evidence to support SI and sensory processing interventions can be found in Watling, Koenig, Davies, and Schaaf (2011) and also in Dunn (2014). Occupational therapy practitioners working in schools use evidence-based sensory-based interventions or a SI approach when sensory-related issues are identified and affect a child's ability to benefit from his or her education.

Studies have identified atypical sensory reactivity within the general population of between 5% and 16.5% (Ahn, Miller, Milberger, & McIntosh, 2004; Ben-Sasson, Carter, & Briggs-Gowan, 2009). The incidence of sensory modulation disorders increases to 35% in a Head Start sample, with 45% of those children showing extreme differences in underresponsive or seeking behaviors (Reynolds, Shepherd, & Lane, 2008). In a study of children with autism spectrum disorder, approximately 95% of the sample demonstrated some degree of sensory processing dysfunction (Tomchek & Dunn, 2007). Given that sensory reactivity is only one of the several patterns of sensory integrative deficits (Parham & Mailloux, 2010), estimates of school-age children with all types of sensory difficulties who require occupational therapy may be even higher. The research suggests that sensory-based interventions may be necessary for these students to participate in school.

Federal and State Mandates for Occupational Therapy Practitioners Working in Public Education

Occupational therapy practitioners working in schools, including preschools, are required to follow federal and state education laws and regulations as well as professional licensure regulations and guidelines. In addition, occupational therapy practitioners are guided by the *Occupational Therapy Practice Framework: Domain and Process* (3rd ed.; AOTA, 2014b), the *Occupational Therapy Code of Ethics (2015)* (AOTA, 2015), and *Standards of Practice for Occupational Therapy* (AOTA, 2010). The *Framework* promotes occupation-based, client-centered, contextual, and evidence-based services. The scope of occupational therapy evaluation and intervention in the school setting includes areas that affect the child's "learning and participation in the context of educational activities, routines, and environments" (AOTA, 2011, p. S49).

---

[1]*Occupational therapists* are responsible for all aspects of occupational therapy service delivery and are accountable for the safety and effectiveness of the occupational therapy service delivery process. *Occupational therapy assistants* deliver safe and effective occupational therapy services under the supervision of and in partnership with an occupational therapist (AOTA, 2014a).
[2]When the term *occupational therapy practitioner* is used in this document, it refers to both occupational therapists and occupational therapy assistants (AOTA, 2006).

Specific to public schools are parameters established by federal laws, including the No Child Left Behind Act of 2001 (NCLB; Pub. L. 107–110); the Individuals With Disabilities Education Improvement Act of 2004 (IDEA 2004; Pub. L. 108–446); and Section 504 of the Rehabilitation Act of 1973, as amended (Pub. L. 93–112, Pub. L. 99–506), mandating a child's right to a free, appropriate public education (FAPE) that includes occupational therapy as a related service. NCLB focuses on improving education for all children, requiring schools to use "effective methods and instructional strategies that are based on scientifically based research" (§ 1114(b)(1)(B)(ii)) and to demonstrate "adequate yearly progress" as measured by annual statewide assessment of student learning.

IDEA establishes the rights of children with disabilities to receive a FAPE in the least restrictive environment (LRE) and reinforces the need for effective instructional practices within special education. A child meeting the eligibility criteria for one of the disability categories identified in IDEA 2004, and also demonstrating a need for specialized instruction, is entitled to special education and related services. The individualized education program (IEP) must contain a statement of special education and related services and supplementary aids and services, based on peer-reviewed research to the extent practical, to be provided to the child, or on behalf of the child, and a statement of the program modifications or supports for school personnel that will be provided to enable the child to attain the annual goals, to be involved in and make progress in the general education curriculum, and to be educated and participate with other children (§300.320(a)(4)).

The LRE mandate within IDEA requires that children with disabilities be educated within the general education environment unless "the nature or severity of the disability is such that education in regular classes with the use of supplementary aids and services cannot be achieved satisfactorily" (§300.114(a)(2)). The IEP must identify the extent to which the child will not participate with other children in the regular classroom and other activities within the educational environment (§300.114(a)(5)), and state departments of education must report to the Office of Special Education Programs the amount of time the child is removed from the classroom (IDEA 2004).

Under IDEA, each state must establish rules and regulations for determining eligibility for special education on the basis of the federal code. Local education agencies (LEAs) have some discretion regarding the provision of services so long as they meet the minimum requirements mandated by the federal and state education agencies. Many state and LEAs provide early intervening services (EIS) under IDEA 2004, which authorizes multitiered systems of support (e.g., Response to Intervention, positive behavior interventions and supports; §1413(f)).

Under EIS, occupational therapy practitioners working in public schools may provide professional development to educators to support the delivery of scientifically based instruction or interventions and, if state professional regulations allow, evaluations, services, and supports to general education children to increase their performance in general education. This encourages occupational therapy practitioners to provide systems (i.e., schoolwide) and team approaches as well as, possibly, individual services to enhance general education performance. For example, an occupational therapist may provide professional development based on SI theory and methods to general education teachers regarding ways to modify or adapt the environment and context to support participation and engagement in the classroom or on the playground.

Under Section 504 of the Rehabilitation Act of 1973, children who are not eligible for specially designed instruction under IDEA but who need supports and accommodations for equal access may be determined by the school district to be eligible for a 504 plan, which identifies the accommodations, modifications, and services needed. Occupational therapy practitioners may be participants in the development and implementation of the 504 plan.

Application of Sensory Integration Theory and Methods in Schools

Clinical and Professional Reasoning

Occupational therapy is provided toward the aim of affording opportunities for full participation in everyday activities and occupations in which individuals choose to engage (Christiansen & Townsend, 2010). The imperative when working in schools is to provide occupational therapy for the purpose of meeting the child's specific needs to support his or her ability to access the curriculum and benefit from his or her education in the LRE. As members of the IEP team, occupational therapists rely on the results of the evaluation to determine the child's needs, to establish goals, and to make recommendations to the IEP team regarding the types and intensity of occupational therapy services the child requires to benefit from the educational program. Through accurate functional baseline data, measurable goals, and data collection to monitor a child's successful participation in the natural environment, occupational therapy practitioners provide accountability for a child's progress in occupational therapy intervention as it relates to education.

Clinical reasoning based on professional training, evidence, and expertise guides the occupational therapist's selection and use of one or more theories on SI (Boyt Schell & Schell, 2008; Burke, 2001; Dunn, 2013; Parham, 1987; Schaaf & Smith Roley, 2006). The child's ability to adapt, organize, and integrate sensory information in school environments and activities is important for performance (Watling et al., 2011).

Evaluation

Occupational therapists evaluate a child's school performance by using "a variety of assessment tools and strategies to gather relevant functional, developmental and academic information including information provided by the parent" (IDEA 2004, § 614(b)(2)(A)). Multiple data sources are used during the evaluation, including review of pertinent medical and educational information; interviews with teachers, parents, and the child; observations in natural settings; and various assessments (Coster & Frolek Clark, 2013).

When referrals or observations suggest sensory, motor, and praxis issues, the occupational therapy evaluation includes assessment of these areas (AOTA, 2014b; Lane, Smith Roley, & Champagne, 2013; Stewart, 2010; Watling et al., 2011). Assessments may include direct observation of the child's performance in a variety of tasks to analyze the demands of the activities (e.g., objects and their properties, space, sequencing, timing), social and physical characteristics of the environments, and effectiveness of the child's performance skills and patterns in those activities and environments. The occupational therapist conducts assessments of sensory and neuromotor functions through observations in various environments and analyzes play performance and functional participation of the child in response to the setting's demands (Blanche, 2002; Blanche, Bodison, Chang, & Reinoso, 2012; Knox, 2008; Lane et al., 2013; Schaaf & Smith Roley, 2006; Skard & Bundy, 2008; Watling et al., 2011; Wilson, Pollock, Kaplan, & Law, 1994). Interventions are then designed on the basis of data analysis, with a focus on assisting the child to benefit from his or her educational program (Schaaf & Blanche, 2012). Several structured screenings and assessments have been developed to assess the child's sensory, motor, and praxis abilities:

- The DeGangi–Berk Test of Sensory Integration (DeGangi & Berk, 1983) is a preschool screening focused on sensory-based postural and motor functions.

- The Sensory Integration and Praxis Tests (SIPT; Ayres, 1989) is a standardized performance measure used to identify sensory integrative dysfunction related to learning and behavior. The SIPT is a series of 17 individual tests that provide information on visual perception; visual–motor and fine motor performance; construction; tactile discrimination; tactile sensitivity; kinesthesia; vestibular functions, including postrotary nystagmus and balance; bilateral motor control; and praxis.

- The Sensory Processing Measure: Home Form (Parham & Ecker, 2007); Sensory Processing Measure: Main Classroom and School Environments Form (Miller-Kuhaneck, Henry, & Glennon, 2007);

Sensory Processing Measure–Preschool: Home Form (Parham & Ecker, 2010); and Sensory Processing Measure–Preschool: Main Classroom and School Environments Form (Miller-Kuhaneck, Henry, & Glennon, 2010) are integrated systems of rating scales that enable assessment on the basis of parent and educational staff report of sensory processing issues, planning and ideas, and social participation in preschool through elementary school-age children.

- The Sensory Profile 2 (Dunn, 2014) includes infant, toddler, child, and school rating forms, and the Adolescent/Adult Sensory Profile (Brown & Dunn, 2002) consists of standardized questionnaires that focus on the student's sensory processing performance patterns within the natural context.

Intervention

Although the scope of occupational therapy services expands far beyond the use of SI methods, if one or more types of SI and praxis deficits are revealed during the evaluation, the use of SI methods is appropriate (Table 1). Occupational therapy practitioners with this focus may use a continuum of intervention approaches and types to enhance the child's ability to be educated and participate in daily occupations with other children. Services may be provided individually (e.g., providing one-on-one intervention to remediate vestibular–ocular difficulties affecting visual tracking and handwriting), through consultation and collaboration with groups (e.g., offering staff in-services on sensory regulatory strategies), or through education and training (e.g., establishing an awareness and understanding of sensory needs addressed through occupational therapy; AOTA, 2014b).

Table 1. Occupational Therapy Approaches in Schools Using SI Theory and Methods

Occupational Therapy Approach	Examples of Pathways to Outcomes
Create and promote health and participation.	• Create a class for parents or educational staff to teach the relationships among sensory processing, learning, and behavior. • Promote increased physical activity for students to improve physical and mental health as well as cognitive and social performance. • Support installation of various equipment available at schools and public playgrounds to promote diversity in sensory play experiences. • Design sensory-enriched classrooms with various seating options as well as opportunities for tactile, movement, and proprioceptive experiences throughout the day.
Establish or restore performance skills and performance patterns.	• Provide controlled sensory input through activities that require increasingly complex adaptive responses to novel activity to support ability to access Common Core curriculum standards and participate in classroom activities. • Design activities rich in tactile, vestibular, and proprioceptive information that increase academic, physical, and social performance skills. • Facilitate development of appropriate SI and motor planning skills needed for organizing materials, completing tasks within an appropriate time frame, and adapting to transitions. • Establish or restore SI and praxis needed for physical, social, and object play.
Maintain student ability to engage in and cope with school-related activities.	• Structure the sensory environment to meet the student's needs, such as reducing sensory distractions and improving the ergonomic comfort of the chair and desk. • Teach sensory self-regulation strategies for academic achievement, social–emotional well-being, physiological homeostasis, positive behavior, and motor performance in play. • Maintain ability to organize behavior by providing scheduled sensory breaks and sensory accommodations, such as changing the size, maneuverability, comfort, and location of the seat and desk. • Maintain peer relationships by supporting and compensating for motor planning needs in age-appropriate games and sports. • Maintain student productivity by providing compensation techniques for sensory and motor planning deficits using study carrels, visual timers, weighted vests, alternate seating arrangements, modified writing tools, and paper and other assistive technology.

(Continued)

Table 1. Occupational Therapy Approaches in Schools Using SI Theory and Methods *(cont.)*

Occupational Therapy Approach	Examples of Pathways to Outcomes
Modify activity to help student compensate for sensory, motor, and praxis deficits.	• Through collaborative consultation with education staff and parents, develop strategies for modifying the sensory, motor, or praxis demands of assignments to increase student productivity. • Support student participation in general curriculum by modifying sensory and motor planning demands of the activity. • Structure or modify the environment to support the student's sensory, motor, motor planning, and self-regulatory capacities and needs.
Prevent barriers to participation and improve safety.	• Prevent inattention, poor posture, and restlessness when sitting for prolonged periods by modifying seating options, allowing sensory breaks, and allowing the student to work in various positions. • Prevent social isolation by providing motor planning and social strategies to participate with peers. • Prevent socially inappropriate behaviors and behavioral distress or disruption by detecting and meeting sensory and self-regulatory needs. • Prevent injury by providing ergonomic seating and safety strategies for students whose nervous systems have reduced registration of sensory information. • Prevent barriers to child participation by increasing the understanding of the school district staff regarding the role that SI and praxis play in influencing learning and behavior.

Note. SI = sensory integration.

Collaboration with school staff and IEP team members provides opportunities for education and training to increase their understanding of the contribution of SI and praxis to participation at school. Collaboration allows the occupational therapy practitioner to advocate for accommodations and modifications that will assist the child's school performance and to model services that enhance participation in physical and social play. Adaptation of the school environment according to children's sensory, motor, and praxis needs has been consistently recognized in the professional literature as a way to support their successful participation. It may include increasing the number of activity breaks and ensuring that all children have access to recess (Pellegrini, 2005). As teachers, administrators, and paraprofessionals better understand sensory-related behaviors, they can implement suggested evidence-based sensory strategies, embedding them in the classroom routine to improve children's ability to learn (Prizant, Wetherby, Rubin, & Laurent, 2003). Table 2 provides case examples of school-based occupational therapy interventions with a preschool child, an elementary school child, and a middle school child.

Table 2. Case Examples Using SI Theory in Schools

The following vignettes are outlined relative to the *Occupational Therapy Practice Framework: Domain and Process* (3rd ed.; AOTA, 2014b) to illustrate occupational therapy using SI theory and methods in schools.

Case 1. Natasha: Preschool-Age Child
Evaluation

Referral: **Natasha** is a **3-year-old child** enrolled in a special education preschool. The IEP team recommended an OT evaluation because Natasha has difficulty with classroom transitions and social interactions.

Occupational Profile

Natasha's family and educational team are seeking OT services because of her difficulty with transitioning and coping in the classroom. Natasha is sensitive to noise; she cries and clings to the aide in the classroom. She performs well at skilled tasks. Additional information was gathered from her medical, developmental, educational, and occupational histories. The priorities listed by the teacher and parents include social interactions (i.e., friendships) and performance within the flow of the classroom (i.e., transitioning).

Analysis of Occupational Performance

Interview Data	Observation Data	Test Data
• *Speech–language therapist report:* Natasha's receptive language is below	• Natasha prefers to sit alone or next to an adult.	• Evaluation of sensory processing using Infant/Toddler Sensory Profile (Dunn, 2002)

(Continued)

Table 2. Case Examples Using SI Theory in Schools *(cont.)*

average and decreases when there is noise in the room. • *Teacher report:* Natasha has difficulty adapting to the flow of classroom activities. She needs an exceptional amount of attention from adults to stay calm. She is able to cognitively perform the tasks but is overwhelmed with the noise and movement in the room. • *Parent report:* The mother is concerned about Natasha's unhappiness at school and inability to play and make friends.	• Natasha needs extra cues to pay attention. Although physically capable, she does not complete a fine motor preschool activity without adult direction. • She does not initiate social interaction with other children and becomes irritable when children come near her. • She cries when entering the lunchroom or when a group of noisy children run past her during recess. • She does not like to go to lunch and refuses to eat anything but chips.	• DeGangi–Berk Test of Sensory Integration (DeGangi & Berk, 1983) • Postrotary Nystagmus Test (Ayres, 1989; Mailloux et al., 2014) • Structured clinical observations (Blanche, 2002) • Evaluation of play skills using Knox Preschool Play Scale (Knox, 2008).

Intervention Examples

IEP Goals	*OT Intervention Plan and Goals*	*OT Intervention Process and Strategies*
Natasha: • Will transition between classroom activities independently 4 of 5 transitions for 3 days. • Will sustain adult-facilitated interaction with her peers during free play for 5 minutes during a 15-minute observation 4 of 5 free play periods. • Will carry out verbal instructions with visual cues 4 of 5 opportunities with 80% accuracy.	OT is to be provided within the classroom setting during routine activities. Natasha's response to intervention in relation to learning, behavior, and adjustment to preschool will be monitored closely for progress and signs of a disorder in SI. Changes to service delivery may be recommended to the IEP team as needed. *OT Goals:* Natasha • Will regulate her responses to environmental stimuli to remain calm during routine class transitions. • Will self-regulate her responses to tactile stimuli to sit next to several peers and focus on the activity during playground and eating activities. • Will motor plan her body movements to engage in preschool play. • Will improve her spatial location of sound relative to the position of her body in the classroom with and without background noise.	The OT practitioner will facilitate and enhance performance through the following therapeutic activities: *Client level:* • Increase sensory modulation through the use of heavy work activities. • Improve vestibular spatial body awareness through moving on swings and locating visual and auditory targets. • Improve adaptive responses and motor planning to increase competence when faced with dynamic activities and in her overall repertoire of play skills. *Activity level:* • Increase texture and weight of materials used during class activities. • Use visual cues for improved independence during familiar sequences and routines. *Environment level:* • Before class, Natasha will arrive early and will enter classroom prior to other children to gradually adjust to the increased noise and pace of the day. • Natasha will receive visual cues and tangible transition prompts, such as a visual schedule, to provide advance notice of classroom activity changes. • Natasha will be provided with a variety of seating options during circle time, such as a bean bag chair, rocking chair, ball chair, or cube seat. • Seating will be arranged near an adult.

Outcomes

Outcomes were reported by members of the IEP team.

Performance Skills

•   Improvement noted in all skill areas—motor, process, and social skills.

Table 2. Case Examples Using SI Theory in Schools *(cont.)*

Performance Patterns

- Easier transitions

- Increased attention

- New friendships

- Sustained participation during classroom activities without withdrawing

- Teacher and parent satisfaction that Natasha is able to participate in her preschool program and appears happier at school.

Participation

- Improved self-regulation and adaptation in the preschool routine.

Case 2. Billy: Elementary School–Age Student
Evaluation

Referral: **Billy** is a **7-year-old student** in a general education classroom environment. The IEP team requested an OT evaluation because of Billy's poor handwriting, aggressive behavior, difficulty completing work, and diagnosis of developmental coordination disorder.

Occupational Profile

Billy's guardians and educational team requested an OT evaluation because of his difficulty with writing, aggressive behavior, and a medical diagnosis of developmental coordination disorder. Information was obtained from Billy's medical, developmental, educational, and occupational histories. Billy receives speech therapy and specialized academic instruction from a resource specialist. He was referred to OT because of increasing aggressive behavior, difficulty beginning and completing work that was modified for his level of ability, and disorganized handwriting with almost no spacing between words. Billy has difficulty with play and social participation on the playground. He has poorly established habits and routines of organizing his belongings and self-care at school, often appearing disheveled. Parental and IEP team priorities include improving Billy's ability to meet the Common Core Standards (through handwriting and work completion) and ability to play more effectively with his peers.

Analysis of Occupational Performance

Interview Data	Test Data

Teacher report:
 	
- Billy has above-average academic ability but completes fewer than half of his assignments in the proper amount of time.
 	
- Billy does not interact with his peers.
 	
- Billy has expressed the concern that as the demands of school increase, he is going to fall further and further behind.
 	
- Billy has poor use of his hands for tasks, such as opening his lunch containers and managing classroom tools.
 	
- Billy's writing is illegible.
 	
Parent report:
 	
- Billy has no friends.
 	
- Billy has difficulty comprehending simple verbal instructions.
 	
- Billy has unusual habits and rituals.
 	
- Billy has poorly established patterns of daily activities, such as getting ready to go to bed or mealtimes.
	- Sensory Integration and Praxis Tests (Ayres, 1989) and clinical observation results were as follows:
	
	   o Visual–perception tests within normal limits
	
	   o Visual–motor tests 1–2 standard deviations below the mean
	
	   o Visual construction test scores in the high-average range
	
	   o Poor bilateral motor control
	
	   o Poor oral praxis and postural praxis
	
	   o Poor tactile discrimination
	
	   o Poor posture and eye control
	
	   o Decreased prone extension and supine flexion
	
	- Sensory Processing Measure–Home Form (Parham & Ecker, 2007) revealed definite differences in social participation, movement, tactile functions, body awareness, and ideas and planning.
	
	- Sensory Processing Measure–Main Classroom and Social Environments Form (Miller-Kuhaneck et al., 2007) revealed definite differences in response to movement and body awareness; Billy is easily overwhelmed with auditory and visual activity in the environment.
	
	- Classroom handwriting portfolio was compared with peers and revealed a discrepancy.

Intervention Examples		
IEP Goals	*OT Intervention Plan and Goals*	*OT Intervention Process and Strategies*

(Continued)

529

Table 2. Case Examples Using SI Theory in Schools *(cont.)*

Billy:		The OT practitioner will facilitate adaptive responses through provision of sensory and motor challenges through the following interventions:
• Will be able to write 3 legible sentences in his journal during a 20-minute writing period 4 of 5 opportunities.	OT is recommended to improve visual–motor control and overall attention.	
	OT is to be provided in a specially equipped environment, and consultation is to be provided to the IEP team members.	
• Will stay on topic and remain in his seat for the duration of a 15-minute social studies lesson 4 of 5 opportunities.	*OT Goals:* Billy	*Client level:*
• Will participate appropriately in a structured playground activity with 1 other child without leaving the activity or arguing with the child for 10 minutes during the recess or lunch break 2 of 3 opportunities.	• Will organize visual–motor information to write legible words.	• Use weight-bearing and heavy work activities to increase strength of Billy's trunk and upper extremities.
	• Will organize somatosensory input from his body to imitate and follow visual directions during structured playground activities.	• Increase Billy's exploration of multiple textures, sizes, and shapes to improve sensitivity and stereognosis in his hands.
	• Will remain comfortably seated and regulate his attention during instruction to remain focused and on task during social studies.	*Activity level:*
	• Will confidently access playground equipment and perform in recess and physical education games with peers.	• Instruct teacher in kinesthetic and visual support method to reteach fundamentals of handwriting.
		• Use weighted pencils, pencil grips, and paper with highlighted areas.
		• Allow Billy to do some of his work while standing, ball-sitting, or lying on his stomach.
		Environment level:
		• Provide written text to copy rather than copying from blackboard.
		• Provide written instructions and pictures of daily sequences of activities with times and locations.
		• Allow structured time for movement throughout the day as needed.

Outcomes

Outcomes were reported by members of the IEP team.

Occupational Performance

• Improved writing and language arts skills.

• Increased ADL and functional independence.

• Improved social participation.

• Independent engagement in structured activities.

• Improved participation and organization of behavior in daily routines.

Case 3. John: Middle School–Age Student

Evaluation

Referral: **John** is **12 years old** and has just entered middle school. The IEP team requested an OT evaluation because John cannot organize his belongings and schedule or find his way around the middle school campus. He is experiencing high anxiety and refusing to go to school. Although psychoeducational assessments reveal adequate cognitive abilities, the IEP team members report escalating concerns related to John's ability to academically and physically keep up with his peers.

Table 2. Case Examples Using SI Theory in Schools *(cont.)*

Occupational Profile

John's family and the educational team requested an OT evaluation because of his difficulty finding his way around his school and resulting anxiety and depression. Additional information from John's medical, developmental, educational, and occupational histories was reviewed. Team priorities include increasing John's confidence and independence in performing school curriculum activities and ability to navigate around school without getting lost.

Analysis of Occupational Performance

Interview Data	Data From Record Review	Test Data
Parent report: • John gets lost easily. • John works best in a self-contained class-room with group transitions; however, the middle school is not structured this way. • John demonstrates poor spatial abilities, such as when he needs to align numbers in math. • John talks his way out of anything he finds difficult. *John's self-report:* • He has anxiety attacks. • He feels sick during rides in the car to school. • He feels stupid. • He wants to be home schooled. • He spends most of his day in sedentary activities. • He cannot tolerate backward movement of his head. • He cannot play desired team sports at the skill level of his peers and as a result feels rejected and humiliated by other children.	The elementary school file indicates that John performed well in academics but rarely finished written work on time in a legible or organized manner. He was well behaved and liked by peers. • John's teacher notes that John does not volunteer for classroom errands on the school grounds unless he could go with a peer. • John often lost his completed assignments in the classroom, later to be found in his messy desk or in unlikely places in the classroom.	• Below age level on VMI visual–motor integration and visual perception (Beery, Buktenica, & Beery, 2010). • Within normal limits on VMI fine motor coordination in tracing precision (Beery et al., 2010). • Poor 2- and 3-dimensional construction ability. • Poor balance with eyes closed. • Self-reports of dizziness on playground swings. • Poor disassociation of his head, neck, and body. • Excessive talking to avoid performing during the evaluation observation. • Inability to locate familiar landmarks (e.g., office).

Intervention Examples

IEP Goals	OT Intervention Plan and Goals.	OT Intervention Process and Strategies
John: • Will arrive at all of his classes independently and on time for 2 weeks. • Will attend school 8 of 10 days with low levels of anxiety, as noted by self-report. • Will show increased tolerance for bus rides as reported by John, parent, and bus driver 4 of 5 days. • Will identify age-appropriate leisure time options that are within his ability and interest level, such as individually oriented community sports and lessons (e.g., karate, yoga, swimming, chess, arts and crafts). • Will explore junior high extracurricular activities and clubs.	OT is recommended in the school setting. *OT Goals:* John • Will identify 1 strategy of 3 options (i.e., map, written sequence, self-instruction) that works best for him to get to familiar places. • Will identify, select, and participate in leisure and extracurricular physical activities. • Will learn to identify antecedents to periods of increased anxiety and use relaxation techniques to remain calm when transitioning from home to school and between classes.	The OT practitioner will facilitate and enhance performance through the following interventions: *Client level:* • Develop various strategies for John to practice to improve his awareness of the geography of the campus. • Provide strategies to help John become aware of and identify his own sensory strengths, sensitivities, and preferences. • Increase proprioceptive heavy work activities to improve John's sense of his body in space. • Educate John to avoid intense vestibular activities.

(Continued)

Table 2. Case Examples Using SI Theory in Schools *(cont.)*

		Activity level: • Provide cues, landmarks, and signs that John can record as he walks to class. • Enroll John in extracurricular activities such as karate, yoga, swimming, or rock climbing. *Environment level:* • Pair John initially with a peer to walk to class. • Make a list of visual details as landmarks, take pictures, or put room numbers on an index card, color-coded for each of John's classes, to enable him to get to different classes.

Outcomes

Outcomes were reported by members of the IEP team.

Participation

- Improved confidence in his own ability to adapt to and meet the everyday spatial demands of school activities, greatly reducing stress at school.
- Increased self-awareness and self-determination in seeking advice to devise strategies to compensate in situations that are uncomfortable or intimidating.
- Improved ability to arrive at class on time.
- Independence in finishing and finding 75% of his assignments.
- Decreased resistance to going to school.
- Increased initiation of participation in leisure activities with peers, such as school clubs.

Client Satisfaction

- Confidence in traveling between classes without assistance.
- Increased parent-reported happiness at home and at school.
- Cessation of reports of depression or anxiety.

Note. ADL = activity of daily living; AOTA = American Occupational Therapy Association; IEP = individualized education program; OT = occupational therapy; SI = sensory integration; VMI = Beery–Buktenica Developmental Test of Visual–Motor Integration.

Occupational therapy services provided to support a child with sensory processing differences may be delivered within multiple contexts that include the variety of educational environments and routines. Two types of commonly applied occupational therapy interventions for children with sensory processing and SI challenges in school-based practice include (1) occupational therapy using sensory-based interventions and (2) occupational therapy using an SI approach.

Occupational Therapy Using Sensory-Based Interventions

Sensory-based interventions focus on how sensory input within the school environment affects student participation (Foster & Cox, 2013). Occupational therapy practitioners use sensory-based interventions to address specific sensory needs related to sensory modulation or sensory discrimination (Watling et al., 2011). Sensory-based interventions used in school settings commonly involve the application of Dunn's (2013) model that organizes sensory processing into four basic patterns of behavioral responses ("seekers," "avoiders," "bystanders," and "sensors"), which depend on individuals' thresholds for sensory input and whether they use active or passive strategies to support self-regulation. Using this strengths-based model, the occupational therapy practitioner designs interventions that consider the sensory needs of the students and teachers within the context (i.e., authentic activity settings and routines). Interventions may include helping school personnel consider sensory processing patterns or factors when addressing student concerns, implementing daily routines that incorporate sensory-based activities, and modifying the environment to match students' sensory needs and support participation. Self-regulation strategies may be taught using the Alert Program (Williams & Shellenberger, 1994) and Zones of Regulation (Kuypers, 2011).

Provision of occupational therapy using sensory-based interventions often involves the use of sensory accommodations or strategies such as the use of mobile-seating options or fidget toys to address single-sensory systems. Some sensory strategies, such as the use of dynamic seating and strategies to increase attention, have shown promising results (Bagatell, Mirigliani, Patterson, Reyes, & Test, 2010; Fertel-Daly, Bedell, & Hinojosa, 2001; Schilling & Schwartz, 2004; Schilling, Washington, Billingsley, & Deitz, 2003). It is important to communicate to the educational team that these strategies must be used within the overall context of an occupational therapy intervention plan. Sensory-based strategies without the oversight of an occupational therapist do not constitute occupational therapy.

Occupational Therapy Using a Sensory Integrative Approach

Occupational therapy using a sensory integrative approach is grounded in the work of A. Jean Ayres, PhD, OTR, and identified by the trademarked term *Ayres Sensory Integration*® (ASI; Fertel-Daly et al., 2001). ASI represents a

- Well-developed theory grounded in basic and applied science (Berthoz, 2002; Berthoz & Petit, 2008; Head, 1920; Sherrington, 1906, 1940; Stein, 2012);

- Model of practice (Ayres, 1972a, 1972b, 1979);

- Set of standardized, structured and unstructured assessments (Ayres, 1989; Blanche, 2002; Davies & Tucker, 2010; Mailloux et al., 2011; Mulligan, 1998; Watling et al., 2011); and

- Replicable intervention, with evidence of its effectiveness (Pfeiffer, Koenig, Kinnealey, Sheppard, & Henderson, 2011; Schaaf et al., 2014; Smith Roley, Mailloux, Miller-Kuhaneck, & Glennon, 2007; Watling et al., 2011).

For school-based practice, difficulties in sensory integration and praxis are predictive of academic achievement in elementary school children (Parham, 1998). A compendium of evidence in SI can be found in Watling and colleagues (2011).

The use of ASI requires additional knowledge and skills, such as administering and interpreting the SIPT (Ayres, 1989). Occupational therapy practitioners gain expertise through workshops, publications, mentoring, pediatric study groups, and postgraduate studies. To ensure implementation of ASI with fidelity, intervention is provided by a skilled occupational therapy practitioner who is guided by the interpretation of a thorough assessment and who provides services within a therapeutically designed setting with appropriate space and equipment. This method relies on interactions between the therapist and child in a sensory-rich environment and uses a collaborative and playful approach, with attention to the child's successful adaptation to a variety of novel challenges, including sensory reactivity, sensory–perceptual and postural skills, and praxis. Collaboration with caregivers is essential, as are the one-to-one interactions with the child (Parham et al., 2011).

Therapy services that support participation in the LRE frequently occur in natural school spaces (e.g., classroom, playground, gym, cafeteria). Provision of SI methods, such as moving through space (e.g., climbing in, over, and under large equipment; swinging on equipment; playing with toys and structures graded for specific needs), may be essential to meet the IEP goals for some children and can be provided on a school campus.

The choice of interventions is guided by the best available research regarding the effectiveness of the intervention related to the identified goals for the child. The efficacy of occupational therapy's use of SI and sensory processing has been investigated by numerous researchers during the past 35 years. The outcome of occupational therapy using SI methods is to improve function in various daily occupations (Ayres, 1979; Bundy, Lane, & Murray, 2002; Dunn, 2001; Parham & Mailloux, 2010; Smith Roley, Blanche, & Schaaf, 2001; Watling et al., 2011). Recent studies adhering to fidelity in ASI intervention have shown promising results (Fazlio lu & Baran, 2008; Pfeiffer et al., 2011; Smith, Press, Koenig, & Kinnealey, 2005). Research supporting the use of SI methods can be found in *Occupational Therapy Practice Guidelines for Children and Adolescents With Challenges in Sensory Processing and Sensory Integration* (Watling et al., 2011). Selected studies supporting projected educational outcomes, by OT focus area, are provided in Table 3.

Table 3. Occupational Therapy Service Continuum Focus Areas, Projected Outcomes, and Research Support for School-Based Practice Using SI Theory and Methods

This table provides samples of studies supporting various SI theory and methods and outcomes in school-based practice. It is not an exhaustive list of the available evidence.

OT Focus Area	Projected Educational Outcomes	Examples of Resources and Evidence
Participation in education Emotional regulation, sensory–perceptual, motor, praxis, and cognitive skills	Students will access general education curriculum and attend to classroom instruction for longer periods of time prior to identification for special education eligibility and formal OT evaluation.	Schilling et al. (2003)
School readiness for education participation Play and leisure Communication and social skills	Students access general education standards and learn adaptive behavior and social skills.	Jarrett & Maxwell (2000) Pellegrini & Smith (1993, 1998)
Self-regulation, including the development of emotional regulation, cognitive, and sensory–perceptual skills	Students build sensory self-awareness and self-regulatory strategies to increase focus of attention and completion of schoolwork.	Wells, Chasnoff, Schmidt, Telford, & Schwartz (2012)
Attention and on-task behavior to improve participation in education	Students increase on-task behavior through classroom modifications, sensory strategies, sensory breaks, and sensory diets integrated into the school routine.	Kinnealey et al. (2012) VandenBerg (2001)
Cognitive, sensory–perceptual, and motor and praxis skills that enhance academic learning	Academic scores are improved through SI methods focusing on eliciting adaptive responses during OT. Gains in language comprehension and on expressive language measures are noted after OT using SI methods.	Ayres (1972a) Ayres & Mailloux (1981)
Sensory functions and sensory–perceptual skills influencing readiness to learn Adaptation	Individuals with hyperresponsiveness such as tactile defensiveness and gravitational insecurity responded better to intervention than those with underresponsiveness or who failed to orient to sensory input.	Ayres & Tickle (1980)
Cognitive, sensory–perceptual, and motor and praxis skills that enhance academic learning and communication and social skills	Following SI intervention, children with decreased cognitive function showed improved spontaneous language, indicating that vestibular activities are effective nonverbal strategies for increasing spontaneous language.	Magrun, Ottenbacher, McCue, & Keefe (1981)
Participation in ADLs and ability to engage in a variety of functional activities	Group who received SI intervention showed reduced self-stimulating behaviors that interfere with participation in functional activities. Study compared an SI approach with tabletop activities in children with pervasive developmental disorder and mental retardation.	Smith, Press, Koenig, & Kinnealey (2005)

Table 3. Occupational Therapy Service Continuum Focus Areas, Projected Outcomes, and Research Support for School-Based Practice Using SI Theory and Methods *(cont.)*

OT Focus Area	Projected Educational Outcomes	Examples of Resources and Evidence
Sensory–perceptual and fine motor skills affecting penmanship and handwriting	Using sensory strategies via classroom consultation and direct intervention related to sensory processing improve visual–motor skills, which support penmanship and writing skills.	Hall & Case-Smith (2007)
Participation in play and leisure, including curiosity and independent learning	SI approaches improve play and interactions with others and with toys and other objects, as well as tolerance for vestibular and proprioceptive sensations, and lead to greater sensory exploration of the environment. Sensory exploration improves as a key feature of independent learning intervention when OT with a SI approach is used to address symptoms related to learning disorders.	Schaaf, Merrill, & Kinsella (1987)
Reading	Smooth eye pursuits, which are important in developing reading skills, improved in this study, which demonstrated a reduction in the number of saccades for the intervention cohort and reduced time necessary to accomplish smooth pursuits.	Horowitz, Oosterveld, & Adrichem (1993)
Academic skills Motor skills	SI intervention methods prove equally as effective as tutoring in improving academic and motor skills, with maintenance of gains in motor skills development. This randomized clinical trial compared OT using SI with tutoring to improve academic and motor skills. Although the SI group did not make greater gains in the initial study, at follow-up 2 years later, only the SI group maintained their gross motor skills.	Wilson, Kaplan, Fellowes, Gruchy, & Faris (1992)
Emotional regulation skills resulting in positive behavior Health and wellness Quality of life	A decrease in disruptive behaviors is noted with improved speech, play, attention, and social dialogue. This single-case study of 2 children demonstrated improvements in social interaction, approach to novel activities, response to affection, and response to movement.	Linderman & Stewart (1999)
Self-advocacy and parent advocacy Quality of life	Parents report increased ability to advocate for their child on the basis of improved understanding of their child's behavior and validation of their parenting efforts. At the clinic site, waiting room interactions allowed parents time to share experiences and resources with others and expand their understanding of their children.	Cohn (2001) Cohn, Miller, & Tickle-Degnen (2000)
Positive behavior Increased engagement Independent work	SI supports behavior in preschool-aged child, including increased engagement, decreased aggression, less need for intense teacher direction, and decreased mouthing of objects. Using a single-case-study design, researchers found that the child benefited from classic ASI, affecting his preschool performance.	Roberts, King-Thomas, & Boccia (2007)
Participation at school	SI supports occupational performance and behavior in a school-age child, improving participation at school, at home, and in the community. Using a single-case-study design, the researchers found that the child benefited from classic ASI, which affected his occupational performance and behavior.	Schaaf & Nightlinger (2007)

(Continued)

Table 3. Occupational Therapy Service Continuum Focus Areas, Projected Outcomes, and Research Support for School-Based Practice Using SI Theory and Methods *(cont.)*

OT Focus Area	Projected Educational Outcomes	Examples of Resources and Evidence
Play Learning	Research suggests that learning is enhanced by emotion, spontaneity, and play, which are the essential ingredients in a SI approach used within OT. Physiological data show increased cortical blood volume during performance of novel integration activities in a spontaneous, playful manner.	Peyton, Bass, Burke, & Frank (2005)
Occupational performance in educational settings observed via academic achievement	Measures of SI in elementary students are significantly related to school achievement concurrently and predictively over a 4-year period, even when controlling for intelligence. A particularly strong link between praxis and math achievement is evident.	Parham (1998)

Note. This table provides examples of studies supporting SI theory, methods, and outcomes in school-based practice. It is not an exhaustive list of the available evidence. ADLs = activities of daily living; ASI = Ayres Sensory Integration®; OT = occupational therapy; SI = sensory integration.

Through accurate functional baseline data, measurable student goals, and data collection to monitor a child's successful participation in the natural environment, occupational therapy practitioners provide accountability for a child's progress in occupational therapy intervention as it relates to education. Goal attainment scaling is a promising method providing practitioners with the possibility of measuring achievement toward customized, participation-based goals (Mailloux et al., 2007).

Summary

AOTA recognizes SI as one of several theories and methods used by occupational therapists and occupational therapy assistants working with children in public and private schools. Regardless of the theories and methods used, occupational therapy practitioners work within the framework of occupational therapy toward the desired outcome of enhancing a person's ability to participate in life through engagement in everyday activities (AOTA, 2014b). When children demonstrate sensory, motor, or praxis deficits that interfere with their ability to access the general education curriculum, occupational therapy using an SI approach is appropriate.

References

Ahn, R. R., Miller, L. J., Milberger, S., & McIntosh, D. N. (2004). Prevalence of parents' perceptions of sensory processing disorders among kindergarten children. *American Journal of Occupational Therapy, 58,* 287–293. http://dx.doi.org/10.5014/ajot.58.3.287

American Occupational Therapy Association. (2006). Policy 1.44: Categories of occupational therapy personnel. In *Policy manual* (2013 ed., pp. 32–33). Bethesda, MD: Author.

American Occupational Therapy Association. (2010). Standards of practice for occupational therapy. *American Journal of Occupational Therapy, 64*(Suppl.), S106–S111. http://dx.doi.org/10.5014/ajot.2010.64S106

American Occupational Therapy Association. (2011). Occupational therapy services in early childhood and school-based settings. *American Journal of Occupational Therapy, 65*(Suppl.), S46–S54. http://dx.doi.org/10.5014/ajot.2011.65S46

American Occupational Therapy Association. (2014a). Guidelines for supervision, roles, and responsibilities during the delivery of occupational therapy services. *American Journal of Occupational Therapy, 68*(Suppl. 3), S16–S22. http://dx.doi.org/10.5014/ajot.2014.686S03

American Occupational Therapy Association. (2014b). Occupational therapy practice framework: Domain and process (3rd ed.). *American Journal of Occupational Therapy, 68*(Suppl. 1), S1–S48. http://dx.doi.org/10.5014/ajot.2014.682006

American Occupational Therapy Association. (2015). Occupational therapy code of ethics (2015). *American Journal of Occupational Therapy, 69*(Suppl. 3), 6913410030. http://dx.doi.org/10.5014/ajot.2015.696S03

Ayres, A. J. (1972a). Improving academic scores through sensory integration. *Journal of Learning Disabilities, 5,* 338–343. http://dx.doi.org/10.1177/002221947200500605

Ayres, A. J. (1972b). Types of sensory integrative dysfunction among disabled learners. *American Journal of Occupational Therapy, 26,* 13–18.

Ayres, A. J. (1979). *Sensory integration and the child.* Los Angeles: Western Psychological Services.

Ayres, A. J. (1989). *Sensory Integration and Praxis Tests manual.* Los Angeles: Western Psychological Services.

Ayres, A. J., & Mailloux, Z. (1981). Influence of sensory integration procedures on language development. *American Journal of Occupational Therapy, 35,* 383–390. http://dx.doi.org/10.5014/ajot.35.6.383

Ayres, A. J., & Tickle, L. S. (1980). Hyper-responsivity to touch and vestibular stimuli as a predictor of positive response to sensory integration procedures by autistic children. *American Journal of Occupational Therapy, 34,* 375–381. http://dx.doi.org/10.5014/ajot.34.6.375

Bagatell, N., Mirigliani, G., Patterson, C., Reyes, Y., & Test, L. (2010). Effectiveness of therapy ball chairs on classroom participation in children with autism spectrum disorders. *American Journal of Occupational Therapy, 64,* 895–903. http://dx.doi.org/10.5014/ajot.2010.09149

Beery, K. E., Buktenica, N. A., & Beery, N. A. (2010). *The Beery–Buktenica Developmental Test of Visual–Motor Integration* (6th ed.). San Antonio, TX: NCS Pearson.

Ben-Sasson, A., Carter, A. S., & Briggs-Gowan, M. J. (2009). Sensory over-responsivity in elementary school: Prevalence and social–emotional correlates. *Journal of Abnormal Child Psychology, 37,* 705–716. http://dx.doi.org/10.1007/s10802-008-9295-8

Berthoz, A. (2002). *The brain's sense of movement: Perspectives in cognitive neuroscience* (G. Weiss, Trans.). Boston: Harvard Press.

Berthoz, A., & Petit, J. (2008). *The physiology and phenomenology of action.* New York: Oxford University Press.

Blanche, E. I. (2002). *Observations based on sensory integration theory.* Torrance, CA: Pediatric Therapy Network.

Blanche, E. I., Bodison, S., Chang, M. C., & Reinoso, G. (2012). Development of the Comprehensive Observations of Proprioception (COP): Validity, reliability, and factor analysis. *American Journal of Occupational Therapy, 66,* 691–698. http://dx.doi.org/10.5014/ajot.2012.003608

Boyt Schell, B. A., & Schell, J. W. (Eds.). (2008). *Clinical and professional reasoning in occupational therapy.* Baltimore: Lippincott Williams & Wilkins.

Brown, C., & Dunn, D. (2002). *Adolescent/Adult Sensory Profile.* San Antonio, TX: Pearson.

Bundy, A. C., Lane, S. J., & Murray, E. A. (2002). *Sensory integration: Theory and practice* (2nd ed.). Philadelphia: F. A. Davis.

Burke, J. (2001). Clinical reasoning and the use of narrative in sensory integration assessment and intervention. In S. Roley, E. Blanche, & R. Schaaf (Eds.), *Understanding the nature of sensory integration with diverse populations* (pp. 203–214). Austin, TX: Pro-Ed.

Christiansen, C. H., & Townsend, E. A. (2010). *Introduction to occupation: The art and science of living* (2nd ed.). Cranbury, NJ: Pearson Education.

Cohn, E. S. (2001). Parent perspectives of occupational therapy using a sensory integration approach. *American Journal of Occupational Therapy, 55,* 285–294. http://dx.doi.org/10.5014/ajot.55.3.285

Cohn, E., Miller, L. J., & Tickle-Degnen, L. (2000). Parental hopes for therapy outcomes: Children with sensory modulation disorders. *American Journal of Occupational Therapy, 54,* 36–43. http://dx.doi.org/10.5014/ajot.54.1.36

Coster, W., & Frolek Clark, G. (2013). Best practices in school occupational therapy evaluation to support participation. In G. Frolek Clark & B. E. Chandler (Eds.), *Best practices for occupational therapy in schools* (pp. 83–93). Bethesda, MD: AOTA Press.

Davies, P. L., & Tucker, R. (2010). Evidence review to investigate the support for subtypes of children with difficulty processing and integrating sensory information. *American Journal of Occupational Therapy, 64,* 391–402. http://dx.doi.org/10.5014/ajot.2010.09070

DeGangi, G. A., & Berk, R. A. (1983). *DeGangi–Berk Test of Sensory Integration kit.* Torrance, CA: Western Psychological Services.

Dunn, W. (2001). The sensations of everyday life: Theoretical, conceptual, and pragmatic considerations (Eleanor Clarke Slagle Lecture). *American Journal of Occupational Therapy, 55,* 608–620. http://dx.doi.org/10.5014/ajot.55.6.608

Dunn, W. (2002). *Infant/Toddler Sensory Profile manual.* San Antonio, TX: Psychological Corporation.

Dunn, W. (2013). Best practices in sensory processing skills to enhance participation. In G. Frolek Clark & B. E. Chandler (Eds.), *Best practices for occupational therapy in schools* (pp. 403–417). Bethesda, MD: AOTA Press.

Dunn, W. (2014). *Sensory Profile 2.* San Antonio, TX: Pearson.

Fazlio lu, Y., & Baran, G. (2008). A sensory integration therapy program on sensory problems for children with autism. *Perceptual and Motor Skills, 106,* 415–422. http://dx.doi.org/10.2466/pms.106.2.415-422

Fertel-Daly, D., Bedell, G., & Hinojosa, J. (2001). Effects of a weighted vest on attention to task and self-stimulatory behaviors in preschoolers with pervasive developmental disorders. *American Journal of Occupational Therapy, 55,* 629–640. http://dx.doi.org/10.5014/ajot.55.6.629

Foster, L., & Cox, J. (2013). Best practices in supporting students with autism. In G. Frolek Clark & B. E. Chandler (Eds.), *Best practices for occupational therapy in schools* (pp. 273–284). Bethesda, MD: AOTA Press.

Hall, L., & Case-Smith, J. (2007). The effect of sound-based intervention on children with sensory processing disorders and visual–motor delays. *American Journal of Occupational Therapy, 61,* 209–215. http://dx.doi.org/10.5014/ajot.61.2.209

Head, H. (1920). *Studies in neurology* (Vol. 2). London: Oxford University Press.

Horowitz, L. J., Oosterveld, W. J., & Adrichem, R. (1993). Effectiveness of sensory integration therapy on smooth pursuits and organization time in children. *Pädiatrie und Grenzgebiete, 31,* 331–344.

Individuals With Disabilities Education Improvement Act of 2004, Pub. L. 108–446, 20 U.S.C. §§ 1400–1483.

Jarrett, O. S., & Maxwell, D. M. (2000). What research says about the need for recess. In R. Clements (Ed.), *Elementary school recess: Selected readings, games, and activities for teachers and parents* (pp. 12–23). Lake Charles, LA: American Press.

Kinnealey, M., Pfeiffer, B., Miller, J., Roan, C., Shoener, R., & Ellner, M. L. (2012). Effect of classroom modification on attention and engagement of students with autism or dyspraxia. *American Journal of Occupational Therapy, 66,* 511–519. http://dx.doi.org/10.5014/ajot.2012.004010

Knox, S. (2008). Development and current use of the revised Knox Preschool Play Scale. In L. D. Parham & L. S. Fazio (Eds.), *Play in occupational therapy for children* (2nd ed., pp. 55–70). St. Louis, MO: Mosby/ Elsevier.

Kuypers, L. (2011). *The zones of regulation.* San Jose, CA: Think Social.

Lane, S. J., Smith Roley, S., & Champagne, T. (2013). Sensory integration and processing: Theory and applications to occupational performance. In B. A. Boyt Schell, G. Gillen, M. E. Scaffa, & E. S. Cohn (Eds.), *Willard and Spackman's occupational therapy* (12th ed., pp. 816–868). Philadelphia: Lippincott Williams & Wilkins.

Linderman, T. M., & Stewart, K. B. (1999). Sensory integrative–based occupational therapy and functional outcomes in young children with pervasive developmental disorders: A single-subject study. *American Journal of Occupational Therapy, 53,* 207–213. http://dx.doi.org/10.5014/ajot.53.2.207

Magrun, W. M., Ottenbacher, K., McCue, S., & Keefe, R. (1981). Effects of vestibular stimulation on spontaneous use of verbal language in developmentally delayed children. *American Journal of Occupational Therapy, 35,* 101–104. http://dx.doi.org/10.5014/ajot.35.2.101

Mailloux, Z., Leão, M., Becerra, T. A., Mori, A. B., Soechting, E., Roley, S. S., . . . Cermak, S. A. (2014). Modification of the Postrotary Nystagmus Test for evaluating young children. *American Journal of Occupational Therapy, 68,* 514–521. http://dx.doi.org/10.5014/ajot.2014.011031

Mailloux, Z., May-Benson, T. A., Summers, C. A., Miller, L. J., Brett-Green, B., Burke, J. P., . . . Schoen, S. A. (2007). The Issue Is—Goal attainment scaling as a measure of meaningful outcomes for children with sensory integration disorders. *American Journal of Occupational Therapy, 61,* 254–259. http://dx.doi.org/10.5014/ajot.61.2.254

Mailloux, Z., Mulligan, S., Roley, S. S., Blanche, E., Cermak, S., Coleman, G. G., . . . Lane, C. J. (2011). Verification and clarification of patterns of sensory integrative dysfunction. *American Journal of Occupational Therapy, 65,* 143–151. http://dx.doi.org/10.5014/ajot.2011.000752

Miller-Kuhaneck, H., Henry, D. A., & Glennon, T. J. (2007). *Sensory Processing Measure: Main classroom and school environments form.* Torrance, CA: Western Psychological Services.

Miller-Kuhaneck, H., Henry, D. A., & Glennon, T. J. (2010). *Sensory Processing Measure–Preschool: Main classroom and school environments form.* Torrance, CA: Western Psychological Services.

Mulligan, S. (1998). Patterns of sensory integration dysfunction: A confirmatory factor analysis. *American Journal of Occupational Therapy, 52,* 819–828. http://dx.doi.org/10.5014/ajot.52.10.819

No Child Left Behind Act of 2001, Pub. L. 107–110, 20 U.S.C. §§ 6301–8962.

Parham, D. (1987). Toward professionalism: the reflective therapist. *American Journal of Occupational Therapy, 41,* 555–561. http://dx.doi.org/10.5014/ajot.41.9.555

Parham, L. D. (1998). The relationship of sensory integrative development achievement in elementary students: Four-year longitudinal patterns. *OTJR: Occupation, Participation and Health, 18,* 105–127. http://dx.doi.org/10.1177/153944929801800304

Parham, L. D., & Ecker, C. (2007). *Sensory Processing Measure: Home form.* Torrance, CA: Western Psychological Services.

Parham, L. D., & Ecker, C. (2010). *Sensory Processing Measure–Preschool: Home form.* Torrance, CA: Western Psychological Services.

Parham, L. D., & Mailloux, Z. (2010). Sensory integration. In J. Case-Smith (Ed.), *Occupational therapy for children* (6th ed., pp. 325–372). St. Louis, MO: Mosby.

Parham, L. D., Roley, S. S., May-Benson, T. A., Koomar, J., Brett-Green, B., Burke, J. P., . . . Schaaf, R. C. (2011). Development of a fidelity measure for research on the effectiveness of the Ayres Sensory Integration® intervention. *American Journal of Occupational Therapy, 65,* 133–142. http://dx.doi.org/10.5014/ajot.2011.000745

Pellegrini, A. D. (2005). *Recess: Its role in education and development.* Mahwah, NJ: Erlbaum.

Pellegrini, A. D., & Smith, P. K. (1993). School recess: Implications for education and development. *Review of Educational Research, 63,* 51–67. http://dx.doi.org/10.3102/00346543063001051

Pellegrini, A. D., & Smith, P. K. (1998). Physical activity play: The nature and function of a neglected aspect of playing. *Child Development, 69,* 577–598. http://dx.doi.org/10.1111/j.1467-8624.1998.tb06226.x

Peyton, J. L., Bass, W. T., Burke, B. L., & Frank, L. M. (2005). Novel motor and somatosensory activity is associated with increased cerebral cortical blood volume measured by near-infrared optical topography. *Journal of Child Neurology, 20,* 817–821. http://dx.doi.org/10.1177/08830738050200100701

Pfeiffer, B. A., Koenig, K., Kinnealey, M., Sheppard, M., & Henderson, L. (2011). Effectiveness of sensory integration interventions in children with autism spectrum disorders: A pilot study. *American Journal of Occupational Therapy, 65,* 76–85. http://dx.doi.org/10.5014/ajot.2011.09205

Prizant, B. M., Wetherby, A. M., Rubin, E., & Laurent, A. (2003). The SCERTS Model: A transactional, family-centered approach to enhancing communication and socioemotional abilities of children with autism spectrum disorder. *Infants and Young Children, 16,* 296–316. http://dx.doi.org/10.1097/00001163-200310000-00004

Rehabilitation Act of 1973, Pub. L. 93–112, 29 U.S.C. §§ 701–7961.

Rehabilitation Act Amendments of 2004, 29 U.S.C. § 794.

Reynolds, S., Shepherd, J., & Lane, S. J. (2008). Sensory modulation disorders in a minority Head Start population: Preliminary prevalence and characterization. *Journal of Occupational Therapy, Schools, and Early Intervention, 1,* 186–198. http://dx.doi.org/10.1080/19411240802589031

Roberts, J. E., King-Thomas, L., & Boccia, M. L. (2007). Behavioral indexes of the efficacy of sensory integration therapy. *American Journal of Occupational Therapy, 61,* 555–562. http://dx.doi.org/10.5014/ajot.61.5.555

Schaaf, R. C., & Blanche, E. I. (2012). Emerging as leaders in autism research and practice: Using the data-driven intervention process. *American Journal of Occupational Therapy, 66,* 503–505. http://dx.doi.org/10.5014/ajot.2012.006114

Schaaf, R. C., Mailloux, Z., Faller, P., Hunt, J., van Hooydonk, E., Freeman, R., . . . Kelly, D. (2014). An intervention for sensory difficulties in children with autism: A randomized trial. *Journal of Autism and Developmental Disorders, 44,* 1493–1506. http://dx.doi.org/10.1007/s10803-013-1983-8

Schaaf, R. C., Merrill, S. C., & Kinsella, N. (1987). Sensory integration and play behavior: A case study of the effectiveness of occupational therapy using sensory integrative techniques. *Occupational Therapy in Health Care, 4*, 61–75.

Schaaf, R. C., & Nightlinger, K. M. (2007). Occupational therapy using a sensory integrative approach: A case study of effectiveness. *American Journal of Occupational Therapy, 61*, 239–246. http://dx.doi.org/10.5014/ajot.61.2.239

Schaaf, R. C., & Smith Roley, S. (2006). *SI: Applying clinical reasoning to practice with diverse populations.* Austin, TX: Pro-Ed.

Schilling, D. L., & Schwartz, I. S. (2004). Alternative seating for young children with autism spectrum disorder: Effects on classroom behavior. *Journal of Autism and Developmental Disorders, 34*, 423–432. http://dx.doi.org/10.1023/B:JADD.0000037418.48587.f4

Schilling, D. L., Washington, K., Billingsley, F. F., & Deitz, J. (2003). Classroom seating for children with attention deficit hyperactivity disorder: Therapy balls versus chairs. *American Journal of Occupational Therapy, 57*, 534–541. http://dx.doi.org/10.5014/ajot.57.5.534

Sherrington, C. (1906). *The integrative action of the nervous system.* New Haven, CT: Yale University Press.

Sherrington, C. (1940). *Man on his nature.* Garden City, NY: Doubleday.

Skard, G., & Bundy, A. C. (2008). Test of Playfulness. In L. D. Parham & L. Fazio (Eds.), *Play in occupational therapy for children* (2nd ed., pp. 71–93). St. Louis, MO: Mosby/Elsevier.

Smith, S. A., Press, B., Koenig, K. P., & Kinnealey, M. (2005). Effects of sensory integration intervention on self-stimulating and self-injurious behaviors. *American Journal of Occupational Therapy, 59*, 418–425. http://dx.doi.org/10.5014/ajot.59.4.418

Smith Roley, S., Blanche, E. I., & Schaaf, R. (Eds.). (2001). *Understanding the nature of sensory integration with diverse populations.* Austin, TX: Pro-Ed.

Smith Roley, S., Mailloux, Z., Miller-Kuhaneck, H., & Glennon, T. (2007). Understanding Ayres Sensory Integration®. *OT Practice, 12*(17), CE-1–CE-8.

Stein, B. (2012). *The new handbook of multisensory processing.* Cambridge, MA: MIT Press.

Stewart, K. B. (2010). Purposes, processes, and methods of evaluation. In J. Case-Smith & J. C. O'Brien (Eds.), *Occupational therapy for children* (pp. 193–215). Maryland Heights, MO: Mosby/Elsevier.

Tomchek, S. D., & Dunn, W. (2007). Sensory processing in children with and without autism: A comparative study using the Short Sensory Profile. *American Journal of Occupational Therapy, 61*, 190–200. http://dx.doi.org/10.5014/ajot.61.2.190

VandenBerg, N. L. (2001). The use of a weighted vest to increase on-task behavior in children with attention difficulties. *American Journal of Occupational Therapy, 55*, 621–628. http://dx.doi.org/10.5014/ajot.55.6.621

Watling, R., Koenig, K. P., Davies, P. L., & Schaaf, R. C. (2011). *Occupational therapy practice guidelines for children and adolescents with challenges in sensory processing and sensory integration.* Bethesda, MD: AOTA Press.

Wells, A. M., Chasnoff, I. J., Schmidt, C. A., Telford, E., & Schwartz, L. D. (2012). Neurocognitive habilitation therapy for children with fetal alcohol spectrum disorders: An adaptation of the Alert Program®. *American Journal of Occupational Therapy, 66*, 24–34. http://dx.doi.org/10.5014/ajot.2012.002691

Williams, M. S., & Shellenberger, S. (1994). *How does your engine run? A leader's guide to the Alert Program for Self-Regulation.* Albuquerque, NM: Therapy Works.

Wilson, B., Kaplan, B., Fellowes, S., Gruchy, C., & Faris, P. (1992). The efficacy of sensory integration intervention compared to tutoring. *Physical and Occupational Therapy in Pediatrics, 12,* 1–37. http://dx.doi.org/10.1080/J006v12n01_01

Wilson, B. N., Pollock, N., Kaplan, B. J., & Law, M. (1994). *Clinical observations of motor and postural skills.* Tucson, AZ: Therapy Skill Builders.

Authors

Susanne Smith Roley, OTD, OTR/L, FAOTA
Julie Bissell, OTD, OTR/L
Gloria Frolek Clark, PhD, OTR/L, FAOTA

for

The Commission on Practice
Debbie Amini, EdD, OTR/L, CHT, *Chairperson*

Adopted by the Representative Assembly Coordinating Council (RACC) for the Representative Assembly, 2015

Note. This document replaces the 2009 document *Providing Occupational Therapy Using Sensory Integration Theory and Methods in School-Based Practice,* previously published and copyrighted by the American Occupational Therapy Association in the *American Journal of Occupational Therapy, 63,* 823–842. http://dx.doi.org/10.5014/ajot.63.6.823

Citation. American Occupational Therapy Association. (2015). Occupational therapy for children and youth using sensory integration theory and methods in school-based practice. *American Journal of Occupational Therapy, 69*(Suppl. 3), 6913410040. http://dx.doi.org/10.5014/ajot.2015.696S04

Occupational Therapy in the Promotion of Health and Well-Being

The purpose of this statement is to describe occupational therapy's contribution in the areas of health promotion and prevention. It is intended for internal and external audiences. The American Occupational Therapy Association (AOTA) supports and promotes involvement of occupational therapists and occupational therapy assistants in the development and provision of programs and services that promote health, well-being, and social participation of all people.

Health Promotion

It is important to frame the discussion of occupational therapy's role in health promotion by first defining the term. The World Health Organization (WHO) provides the following definition in the *Ottawa Charter for Health Promotion*:

> *Health promotion* is the process of enabling people to increase control over, and to improve, their health. To reach a state of complete physical, mental, and social well-being, an individual or group must be able to identify and realize aspirations, to satisfy needs, and to change or cope with the environment. Health is, therefore, seen as a resource for everyday life, not the objective of living. Health is a positive concept emphasizing social and personal resources, as well as physical capacities. Therefore, health promotion is not just the responsibility of the health sector, but goes beyond healthy lifestyles to well-being. (WHO, 1986, para. 2, italics added)

Trentham and Cockburn (2005) expand on this definition by stating that

> *health promotion* is equally and essentially concerned with creating the conditions necessary for health at individual, structural, social, and environmental levels through an understanding of the determinants of health: peace, shelter, education, food, income, a stable ecosystem, sustainable resources, *social justice,*[1] and equity. (p. 441, italics added)

Since 1980, the U.S. Department of Health and Human Services (HHS) has established health promotion and disease prevention objectives to facilitate and measure improvement in health (HHS, 1980, 1990, 2000, 2010). The vision of Healthy People 2020 is the realization of "a society in which all people live long, healthy lives" (HHS, 2010, p. 2). *Healthy People 2020* has four major goals:

1. "Attain high-quality, longer lives free of preventable disease, disability, injury, and premature death."

2. "Achieve health equity, eliminate disparities, and improve health of all groups."

3. "Create social and physical environments that promote good health for all."

4. "Promote quality of life, healthy development, and healthy behaviors across all life stages." (p. 5)

Active engagement in life and overall health status and not just longevity is emphasized. From an individual perspective, a healthy life means the use of capacities and adaptations across the life span, allowing people to enter into satisfying relationships with others, to work, and to play. From a national

---

[1]Some italicized terms in this statement are defined in the glossary.

perspective, a healthy life means vital, creative, and productive citizens and residents contributing to flourishing communities and a thriving nation.

Health Disparities

It is important from a health promotion perspective to differentiate between the constructs of health and functional status. Many assessments of health status include items that measure function. As a result, these tools are negatively biased against persons with disabilities. It is possible to be physically and mentally healthy and have a high quality of life in spite of disability and functional limitations (Krahn, Fujiura, Drum, Cardinal, & Nosek, 2009). As noted earlier, one goal of *Healthy People 2020* is to eliminate health disparities (HHS, 2010).

The term *health disparities* refers to population-specific differences in disease rates, health outcomes, and access to health care services. Addressing health disparities is consistent with the occupational therapy profession's official document on nondiscrimination and inclusion, which states, "Inclusion requires that we ensure not only that everyone is treated fairly and equitably but also that all individuals have the same opportunities to participate in the naturally occurring activities of society" (AOTA, 2009b, p. 819).

Persons with disabilities may be the largest population experiencing health disparities. "The differences in health status between people with disabilities and without disabilities are increasingly recognized as preventable and therefore unacceptable" (Krahn, Putnam, Drum, & Powers, 2006, p. 18). Persons with disabilities are at risk for developing secondary conditions that are physical and mental as well as social health problems that are the direct or indirect consequence of the disability. The five most frequent secondary conditions identified in a study by Kinne, Patrick, and Doyle (2004) are (1) chronic muscle and joint pain, (2) sleep disturbances, (3) extreme fatigue, (4) weight or eating problems, and (5) depression.

The prevalence of these conditions was 2 to 3 times higher among adults with disabilities than among adults without disabilities. In addition, persons with disabilities often have higher rates of diabetes, obesity, anxiety, social isolation, and unemployment (Drum, Krahn, Culley, & Hammond, 2005) and less satisfaction with care within the health system (Krahn et al., 2006) than their able-bodied counterparts. Secondary conditions, many of which are preventable, are often considered the primary cause of health disparities for this population.

Health promotion programs and services may target individuals, communities, and populations as well as policymakers. The focus of these programs is to

- Prevent or reduce the incidence of illness or disease, accidents, and injuries in the population;

- Reduce health disparities among racial and ethnic minorities and other underserved populations;

- Enhance mental health, resiliency, and quality of life;

- Prevent secondary conditions and improve the overall health and well-being of people with chronic conditions or disabilities and their caregivers; and

- Promote healthy living practices, social participation, *occupational justice,* and healthy communities, with respect for cross-cultural issues and concerns.

Prevention Strategies

A key purpose of health promotion is improved well-being, quality of life, and social participation for individuals and populations. Health management and maintenance for persons with or without disabilities require the implementation of prevention strategies. Prevention is generally categorized into three levels: (1) primary, (2) secondary, and (3) tertiary.

Primary prevention is defined as education or health promotion efforts designed to prevent the onset and reduce the incidence of unhealthy conditions, diseases, or injuries. Primary prevention attempts to identify, reduce, or eliminate risk factors for disease and injury. For persons with disabilities, primary prevention may include modifying the physical and social environment to address the special needs resulting from the disability. Strategies for improving nutrition; increasing physical activities; smoking cessation; weight management; and screening for heart disease, diabetes, and cancer are important for persons with disabilities as well as the general population.

Secondary prevention typically includes screening, early detection, and intervention after disease has occurred; it is designed to prevent or disrupt the disabling process. For persons with disabilities, secondary prevention involves limiting the development of secondary conditions and their subsequent impact on function and quality of life.

Tertiary prevention refers to services designed to prevent the progression of a condition. Tertiary prevention for persons with disabilities should also include strategies to promote equal opportunity, full participation, independent living, and economic self-sufficiency (Patrick, Richardson, Starks, Rose, & Kinne, 1997).

Population Health Approach

Population health focuses on *aggregates,* or communities of people, and the many factors that influence their health. A population health approach strives to identify and reduce health disparities as well as enhance the overall health and well-being of a population (Finlayson & Edwards, 1997). In addition to providing occupational therapy interventions for individuals, occupational therapy practitioners can develop and implement occupation-based population health approaches to enhance occupational performance and participation, quality of life, and occupational justice.

Health Promotion and Occupation

Healthy People 2020 and the Ottawa Charter for Health Promotion parallel occupational therapy's belief that engagement in meaningful occupations supports health and leads to a productive and satisfying life. Wilcock (2006) stated that

> Following an occupation-focused health promotion approach to well-being embraces a belief that the potential range of what people can do, be, and strive to become is the primary concern and that health is a by-product. A varied and full occupational lifestyle will coincidentally maintain and improve health and well-being if it enables people to be creative and adventurous physically, mentally, and socially. (p. 315)

According to Christiansen (1999), "Health enables people to pursue the tasks of everyday living that provide them with the life meaning necessary for their well-being" (p. 547). *Well-being* is a state of flourishing that consists of the following elements: positive emotion, engagement or flow, *meaning* (i.e., a sense of belonging to or serving something larger than oneself), positive relationships, and accomplishment or achievement (Seligman, 2011).

Occupational therapy services are provided to clients of all age groups, infants through older adults, from a variety of socioeconomic, cultural, and ethnic backgrounds, who possess or who are at risk for impairments, activity limitations, or participation restrictions. According to AOTA (2008), occupational therapy practitioners[2] recognize that health is supported when individuals are able to engage in occupations and activities that allow them to achieve the desired outcome of participation in their chosen environments. The essence of occupational therapy is "supporting health and participation in life through engagement in occupation" (p. 626). This focus on engagement in occupation is interwoven through the delivery of service, beginning with evaluation and continuing through the intervention phase. Health management and maintenance are included within the domain of occupational therapy as an instrumental activity of daily living; health promotion and prevention are identified as occupational therapy

---

[2]When the term *occupational therapy practitioner* is used in this document, it refers to both occupational therapists and occupational therapy assistants (AOTA, 2006).

intervention approaches; and health and wellness, quality of life, and occupational justice are potential outcomes of occupational therapy services (AOTA, 2008).

Occupations are purposeful and meaningful daily activities that fill a person's time and are typically categorized as self-care, work, play or leisure, and rest (AOTA, 1995; Meyer, 1922). A natural, balanced pattern of occupations is believed to be health enhancing and fulfills both the needs of the individual and the demands of the environment (Kielhofner, 2004; Meyer, 1922). This belief has been supported in studies with well elderly individuals in urban communities (Clark et al., 1997, 2001, 2012).

By engaging clients in everyday occupations, occupational therapy practitioners promote physical and mental health and facilitate well-being for persons with and without disabilities. Occupational therapy practitioners promote positive mental health through competency enhancement strategies, such as skill development, environmental supports, and task adaptations, and they prevent mental illness through risk reduction strategies, such as establishing healthy habits and routines and providing training in relaxation and coping techniques (AOTA, 2010).

Occupational imbalance, deprivation, and *alienation* are risk factors for health problems in and of themselves. They may also result from or lead to the development of other risk factors, which can in turn result in larger health and social problems. Causes are varied (e.g., unanticipated caregiving responsibilities, losses in employment or housing) and can lead to occupational imbalance, deprivation, and alienation, which can then lead to individual health problems such as stress, sleep disturbance, and depression (Wilcock, 2006).

Belle et al. (2006) demonstrated that caregivers of people with dementia experienced significant improvement in quality of life and a decrease in depression after intervention that included stress management; strategies for engaging in pleasant events; and teaching of healthy behaviors, communication skills, and problem-solving skills regarding behavior management of care recipients' difficult behaviors. Elliott, Burgio, and DeCoster (2010) similarly found that a caregiver intervention enhances health and decreases depression, resulting in a decrease in perceived burden. Occupational therapy practitioners are in a prime position to recognize the occupation and health problems inherent with caregiving and offer interventions such as those described in the cited research as well as additional interventions from an occupation lens, such as task analysis and modification to minimize the physical and emotional stresses of caregiving.

Role of Occupational Therapy in Health Promotion

Occupational therapy practitioners have three critical roles in health promotion and prevention:

1. To promote healthy lifestyles;

2. To emphasize occupation as an essential element of health promotion strategies; and

3. To provide interventions, not only with individuals but also with populations.

It is important that occupational therapy practitioners promote a healthy lifestyle for all individuals and their families, including people with physical, mental, or cognitive impairments. An occupation-focused approach to prevention of illness and disability has been defined by Wilcock (2006) as

> the application of medical, behavioral, social, and *occupational science* to prevent physiological, psychological, social, and occupational illness; accidents; and disability; and to prolong quality of life for all people through advocacy and mediation and through occupation-focused programs aimed at enabling people to do, be, and become according to their natural health needs. (p. 282, italics added)

The roles of occupational therapy practitioners in evaluation and intervention in health promotion practice are based on the *Guidelines for Supervision, Roles, and Responsibilities During the Delivery of Occupational Therapy Services* (AOTA, 2009a). Occupational therapy practitioners possess the basic knowledge and skills to carry out health promotion interventions to prevent injury and maximize well-being. However, this area of practice is very broad, and practitioners need to continually expand their knowledge in health promotion to be effective and competent members of the team.

While recognizing the unique role of occupational therapy in health promotion and prevention, it is also important to acknowledge and respect the contributions of other health care professions in this arena. Occupational therapy practitioners should operate within their scope of practice and training and partner with other health promotion disciplines with specialized expertise such as in the areas of public health, health education, nutrition, and exercise science.

As in all other areas of practice, health promotion services should be based on the best available evidence. Law, Steinwender, and LeClair (1998) conducted an extensive review of the literature on the relationship between occupation and health. The longitudinal studies that were reviewed found that activity participation had a significant effect on perceived health. Maintenance of everyday activities, social interactions, and community mobility influenced self-reported quality of life.

A long-term benefit attributable to preventive occupational therapy was shown by Clark et al. (2001) when they reevaluated participants from the Well Elderly Study and found that 90% of therapeutic gain observed after intervention was retained at the 6-month follow-up. The Well Elderly Study was replicated through the Well Elderly Trial 2 with participants from a wider array of economic and ethnic backgrounds. Occupational therapy health promotion was once again found to be a cost-effective method to enhance health and well-being among older adults in an urban context (Clark et al., 2012).

Interventions With Individuals

The following are examples of occupation-based primary prevention intervention that target individuals:

- Musculoskeletal injury prevention and management programs

- Anger management and conflict resolution training for parents, teachers, and school-aged youth to reduce the incidence of bullying and other violence

- Parenting skills training to enhance family health and decrease potential for abuse

- Fall prevention programs for community-dwelling seniors

- Ensuring health literacy for non–English-speaking populations.

Examples of secondary prevention carried out by occupational therapy practitioners may include

- Education and training regarding eating habits, activity levels, and prevention of secondary disability subsequent to obesity;

- Education and training on stress management and adaptive coping strategies to enhance resilience for persons with mood disorders and posttraumatic stress disorder; and

- Osteoporosis prevention and management classes for individuals recently diagnosed with or at high risk for this condition.

Examples of occupation-based tertiary prevention intervention may include

- Transitional or independent-living skills training for people who have mental illness and those with cognitive impairments;

- Leisure participation groups for older adults with dementia to prevent depression, enhance socialization, and improve quality of life;

- Social participation activities at a drop-in center for adults with severe mental illness; and

- Stroke support groups for survivors and caregivers.

Occupational therapy practitioners have an opportunity to complement existing health promotion efforts by adding the contribution of occupation to programs developed by experts in health education, nutrition, exercise, and so forth. For example, when working with a person with a lower extremity amputation due to diabetes, the occupational therapy practitioner may focus on the occupation of meal preparation using foods and preparation methods recommended in the nutritionist's health promotion program. This focus enables achievement of the occupational therapy goal of functional independence in the kitchen and reinforces the importance of proper nutrition for the prevention of further disability (Scaffa, 2001).

Interventions With Populations

To be effective, health promotion efforts cannot focus only on intervention at the individual level. Because of the inextricable and reciprocal links between people and their environments, larger groups, organizations, communities, and populations may also benefit from occupational therapy intervention (AOTA, 2008; Law, 1991; Wilcock, 2006).

Examples of interventions through the intermediary of organizations include

- Consultation to businesses to promote well-being of workers through identification of problems and solutions for balance among work, leisure, and family life;

- Consultation to schools regarding implementation of Americans With Disabilities Act of 1990 (ADA; Pub. L. 101–336) requirements;

- Education for day care staff regarding normal growth and development, handling behavior problems, and identifying children at risk for developmental delays; and

- Promotion of ergonomically correct workstations in schools and offices.

Community or population-level interventions may include

- Consulting with the local transportation authority regarding accessible public transportation;

- Consulting with contractors, architects, and city planners regarding accessibility and universal design;

- Implementing a community-wide screening program for depression at nursing homes, assisted living facilities, and senior centers for the purpose of developing group and individual prevention and intervention programs;

- Conducting needs assessments and implementing intervention strategies to reduce health disparities in communities with high rates of disease or injury, such as lifestyle management programs addressing hypertension, diabetes, and obesity;

- Addressing the health and occupation needs of the homeless population by eliminating barriers and enhancing opportunities for occupational engagement; and

- Training volunteers to function effectively in special needs shelters during disasters.

Governmental or policy-level interventions may include

- Promoting policies that offer affordable, accessible health care to everyone, including people with disabilities;

- Promoting barrier-free environments for all ages, including aging in place and universal design;

- Supporting full inclusion of children with disabilities in schools and day care programs;

- Lobbying for public funds to support research and program development in areas related to improvement in quality of life for people at risk and those with disabilities; and

- Promoting policies that establish opportunities for rehabilitation in the community for people discharged from inpatient psychiatric programs.

Opportunities for Occupational Therapy in Health Promotion

Funding for health promotion programs can come from governmental agencies, foundations, nonprofit organizations, insurance companies, and large corporations, among others. In addition, fee for service is an option. Typically, health promotion and prevention programs do not rely on a single source of funding (Brownson, 1998; Scaffa, 2001).

Changes in health care brought about by the 2010 Patient Protection and Affordable Care Act (ACA; Pub. L. 111–148) have already and will continue to have an impact on health promotion, prevention, and public health service provision. Although the ACA is designed to improve individual health by increasing access to health insurance and health care, several provisions relate directly to health promotion. Specifically, Title IV calls for

- Increasing funding for prevention and public health programs;

- Providing education and outreach related to health promotion and disease prevention;

- Reviewing evidence related to preventive services and the development of recommendations;

- Providing Medicare coverage of annual well care visits and the development of personalized prevention plans;

- Improving access to preventive services for eligible adults in Medicaid;

- Eliminating patient copays for prevention services;

- Dispersing incentives for prevention of chronic diseases in Medicaid;

- Evaluating outcomes of community-based prevention and wellness programs for Medicare beneficiaries;

- Removing barriers and improving access to health promotion services for individuals with disabilities;

- Providing grants for employer-based wellness programs; and

- Funding for childhood obesity demonstration project (Kaiser Family Foundation, 2011; Network for Public Health Law, 2011).

Occupational therapy practitioners can seize opportunities to participate in the provision of health promotion and prevention services under the ACA by becoming a member of the primary care team and the patient's medical home. Failure to integrate occupational therapy into these arenas could severely limit the profession's future growth.

Case Studies

The following case studies provide examples of the role of occupational therapy in health promotion and prevention of disease and injuries.

Primary Prevention—Working With a Family

A retired couple consult an occupational therapist about a home safety assessment for the purpose of remaining in their home as they age.

Assessment

The occupational therapist develops an occupational profile (AOTA, 2008) using a semistructured interview format. She gathers information about the couple's goals, occupational history, health, occupational performance, and satisfaction level within the various performance areas, as well as social connectedness and overall life satisfaction.

Both spouses are healthy and able to perform daily tasks with a high level of satisfaction. They have a strong social support network and report being very satisfied with their lives. The occupational therapist also explores the health history of their parents and learns of a history of Alzheimer's disease and diabetes. She assesses the environment (i.e., home, yard, neighborhood) for accessibility and safety using the

Safety Assessment of Function and the Environment for Rehabilitation (SAFER) tool (Oliver, Blathwayt, Brackley, & Tamaki, 1993).

The occupational therapist notes that the living area is on three levels (several steps have no railings); rooms and hallways are generally poorly lit; and the rooms have too much furniture, leaving narrow or obstructed passageways. The yard has uneven and poorly defined walkways. The couple lives in a residential neighborhood with a distance of 3 miles to shopping. No public transportation is available, even for people with mobility impairments.

Intervention

For immediate consideration, the occupational therapist recommends that the couple install railings near all stairs, increase the level of lighting, and decrease the amount of furniture. She works with them to find the best configuration of furniture placement to maximize safety when walking in a room. She recommends that they consider changing the landscape to include clearly defined and level walkways that will also accommodate wheeled mobility, should that ever be needed.

A second set of recommendations includes how to retrofit the house if mobility impairments preclude climbing stairs in the future. The therapist describes optimal placement of an elevator from the first to the second floor. There is not an easy placement of an elevator from the basement to the first floor, so the therapist describes how the occupations now performed in the basement (e.g., exercise, laundry, computer use) may be transferred to the other two floors. The therapist works with the couple on problem solving around transportation, should driving become difficult.

Primary Prevention—Working With a Business

A commercial bakery contacts an occupational therapist to assess the various workstations in the bakery and make recommendations for improvements. Management goals include increasing productivity and decreasing sick days and worker compensation claims.

Assessment

The occupational therapist observes the work performed at the various workstations and interviews the workers. He notes body mechanics, repetitive motions, machine design, layout of workstations with travel distances, weights lifted and number of lifts per time unit, work speed and load, noise, temperature, air quality, clothing comfort, and length and frequency of rest breaks. He also notes worker-to-worker interaction and interaction among workers, supervisors, and management. In general, the supervisors and management seem approachable and open to suggestions from the workers.

The occupational therapist identifies a high frequency of lifting and repetitive motion done by the workers. Workstations require a significant amount of static standing, which can contribute to many musculoskeletal problems. Travel distances are long, work speed is rapid, noise level is high in certain parts of the factory, and the temperature is uncomfortably warm.

Intervention

The occupational therapist recommends ergonomically designed workstations that can decrease the amount of static work, time standing, travel, or lifting and that can improve working positions. Because some jobs involve repetitive motions that may not be avoided, the therapist instructs the managers in the benefits of rest breaks and instructs the workers in stretching exercises. Each worker is also instructed in proper body mechanics at his or her workstation. The therapist works with the management to design a daily schedule that allows for an even workflow to decrease times of high stress. The therapist is asked to return every 6 months to reassess and instruct new employees.

Primary Prevention—Working With a School

An elementary school is planning a new playground, which must be accessible to every child in the school. An occupational therapist is consulted for input on design features that will make the playground aesthetically pleasing, fun, and challenging to use for children of all abilities.

Assessment

The occupational therapist surveys the area where the school is planning to locate the playground. He uses the guidelines for play areas developed by the U.S. Access Board (2007) to ensure minimum requirements are met. He then researches commercially available playground equipment to find equipment that will be fun and challenging to use for all populations in the school as well as encourage interaction among the children.

Intervention

The occupational therapist provides the school with a report detailing his recommendations for important features in the playground equipment and the layout of the playground. He is careful to identify all safety issues and suggests ways to make the playground as safe as possible. The report also includes recommendations for landscaping so that children using wheeled mobility can easily navigate around the playground. The therapist remains on the design team for consultation until the playground is completed.

Secondary Prevention—Working With a Local Governmental Agency

An occupational therapist working in home health has noticed that her elderly clients who no longer drive because of a variety of functional limitations have no other means of transportation to go grocery shopping, run errands, and visit friends. The therapist reviews the literature for evidence and locates the special issue of the *American Journal of Occupational Therapy* that includes several systematic reviews on the relationship between occupation and productive aging (Leland & Elliott, 2012), and she commits to taking action.

Assessment

To determine the need for alternative means of transportation, the occupational therapist conducts a needs assessment, gathering existing data from several sources, including state and local census data and information from community organizations that provide services to older adults.

Intervention

The occupational therapist contacts the county office on aging to discuss her findings and concerns. She conducts a brief presentation, including data she collected about the local community and evidence from the systematic reviews. A joint task force is formed with local senior centers to further study the transportation experience of elderly county residents and make recommendations. Cognizant of the need to balance the fiscal resources of the county with the needs of aging county residents, the task force develops a proposal for extending one bus route and including three additional stops on two other bus routes during the weekday non–rush hour time period. The proposal emphasizes the importance of transportation and social participation to the health and well-being of elders.

Tertiary Prevention—Working With a Group

A rehabilitation unit in a hospital decides to offer health promotion classes to former patients with chronic conditions. An occupational therapy assistant is chosen to lead a class for patients with chronic obstructive pulmonary disease.

Assessment

The occupational therapy assistant researches information on the disease, existing programs, and their content and outcomes. He researches optimal group size, length of each session, session frequency, and number of sessions.

Intervention

Using the assessment information, the supervising occupational therapist works with the occupational therapy assistant and a respiratory therapist to develop the health promotion class, including number of participants, length of session, and topics offered. It is decided that a maximum of 15 participants will meet monthly for 1½ hours for a total of 12 sessions. Topics include self-management, assertive communication, information-seeking, and problem-solving skills. The group will also function as a support group. The occupational therapist collects data to determine the effectiveness of the program in preventing secondary conditions associated with chronic obstructive pulmonary disease and promoting independent living and quality of life.

Summary

Through this statement, the AOTA described the role of occupational therapy in the promotion of health and well-being among individuals, families, communities, and populations. Three levels of prevention services were defined, and potential contributions by occupational therapy practitioners were detailed at each level.

The examples provided are just a few of the extensive, rich, and varied occupation-based approaches that can facilitate the achievement of the national goals outlined in Healthy People 2020. These approaches include, but are not limited to, the creation of health-promoting social and physical environments, improved quality of life, healthy development, and health equity for all.

References

American Occupational Therapy Association. (1995). Occupation: A position paper. *American Journal of Occupational Therapy, 49,* 1015–1018. http://dx.doi.org/10.5014/ajot.49.10.1015

American Occupational Therapy Association. (2006). Association policies: Policy 1.44: Categories of occupational therapy personnel. *American Journal of Occupational Therapy, 60,* 683–684. http://dx.doi.org/10.5014/ajot.60.6.681

American Occupational Therapy Association. (2008). Occupational therapy practice framework: Domain and process (2nd ed.). *American Journal of Occupational Therapy, 62,* 625–683. http://dx.doi.org/10.5014/ajot.62.6.625

American Occupational Therapy Association. (2009a). Guidelines for supervision, roles, and responsibilities during the delivery of occupational therapy services. *American Journal of Occupational Therapy, 63,* 797–803. http://dx.doi.org/10.5014/ajot.63.6.797

American Occupational Therapy Association. (2009b). Occupational therapy's commitment to non-discrimination and inclusion. *American Journal of Occupational Therapy, 63,* 819–820. http://dx.doi.org/10.5014/ajot.63.6.819

American Occupational Therapy Association. (2010). Specialized knowledge and skills in mental health promotion, prevention, and intervention in occupational therapy practice. *American Journal of Occupational Therapy, 64*(6, Suppl.), S30–S43. http://dx.doi.org/10.5014/ajot.2010.64S30

Americans With Disabilities Act of 1990, Pub. L. 101–336, 42 U.S.C. § 12101.

Belle, S. H., Burgio, L., Burns, R., Coon, D., Czaja, S. J., Gallagher-Thompson, D., . . . Zhang, S. (2006). Enhancing the quality of life of dementia caregivers from different ethnic or racial groups. *Annals of Internal Medicine, 145,* 727–738. http://dx.doi.org/10.7326/0003-4819-145-10-200611210-00005

Brownson, C. A. (1998). Funding community practice: Stage 1. *American Journal of Occupational Therapy, 52,* 60–64. http://dx.doi.org/10.5014/ajot.52.1.60

Christiansen, C. H. (1999). Defining lives: Occupation as identity: An essay on competence, coherence, and the creation of meaning. *American Journal of Occupational Therapy, 53,* 547–558. http://dx.doi.org/10.5014/ajot.53.6.547

Clark, F., Azen, S. P., Carlson, M., Mandel, D., LaBree, L., Hay, J., . . . Lipson, L. (2001). Embedding health-promoting changes into the daily lives of independent-living older adults: Long-term follow-up of occupational therapy intervention. *Journals of Gerontology, Series B: Psychological Sciences and Social Sciences, 56,* 60–63. http://dx.doi.org/10.1093/geronb/56.1.P60

Clark, F., Azen, S. P., Zemke, R., Jackson, J., Carlson, M., Mandel, D., . . . Lipson, L. (1997). Occupational therapy for independent-living older adults: A randomized controlled trial. *JAMA, 278,* 1321–1326.

Clark, F., Jackson, J., Carlson, M., Chou, C., Cherry, B. J., Jordan-Marsh, M., . . . Azen, S. P. (2012). Effectiveness of a lifestyle intervention in promoting the well-being of independently living older people: Results of the Well Elderly 2 randomised controlled trial. *Journal of Epidemiology and Community Health, 66,* 782–790. http://dx.doi.org/10.1136/jech.2009.099754

Drum, C. E., Krahn, G., Culley, C., & Hammond, L. (2005). Recognizing and responding to the health disparities of people with disabilities. *Californian Journal of Health Promotion, 3,* 29–42.

Elliott, A. F., Burgio, L. D., & DeCoster, J. (2010). Enhancing caregiver health: Findings from the Resources for Enhancing Alzheimer's Caregiver Health II Intervention. *Journal of the American Geriatrics Society, 58,* 30–37. http://dx.doi.org/10.1111/j.1532-5415.2009.02631.x

Finlayson, M., & Edwards, J. (1997). Evolving health environments and occupational therapy: Definitions, descriptions, and opportunities. *British Journal of Occupational Therapy, 60,* 456–460.

Kaiser Family Foundation. (2011). *Summary of new health reform law.* Retrieved from www.kff.org/healthreform/8061.cfm

Kielhofner, G. (2004). *Conceptual foundation of occupational therapy* (3rd ed.). Philadelphia: F. A. Davis.

Kinne, S., Patrick, D. L., & Doyle, D.L. (2004). Prevalence of secondary conditions among people with disabilities. *American Journal of Public Health, 94,* 443–445. http://dx.doi.org/10.2105/AJPH.94.3.443

Krahn, G. L., Fujiura, G. T., Drum, C. E., Cardinal, B. J., & Nosek, M. A.; RRTC Expert Panel on Health Measurement. (2009). The dilemma of measuring perceived health status in the context of disability. *Disability and Health Journal, 2,* 49–56. http://dx.doi.org/10.1016/j.dhjo.2008.12.003

Krahn, G. L., Putnam, M., Drum, C. E., & Powers, L. (2006). Disabilities and health. *Journal of Disability Policy Studies, 17,* 18–27. http://dx.doi.org/10.1177/10442073060170010201

Law, M. (1991). The environment: A focus for occupational therapy [Muriel Driver Memorial Lecture]. *Canadian Journal of Occupational Therapy, 58,* 171–179. http://dx.doi.org/10.1177/000841749105800404

Law, M., Steinwender, S., & LeClair, L. (1998). Occupation, health, and well-being. *Canadian Journal of Occupational Therapy, 65,* 81–91. http://dx.doi.org/10.1177/000841749806500204

Leland, N. E., & Elliott, S. J. (2012). Special issue on productive aging: Evidence and opportunities for occupational therapy practitioners. *American Journal of Occupational Therapy, 66,* 263–265. http://dx.doi.org/10.5014/ajot.2010.005165

Meyer, A. (1922). The philosophy of occupation therapy. *Archives of Occupational Therapy, 1,* 1–10.

Network for Public Health Law. (2011). *Public health provisions of the Patient Protection and Affordable Care Act: Issue brief.* Retrieved from www.networkforphl.org/_asset/x4mc6h/ACA-chart-formatted-FINAL.pdf

Oliver, R., Blathwayt, J., Brackley, C., & Tamaki, T. (1993). Development of the Safety Assessment of Function and the Environment for Rehabilitation (SAFER) tool. *Canadian Journal of Occupational Therapy, 60,* 78–82. http://dx.doi.org/10.1177/000841749306000204

Patient Protection and Affordable Care Act, Pub. L. 111–148, § 3502, 124 Stat. 119, 124 (2010).

Patrick, D. L., Richardson, M., Starks, H. E., Rose, M. A., & Kinne, S. (1997). Rethinking prevention for people with disabilities, Part II: A framework for designing interventions. *American Journal of Health Promotion, 11,* 261–263. http://dx.doi.org/10.4278/0890-1171-11.4.261

Scaffa, M. E. (2001). *Occupational therapy in community-based practice settings.* Philadelphia: F. A. Davis.

Seligman, M. (2011). *Flourish: A visionary new understanding of happiness and well-being.* New York: Free Press.

Trentham, B., & Cockburn, L. (2005). Participatory action research: Creating new knowledge and opportunities for occupational engagement. In F. Kronenberg, S. Simó Algado, & N. Pollard (Eds.), *Occupational therapy without borders: Learning from the spirit of survivors* (pp. 440–453). Philadelphia: Churchill Livingstone.

U.S. Access Board. (2007). *Accessible play areas: A summary of accessibility guidelines for play areas.* Retrieved from www.access-board.gov/play/guide/guide.pdf

U.S. Department of Health and Human Services. (1980). *Promoting health/preventing disease: Objectives for the nation.* Washington, DC: U.S. Government Printing Office.

U.S. Department of Health and Human Services. (1990). *Healthy People 2000.* Washington, DC: U.S. Government Printing Office.

U.S. Department of Health and Human Services. (2000). *Healthy People 2010: Understanding and improving health* (2nd ed.). Washington, DC: U.S. Government Printing Office.

U.S. Department of Health and Human Services. (2010). *Healthy People 2020* [Brochure]. Retrieved from www.healthypeople.gov/2020/TopicsObjectives2020/pdfs/HP2020_brochure_with_LHI_508.pdf

Wilcock, A. A. (2006). *An occupational perspective of health* (2nd ed.). Thorofare, NJ: Slack.

World Health Organization. (1986). *The Ottawa Charter for health promotion.* Retrieved from www.who.int/healthpromotion/conferences/previous/ottawa/en/

Zemke, R., & Clark, F. (1996). *Occupational science: The evolving discipline.* Philadelphia: F. A. Davis.

Authors
S. Maggie Reitz, PhD, OTR/L, FAOTA
Marjorie E. Scaffa, PhD, OTR/L, FAOTA

for

The Commission on Practice
Debbie Amini, EdD, OTR/L, CHT, *Chairperson*

Adopted by the Representative Assembly Coordinating Council (RACC) for the Representative Assembly

Note. This document replaces the 2007 Statement *Occupational Therapy in the Promotion of Health and the Prevention of Disease and Disability,* previously published and copyrighted in 2008 by the American Occupational Therapy Association in the *American Journal of Occupational Therapy, 64,* 694–703.

Appendix. Glossary of Health Promotion Terms

Occupational alienation—"Sense of isolation, powerlessness, frustration, loss of control, and estrangement from society or self as a result of engagement in occupation that does not satisfy inner needs" (Wilcock, 2006, p. 343).

Occupational deprivation—"Deprivation of occupational choice and diversity because of circumstances beyond the control of individuals or communities" (Wilcock, 2006, p. 343).

Occupational imbalance—"A lack of balance or disproportion of occupation resulting in decreased well-being" (Wilcock, 2006, p. 343).

Occupational justice—"The promotion of social and economic change to increase individual, community, and political awareness, resources, and equitable opportunities for diverse occupational opportunities that enable people to meet their potential and experience well-being" (Wilcock, 2006, p. 343).

Occupational science— "An interdisciplinary academic discipline in the social and behavioral sciences dedicated to the study of the form, the function, and the meaning of human occupations" (Zemke & Clark, 1996, p. vii).

Social justice—"The promotion of social and economic change to increase individual, community, and political awareness, resources, and opportunity for health and well-being" (Wilcock, 2006, p. 344).

Well-being—A state of flourishing that consists of the following elements: positive emotion, engagement or flow, *meaning* (a sense of belonging to or serving something larger than oneself), positive relationships and accomplishment or achievement (Seligman, 2011).

Occupational Therapy Services for Individuals Who Have Experienced Domestic Violence

The primary purpose of this statement is to define the role of occupational therapy and the scope of services available for survivors and families who have experienced domestic violence. The American Occupational Therapy Association (AOTA) supports and promotes the use of this document by occupational therapists, occupational therapy assistants, and individuals interested in this topic as it relates to the profession of occupational therapy.

Domestic Violence

Prevalence

Domestic violence is a societal problem in the United States and internationally that affects not only the survivor of the violence but also the children witnessing it, the family and friends of the survivor, and the communities in which it occurs. In 2008, there were approximately 552,000 reported cases of non-fatal domestic violence against females and approximately 101,000 reported cases against males (U.S. Department of Justice [USDOJ], 2011). These are the reported cases; it is estimated that the numbers are much higher because many cases of abuse are unreported (National Coalition Against Domestic Violence [NCADV], 2007; Centers for the Disease Control and Prevention [CDC], 2010).

Definitions

The term *victim* is sometimes used to describe individuals who are or have been in an abusive relationship. The term *survivor* is used to describe individuals who are currently in the abusive relationship or who have overcome the abuse. We choose to use the term survivor because it is more empowering and denotes the strength and courage needed to endure as well as leave the abusive relationship.

There are numerous definitions of domestic violence depending on the state and organization. This document defines *domestic violence* as a pattern of "coercive behavior designed to exert power and control over a person in an intimate relationship through the use of intimidating, threatening, harmful, or harassing behavior" (Office for Victims of Crime [OVC], 2002). The emphasis is on a *pattern* of abuse and violence that becomes part of their lives, leaving lasting effects on the survivor and children. *Domestic violence* often is used more globally to account for the broad impact it has on the family, whereas the term *intimate partner violence (IPV)* specifically refers to the violence between a former or current partner or spouse (National Institute of Justice [NIJ], 2007).

For the purposes of this paper, the term *domestic violence* is used because of its broader connotation. Although women are abused in 85% to 95% of the reported domestic violence cases (Fisher & Shelton, 2006), men also are abused and face an additional stigma of gender roles, which often prevents them from coming forward (OVC, 2002). Therefore, it is important to view domestic violence as an issue of obtaining power and control over a partner without assuming that the partner is female.

Survivor Characteristics

Domestic violence occurs in both heterosexual and homosexual relationships at nearly the same rate (National Coalition of Anti-Violence Programs, 1998). In a national study, Tjaden and Thoennes (2000a) indicated that 11% of lesbians reported violence by their female partner and 15% of gay men who had lived with a male partner reported being victimized by that partner. Survivors of domestic violence in a homosexual relationship may have more difficulty accessing services and may face further stigma and marginalization due to their sexual orientation.

Domestic violence knows no boundaries; it crosses into all socioeconomic classes, races, societies, and ages, regardless of the sexual orientation that defines the relationships. The key issue in domestic violence is the use of a pattern of abusive behavior by the abuser to establish fear, power, and control over an intimate or formerly intimate partner.

Women with disabilities who are abused may face additional barriers that make it more difficult to leave the abusive relationship and access services. Although there are inconsistent findings regarding the incidence of abuse of women with disabilities, several sources indicate that women with disabilities are assaulted, raped, and abused at a rate twice that of women without disabilities (Brownridge, 2006; Helfrich, Lafata, MacDonald, Aviles, & Collins, 2001; Milberger et al., 2002; NIJ, 2000; Nosek, Hughes, Taylor, & Taylor, 2006). Analysis of data from the 2007 National Crime Victimization Survey indicated that the rates of violence against women with disabilities was highest among women with cognitive disabilities (Rand & Harrell, 2009).

Women with disabilities may be dependent on their partners for financial, physical, and/or medical support and thus may stay in abusive relationships for longer periods of time (Helfrich et al., 2001; NIJ, 2000). Their abusers may withhold necessary equipment such as wheelchairs, braces, medications, and transportation as a means to control them (NIJ, 2000).

Domestic violence also affects older adults. Domestic violence in older adults has unique considerations due to the chronic exposure to abuse over a lifetime (Jacobson, Pabst, Regan, & Fisher, 2006; Zink, Regan, Jacobson, & Pabst, 2003). The couple may experience feelings of guilt mixed with responsibility, particularly when the abuser is also the caregiver or when the caregiver needs to care for the abuser. As the couple gets older and experiences changes in their health, the violence may be masked by conditions such as Alzheimer's disease, or it may be heightened by the added stress that caregiving brings to the relationship (National Coalition Against Domestic Violence, n.d.; Zink et al., 2003).

Causes and Contributing Factors

Factors that cause or contribute to domestic violence have been discussed and contested by social scientists for decades, with little agreement about the commonalities (Jewkes, 2005). The exception is poverty, which is the only factor that consistently has been found to be a key contributor to domestic violence (Davies, 2008; Jewkes, 2005; Josephson, 2005; Lyon, 2000, 2002; Sokoloff & Dupont, 2005). The most recent USDOJ (2007) statistics from an analysis of reported and unreported family violence indicate that persons in households with annual incomes less than $7,500 (below the U.S. poverty threshold) have higher rates of assault than do persons in households with higher income levels. Furthermore, the data also indicate that social class appears to be inversely related to the severity of the violence; more severe domestic violence occurs against women within the lowest socioeconomic group (Bograd, 2005; Browne & Bassuk, 1997; Davies, 2008; Lyon, 2000, 2002; Rank, 2004; Rice, 2001).

Limited education and being a victim of child maltreatment, especially sexual abuse, also have been found to be strong links to subsequent victimization (Browne & Bassuk, 1997; Tjaden & Thoennes, 2000b). Being verbally abused has been found to be a highly predictive variable for abuse by an intimate partner (Tjaden & Thoennes, 2000b).

Being economically poor also has serious implications in terms of whether a woman stays in an abusive relationship. Studies of female survivors of domestic violence have consistently indicated that a survivor's ability to earn an independent source of income that allows her to successfully sustain her family is the most significant indicator that she will be able to permanently leave the abusive relationship (Economic Stability Working Group, 2002; Waldner, 2003). It makes sense, then, that the lack of a sustainable income is a significant reason why, on average, survivors return to abusive relationships 5–7 times (Adair, 2003; Brush, 2003; Harris, 2003).

Childhood Exposure

Between 7 and 14 million children and youth are exposed to adult domestic violence each year (Edleson et al., 2007). In addition to witnessing the violence between their parents or a parent and partner, it is estimated that child abuse occurs in 30% to 60% of domestic violence cases (Appel & Holden, 1998; McKibben, DeVos, & Newberger, 1998). Children who grow up in a domestic violence household often have low self-esteem, psychosomatic complaints, nightmares, impaired social skills, and poor academic performance. As a result, they may be aggressive, withdrawn, anxious, depressed, and even suicidal (Israel & Stover, 2009; OVC, 2002). In families where there is domestic violence, young boys may model their father's behavior, while girls may model their mother's behavior and show more signs of withdrawal and isolation (Cummings, Peplar, & Moore, 1999; Holt, Buckley, &Whelan, 2008; Huth-Beck, Levendosky, & Semel, 2001; Stiles, 2002).

Some children may have difficulty expressing their feelings and stress and may exhibit aggressive behaviors as a way to try to communicate with their mother. Studies of children exposed to domestic violence indicate that they also may have difficulty with self-calming, sleeping, and eating activities; may demonstrate developmental delays or maladaptive behaviors; and may have poor verbal and social skills that negatively affect their academic performance. They may have higher rates of somatic complaints and interpersonal problems (Cummings et al., 1999; Huth-Beck et al., 2001; Norwood, Swank, Stephens, Ware, & Buzy, 2001; Sternberg et al., 1993; Stiles, 2002).

Types of Violence

Abuse in domestic violence comes in many forms; it may be physical, psychological, sexual, or economic. *Physical violence* may include such behaviors as hitting, slapping, punching, or stabbing. *Psychological violence* may take the form of verbal abuse, harassment, possessiveness, destruction of personal property, cruelty to pets, and isolation (OVC, 2002; USDOJ, n.d.). The abuser often isolates the victim from family and friends, thus limiting access to support systems. *Sexual abuse* can occur between two intimate partners when the abuser forces or coerces the victim into a sexual act. Survivors also may experience *economic abuse* in which the abuser controls the finances, leaving the victim with no money or a limited allowance.

Challenges With Occupation or Activities

Research indicates that women who are survivors of domestic violence may struggle when performing several of their daily life occupations or activities, particularly work performance, educational participation, home management, parenting, and leisure participation (Gorde, Helfrich, & Finlayson, 2004; Helfrich & Rivera, 2006; Javaherian, Krabacher, Andriacco, & German, 2007). They may experience problems with money management, task initiation, self-confidence, coping skills, stress management, and interpersonal relationships (Carlson, 1997; D'Ardenne & Balakrishna, 2001; Helfrich, Aviles, Badiani, Walens, & Sabol, 2006; Levendosky & Graham-Bermann, 2001; Monahan & O'Leary, 1999). They may have difficulty with higher level mental functions, including decision making, judgment, problem solving, and direction following.

Survivors of domestic violence often face challenges sustaining employment (Josephson, 2005; Riger & Staggs, 2004; Tolman & Raphael, 2000). One common reason is that abuse, including stalking and excessive phone calls or other forms of contact, often happens at the workplace (Corporate Alliance to End Partner Violence, 2002–2008). Survivors' inconsistent work histories can cause difficulties with finding a job once they have left the abusive relationship.

In addition, leaving an abusive relationship and becoming a single parent can increase the risk of being unemployed or among the working poor in the United States. The jobless rate for unmarried mothers is almost 3 times that of married mothers, 8.5% as compared to 3.1% (U.S. Department of Labor, 2010).

Occupational Therapy and Domestic Violence

In its broadest sense, the domain of occupational therapy is the facilitation of people's ability to engage in meaningful, daily life activities, or occupations in a manner that supports their full participation in various contexts and positively affects health, well-being, and life satisfaction (AOTA, 2008). Occupational therapists and occupational therapy assistants view occupations as central to a person's identity and competence, influencing how a person spends time and makes decisions (AOTA, 2008). Domestic violence negatively affects the ability of the survivors and their families to engage in their daily life occupations in a competent, healthy, and satisfying manner. Consequently, in the spirit of social and occupational justice, occupational therapy practitioners[1] focus on developing or restoring these abilities. Specifically, occupational therapy practitioners focus on enhancing the ability of the survivors and their families to participate in activities of daily living (ADLs), instrumental activities of daily living (IADLs), rest and sleep, education, work, leisure, play, and social participation for the purpose of gaining skills and abilities needed to take control of their lives, find purpose, and develop a healthy independent lifestyle.

Occupational therapy practitioners work directly and indirectly with survivors of domestic violence and their families in a variety of settings such as hospitals, rehabilitation centers, skilled nursing facilities, outpatient therapy clinics, mental health facilities, school systems, shelters, home health care, and other community programs. Occupational therapy practitioners may work with survivors and family members who have

- Sustained injuries or disabilities as a result of domestic violence,

- Chosen to remain in and rebuild a relationship in which abuse has occurred, or

- Decided to leave the abusive relationship and reconstruct their lives.

In the course of their practice, occupational therapy practitioners also may work with individuals whom they suspect or discover are victims or survivors of domestic violence but who have not reported the domestic violence. In such cases, occupational therapy practitioners have a professional and ethical responsibility to take action that promotes the health and safety of these individuals. As health care professionals, occupational therapy practitioners are mandated to report suspected child abuse. Some states also mandate that they report suspected abuse in adults, particularly in older adults or adults who have intellectual disabilities.

Occupational therapy practitioners need to consult their state regulations and facility guidelines regarding procedures to follow when they suspect or know that domestic violence has occurred. Actions that practitioners may take include

---

[1]When the term *occupational therapy practitioner* is used in this document, it refers to both occupational therapists and occupational therapy assistants (AOTA, 2006). *Occupational therapists* are responsible for all aspects of occupational therapy service delivery and are accountable for the safety and effectiveness of the occupational therapy service delivery process. *Occupational therapy assistants* deliver occupational therapy services under the supervision of and in partnership with an occupational therapist (AOTA, 2009).

- Filing a report to the local law enforcement agency or children's protective services;

- Interviewing, evaluating, and providing interventions without the abuser present to allow the client the opportunity to discuss the situation in relative safety;

- Identifying and assessing injuries and their potential cause;

- Talking to the client about healthy relationships and addressing areas of occupation and performance patterns and skills that may have been affected by the abusive relationship, such as leisure, IADLs, work, and ADLs;

- Respecting the client's perception of the relative danger of the situation to his or her life and the well-being of other family members and remaining empathetic and nonjudgmental about the client's decision to remain in or leave the abusive situation;

- Providing the client with contact information for the local domestic violence hotline; and

- Following safety precautions to determine if it is appropriate to conduct home visits.

Occupational Therapy Evaluation and Intervention

The occupational therapy service delivery process occurs in collaboration with the survivors of domestic violence, their family members, and other service providers. Throughout the occupational therapy evaluation, intervention, and assessment of outcomes, occupational therapy practitioners value and consider the desires, choices, needs, personal and spiritual values, and sociocultural backgrounds of the survivors and their family members. Practitioners also consider the service delivery context. Important outcomes of occupational therapy service provision include, but are not limited to, facilitating the ability of the survivors and their family members to consistently engage in and perform their daily activities, achieving personal satisfaction and role competence, developing healthy performance patterns, and improving their quality of life.

The occupational therapy evaluation is focused on determining what the survivors and their family members want and need to do and identifying the factors that act as supports or barriers to performance of the desired occupations (AOTA, 2008). Occupational performance; routines, roles, and habits; activity demands; sociocultural beliefs/expectations; spirituality; and physical, cognitive, and psychosocial factors are addressed during the evaluation process. Evaluations and assessments that are client-centered and occupation-based are effective for this population.

Occupational therapy service delivery is based on findings from the evaluation and the survivors' and the family members' stated priorities. Interventions with adults who are survivors of domestic violence focus on empowerment and active participation in healthy occupations or daily life activities. Findings from several studies of survivors have indicated that during the early period after leaving the abusive situation, survivors continue to devote themselves to the care of others, especially their children, while often not taking care of themselves (Giles & Curreen, 2007; Underwood, 2009; Wuest & Merritt-Gray, 1999).

Occupational therapy interventions with adult women survivors may include working on the development of a realistic budget; facilitating the use of effective decision-making skills regarding employment opportunities; learning parenting skills and calming techniques to use with their children; encouraging and supporting efforts to attain further education; learning assertiveness skills; and teaching stress management and relaxation techniques to improve sleep patterns (Gorde et al., 2004; Helfrich et al., 2006; Helfrich & Rivera, 2006; Javahcrian et al., 2010). Therapy sessions focused on performance patterns may be helpful, because findings from several studies have indicated that survivors are constantly juggling family, work, and possibly school responsibilities without a significant other to assist them with their obligations (Butler & Deprez, 2002; Jones-DeWeever & Gault, 2006; Underwood, 2009).

Interventions with children who have witnessed domestic violence may include facilitation of developmentally appropriate play skills, social skills training, the use of techniques for improving concentration and attention span during school activities, and assistance with the organization of study habits and school materials. Adolescents may benefit from interventions addressing relationship skills, life skills, stress management, and coping strategies (Javaherian-Dysinger et al., 2011).

Occupational therapy practitioners focus on outcomes throughout the occupational therapy service delivery process. Assessing outcome results assists occupational therapy practitioners with making decisions about future directions of interventions at the individual as well as at the organizational or population level (AOTA, 2008). At the individual level, the selection of outcomes is based on the survivors' priorities and may be modified based on changing needs, contexts, and performance abilities (AOTA, 2008). For example, an occupational therapy practitioner may work with a woman who is a survivor of domestic violence on her goal of obtaining housing. After the woman moves into the new living situation, the practitioner may help the woman work on her goal of maintaining a healthy home environment for herself and her children.

At the organizational or population level, data about targeted outcomes can be aggregated and reported to boards of directors of community agencies, state and federal regulators, and funding agencies. An example of this type of outcome assessment would be the reporting of the number of children who demonstrated difficulty participating in their daily life activities at home, at school, and in their communities because of exposure to domestic violence and the progress they have made during the occupational therapy intervention to increase their level of healthy participation.

Occupational therapy practitioners also may work with the abusers in collaboration with other professionals such as psychologists, social workers, and pastoral counselors. Sometimes the judicial system issues a court order for the abuser to participate in a formal program to address the violent behaviors. These programs are generally based on six principles: (1) the abuser is responsible for the behavior; (2) provocation does not justify violence; (3) violent behavior is a choice; (4) there are nonviolent alternatives; (5) violence is a learned behavior; and (6) domestic violence affects the entire family, whether it is directly or indirectly witnessed (OVC, 2002). Occupational therapy interventions with the abuser may include training in social skills, assertiveness, anger management, stress management, parenting, and spiritual exploration as related to daily occupations.

Education, Training, and Competencies

Occupational therapists and occupational therapy assistants are educationally prepared to address the various occupation-related concerns of survivors of domestic violence. The Accreditation Council for Occupational Therapy Education (ACOTE) standards for educational programs require content related to daily life occupations, human development, human behavior, sociocultural issues, diversity factors, medical conditions, theory, models of practice, evaluation, and techniques for the development and implementation of intervention plans under the scope of occupational therapy (ACOTE, 2010). Occupational therapy practitioners are competent to address life skills, lifestyle management, adaptive coping strategies, adaptation, time management, and values clarification that affect the ability of survivors of domestic violence to participate in their ADLs, IADLs, education, work, play, leisure, and social participation activities. In addition, occupational therapy practitioners have the expertise to work with individuals, organizations, and populations.

Occupational therapists and occupational therapy assistants who are supervised by an occupational therapist are competent in the following areas:

- Establishing and maintaining therapeutic relationships;

- Conducting interviews;

- Administering functional assessments to determine occupational performance needs and to develop an intervention plan;

- Utilizing interpersonal communication skills;

- Designing and facilitating therapeutic groups;

- Developing individualized teaching and learning processes with clients, family, and significant others;

- Coordinating program interventions in collaboration with clients, caregivers, families, and communities grounded in evidence-based practice;

- Developing therapeutic programs;

- Promoting health and wellness through engagement in meaningful occupations; and

- Understanding the effects of health, disability, and social conditions on the individual within the context of family and society (ACOTE, 2010).

Participating in continuing education initiatives advances occupational therapy practitioners' understanding of and capacity to provide interventions that address domestic violence.

Supervision of Other Personnel

When provided as part of an occupational therapy program, the occupational therapist is responsible for all aspects of the service delivery and is accountable for the safety and effectiveness of the service delivery process. The occupational therapy assistant delivers occupational therapy services under the supervision of and in partnership with the occupational therapist (AOTA, 2009). The education and knowledge of occupational therapy practitioners also prepare them for employment in arenas other than those related to traditional delivery of occupational therapy. In these circumstances, the occupational therapy practitioner should determine whether the services they provide are related to the delivery of occupational therapy by referring to their state practice acts, regulatory agency standards and rules, domain of occupational therapy practice, and written or verbal agreement with the agency or payer about the services provided (AOTA, 2009). Occupational therapy practitioners should obtain and use credentials and a job title commensurate with their roles in the specific arena. In such arenas, non–occupational therapy professionals may provide the supervision of occupational therapy assistants.

Case Studies

The following case studies provide examples of the role of occupational therapy in domestic violence.

Adult Case Study: Maria

An occupational therapist working in a shelter for survivors of domestic violence was asked to assess Maria, a 28-year-old mother of two children.

Evaluation

Using the Canadian Occupational Performance Measure (Law et al., 2005), Maria identifies the occupational performance areas are the most important to her. She would like to feel competent in her ability to take care of a house, parent her children, and keep them safe. She also wants to work with the occupational therapist on finding and maintaining a job, budgeting, and completing her GED. Maria rates her performance as 1—*unable to do it* and her satisfaction levels as 1—*not satisfied at all* for these performance areas.

When budgeting is discussed, Maria states that she had never been responsible for money management. She went straight from her parent's home into her marriage at age 17, and her husband would not allow her to have anything to do with the money. He constantly told her that she was "too stupid" to take care of money. She was not allowed to work outside the home, so she was dependent on her husband for money.

Intervention

The occupational therapist helps Maria procure and complete job applications and practice job interviewing skills. After Maria finds a steady job, she and her children move into the shelter's transitional living program. To stay in this program, Maria needs to put a certain amount of money into a savings account on a monthly basis to secure a home for her and her children. Following her first paycheck, the occupational therapist meets with Maria to project a budget for her expenses and savings. Maria asks the occupational therapist to develop her budget for her because she "isn't smart enough to do it herself." She states that math was her worst subject in school. The occupational therapist grades the complexity of the task to enable Maria to develop problem-solving skills and reasoning abilities for budgeting.

The occupational therapist then models for Maria how to contact community agencies to obtain information about GED programs. They determine a daily schedule and identify support networks so that Maria can work, complete her studies, and care for her children.

Older Adult Case Study: Mr. Lee

An occupational therapist in an outpatient clinic receives a referral to provide occupational therapy services to Mr. Lee, a 72-year-old man with a right distal radius fracture and a boxer's fracture. Mr. Lee has chronic obstructive pulmonary disease (COPD) and uses a wheelchair for mobility. He has been living with his current partner for the past 10 years.

Evaluation

During the evaluation the occupational therapist asks Mr. Lee to explain how the injury occurred. He is vague in his responses and simply states that he became weak and fell out of his wheelchair. Over the next few sessions, while providing interventions to address Mr. Lee's hand injuries and COPD, the occupational therapist notices additional bruises on his arms and suspects that he is involved in an abusive relationship.

Intervention

Because the occupational therapist lives in a state that mandates reporting of abuse in adults, she files a report to the appropriate law enforcement agency. She lets Mr. Lee know that law requires such action. The therapist then initiates conversation about domestic violence. Research (Bacchus, 2003; McCauley, 1998) has shown that victims of domestic violence want their health care provider to ask them about domestic violence, thereby creating a venue for them to open up as they feel able.

While continuing to provide interventions related to hand function and energy management, the occupational therapist also reassesses Mr. Lee's areas of occupation, performance skills, and performance patterns to identify additional home and community supports he may need because of the domestic violence. She provides Mr. Lee with resources on domestic violence and the local crisis center's contact information. She includes interventions to focus on building self-esteem and empowerment.

Adolescent Case Study: Heang

Heang is a 16-year-old girl in 10th grade. For the past 2 months she has dated a popular young man who is in the 11th grade. Heang initially thought that his frequent phone calls and text messages throughout the day were very romantic. He started telling her that he did not want her to go out with her friends and got into several fights with Heang's male classmates. After dating for about 1 month, he began to slap and punch her. The next day he would bring her flowers. Rather than tell anyone, Heang withdrew from her friends and after-school activities; she did not socialize with other boys at school or work.

A representative from the local women's shelter spoke to Heang's 10th-grade class about teen dating violence. Realizing that she was a victim of this violence, Heang spoke to her guidance counselor. The counselor referred her to a teen dating violence group run by the school occupational therapist.

Evaluation

The occupational therapist conducts an initial evaluation to assess Heang's occupational needs, problems, and concerns. The therapist analyzes Heang's occupational performance skills, performance patterns, context, and activity demands (AOTA, 2008). After reviewing the results of the evaluation, the therapist develops collaborative goals with Heang related to her school and after-school activities, social participation, leisure activities, and job.

Intervention

Using a cognitive–behavioral approach, the occupational therapist helps Heang explore the impact that the dating violence has had on her school and work performance, social participation, and sense of identity. She encourages Heang to identify the importance of social participation in the development of self-esteem, friendships, health, and identity. Together they develop a plan for Heang to participate again in familiar leisure occupations as well as in new ones.

Infant Case Study: Jonella and Kia

Jonella brought her 4-month-old daughter Kia to an occupational therapist as part of an early intervention service for infants and toddlers. Jonella tells the occupational therapist that she is concerned about Kia, who sleeps only 30 minutes at a time and consistently wakes up screaming. Jonella explains that she and Kia have just left an abusive relationship and now live with friends. Since infancy, Kia has been awakened many times because of the shouting and physical violence. In addition, Jonella could not establish a daily nap and sleep routine for Kia because she frequently had to rush Kia out of the house to keep her safe.

Evaluation

The occupational therapist administers the Test of Sensory Functions in Infants (DeGangi & Greenspan, 1989) and the Transdisciplinary Play-Based Assessment (Linder, 2008) to Kia to assess for sensory issues focusing on self-regulation and for potential developmental complications.

Intervention

The occupational therapist and Jonella collaborate to identify strategies for establishing a consistent nap and sleep routine for Kia. The occupational therapist models strategies that Jonella can use to help calm Kia and modulate the amount of sensory input she receives. They also identify strategies for modifying the environment in the room where Kia sleeps and for helping Jonella relax with Kia before putting her to bed.

Child Case Study: Daniel

A school system occupational therapist is asked to assess Daniel, a 5-year-old student who has an individual education program (IEP), to address learning challenges. His teacher states that Daniel is having extreme problems with manipulating crayons and performing gross motor activities. The teacher informs the therapist that his mother has just left an abusive situation. His mother has stated that Daniel's father would not let her place Daniel in a preschool or in a Mother's Morning Out program. She was not allowed to take Daniel outside to play. In addition, when his father was home, Daniel was expected to sit quietly and not play with toys. In spite of these restrictions, Daniel's mother did her best to expose her son to books and songs and teach him ways to play with household materials.

Evaluation

The occupational therapist performs the Quick Neurological Screening Test II (QNST–II; Mutti, Sterling, Spalding, & Spalding, 1998) and sends the Sensory Profile (Dunn, 1999) home with Daniel for his mother to complete. Daniel scores within the "Definite Difference" range on the following factors on the Sensory Profile: Emotionally Reactive, Oral Sensory Sensitivity, Inattention/Distractibility, Auditory Processing, Vestibular Processing, and Multisensory Processing. As measured by the QNST–II, Daniel also has difficulty with gross motor skills, balance, tactile processing, visual tracking, motor planning, impulsivity, and anxiety.

Intervention

The occupational therapist observes Daniel in the classroom and makes recommendations for strategies that the teacher can use to decrease Daniel's distractibility and to increase his attention and participation at school. The occupational therapy assistant works with Daniel for 45 minutes twice a week, with time divided between intervention in the classroom to address cutting and drawing activities and outside the classroom to increase motor control, sensory awareness, and problem-solving skills.

Family Case Study: Herminie's Family

An occupational therapist is part of a treatment team for individuals who have diabetes. The physician wants the therapist to assess and provide services to Herminie, a 34-year-old woman who is not routinely checking her glucose levels or taking her insulin. Because Herminie speaks limited English, her sister accompanies her to the session and translates for her.

Evaluation

During the interview, Herminie shares that her 13-year-old daughter has taken on the responsibility for prompting Herminie to perform the techniques necessary to keep the diabetes under control. The 13-year-old daughter also takes care of her 7-year-old brother while Herminie works. Herminie left home with her children a year ago because her husband was physically and emotionally abusive to her. According to Herminie's sister, as a result of witnessing the abuse, the daughter is continually afraid that something is going to happen to her mother and brother. She is afraid to leave the house, except to go to school, and does not socialize with friends.

Intervention

With the aid of Herminie's sister, who provides verbal and written translation, the occupational therapist develops a daily checklist that Herminie can use to prompt herself to independently check her glucose levels and take her insulin. She discusses with Herminie how important it is for her, rather than her daughter, to be responsible for managing her diabetes. The occupational therapist meets with Herminie and her daughter weekly for several weeks to reinforce and monitor the progress that Herminie is making and to assist the daughter with reducing her anxiety. With Herminie's and her daughter's permission, the therapist called the daughter's school guidance counselor to discuss the situation and request help with decreasing the daughter's anxiety while facilitating increased socialization. In addition, the occupational therapist recommends that Herminie participate in a domestic violence counseling program.

References

Accreditation Council for Occupational Therapy Education. (2010). *ACOTE standards and interpretive guidelines.* Available online at http://www.aota.org/Educate/Accredit/StandardsReview/guide/42369.aspx?FT=.pdf

Adair, V. (2003). Fulfilling the promise of higher education. In V. Adair & S. Dahlberg (Eds.), *Reclaiming class: Women, poverty, and the promise of higher education in America* (pp. 240–265). Philadelphia: Temple University.

American Occupational Therapy Association. (2006). Policy 1.44: Categories of occupational therapy personnel. In *Policy manual* (2009 ed.). Bethesda, MD: Author.

American Occupational Therapy Association. (2008). Occupational therapy practice framework: Domain and process (2nd ed.). *American Journal of Occupational Therapy, 62*(6), 625–683.

American Occupational Therapy Association. (2009). Guidelines for supervision, roles, and responsibilities during the delivery of occupational therapy services. *American Journal of Occupational Therapy, 63*(6), 796–803.

Appel, A., & Holden, G. (1998). The co-occurrence of spouse and physical child abuse: A review and appraisal. *Journal of Family Psychology, 12*, 578–599.

Bacchus, L. (2003). Experiences of seeking help from health professionals in a sample of women who experienced domestic violence. *Health and Social Care in the Community, 11*, 10–18.

Bograd, M. (2005). Strengthening domestic violence theories: Intersections of race, class, sexual orientation, and gender. In N. J. Sokoloff (Ed.), *Domestic violence at the margins: Readings on race, class, gender, and culture* (pp. 25–38). New Brunswick, NJ: Rutgers University.

Browne, A., & Bassuk, S. (1997). Intimate violence in the lives of homeless and poor housed women: Prevalence and patterns in an ethnically diverse sample. *American Journal of Orthopsychiatry, 6*(2), 261–278.

Brownridge, D. A. (2006). Partner violence against women with disabilities: Prevalence, risk, and explanations. *Violence Against Women, 12*, 805–822. doi:10.1177/1077801206292681

Brush, L. (2003). "That's why I'm on Prozac": Battered women, traumatic stress, and education in the context of welfare reform. In V. Adair & S. Dahlberg (Eds.), *Reclaiming class: Women, poverty, and the promise of higher education in America* (pp. 215–239). Philadelphia: Temple University.

Butler, S., & Deprez, L. (2002). Something worth fighting for: Higher education for women on welfare. *Afflia, 17*(1), 30–54.

Carlson, B. (1997). A stress and coping approach to intervention with abused women. *Family Relations, 46*, 291–298.

Centers for Disease Control and Prevention. (2010). *Intimate partner violence: Consequences.* Retrieved from http://www.cdc.gov/violenceprevention/intimatepartnerviolence/consequences.html.

Corporate Alliance to End Partner Violence. (2002–2008). *Workplace statistics.* Available online at http://www.caepv.org/getinfo/facts_stats.php?

Cummings, J., Peplar, D., & Moore, T. (1999). Behavior problems in children exposed to wife abuse: Gender differences. *Journal of Family Violence, 14*, 133–156.

D'Ardenne, P., & Balakrishna, J. (2001). Domestic violence and intimacy: What the relationship therapist needs to know. *Sexual and Relationship Therapy, 16*, 229–246.

Davies, J. (2008). *Building comprehensive solutions to domestic violence Publication 20: Policy blueprint on domestic violence and poverty: When battered women stay: Advocacy beyond leaving.* Retrieved February 24, 2011, from National Resource Center on Domestic Violence at http://new.vawnet.org/Assoc_Files_VAWnet/BCS20_Staying.pdf

DeGangi, G. A., & Greenspan, S. I. (1989). *Test of Sensory Function in Infants: Manual.* Los Angeles: Western Psychological Services.

Dunn, W. (1999). *Sensory Profile: User's manual.* San Antonio, TX: Psychological Corporation.

Economic Stability Working Group of the Transition Subcommittee of the Governors' Commission on Domestic Violence. (2002, October). *Voices of survival: The economic impacts of domestic violence, A blueprint for action.* Available online at http://www.harborcov.org/pages/publications/voices_of_survival.pdf

Edleson, J. L., Ellerton, A. L., Seagren, E. A., Kirchberg, S. L., Schmidt, S. O., & Ambrose, A. T. (2007). Assessing child exposure to adult domestic violence. *Children and Youth Services Review, 29*(7), 961–971. doi:10.1016/j.childyouth.2006.12.009

Fisher, J., & Shelton, A. (2006). Survivors of domestic violence: Demographics and disparities in visitors to an interdisciplinary specialty clinic. *Community Health, 29*, 118–130.

Giles, J., & Curreen, H. (2007). Phases of growth for abused New Zealand women: A Comparison with other studies. *Afflia, 22*(4), 371–384.

Gorde, M. W., Helfrich, C. A., & Finlayson, M. L. (2004). Trauma symptoms and life skills needs of domestic violence victims. *Journal of Interpersonal Violence, 19*, 691–708.

Harris, A. (2003). Choosing the lesser evil: The violence of the welfare stereotype. In V. Adair & S. Dahlberg (Eds.), *Reclaiming class: Women, poverty, and the promise of higher education* (pp. 131–138). Philadelphia: Temple University.

Helfrich, C. A., Aviles, A. M., Badiani, C., Walens, D., & Sabol, P. (2006). Life skill interventions with homeless youth, domestic violence victims, and adults with mental illness. *Occupational Therapy in Health Care, 20*(3/4), 189–207.

Helfrich, C. A., Lafata, M. J., MacDonald, S. L., Aviles, A., & Collins, L. (2001). Domestic abuse across the lifespan: Definitions, identification, and risk factors for occupational therapists. In C. A. Helfrich (Ed.), *Domestic violence across the lifespan. The role of occupational therapy* (pp. 5–34). Binghamton, NY: Haworth Press.

Helfrich, C. A., & Rivera, Y. (2006). Employment skills and domestic violence survivors: A shelter-based intervention. *Occupational Therapy in Mental Health, 22*(1), 33–48. doi:10.1300/J004v22n01_03

Holt, S., Buckley, H., & Whelan, S. (2008). The impact of exposure to domestic violence on children and young people: A review of the literature. *Child Abuse and Neglect, 32*(8), 797–810. doi:10.1016/j.chiabu.2008.02.004

Huth-Beck, A., Levendosky, A., & Semel, M. (2001). The direct and indirect effects of domestic violence on young children's intellectual functioning. *Journal of Family Violence, 16*, 269–290.

Israel, E., & Stover, C. (2009). Intimate partner violence: The role of the relationship between perpetrators and children who witness violence. *Journal of Interpersonal Violence, 24*(10), 1755–1764. doi:10.1177/0886260509334044

Jacobson, C. J., Pabst, S., Regan, S., & Fisher, B. (2006). A lifetime of intimate partner violence: Coping strategies of older women. *Journal of Interpersonal Violence, 21*(5), 634–651. doi:10.1177/0886260506286878

Javaherian, H., DeBrun, J., Moesser, A., Murphy, R., Salvati, B., & Shaffer, T. (2010). *The Mothering experiences of survivors of domestic violence: An in-depth analysis.* Loma Linda, CA: Loma Linda University, Department of Occupational Therapy.

Javaherian, H., Krabacher, V., Andriacco, K., & German, D. (2007). Surviving domestic violence: Rebuilding one's life. *Occupational Therapy in Health Care, 21*(3), 35–59.

Javaherian-Dysinger, H., Cameron, K., Harding, K., Hedgecock, A., Lopez, A., & Unterseher, R. (2011). *Occupational experiences of youth exposed to domestic violence.* Loma Linda, CA: Loma Linda University, Department of Occupational Therapy.

Jewkes, R. (2005). Domestic violence has many causes. In H. Cothran (Series Ed.) & D. Haugen (Vol. Ed.), *Opposing Viewpoints Series: Domestic violence* (pp. 104–114). Farmington Hills, MI: Thomson Gale.

Jones-DeWeever, A. A., & Gault, B. (2006). *Resilient and reaching for more: Challenges and benefits of higher education for welfare participants and their children.* Available online from Institute for Women's Policy Research at www.iwpr.org/publications

Josephson, J. (2005). The intersectionality of domestic violence and welfare in the lives of poor women. In N. Sokoloff (Ed.), *Domestic violence at the margins: Readings on race, class, gender, and culture* (pp. 83–100). New Brunswick, NJ: Rutgers University.

Law, M., Baptiste, S., Carswell, A., McColl, M. A., Polatajko, H., & Pollock, N. (2005). *Canadian Occupational Performance Measure.* Ottawa, ON: CAOT Publications ACE.

Levendosky, A., & Graham-Bermann, S. (2001). Parenting in battered women: The effects of domestic violence on women and their children. *Journal of Family Violence, 16*, 171–192.

Linder, T. (2008). *Transdisciplinary Play-Based Assessment* (2nd ed.). Baltimore: Paul H. Brookes.

Lyon, E. (2000, October). *Welfare, poverty, and abused women: New research and its implications* (Pub. No. 10). Available online at http://new.vawnet.org?Assoc_Files_VAWnet?BCS10_POV.pdf

Lyon, E. (2002, August). *Welfare and domestic violence against women: Lessons from research.* Retrieved February 24, 2010, from National Resource Center on Violence Against Women at http://new.vawnet.org/category/Main_Doc.php?docid=317

McCauley, J. (1998). Abused women's experiences with clinicians and health services. *Journal of General Internal Medicine, 13*, 549–555.

McKibben, L., DeVos, E., & Newberger, E. (1998). Victimization of mothers of abused children: A controlled study. *Pediatrics, 84*, 531–535.

Milberger, S., LeRoy, B., Martin, A., Israel, N., Potter, L., & Patchak-Schuster, P. (2002). *Michigan study on women with physical disabilities* (Final Report, National Institute of Justice Grant 2000-WT-VX-0018). Available online at http://www.ncjrs.gov/pdffiles1/nij/grants/193769.pdf

Monahan, K., & O'Leary, K. D. (1999). Health injury and battered women: An initial inquiry. *Health and Social Work, 24*, 269–279.

Mutti, M., Sterling, H., Spalding, M., & Spalding, N. (1998). *Quick Neurological Screening Test II (QNST–II)*. Los Angeles: Western Psychological Assessment.

National Coalition Against Domestic Violence. (2007). *Domestic violence facts.* Available online at http://www.ncadv.org/files/DomesticViolenceFactSheet(National).pdf

National Coalition Against Domestic Violence. (n.d.). *The problem: What is battering?* Available online at http://www.ncadv.org/learn/TheProblem.php

National Coalition of Anti-Violence Programs. (1998). *Annual report on lesbian, gay, bisexual, transgender domestic violence.* Available online at http://www.mincava.umn.edu/documents/glbtdv/glbtdv.html

National Institute of Justice. (2000). *Extent, nature, and consequences of intimate partner violence.* Washington, DC: U.S. Department of Justice.

National Institute of Justice. (2007). *Intimate partner violence.* Available online at http://www.ojp.usdoj.gov/nij/topics/crime/intimate-partner-violence/welcome.htm

Norwood, W., Swank, P., Stephens, N., Ware, H., & Buzy, W. (2001). Reducing conduct problems among children of battered women. *Journal of Counseling and Clinical Psychology, 69*, 774–785.

Nosek, M., Hughes, R. B., Taylor, H., & Taylor, P. (2006). Disability, psychosocial, and demographic characteristics of abused women with physical disabilities. *Violence Against Women, 129*, 823–837. doi:10.1177/1077801206292671

Office for Victims of Crime. (2002). *National Victim Assistance Academy: Foundations in victimology and victims' rights and services* (Ch. 9. Domestic Violence). Retrieved February 25, 2011, from http://www.valor-national.org/ovc/chapter9.html.

Rand, M., & Harrell, E. (2009, October). *National Crimes Victimization Survey: Crime against people with disabilities, 2007.* Available online at http://bjs.ojp.usdoj.gov/content/pub/pdf/capd07.pdf

Rank, M. (2004). *One nation underprivileged: Why American poverty affects us all.* New York: Oxford University.

Rice, J. (2001). Poverty, welfare, and patriarchy: How macro-level changes in social policy can help low income women. *Journal of Social Issues, 57*(2), 355–374.

Riger, S., & Staggs, S. (2004). Welfare reform, domestic violence, and employment: What do we know and what do we need to know? *Violence Against Women, 10*, 961–990.

Sokoloff, N., & Dupont, I. (2005). Domestic violence: Examining the intersections of race, class, and gender—An introduction. In N. Sokoloff (Ed.), *Domestic violence at the margins: Readings on race, class, gender, and culture* (pp. 1–13). Piscataway, NJ: Rutgers University.

Sternberg, K., Lamb, M., Greenbaum, C., Cicchetti, D., Dawud, S., Cortes, R., et al. (1993). Effects of domestic violence on children's behavior problems and depression. *Developmental Psychology, 29*, 44–52.

Stiles, M. (2002). Witnessing domestic violence: The effect on children. *American Family Physician, 66*, 2052–2058.

Tjaden, P., & Thoennes, N. (2000a, July). *Extent, nature and consequences of intimate partner violence: Findings from the National Violence Against Women Survey* (NCJ 181867). Available online at http://www.ncjrs.gov/pdffiles1/nij/181867.pdf

Tjaden, P., & Thoennes, N. (2000b, November). *Full report of the Prevalence, Incidence, and Consequences of Violence Against Women: Findings From the National Violence Against Women Survey* (NCJ 183781). Available online at http://www.ojp.usdoj.gov/nij/pubs-sum/183781.htm

Tolman, R. M., & Raphael, J. (2000). A review of research on welfare and domestic violence. *Journal of Social Issues, 56,* 644–682.

Underwood, R. (2009). *Care of self: Construction of subjectivities of low-income, female survivors of domestic violence as they pursue postsecondary education.* Unpublished doctoral dissertation, University of Georgia, Athens.

U.S. Department of Justice, Office of Justice Programs, Bureau of Justice Statistics. (2007, December 19). *Intimate partner violence in the U.S.* Available online at http://www.ojp.usdoj.gov/nij/topics/crime/intimate-partner-violence/welcome.htm

U.S. Department of Justice, Office of Justice Programs, Bureau of Justice Statistics. (2011). *Intimate partner violence.* Retrieved from http://bjs.ojp.usdoj.gov/index.cfm?ty=tp&tid=971#summary.

U.S. Department of Justice. (n.d.). *About domestic violence.* Available online at http://www.ovw.usdoj.gov/domviolence.htm

U.S. Department of Labor. (2010). *Employment characteristics of families summary.* Retrieved February 25, 2011, from http://www.bls.gov/news.release/famee.nr0.htm

Waldner, L. (2003). If you want me to pull myself up, give me bootstraps. In V. Adair & S. Dahlberg (Eds.), *Reclaiming class: Women, poverty, and promise of higher education in America* (pp. 97–110). Philadelphia: Temple University.

Wuest, J., & Merritt-Gray, M. (1999). Not going back: Sustaining the separation in the process of leaving abusive relationships. *Violence Against Women, 5*(2), 110–134.

Zink, T., Regan, S., Jacobson, C. J., & Pabst, S. (2003). Cohort, period, and aging effects: A qualitative study of older women's reasons for remaining in abusive relationships. *Violence Against Women, 9*(12), 1429–1441. doi:10.1177/1077801203259231

Authors

Heather Javaherian-Dysinger, OTD, OTR/L
Robin Underwood, PhD, OTR/L

for

The Commission on Practice
Janet V. DeLany, DEd, MSA, OTR/L, FAOTA, *Chairperson*

Adopted by the Representative Assembly Coordinating Council (RACC) for the Representative Assembly
Revised by the Commission on Practice 2011

Note. This revision replaces the 2006 document *Occupational Therapy Services for Individuals Who Have Experienced Domestic Violence,* previously published and copyrighted in 2007 by the American Occupational Therapy Association in the *American Journal of Occupational Therapy, 61,* 704–709.

Occupational Therapy Services in Early Childhood and School-Based Settings

The primary purpose of this document is to describe how occupational therapy supports children's and youth's learning and development in early childhood and school-based settings. This document is intended for occupational therapists and occupational therapy assistants in practice, academia, research, advocacy, and administrative positions. Other audiences for this statement include regulatory and policymaking bodies, provider groups, accreditation agencies, other professionals, and the general public who may be seeking clarification about occupational therapy's scope of practice and domain of concern related to this topic. The American Occupational Therapy Association (AOTA) provides information and resources to support occupational therapists and occupational therapy assistants in the delivery of effective services for children and youth in a variety of settings, including school-based and early intervention programs, child care, Head Start and Early Head Start, preschool and pre-kindergarten programs, and at home.

Occupational therapists and occupational therapy assistants[1] work with children and youth, parents, caregivers, educators, and other team members to facilitate children's and youth's ability to participate in everyday activities, or *occupations*. Occupations are "activities…of everyday life, named, organized, and given value and meaning by individuals and a culture" (Law, Polatajko, Baptiste, & Townsend, 1997, p. 34). Occupations are meaningful for the child and are based on social or cultural expectations or peer performance. In early childhood (birth–8 years of age) and school-based settings, occupational therapy practitioners[2] use their unique expertise to help children and youth with and without challenges prepare for and perform important learning and developmental activities within their natural environment. Occupational therapy services support a child's participation in activities of daily living (ADLs), instrumental activities of daily living (IADLs), education, work, play, leisure, rest and sleep, and social participation.

Occupational therapists have knowledge and skills in the biological, physical, social, and behavioral sciences to evaluate and intervene with individuals across the life course. Occupational therapy practitioners apply evidence-based research ethically and appropriately to the evaluation and intervention process following professional *Standards of Practice* (AOTA, 2010b) and the *Occupational Therapy Code of Ethics and Ethics Standards* (AOTA, 2010a).

Legislative Influences on Service Delivery

Occupational therapy practice in schools and early childhood settings is affected by many federal and state laws and regulations, as well as local policies and procedures. Table 1 summarizes some of the policies that directly affect the provision of occupational therapy for children and youth. Additional

---

[1]*Occupational therapists* are responsible for all aspects of occupational therapy service delivery and are accountable for the safety and effectiveness of the occupational therapy service delivery process. *Occupational therapy assistants* deliver occupational therapy services under the supervision of and in partnership with an occupational therapist (AOTA, 2009).

[2]When the term *occupational therapy practitioner* is used in this document, it refers to both occupational therapists and occupational therapy assistants (AOTA, 2006).

Table 1. Federal Laws and Their Influence on Occupational Therapy Services

Law	Influence on Occupational Therapy Services
Individuals with Disabilities Education Improvement Act (IDEA), P.L. 108-446	Federal legislation that specifically includes occupational therapy as a related service for eligible students with disabilities, ages 3–21 years, to benefit from special education (Part B) or as a primary service for infants and toddlers who are experiencing developmental delays (Part C).
	IDEA may be reauthorized and amended in 2011.
Elementary and Secondary Education Act (ESEA) Amendments, No Child Left Behind Act (NCLB), P.L. 107-110	Federal legislation that requires public schools to raise the educational achievement of all students, particularly those from disadvantaged backgrounds, students with disabilities, and those with limited English proficiency, and that states establish high standards for teaching and student learning. While not specifically mentioned in the statute, occupational therapy is generally considered to be a pupil service under ESEA.
	ESEA may be reauthorized and amended in 2011.
Section 504 of the Rehabilitation Act of 1973, as amended, 29 U.S.C. 794; Americans with Disabilities Act (ADA, as amended); Americans with Disabilities Act Amendments Act of 2008 (ADAAA), P.L. 110-325	Civil rights statutes that prohibit discrimination on the basis of disability by programs receiving federal funds (Section 504) and by services and activities of state and local government (ADA and ADAAA). Disability here is defined more broadly than in IDEA. Children and youth who are not eligible for IDEA may be eligible for services under Section 504 or the ADA, such as for environmental adaptations and other reasonable accommodations, to help them access and succeed in the learning environment. Each state or local education agency determines eligibility procedures for children and youth served under Section 504 or the ADA.
Title XIX of the Social Security Act of 1965, as amended; Medicaid, P.L. 89-97	Federal–state match program that provides medical and health services for low-income children and adults. Occupational therapy is an optional service under the state plan but mandatory for children and youth under the Early Periodic Screening, Diagnosis and Treatment (EPSDT) services mandate.
	Occupational therapy services provided in early intervention programs are frequently covered by Medicaid. School-based services also may be covered by Medicaid but also must meet applicable medical necessary requirements as well as be educationally relevant.
Improving Head Start for School Readiness Act of 2007, P.L. 110-134	Federal program that provides comprehensive child development services to economically disadvantaged children (ages birth–5 years) and their families, including children with disabilities. Early Head Start serves children up to 3 years of age. Occupational therapy may be provided in these settings under the Head Start requirements or under IDEA.
Assistive Technology Act of 2004, P.L. 108-364, as amended	Federal program that promotes access to assistive technology for persons with disabilities so that they can more fully participate in education, employment, and daily activities.
U.S. Department of Agriculture Food and Nutrition Service (USDA, 2001)	National School Breakfast and Lunch Programs are required to provide food substitutions and modifications of school meals for students whose disabilities restrict their diets, as determined by a doctor.

information about these laws is provided in *Occupational Therapy Services for Children and Youth Under IDEA* (Jackson, 2007).

AOTA believes that occupational therapy practitioners working in early childhood and school settings should have working knowledge of the federal and state requirements to ensure that their program policies are in compliance. Occupational therapy practitioners also should be familiar with their state's occupational therapy practice act and related rules and regulations to ensure that occupational therapy services are provided accordingly.

Occupational Therapy Domain and Process

Occupational therapy supports client health and participation in life through engagement in occupations (AOTA, 2008). Occupational therapy focuses on the following occupations: ADLs, IADLs, education, leisure, play, social participation, work, and rest and sleep.

Occupational therapy practitioners provide services that enable children and youth to organize, manage, and perform their daily life occupations and activities. For example, a middle-school-age child with physical limitations may have difficulty completing written work. The occupational therapy practitioner collaborates with the student, parents, and educators to identify the skills of the student, the demands of the environment, and appropriate solutions for interventions. Another example is the family of a newborn baby with poor feeding skills. The occupational therapist may provide training and support for the family to enhance the baby's ability to drink from a bottle.

In early childhood and school-based practice, occupational therapy clients include individuals (e.g., child, family, caregivers, teachers), organizations (e.g., school districts, community preschools, Head Start), and populations within a community (e.g., homeless children, children at risk for social–emotional difficulties). Occupational therapy services are directed toward facilitating the client's participation in meaningful occupations that are desired and important in the school, family, and community contexts.

Occupational therapy services include evaluation, intervention, and documenting outcomes. During the evaluation, the occupational therapist gains an understanding of the client's priorities and his or her problems when engaging in occupations and activities. Evaluation and intervention address factors that influence occupational performance, including

- Performance skills (e.g., motor and praxis skills, sensory–perceptual skills, emotional regulation skills, cognitive skills, communication and social skills);

- Performance patterns (e.g., as habits, routines, rituals, roles);

- Contexts and environments (e.g., physical, social, cultural, virtual, personal, temporal);

- Activity demands (e.g., required actions, body functions); and

- Client factors (e.g., values and beliefs; mental, neuromuscular, sensory, visual, perceptual, digestive, cardiovascular, and integumentary functions and structures).

Desired outcomes are identified to guide future actions with the client. They also are a means for evaluating the effectiveness of occupational therapy services.

Occupational Therapy Service Provision

Occupational therapy practitioners provide early childhood services in children's homes, child care centers, preschools, Early and Head Start programs, early intervention programs, and clinical settings. Occupational therapy practitioners provide school-based services in both public and private facilities. Funding sources for occupational therapy services vary and may include federal and state funding (e.g., funding through state agencies, Medicaid), insurance, and self-pay.

Children and adolescents may be served under the Individuals with Disabilities Education Act (IDEA) Part C, if they are ages 3 years or younger, or Part B, if they are between the ages of 3 and 21 years. Some states are extending their Part C program to include preschool-age children.

Early Intervention (IDEA Part C; Birth Through Age 2 Years)

Early intervention occupational therapy services are provided to infants and toddlers with developmental delays, with diagnosed physical or mental conditions, or who are at risk for having a developmental delay in order to enhance the family's ability to care for their child with a disability. To be eligible for early intervention services under Part C, a child must have a delay in one or more of five developmental areas: (1) physical (including vision and hearing), (2) cognitive, (3) communication, (4) social–emotional, and (5) adaptive. When evaluating infants or toddlers, the occupational therapist considers aspects of the child's performance that are strengths or barriers to participation within the natural environment and daily routines. The occupational therapist's knowledge of brain development, assessment, and intervention across developmental domains, early literacy, and feeding/eating skills enables them to work with children with disabilities and their families. Infants and toddlers with significant medical or developmental concerns (e.g, feeding, neurological) should receive services from trained professionals, as they are vulnerable and require ongoing evaluation.

IDEA requires that child and family outcomes and services be developed in collaboration with the child's caregivers, other members of the team, and community agencies. These services become part of the individualized family service plan (IFSP). Some examples of occupational therapy services for the five developmental domains are listed in Table 2.

In Part C programs, occupational therapy is a primary service. The occupational therapist may be the sole service provider but most often is part of a collaborative team that works to enhance the family's capacity to care for the child's health and development within daily routines and natural environments. An occupational therapist may serve as the service coordinator to monitor the implementation of the IFSP and coordinate services with other team members and agencies. When the child is turning 3 years of age, the occupational therapist works collaboratively with the IFSP team to transition children to appropriate community-based programs or to preschool special education services, as applicable.

School Age (IDEA Part B; Ages 3–21 Years)

The local school district is responsible for determining whether school-age children and youth with disabilities, including preschool children from ages 3 to 5 years, qualify for special education and related services under IDEA Part B (§602(3)(A)(ii)). A full and individual evaluation is conducted, and an individualized education program (IEP) is developed if the student is eligible for services. Students with disabilities may be eligible for IDEA if they meet one or more of 10 disability categories:

1. Mental retardation;

2. Hearing impairments, including deafness;

3. Speech or language impairments;

4. Visual impairments, including blindness;

5. Serious emotional disturbance;

6. Orthopedic impairment;

7. Autism;

8. Traumatic brain injury;

9. Other health impairment; or

10. Specific learning disabilities (see §602(3)(A)).

Occupational therapy is one of the related services that may be provided to IDEA-eligible students who are receiving special education in schools; homes; hospitals; and other settings, including juvenile justice and alternative education settings. Related services are "transportation, and such developmental, corrective, and other supportive services (including…occupational therapy)…as may be required to assist a child with a disability to benefit from special education, and includes early identification and assessment of disabling conditions in children" (see §602(26)(A)). As such, occupational therapy is a support service for students and teachers.

When an occupational therapy evaluation is required, data collection is focused on identifying the academic, developmental, and functional needs of the student (see §614(d)(3)(A)(iv)). Information is sought regarding the student's strengths and factors that may be interfering with his or her learning and participation in the context of the educational activities, routines, and environments. Observations are made

Table 2. Occupational Therapy's Role in Early Intervention Developmental Areas

Developmental Area	Occupational Therapy's Role
Adaptive	Promote independence in self-care, such as eating and drinking, dressing, and grooming; collaborate with parents about safe positioning and modification of food textures to enhance eating
Cognitive	Promote ability to notice and attend to objects and people in the environment; promote ability to sort and classify objects and to generalize learning to new daily living tasks; promote ability to sequence steps to complete daily living occupations
Communication	Facilitate language development through social interactions, assistive communication devices, switches, toys
Physical	Promote movement for exploration of the environment, facilitate use of arms and hands to handle and manipulate objects, educate caregivers in handling and positioning techniques
Social–emotional	Foster self-regulation, social participation, and play through interactions with peers and adults

where and when difficulties occur at school (i.e., at the times and in the location in which the student normally engages in the activities and is demonstrating behaviors that are of concern). These locations include the classroom, hallways, cafeteria, restrooms, gym, and playground. The student's work, participation, and behaviors are compared with other students in the same environments and situations. Curricular demands and existing task and environmental modifications are reviewed.

Interviews with instructional personnel, the student, and family members are conducted to gather information about the student's participation and performance. Cultural differences that may exist between home and school are explored. Existing special education supports and services, including strategies utilized to improve performance, are reviewed. Practices consistent with universal design for learning (UDL) guidelines (CAST, 2008) and the availability of assistive technologies to support school performance are assessed. Standardized testing may be conducted when needed to gather additional data.

Occupational therapy evaluation results then are shared with the parents and the multidisciplinary IEP team. According to Nolet and McLaughlin (2005), decisions about an IEP are individualized but "start from the expectation that the student is to learn the general education curriculum, and special education's role is to help the student learn and progress in that curriculum" (p. 14). Annual goals for special education instruction are determined by the IEP team, as well as the accommodations and services and supports required to help the student access and progress in the general curriculum. Occupational therapy practitioners collaborate with the IEP team regarding the educational need for occupational therapy services.

On the basis of current occupational therapy evaluation data; the occupational therapist's professional judgment; and other available information about the student's skills, abilities, goals, and objectives to be achieved, the IEP team decides whether occupational therapy services are needed. The development of the IEP is a collaborative process with participation from all team members. The team determines when the student goals need the expertise of an occupational therapy practitioner, as well as the amount of time, frequency, duration, and location of those services. The team meets regularly (at least annually) to assess whether the student is making progress toward achieving his or her goals and whether special education and/or related services (including occupational therapy) need to be continued, modified, or discontinued.

Intervention can be directed toward individuals (including teachers and other adults working with the child), groups, environmental factors, and programmatic needs (see Table 3). According to Brannen et al. (2002), effective implementation includes consultation, collaboration, and teamwork. Throughout the intervention process, the occupational therapy practitioner works collaboratively with the client and other team members such as family members, instructional personnel, school administrators, and private practitioners who may serve the student. Interventions are respectful of the customs, beliefs, activity

Table 3. Occupational Therapy Services and Supports for Students 3–21 Years Under IDEA Part B

IDEA Part B Performance Areas	Occupational Therapy Services and Supports
Academic	Provide consultation with curriculum planners to support academic achievement by identifying needed curriculum accommodations and modifications for standardized testing; suggest adaptations to curriculum materials, methods, processes, and production; identify and provide needed transition supports and services targeting post-secondary goals
Developmental	Foster development of pre-academic skills, including prewriting and pre-scissor skills, toileting skills, eating and drinking skills, dressing and grooming tasks, communication skills, management of sensory needs, social skills
Functional	Facilitate use and management of school-related materials; daily routines/schedule; written school work; task/activity completion; transitions among activities and persons; adherence to rules; self-regulation; interactions with peers and adults; participation in leisure and recreational occupations at home, school, and the community; use of adaptive and assistive technology to support participation and performance
	Assist school in locating driver education training for students with disabilities. Collaborate with family and school staff in the development and implementation of transition programs, including preschool and high school transition. Collaborate with school personnel in the design and implementation of positive mental health programs and positive behavioral support systems

patterns, behavior standards, and expectations accepted by the society of which the client is a member. Along with the provision of strategies and techniques that assist the child with making progress, education and training of other team members also is an important service that occupational therapy practitioners provide. Interventions are provided in natural school environments (e.g., classroom, playground, cafeteria), occurring in the time and place that is most beneficial for the student. As noted in Hanft and Shepherd (2008), the primary setting for occupational therapy services incorporates daily routine and contexts important to the student.

Outcomes are measured by student achievement of the IEP goals and other educational objectives such as curriculum expectations. Outcome measurement for instruction may include participation on national, state, and/or district-wide assessments that are supported by services provided by the occupational therapy practitioner. Outcome measurement for occupations such as self-care, play, leisure, social participation, and work transition that typically are addressed by occupational therapy practitioners in the school setting is accomplished by monitoring progress on IEP goals focused on these areas. Data collected on identified outcomes is reviewed by the IEP team to assist with determining present levels of academic achievement and functional performance and is reported during the required annual review.

Section 504/Americans with Disabilities Act

Section 504 of the Rehabilitation Act prohibits discrimination on the basis of disability for any program receiving federal funds, including schools, early intervention, and Head Start programs. The Americans with Disabilities Act also prohibits discrimination on the basis of disability in education, employment, transportation, health care, and a host of other services and activities of state and local governments, including child care. Students with disabilities who are not eligible for services under IDEA may be eligible under Section 504 or the ADA if the disability is such that it significantly limits "one or more major life activities." Examples include students who have HIV/AIDS, asthma, arthritis, attention deficit disorder/ attention deficit hyperactivity disorder, traumatic brain disorder, conduct disorder, or depression.

Occupational therapists may be asked to help local school district teams determine student eligibility under Section 504 and to assist in the identification of services and development of the 504 plan. If the 504 committee determines that an educational need for occupational therapy exists, services may be provided directly to a child or as a necessary accommodation. While no additional federal funds are available for services under Section 504 or the ADA, compliance with the requirements are mandatory for early childhood and school settings.

Response to Intervention and Early Intervening Services

Two provisions in the 2004 reauthorization of IDEA provide additional opportunities for occupational therapy practitioners to contribute to the success of general education students who are struggling with learning or behavior. The first of these provisions, *Early Intervening Services (EIS)*, provides supports for students in kindergarten through 12th grade who are struggling with learning or behavior. School districts can use a portion of their IDEA funds to provide professional development for teachers and other staff and to provide direct services such as educational and behavioral evaluations, behavioral interventions, small group instruction, and instruction in the use of adaptive and instructional software for students who "need additional academic and behavioral supports to succeed in the general education environment" (see §613(f)(1)).

The second provision, *Response to Intervention (RtI)*, is a systematic process that closely monitors how students respond to different types of services and instruction. In the RtI process, increasingly intense levels of support are provided. Decisions about which supports to provide and at what level of intensity are made through progress monitoring and data analysis. At each step of the process, monitoring and record keeping provide critical information about the student's ongoing instruction and intervention needs.

Both EIS and RtI are preventative, proactive strategies aimed at minimizing the occurrence of behavior and learning problems as early as possible, thereby reducing the need for more intensive services later. When these approaches are used, occupational therapy practitioners implement strategies that can be used throughout a school. For example, suggestions might include the use of wide-lined paper or a pencil grip to support improvements in handwriting, modification of the classroom environment to increase accessibility, use of elastic-waist pants for a child unable to fasten clothing after toileting, strategies to deal with a child who hits others on the playground when he or she becomes frustrated, or general strategies for breaking down steps for jumping rope so that a child struggling with this skill can be successful in physical education. In addition, occupational therapy practitioners may collaborate with other professionals to design school-wide positive mental health programs, positive behavioral support services, and anti-bullying campaigns.

The occupational therapy role in EIS and RtI will vary from state to state and from district to district depending on how these provisions are implemented. Because both initiatives are targeted toward general education, school-based practitioners may need to educate student support teams on how occupational therapy helps meet student's learning and behavioral needs in those environments. In addition, practitioners should participate in state and district professional development activities related to EIS and RtI and become full participants on the local teams considering interventions and supports students need to succeed in school (Clark, 2008; Clark & Polichino, 2008; Jackson, 2007).

OT and OTA Partnerships

Occupational therapists and occupational therapy assistants work together in early childhood and school settings to deliver needed services. Occupational therapists are responsible for formal evaluation and also are accountable for the safety and effectiveness of the service delivery process, including intervention planning, implementation, outcome review, and dismissal/discharge. The occupational therapy assistant implements the intervention plan under the supervision of and in partnership with the therapist. State occupational therapy regulatory agencies determine supervision frequency, methods, and documentation.

Supervision of Other Personnel

Many early intervention programs, schools, or community agencies employ paraprofessionals to assist in the classroom or to provide direct support to some students. The occupational therapist may utilize these individuals, as allowed by state law and regulation, to carry out selected aspects of a service. Paraprofessionals must be properly trained and carefully supervised at all times to assist with the provision of selected activities or programming that will enhance the student's ability to achieve his or her IEP goals or IFSP outcomes. Paraprofessionals do not provide skilled occupational therapy, nor are they substitutes for the occupational therapist. Paraprofessionals perform only those tasks that can be safely performed within the child's routine and do not require the expertise of an occupational therapist or occupational therapy assistant.

The tasks delegated to a paraprofessional should be documented. A plan to train and supervise the paraprofessional must be developed by the occupational therapist. An occupational therapy assistant may train and supervise a paraprofessional in specifically delegated tasks; however, the occupational therapist is ultimately responsible for monitoring programs carried out by paraprofessionals and occupational therapy assistants.

Conclusion

Occupational therapists and occupational therapy assistants provide services to children and youth, families, caregivers, and educational staff within a variety of programs and settings. The ultimate outcome of occupational therapy services in early childhood and school programs is to enable the child to participate in ADLs, education, work, play, leisure, and social interactions.

References

American Occupational Therapy Association. (2006). Policy 1.44: Categories of occupational therapy personnel. In *Policy manual* (2009 ed., pp. 33–34). Bethesda, MD: Author.

American Occupational Therapy Association. (2008). Occupational therapy practice framework: Domain and process (2nd ed.). *American Journal of Occupational Therapy, 62*, 625–683.

American Occupational Therapy Association. (2009). Guidelines for supervision, roles, and responsibilities during the delivery of occupational therapy. *American Journal of Occupational Therapy, 63*(6), 797–803.

American Occupational Therapy Association. (2010a). Occupational therapy code of ethics and ethics standards (2010). *American Journal of Occupational Therapy, 64*(Suppl.), S17–S26.

American Occupational Therapy Association. (2010b). Standards of practice for occupational therapy. *American Journal of Occupational Therapy, 64*(Suppl.), S106–S111.

Americans with Disabilities Act of 1990, Pub. L. 101-336, 104 Stat. 327.

Americans with Disabilities Act Amendments Act of 2008, Pub. L. 110-325, 122 Stat. 3553.

Assistive Technology Act of 2004, Pub. L. 108-364, 118 Stat. 1707.

Brannen, S. J., Cooper, E. B., Dellegrotto, J. T., Disney, S. T., Eger, D. L., Ehren, B. J, et al. (2002). *Developing educationally relevant IEPs: A technical assistance document for speech–language pathologists.* Reston, VA: Council for Exceptional Children.

CAST. (2008). *Universal design for learning guidelines, version 1.0.* Wakefield, MA: Author.

Clark, G. F. (2008). Getting into a collaborative school routine. In B. Hanft & J. Shepherd (Eds.), *Collaborating for student success: A guide for school-based occupational therapy* (pp. 105–137). Bethesda, MD: AOTA Press.

Clark, G. F., & Polichino, J. (2008). *FAQ on response to intervention for school-based occupational therapists and occupational therapy assistants*. Bethesda, MD: American Occupational Therapy Association.

Hanft, B., & Shepherd, J. (2008). *Collaborating for student success: A guide for school-based occupational therapy*. Bethesda, MD: AOTA Press.

Improving Head Start for School Readiness Act of 2007, Pub. L. 110-134, 121 Stat. 1363, 42 U.S.C. 9801 *et seq.*

Individuals with Disabilities Education Improvement Act of 2004, Pub. L. 108-446, 20 U.S.C. §1400 *et seq.*

Jackson, L. (Ed.). (2007). *Occupational therapy services for children and youth under IDEA* (3rd ed.). Bethesda, MD: AOTA Press.

Law, M., Polatajko, H., Baptiste, W., & Townsend E. (1997). Core concepts of occupational therapy. In E. Townsend (Ed.), *Enabling occupation: An occupational therapy perspective* (pp. 29–56). Ottawa, ON: Canadian Association of Occupational Therapists.

No Child Left Behind Act of 2001, Pub. L. 107-110, 116 Stat. 3071.

Nolet, V., & McLaughlin, M. J. (2005). *Accessing the general curriculum: Including students with disabilities in standards-based reform* (2nd ed.). Thousand Oaks, CA: Corwin Press.

Rehabilitation Act Amendments of 2004, 29 U.S.C. §794.

Social Security Act of 1965, Pub. L. 89-97, 79 Stat. 286, Title XIX.

U.S. Department of Agriculture Food and Nutrition Service. (2001). *Accommodating children with special dietary needs in the school nutrition programs: Guidance for school food service staff*. Washington, DC: Author.

Authors
Gloria Frolek Clark, MS, OTR/L, BCP, FAOTA
Leslie Jackson, MEd, OT, FAOTA
Jean Polichino, MS, OTR, FAOTA

for

The Commission on Practice
Janet V. DeLany, DEd, MSA, OTR/L, FAOTA, *Chairperson*

Adopted by the Representative Assembly Coordinating Council (RACC) for the Representative Assembly

Revised by the Commission on Practice 2011

Note. This revision replaces the 2004 document *Occupational Therapy Services in Early Childhood and School-Based Settings,* previously published and copyrighted in 2004 by the American Occupational Therapy Association in the *American Journal of Occupational Therapy, 58,* 681–685.

Occupational Therapy Services in Facilitating Work Performance

The purpose of this statement is to describe for external audiences the role of occupational therapists and occupational therapy assistants[1] in facilitating successful engagement of people in their chosen work activities and in meaningful work roles. The overarching goal of occupational therapy is to support people's "health and participation in life through engagement in occupation" (American Occupational Therapy Association [AOTA], 2008, p. 626). Work is one of eight areas of occupation[2] categorized with the domain of occupational therapy practice (AOTA, 2008). The *Occupational Therapy Practice Framework: Domain and Process, 2nd Edition* defines *work* as "activities needed for engaging in remunerative employment or volunteer activities . . . [and includes] identifying and selecting work opportunities, employment seeking and acquisition tasks, job performance issues, retirement preparation and adjustment, volunteer exploration and volunteer participation" (AOTA, 2008, p. 632). Work performance supports meaningful participation and attainable productivity, which are essential for people's health and well-being.

Occupational therapy practitioners[3] provide services to clients at the individual, organizational, and population level who are experiencing problems or who have concerns for potential problems for engaging in work-related occupations. Difficulties or potential difficulties in work performance may arise from challenges the client is experiencing related to motor, sensory–perceptual, emotional regulation, cognitive, or communication and social performance skills or from those associated with performance patterns, the activity demands, or the context and environment. Occupational therapy practitioners provide work-related services in a variety of settings, including, but not limited to, business and industrial environments, acute care and rehabilitation facilities, psychiatric centers, sheltered workshops, schools, and community settings. Within these settings occupational therapy practitioners provide services that address work hardening/conditioning, pre-work screening, functional capacity assessment and ergonomics, pre-vocational assessment and training, sheltered employment, supported employment, and transition from school to work. The occupational therapy process includes evaluation; intervention planning, implementation, and review; and outcome monitoring. The key services include wellness and prevention services, restorative and compensatory interventions, consultation, education, advocacy, and case management.

Occupational Therapy Evaluation in Work Programs

Using a client-centered approach, the occupational therapist develops an occupational profile to understand the client's occupational history and reasons for seeking services. As part of the process, the occupational therapist gathers information about the client's capacities and needs, values and interests, priorities, and desired outcomes. The occupational therapist then analyzes information about the client's occupa-

---

[1]*Occupational therapists* are responsible for all aspects of occupational therapy service delivery and are accountable for the safety and effectiveness of the occupational therapy service delivery process. *Occupational therapy assistants* deliver occupational therapy services under the supervision of and in partnership with an occupational therapist (AOTA, 2009).

[2]Areas of occupation include "Activities of daily living, instrumental activities of daily living, rest and sleep, education, work, play, leisure, and social participation" (AOTA, 2008, p. 630).

[3]When the term *occupational therapy practitioner* is used in this document, it refers to both occupational therapists and occupational therapy assistants (AOTA, 2006).

tional performance gathered through formal evaluation, record review, interview, and observations related to the client's body functions, performance skills, performance patterns, the demands of the work activity, and the context and environment of the work occupation (AOTA, 2008). The occupational therapy evaluation may include data collection in the following areas:

- Job analysis to identify the required activity demands of the work tasks and possibilities for assistive technologies, job adaptations, or work accommodations;

- Evaluation of work and productive tasks, including work routines, tools and equipment, ergonomic considerations, and accessibility;

- Evaluation of work organizational culture, including psychological and social factors, and productivity expectations and job requirements both internal and external to the organization, including regulatory issues (Gupta & Sabata, 2010);

- The client's social and communication skills; functional abilities; potential for improvement; and need for adaptation, compensation, or occupational change; and

- The client's vocational aptitudes and interests necessary for development of transition plan from school to work preparation.

This information is synthesized to develop a plan of intervention that addresses the client's work participation needs, desired outcomes, and performance goals.

Occupational Therapy Intervention in Work Programs

Occupational therapy practitioners provide services to develop or increase the ability of the client to participate in and manage productive work, maintain health, adhere to safe work practices, and prevent work-related disability. Using the information gathered in the evaluation process, the occupational therapy practitioner collaborates with the client and other team members (e.g., employers, case managers, family members) or agencies (e.g., educational, local/state, vocational rehabilitation and social services departments and programs) to plan and implement intervention strategies. When developing these intervention strategies, occupational therapy practitioners consider the client's age, interests, values, beliefs, culture, skills and abilities, motivation, and psychological and social status. They address issues of worker role, task demands, work context, and work culture, as well as identify available resources. Intervention strategies are designed to identify, explore, and expand work options; enhance or develop work-related abilities (e.g., improve physical capacities, improve health and safety performance, develop skills and ability to participate); and obtain or retain employment. The following are some examples of occupational therapy interventions aimed at improving work performance and facilitating safe participation in work activities:

- Education related to health, safety and injury prevention, proper body mechanics, postural awareness, joint protection, ergonomic considerations, symptom awareness, and stress and pain management strategies applicable to work and productive activities;

- Adaptations to work activities, the work environment, and work demands and the use of assistive technologies that support the client's participation in the desired work activities;

- Strategies to improve social, communication, emotional regulation, and coping skills;

- Strategies to improve foundational work behaviors and work skills;

- Development of programs that incorporate graded activity, simulated activity, and work activity trials to allow for the gradual return to full work activity after illness or injury;

- Development of occupational activities to develop, increase, or improve productive work behaviors and skills;

- Development of work transition programs, job modifications, or job adaptations to facilitate successful work performance;

- Development of individualized plans for the transition of individuals with disabilities from school to work;

- Consultation and collaboration with clients about adaptations of work tasks, tools, equipment, and the work environment;

- Consultation with clients regarding injury management and prevention to reduce the incidence of disability-related injury;

- Collaboration with other team members, employers, services, and agencies to coordinate restorative and prevention services provided to the worker; and

- Case management services to assist in the coordination and planning for beginning or returning to work.

Table 1 provides examples of how performance related to work may be compromised and how occupational therapy practitioners may assist clients in participating in meaningful and productive work activities.

Funding Sources

Reimbursement for services related to occupational performance is dependent upon the type of services provided, the beneficiary of the services, and the setting where services are provided. Reimbursement may include, but may not be limited to,

- Direct reimbursement by employers or agencies for services to individuals or populations such as job analysis for a population; development of pre-work screens; ergonomic assessment of work, worker, and workplace; and educational programs for health, safety, and injury prevention.

- Local, state, or federally related program including workers' compensation, special education, Social Security Disability Insurance, and Medicare or medical assistance (see Appendix A for an overview of relevant legislation affecting rehabilitation services for the worker).

- Community agency resources using funds secured through federal or state monies, community or private grants, or other philanthropic donations. This often includes services provided to sheltered workshops, supported employment programs, and programs supporting individuals who are at a socioeconomic disadvantage (see Appendix B).

Table 1. Selected Case Examples

Descriptions of Client Work Performance	Occupational Therapy Evaluation	Occupational Therapy Intervention

Industrial Site—Strains and Sprains
 	
An employer in a heavy equipment manufacturing plant has recently noted a decrease in productivity and an increase in workers' compensation claims in the maintenance department. Further investigation revealed a high incidence of upper-extremity and low-back muscle strains and sprains among the maintenance crew.
 	
The employer contacts an occupational therapist for consultation to help address the problem.
 	
The employer's goals are to reduce strains and sprains, lost days of work, and costs associated with workers' compensation claims. He also is interested in promoting a safer workplace and improving employee job satisfaction and security.
	• Conduct preliminary onsite inspection of department to identify triggers such as makeshift changes to equipment and signs of worker movement and positional discomfort that could be contributing to upper-extremity and back complaints.
	• Interview employees to gain their perspective on incidence of injuries, probable causes, and suggested remedies.
	• Perform a functional job task analysis, including identification of the physical job demands and ergonomic considerations for the different maintenance activities, including
	  ○ Materials handling, equipment operations, and tools usage;
	  ○ Postural considerations;
	  ○ Work environment;
	  ○ Stress factors such as force, repetition, hold time/rest time, angle/twist/body mechanics, impact, vibration, acceleration, and work time duration.
	• Analyze the data from the work site.
	• Determine areas requiring intervention.
	• Evaluate potential modifications to job, environment, tools, or client functions.
		• Collaborate with the employer to identify and implement ergonomic changes in specific work areas to minimize risk factors associated with equipment, required body positions, and the environment (Chiarello, 2003).
		• Develop an in-service education program for the maintenance department to address risk factor reduction strategies and body mechanics.
		• Develop a wellness program that includes daily flexibility and stretching sessions in addition to worker-centered lifestyle choice classes (e.g., smoking cessation, weight control, stress reduction; Gupta, 2008).
		• Cross-train workers to ensure adequate staffing coverage in the event of absenteeism as well as job rotation to allow a variety of positions, physical exertions, and equipment usage.
		• Institute an annual onsite evaluation to monitor modifications and programs.

Repetitive Strain Injury—Factory Worker
 	
Carla is a 43-year-old woman working as a sewing machine operator and fabric cutter in a garment factory. For the past several months, she has worked 8 hours per day, 5 days per week, plus 4 hours of overtime 2–3 days per week.
 	
She recently was diagnosed with right-dominant-hand deQuervain's tenosynovitis and has been off work for 2 months. Her case manager reports that she has experienced improvement in her wrist and hand function since undergoing treatment but is reluctant to return to work due to concerns she will have a relapse and not be able to do her job.
 	
The employer is willing to consider a transitional return-to-work option. The physician refers the employee to an occupational therapist to determine her functional abilities and potential for successful return to work.
	• Conduct a functional capacity evaluation to determine the physical and functional abilities of the client, including upper-extremity strength and overall endurance to perform work task.
	• Assess worksite, and offer employer suggestions to reduce risk to client.
	• Assess body mechanics and risk for repeated injury associated with
	  ○ Repetitive cutting through several layers of fabric and
	  ○ Static positioning of wrists and fingers when guiding material through an industrial sewing machine.
		• Instruct client with incorporating proper body mechanics and use of ergonomic scissors when cutting layers of fabric.
		• Provide employer with strategies regarding institution of job rotation program and incorporation of improved positioning and work techniques for all employees (Jaegers, 2008).
		• Implement a work conditioning program that includes education, flexibility and stretching, work simulation, and strengthening activities.
		• Collaborate with client and employer to identify ergonomic changes and accurate job placement for safe, productive, functional work performance (Sandqvist & Henriksson, 2004).

Developmental Disabilities **Mark is an 18-year-old high school senior with Down Syndrome** resulting in mild intellectual disability. Mark lives with his parents, who drive him to and from school. He wants to seek employment after graduation. Mark received occupational therapy services during his elementary and middle school years. The focus of occupational therapy was on	• Review Mark's records and interview Mark and his parents to learn about his occupational performance related to work, and identify his perceived needs as he moves forward (Sabata & Endicott, 2005). • Determine a work transition plan that addresses work behaviors, communication skills, and social interaction skills.	• Educate Mark and his family about pertinent laws, community agencies, and resources available to assist him in seeking gainful employment (Sabata & Endicott, 2007; Vogtle & Brooks, 2005). • Collaborate with speech–language pathologist to incorporate peer buddy system to strengthen social and communication skills.

Table 1. Selected Case Examples *(cont.)*

Descriptions of Client Work Performance	Occupational Therapy Evaluation	Occupational Therapy Intervention
Developmental Disabilities *(cont.)* independence in daily living skills and the development of appropriate social behaviors. The goal was to maximize classroom learning and interaction with his classmates, ultimately affording Mark the skills to participate in his community (AOTA, 2008). Mark has not worked outside the home and has not had the opportunity to develop work skills or work behaviors. He has difficulty with time management, attention span, and sustained focus on a task.	• Assess the level of difficulty he has with time management, especially with his morning routine. • Assess his pre-work skills, including concentration span, attention to task, and organizational skills; ability to follow written and verbal directions; and ability to communicate his ideas to others. • Determine performance skills in the area of community mobility and transportation usage (AOTA, 2008).	• Instruct Mark on the use of a visual calendar to help him stay focused and complete his morning routines in a timely manner. • Assist Mark in mastering the steps necessary to ride the city bus as a means to travel to and from a job.
Mental Health—Schizophrenia **Natalie, a 27-year-old woman** with a history of schizophrenia, is a consumer at a community support day program. She lives in a subsidized apartment with two other individuals who also have been diagnosed with a mental illness. In the past Natalie has not been able to secure a job due to disorganized thinking, which affected her concentration and follow-through. Based on recent positive response to antipsychotic medication and success in volunteer work at the day program, Natalie has identified a goal of acquiring part-time office work and getting an apartment of her own. Natalie states that she lacks self-confidence related to working and that she is afraid she will not remember how to use a computer or be able to keep up with everyone else at a job. Her case worker has sought the services of an occupational therapist to assist in the work transition process.	Administer an occupational profile to determine Natalie's occupational history, work experiences, interests, patterns of daily living, and meaningful occupations (AOTA, 2008). Assess Natalie's abilities in the following areas: • Problem-solving skills • Independence in daily living activities • Use of public transportation • Medication management • Seeking help and advocating for her needs. Determine her work readiness skills development in task organization and time management.	• Collaborate with Natalie to locate and select appropriate resources and support systems to help her seek, obtain, and sustain gainful part-time employment (Liu, Hollis, Warren, & Williamson, 2007). • Assist Natalie with experiential exploration of potential jobs of interest. • Collaborate with a vocational counselor to set up a supported employment program (Liu et al., 2007). • Work with employer on reasonable accommodations per Natalie's ability to perform the essential functions of a given job (Americans with Disabilities Act, 1990). • Meet with job coach and Natalie to provide specific strategies for work skills development while building on her current skills and strengths (Sabata & Endicott, 2007).
Rheumatoid Arthritis **Sarah, a 45-year-old woman** with rheumatoid arthritis, is employed as a housekeeper at a hotel. She is unable to perform her work tasks due to exacerbation of her rheumatoid symptoms. She presents with decreased gross grasp, decreased pinch strength, difficulty reaching above shoulder height, and poor endurance for continuous work activity over 4 hours.	The occupational therapist observes performance and analyzes activities to determine points of difficulty. In collaboration with Sarah, the therapist concludes that dusting and washing pictures, mirrors, and door frames above shoulder level are no longer possible without adaptation of the equipment used to perform these tasks. Grasp of smaller items (e.g., dusters with ½" handles and mops with 1" handles) is particularly difficult for Sarah in her work. She demonstrates difficulty changing toilet paper roles that require lateral and three-point pinch. Sarah uses her arms to lift bed linens and has difficulty grasping the material as she makes beds. She requires a rest period after cleaning each room.	• Work with Sarah and her employer to identify and prioritize work activities. • Recommend adaptations and modifications in processes, approaches, and the contexts of required housekeeping tasks to support improved performance. • Recommend ergonomic changes to the tools and materials needed to do her job. • Train Sarah in work simplification and adapted techniques. • Work with Sarah to identify alternate work options, including training at a local community college in a career that requires less physical effort and stress upon the body.

(Continued)

Table 1. Selected Case Examples *(cont.)*

Descriptions of Client Work Performance	Occupational Therapy Evaluation	Occupational Therapy Intervention
Older adults seeking volunteer activities **A group of senior citizens** who attend a weekly "Dine and Learn" lunch program at a local senior center were discussing their interest in volunteering in their community. They are interested in volunteerism as a way to stay physically and mentally active. The seniors have not had previous volunteer experience and are not certain where to begin to find a suitable venue and offer their services.	The occupational therapist uses a leisure activity check list to begin identifying areas of potential interest, such as woodworking, home repairs, working with adolescents, and financial consultation. As a result of an Internet search, the seniors identify local organizations and programs in need of volunteers that could benefit from their expertise. Settings include a Boys Club program teaching inner-city youth to make small furniture and decorative items, a service run by an area church to assist elders completing complex tax returns, and the local chapter of Habitat for Humanity.	• Establish a data bank and referral system that matches interests of group members with related volunteer opportunities. • Organize a volunteer fair for the seniors to connect with and learn about the community organizations volunteer needs. • Develop a training program within the senior center to prepare the seniors to match their skills with the specific needs and interests of the organizations.

References

American Occupational Therapy Association. (2006). Policy 1.44: Categories of occupational therapy personnel. In *Policy manual* (2007 ed., pp. 33–34). Bethesda, MD: Author.

American Occupational Therapy Association. (2008). Occupational therapy practice framework: Domain and process (2nd ed.). *American Journal of Occupational Therapy, 62*, 625–683.

American Occupational Therapy Association. (2009). Guidelines for supervision, roles, and responsibilities during the delivery of occupational therapy services. *American Journal of Occupational Therapy, 63*, 797–803.

Americans with Disabilities Act of 1990, P. L. 101-336, 104 Stat. 327.

Chiarello, B. (2003). Does ergonomics improve productivity? An evidenced–based review. *Work Programs Special Interest Section Quarterly, 17*(4), 1–4.

Gupta, J. (2008). Promoting wellness at the workplace. *Work and Industry Special Interest Section Quarterly, 22*(2), 1–4.

Gupta, J., & Sabata, D. (2010). Older workers: Maintaining a worker role and returning to the workplace. In B. Braveman & J. J. Page (Eds.), *Work: Occupational therapy intervention to promote participation and productivity*. Philadelphia: F. A. Davis.

Jaegers, L. (2008). Ergonomics, health, and wellness in industry. A holistic approach. *Work Programs Special Interest Section Quarterly, 22*(3), 4.

Liu, K. W. D., Hollis, V., Warren, S., & Williamson, D. L. (2007). Supported-employment program processes and outcomes: Experiences of people with schizophrenia. *American Journal of Occupational Therapy, 61*, 543–554.

Sabata, D., & Endicott, S. (2007). Workplace changes: Seizing opportunities for persons with disabilities in the workplace. *Work Programs Special Interest Section Quarterly, 21*(2), 1–3.

Sandqvist, J. L., & Henriksson, C. M. (2004). Work functioning: A conceptual framework. *Work: A Journal of Prevention, Assessment, and Rehabilitation, 23*, 147–157.

Vogtle, L. K., & Brooks, B. (2005). Common issues for adults with DD. *OT Practice, 10*, 8–12.

Additional Readings

Aja, D. (2004, March). Using a functional capacity evaluation as a successful benchmark in the life care plan process. *Work Programs Special Interest Section Quarterly, 18*(1), 1–4.

American Medical Association. (2008). *International classification of diseases* (9th rev., Clinical Modification, Hospital, Vols. 1–3). Chicago: Author.

Gibson, L., Strong, L., & Wallace, B. (2005). Functional capacity evaluation as a performance measure: Evidence for a new approach for clients with chronic back pain. *Clinical Journal of Pain, 21*, 207–215

Glass, L. S. (Ed.). (2004). *Occupational medicine practice guidelines* (2nd ed.). Beverly Farms, MA: OEM Press.

Gross, D. P., & Battie, M. C. (2003). Construct validity of a kinesiophysical functional capacity evaluation administered within a worker's compensation environment. *Journal of Occupational Rehabilitation, 13*, 287–295.

Gross, D. P., Battie, M. C., & Cassidy, D. (2004). The prognostic value of functional capacity evaluation in patients with chronic low back pain: Part 1. Timely return to work. *Spine, 29*, 914–919.

Haldorsen, E. M., Grasdal, A. L., Skouen,. S., Risa, A. E., Skronholm, K., & Ursin, H. (2002). Is there a right treatment for a particular patient group? Comparison of ordinary treatment, light multidisciplinary treatment, and extensive multidisciplinary treatment for long-term sick-listed employees with musculoskeletal pain. *Pain, 95*, 49–63.

Hayden, J., van Tulder, M., Malmivaara, A., & Koes, B. (2005). Meta-analysis: Exercise therapy for nonspecific low back pain. *Annals of Internal Medicine, 142*, 765–775.

Heymans, M., van Tulder, M., Esmail, R., Bombardier, C., & Koes, B. (2004). Back schools for non-specific low-back pain. *Cochrane Database of Systematic Reviews, 3*, CD000261.

Howard, N., Spielholz, P., Bao, S., Silverstein, B., & Fan, Z. (2009). Reliability of an observational tool to assess the organization of work. *International Journal of Industrial Ergonomics, 39*, 260–266.

Innes, E. (2006). Reliability and validity of functional capacity evaluations: An update. *International Journal of Disability Management Research, 135*, 135–148.

Innes, E., & Straker, L. (2003). Attributes of excellence in work-related assessment. *Work: A Journal of Prevention, Assessment and Rehabilitation, 20*(1), 63–76.

Jacobs, K. (2008). *Ergonomics for therapists* (3rd ed.). St. Louis, MO: Mosby.

Kaskustas, V., & Snodgrass, J. (2009). *Occupational therapy practice guidelines for individuals with work-related injuries and illnesses.* Bethesda, MD: AOTA Press.

Larson, B. A., & Ellexson, M. T. (2000). Blueprint for ergonomics. *Work: A Journal of Prevention, Assessment, and Rehabilitation, 15*, 107–112.

Larson, B. A., & Ellexson, M. T. (2009). Industrial rehabilitation and work injury prevention. In I. Söderback (Ed.), *International handbook of occupational therapy interventions.* New York: Springer.

Maher, C., & Bear-Lehman, J. (2008). Orthopaedic conditions. In M. V. Radomski & C. A. Trombly Latham (Eds.), *Occupational therapy for physical dysfunction* (6th ed., pp. 1106–1130). Baltimore: Lippincott Williams & Wilkins.

Maloney, C. C. (2003, September). Work simulation strategies in work programs. *Work Programs Special Interest Section Quarterly, 17*(3), 1–3.

Matheson, L. (2003). Functional capacity evaluation. In G. Andersson, S. Demeter, & G. Smith (Eds.), *Disability evaluation* (2nd ed.). Chicago: Mosby.

Meyer, K., Fransen, J., Huwiler, J., Uebelhart, T., & Klipstein, A. (2005). Feasibility and results of a randomized pilot-study of a work rehabilitation programme. *Journal of Back and Musculoskeletal Rehabilitation, 18,* 67–78.

Miller, D. M. (2004, February 9). Psychosocial issues and the return-to-work process. *OT Practice, 9*(3), 16–20.

Moyers, P. A., & Dale, L. M. (2007). *The guide to occupational therapy practice* (2nd ed.). Bethesda, MD: AOTA Press.

Musich, S., Napier, D., & Edington, D. W (2001). The association of health risks with workers' compensation costs. *Journal of Occupational and Environmental Medicine, 43*(6), 534–541.

National Committee on Vital and Health Statistics. (2002). *Classifying and reporting functional status* (Report of the Subcommittee on Population). Retrieved February 8, 2009, from http://ncvhs.hhs.gov/ 020211mn. htm

Sanders, M. J. (Ed.). (2003). *Management of musculoskeletal disorders.* Newton, MA: Butterworth Heinemann.

Siporin, S., & Lysack, C. (2004). Quality of life and supported employment: A case study of three women with developmental disabilities. *American Journal of Occupational Therapy, 58,* 455–465.

Soer, R., van der Scnans, C., Groornoff, J. W. Ceenzen, J. H., & Reneman, M. E. (2008). Towards consensus in operational definitions in functional capacity evaluation: A Delphi survey. *Journal of Occupational Rehabilitation, 18,* 389–400.

Stutzman, L. (2001, August). Evidence-based return to work guidelines. *CWCE Magazine,* pp. 36–38.

U.S. Bureau of Labor Statistics. (2008). *Nonfatal occupational injuries and illnesses requiring days away from work, 2007* [Press release from the U.S. Department of Labor, No. 08-1716]. Washington, DC: Author.

World Health Organization. (2003). *The burden of musculoskeletal conditions at the start of the new millennium* (WHO Technical Report Series). Geneva, Switzerland: Author.

Authors

Melanie Ellexson, MBA, OTR/L, FAOTA
Barbara Larson, MA, OTR, FAOTA

for

The Commission on Practice
Janet V. DeLany, DEd, OTR/L, FAOTA, *Chairperson*

Adopted by the Representative Assembly Coordinating Council (RACC) for the Representative Assembly

Revised by the Commission on Practice 2011

Note. This revision replaces the 2005 document *Occupational Therapy Services in Facilitating Work Performance,* previously published and copyrighted in 2005 by the American Occupational Therapy Association in the *American Journal of Occupational Therapy, 59,* 676–679.

Appendix A. Selected Work Legislation

Legislation	Scope
Federal Employees Liability (FELA) Act, 1908 (45 U.S.C. 51 et seq.)	Established the no-fault insurance system that pays benefits to employees for accidental injuries or diseases that are work related.
Vocational Rehabilitation Act Amendments of 1943 (P.L. 78–113)	Changed the original provision of the Vocational Rehabilitation Act of 1920 (P.L. 66–236). Added people with physical disabilities, blindness, developmental delays, and psychiatric disabilities to those served. Established the Office of Vocational Rehabilitation. Put a new emphasis on activities of daily living and adaptation. Removed ceiling on appropriation.
Vocational Rehabilitation Act Amendments (Hill–Burton Act) of 1954 (P.L. 86–565)	Authorized greater financial support, research and demonstration grants, professional preparation grants, state agency expansion and improvements grants, and grants to expand rehabilitation facilities.
Vocational Rehabilitation Act Amendments of 1965 (P.L. 89–333)	Increased services for several types of people with disabilities and social handicaps. Made construction money available for rehabilitation centers and workshops.
Architectural Barriers Act of 1968 (P.L. 90–48)	Led the way to changes in access for people with disabilities.
Developmental Disabilities Services and Facilities Construction Act of 1970 (P.L. 91–517)	Gave states broad responsibility for planning and implementing a comprehensive program of services to people with developmental delays, epilepsy, cerebral palsy, and other neurological impairments.
Occupational Safety and Health Act of 1970 (P.L. 91–596)	Mandated that the employer provide employment free from recognized hazards that are likely to cause death or serious harm to workers.
Rehabilitation Act of 1973 (P.L. 93–112)	Expanded services to people with more severe disabilities. Provided for affirmative action in employment (Section 503) and nondiscrimination in facilities (Section 504) by federal contractors and grantees.
Rehabilitation Act Amendments of 1986 (P.L. 99–506)	Clarifications included that in evaluating rehabilitation potential, one must consider recreation, employability, and rehabilitation engineering needs.
Education of the Deaf Act (EDA) of 1986 (P.L. 99–371)	Extended statutory authority of the National Technical Institute of the Deaf to provide technical training and education to prepare deaf people for employment.
Omnibus Budget Reconciliation Act of 1987 (P.L. 100–203)	Permitted states to offer prevocational, educational, and supported employment services to people deinstitutionalized at any time before the waiver program.
Americans with Disabilities Act (ADA) of 1990 (P.L. 101–336)	Prevented discrimination against individuals with disabilities. Guaranteed equal protection for individuals with disabilities in employment, public accommodations, transportation, state and local government, and telecommunications.
Ticket-to-Work and Work Incentives Improvement Act of 1999 (P.L. 106–170)	Established to increase opportunities and choices for Social Security disability beneficiaries to obtain employment, vocational rehabilitation, and other support services from public and private providers, employers, and other organizations.
Americans with Disabilities Act Amendments Act (ADAAA) of 2008 (P.L. 110-325)	Focuses on the discrimination at issue instead of the individual's disability. Makes important changes to the definition of the term *disability* by rejecting the holdings in several Supreme Court decisions and portions of Equal Employment Opportunity Commission's (EEOC) ADA regulations. Retains the ADA's basic disability definition as an impairment that substantially limits one or more major life activities, a record of such an impairment, or being regarded as having such an impairment.

Appendix B. Internet Resources

American National Standards Institute	www.ansi.org
Board of Certification in Professional Ergonomics	www.bcpe.org
California Code of Regulations, Title 8, § 5110. Repetitive Motion Injuries	www.dir.ca.gov/title8/5110.html
California Department of Industrial Relations	www.dir.ca.gov
Canadian Centre for Occupational Health and Safety	www.ccohs.ca
Centers for Disease Control and Prevention	www.cdc.gov
Ergoweb	www.ergoweb.com
Foundation for Professional Ergonomics	www.ergofoundation.org
Health calculator page	www.halls.md/index.htm
Human Factors and Ergonomics Society	www.hfes.org
IIEE Applied Ergonomics Community	www.appliedergo.org
Institute for Work and Health	www.iwh.on.ca
International Ergonomics Association	www.iea.cc
International Society for Occupational Ergonomics and Safety	www.isoes.info
National Safety Council	www.nsc.org/Pages/Home.aspx
National Institute for Occupational Safety and Health	www.cdc.gov/niosh/homepage.html
Occupational Safety and Health Administration	www.osha.gov
The (Ontario, Canada) Workplace Safety and Insurance Board	www.wsib.on.ca/wsib/wsibsite.nsf/public/homepage
U.S. Department of Labor	www.dol.gov

Occupational Therapy Services in the Promotion of Mental Health and Well-Being

Introduction and Purpose

This statement describes the role of occupational therapists and occupational therapy assistants[1] in addressing the psychological and social aspects of human performance as they influence health, well-being, and participation in occupations. Psychological and social health is necessary for a positive sense of well-being and transcends all practice areas or medical diagnoses. The impact of social and psychological health is a consideration in all occupational therapy interventions and ensures that all persons are afforded opportunities to participate in life through engagement in meaningful occupations.

The occupational therapy profession is rooted in the belief that "Man, through the use of his hands as energized by mind and will, can influence the state of his own health" (Reilly, 1962, p. 2). Although challenges to occupational performance related to psychological and social factors may not be the primary reason why some clients (e.g., persons, groups, populations) receive occupational therapy services, the relationship between these factors and occupational performance is central to their successful engagement in desired and needed occupations (American Occupational Therapy Association [AOTA], 1997). The World Health Organization (WHO; 2004) described *mental health* not merely as the absence of mental illness but as the presence of "a state of well-being in which the individual realizes his or her own abilities, can cope with the normal stresses of life, can work productively and fruitfully, and is able to make a contribution to his or her community" (p. 12). The *Occupational Therapy Practice Framework: Domain and Process* (AOTA, 2014b, p. S4) defines *well-being* as contentment with one's health, self-esteem, sense of belonging, security, and opportunities for self-determination, meaning, roles, and helping others.

Audience

This statement is intended for occupational therapists and occupational therapy assistants in practice, academia, research, advocacy, and administrative positions. Other audiences for this statement include regulatory and policymaking bodies, provider groups, accreditation agencies, other professionals, and the general public who may be seeking clarification about occupational therapy's scope of practice and domain of concern related to this topic.

Definitions

In *Healthy People 2020*, mental health is defined as "a state of successful performance of mental function, resulting in productive activities, fulfilling relationships with other people, and the ability to adapt to change and to cope with challenges (U.S. Department of Health and Human Services, 2016, para. 2). Psychological and social well-being contribute to mental health and to successful engagement in meaningful occupations and roles. Psychological factors include individual beliefs, values, and a person's unique perspective of the world. What a person chooses to value and their beliefs influence choices in occupations and relationships (Christiansen & Townsend, 2010). As described within the *International Classification of Functioning, Disability and Health* (WHO, 2004), psychological factors are global mental functions related to

---

[1]*Occupational therapists* are responsible for all aspects of occupational therapy service delivery and are accountable for the safety and effectiveness of the occupational therapy service delivery process. *Occupational therapy assistants* deliver occupational therapy services under the supervision of and in partnership with an occupational therapist (AOTA, 2014a).

the experience of self, time, and emotion; they also include energy, drive, temperament, and personality. They also can be described as motivation for personal growth, impulse control, emotional stability, body image, self-concept, self-esteem, coping, sense of life purpose, sense of autonomy over personal choices and environmental demands, and behavioral regulation (Keyes, 2009).

Social factors occur at both the personal and environmental levels. At the personal level, these factors include the ability of clients to communicate and interact with others. People exhibiting social well-being will demonstrate empathy, affection, and intimacy, as well as the ability to maintain caring relationships. Having a positive worldview, caring about society, having a sense of belonging, accepting the contributions of others, and valuing one's efforts to support the greater good contribute to one's mental health (Keyes, 2009).

At the environmental level, social factors are external to clients and reflect the connection to the surrounding world. Factors include the availability, attitudes, and values of social support systems at the family, community, and societal levels. Social environments that allow for successful engagement in life may include supportive families and friends, spiritual activities, support groups, clubs, available housing, fiscal resources, and inclusive policies and regulations (AOTA, 2014b; Bonder, 1993; WHO, 2004).

Positive psychological and social factors of mental health such as intact self-concept, motivation, and resilience can assist clients who are experiencing challenges with daily life by providing the internal foundation necessary for coping, goal setting, and behaviors leading to personal and environmental/contextual adaptations. The ability to acknowledge, accept, and ultimately adapt to real or perceived challenges enhances clients' sense of self- worth and self-efficacy, which in turn contributes to the maintenance, restoration, or creation of intact psychosocial functioning (Bandura, 1994; Drench, Noonan, Sharby, & Ventura, 2011; Livneh & Antonak, 2005).

Clients demonstrate positive *social aspects of mental well-being* through performance of skills, including those related to communication, expression, and regulation of emotions. They demonstrate their *social abilities* through how they initiate and maintain relationships, interpret and respond to verbal and nonverbal forms of communication, respond to the thoughts and emotions of others, communicate their needs, and choose socially appropriate responses. These abilities translate into positive interactions within clients' social networks (AOTA, 2014b). Clients demonstrate positive *psychological aspects of mental well-being* through display of affect, behavior, and description of their thoughts, feelings, and concerns (Bonder, 1993).

Both psychological and social factors and performance skills influence and are influenced by the supports and challenges clients experience in day-to-day living. Clients who exhibit self-efficacy, hopefulness, and motivation are able to successfully adapt to change and engage appropriately in desired socially constructed activities and situations. In contrast, clients struggling to successfully engage in their daily occupations may be experiencing psychosocial difficulties.

Rationale and Significance

Occupational therapy practitioners[2] recognize that mental well-being is an integral part of the ability of all people to engage in desired and necessary life occupations regardless of physical and social situation or context. Practitioners also understand that challenges to subjective well-being can occur because of a variety of circumstances, such as when clients face major life changes due to acquired illness or disability; face unique functional challenges due to congenital or developmental disabilities; or cope with anticipated change in habits, routines, and roles resulting from a move or loss of a significant other (Pendleton & Schultz-Krohn, 2013). Occupational therapy practitioners understand that clients' ongoing occupational

---

[2]When the term *occupational therapy practitioner* is used in this document, it refers to both occupational therapists and occupational therapy assistants (AOTA, 2015).

performance is sustained by the interrelationship of patterns of daily living, personal history, experiences, interests, values, beliefs, and needs.

Taking the time to understand what is currently important and meaningful to clients as well as understanding past roles, experiences, strengths, and patterns of coping sheds light on how current issues and problems are affecting clients' health and participation in desired occupations (Bonder, 1997; Nilsson & Townsend, 2010; Pendleton & Schultz-Krohn, 2013). Occupational therapy practitioners collaborate with clients in achieving adaptation to actual or potential life changes through (1) provision of activities and occupations that assist with future goal setting; (2) occupational engagements that allow clients to demonstrate abilities, recognize assets, and understand continuing challenges; and (3) adaptations to the physical and social environment (Pendleton & Schultz-Krohn, 2013)

Background and Historical Perspective

Attention to the psychological and social factors influencing mental well-being and occupational performance is grounded in the historical roots of the occupational therapy profession. Its founders were concerned with the negative effects of inactivity on individuals. They envisioned occupational therapy as a holistic profession, focusing on the mind–body interrelationship and the importance of occupations in helping those with physical, psychological, and social challenges maintain a positive life orientation (Mosey, 1996).

The founders believed that humans beings brought to their occupations a complex mix of personal, physical, psychological, and social factors and also were influenced by cultural, social, environmental, and political variables (Kielhofner, 2009). "This founding vision had at its center a profound belief in the value of therapeutic occupations as a way to remediate illness and maintain health." (Slagle, 1924, as cited in AOTA, 2014b, p. S3). It emphasized the importance of establishing a therapeutic relationship and collaborating with the client in designing interventions from a holistic perspective incorporating all aspects of the client and environment (AOTA, 2014b; Meyer, 1922).

Today occupational therapy remains a holistic profession, committed to supporting clients' health, well-being, and participation in life through addressing the constellation of contextual, environmental, physical, psychological, and social factors that support engagement in desired occupation.

Relationship to the Occupational Therapy Domain and Process

Clients' engagement and performance in meaningful occupations is a result of personal choices and motivation, within a collaborative and supportive context and environment. Engagement includes both *objective* (physically observable) and *subjective* (emotional and psychological) aspects of the clients' experiences and involves the transactional interaction of the mind, body, and spirit (AOTA, 2014b). During the evaluation and intervention process, occupational therapy practitioners collaborate with clients to consider the interrelated personal, contextual, and environmental factors that support performance and are pertinent to their occupational needs (Egan & Dubouloz, 2014). Identifying the psychological attributes and social capacities supports a holistic view of clients and contributes to the design of client-centered interventions that promote health, well-being, and participation in life through successful engagement in desired and meaningful occupations.

Occupational Therapy Practice, Practice Settings, and Related Issues

Interventions

The overarching goal of occupational therapy is to support clients in "achieving health, well-being, and participation in life through engagement in occupation" (AOTA, 2014b, p. S4). *Clients* include persons, groups, and populations. Their engagement in occupations can occur in any setting in which clients participate in work, play, education, leisure, rest and sleep, activities of daily living, and instrumental activities of daily living. Examples of settings include home, work, community, hospitals and rehabilitation facilities, and schools.

Clients receive occupational therapy services when they have experienced a disruption in their ability to participate in meaningful occupations, or they may receive services as part of an early intervention or health promotion program. Addressing psychological and social factors of mental health through interventions designed to enhance or restore well-being, occupational balance, and occupational engagement is a critical component of the therapeutic process (Hocking, 2014; Nilsson & Townsend, 2010). Occupational therapy practitioners are educated to use occupations and therapeutic relationships. Practitioners may use conditional and interactive reasoning (Schell & Schell, 2008), communicate within and through occupation, and administer standardized and non- standardized assessments to evaluate the impact of psychological and social factors on clients' engagement in occupation. Specific strategies used to elicit strengths and needs may include engaging in therapeutic use of self, using active listening, developing opportunities for choices and personal narratives, facilitating problem solving, modeling, and supporting effective communication strategies (Keyes, 2009; Taylor, 2008).

Therapeutic use of self is an integral part of the process of occupational therapy and is used with all clients in all settings. Occupational therapy practitioners develop and manage their therapeutic relationship with clients by using narrative and clinical reasoning; empathy; and a client-centered, collaborative approach to service delivery (adapted from Taylor & Van Puymbroeck, 2013, as cited in AOTA, 2014b). *Therapeutic use of self* includes interpersonal methods and skills necessary to respond to clients; characteristics to model; levels of active engagement; effective use of personal attributes; and approaches that motivate, guide, and promote confidence in clients. Therapeutic use of self contributes to client-centered collaboration, caring, and empathy and the integration of multiple methods of clinical reasoning, in particular, narrative reasoning. The integration of the elements of therapeutic use of self within occupational engagement provides for a dynamic and powerful therapeutic process (Taylor, 2008).

Occupational therapy practitioners may provide additional interventions for clients struggling with psychological and social challenges through the therapeutic use of occupations, activities, and preparatory methods; education and training; advocacy; and group interventions. Practitioners use occupations, activities, and preparatory methods as a means of enhancing psychological and social aspects of clients' mental well-being and for improving engagement in satisfying life experiences (AOTA, 2014b). Practitioners also recognize the interrelated nature of clients' mental well-being and occupational engagement and seek to improve both while addressing them simultaneously. The therapeutic use of occupations includes opportunities for

- *Mastery experiences,* in which occupational engagement allows clients to demonstrate abilities, recognize assets, and understand and adapt to continuing challenges, and

- *Role modeling,* in which clients learn to effectively problem solve and engage in occupations by observing the occupational therapy practitioner.

Occupational therapy practitioners may adapt the physical and social environment and the demands of the activity to support clients' successful engagement in the desired activities and occupations. Practitioners may recommend strategies and resources for clients to minimize physical and psychological challenges that affect occupational engagement.

Occupational therapy practitioners may *educate* clients about goal setting and communication strategies and provide *training* to facilitate skill development (AOTA, 2014b). Goal setting can enhance a sense of hopefulness and motivation to work for positive future outcomes. Practitioners facilitate the goal-setting process through assisting with values clarification, identification, and acknowledgment of future desires and with the process of self-reflection (Drench et al., 2011). Communication and adaptation to the social environment involves educating and providing specific training and skill development about interpersonal communication, including verbal and nonverbal behaviors and socially appropriate behaviors when in various life contexts such as on-on-one situations with friends and significant individuals within the home, school, work, social situations, and public places. Practitioners also provide education to caregivers and others who work with clients experiencing psychological and social difficulties to address how to use occupations to promote positive self-concept, motivation, and mood and to assist clients in developing resiliency and in adapting to challenges (AOTA, 2014b; Burnett, 2013; Crist, 2011; Graff et al., 2006; Nilsson & Townsend, 2010).

Occupational therapy practitioners can be *advocates,* working on behalf of clients who may be experiencing occupational deprivation or injustices that limit their ability to engage in meaningful and relevant occupations. *Advocacy* efforts are directed toward prompting occupational justice and empowering clients to seek out and obtain resources to fully participate in daily life occupations. Advocacy also includes practitioners working within groups and populations to address policies and practices that promote positive mental well-being that otherwise would adversely affect occupational performance. Outcomes of advocacy and self-advocacy support health, well-being, and occupational participation at the individual or systems level. Addressing these concerns can lead to enhanced self-efficacy and success of the individual facing challenges (Crist, 2011; Nilsson & Townsend, 2010).

Occupational therapy practitioners also use their unique knowledge and skills in *group interventions* as a method of service delivery. The dynamics of social interactions inherent in a group setting facilitates learning and allows clients to explore and develop skills for participation with others in meaningful occupations (AOTA, 2014b). Table 1 provides case examples of occupational therapy interventions for the promotion of psychological and social aspects of mental well-being in a variety of practice settings.

Outcomes

"The benefits of occupational therapy are multifaceted and may occur in all aspects of the domain of concern" (AOTA, 2014b, p. S16). Improved occupational performance contributes to self-efficacy and hopefulness about the future. Clients' subjective impressions related to goal attainment may include improved outlook, confidence, hope, playfulness, self-efficacy, sustainability of valued occupations, resilience, and perceived well-being. These examples of subjective and observable outcomes contribute to improved occupational performance and support health, well-being, and participation in life through engagement in occupation (AOTA, 2014b).

Achievement of psychological and social aspects of mental well-being through adaptation to change by clients receiving occupational therapy services is a dynamic, nonlinear process that includes working through the initial responses of shock, anger, depression, and hostility and the intermediate coping strategy of denial. Positive mental well-being occurs when clients are able to acknowledge and positively adjust to their current situation. In cases in which changes in physical, mental, social, environmental, or health status are permanent, those individuals who can acknowledge and accept their new state, gain a new sense of self-concept, reappraise life value, and seek new meanings and goals will achieve the ultimate goal of adjustment. It is necessary for individuals to reestablish a positive sense of self-worth, realize the existence of remaining and newly discovered potentialities, actively pursue and implement social and vocational goals, and overcome obstacles while working toward those goals (Livneh & Antonak, 2005).

Occupational Therapy Education and Training

Occupational therapists and occupational therapy assistants complete nationally accredited educational programs that prepare them to address the psychological and social aspects of mental well-being of all their clients. The Accreditation Council for Occupational Therapy Education® (ACOTE®) standards for accreditation requirements of occupational therapy and occupational therapy assistants educational programs stipulate coursework that will enable practitioners to demonstrate knowledge and understanding of (1) human behavior, including behavioral and social sciences; (2) support for the quality of life, well-being, and occupation of the individual, group, or population to promote physical and mental health; and (3) the ability to use the therapeutic use of self, which includes one's personality, insights, perceptions, and judgments as part of the therapeutic process (ACOTE, 2012). Relevant coursework and clinical experiences promote an understanding of health and wellness, including ethical and practical considerations within cultural, personal, temporal, and virtual contexts. Foundational to the practice of occupational therapy is the application of evidence-based intervention, review of theoretical perspectives to support intervention, and training in assessment and evaluation (ACOTE, 2012). In addition, many occupational therapy practitioners complete fieldwork training in areas in which psychological and social factors are explicitly addressed. These settings include psychiatric units and hospitals, substance abuse facilities, prisons, juvenile detention centers, adult day care facilities, community practice, and school systems.

Summary and Conclusion

Supporting clients' engagement in meaningful occupations and routines involves understanding and harnessing individual psychological and social factors to promote mental and physical health and recovery and adaptation to their current life situation. An appreciation of the impact of psychological attributes and social capacities within the environments and contexts of clients is the foundation on which all occupational therapy evaluation, intervention, and outcomes are based. The efficacy of occupational therapy intervention is measured by these principles and beliefs in supporting health and participation in life regardless of diagnosis or practice setting (Pendleton & Schultz-Krohn, 2013; Yerxa, 1967).

Table 1. Case Examples of Occupational Therapy Interventions With a Focus on Mental Health

Case Example	Challenges to Occupational Performance and Mental Health	Occupational Therapy Interventions, With a Focus on Mental Health
Abby, age 8, has been having difficulty in school with reading, writing, and math. She tends to reverse her letters when writing, and her hand hurts after writing her name. She previously received speech therapy at school but has recently been discharged from school speech services. Her parents report that Abby is highly anxious. The school psychologist has suggested that Abby may have obsessive–compulsive disorder. Her parents do not think she has OCD, but they recognize that she tends to like to control her environment whenever possible, to the detriment of her participation in play and ADLs. When she is successful at a task or game, she will perform it the same way every time to ensure that success. For example, if she was able to tie her shoes successfully when she sat on the third step of the stairs, she will put her shoes on only when she is sitting on the third step. She likes to be in charge when she plays with her peers, telling them what to do and where to stand, and she refuses to play when they do not listen to her. An occupational therapy evaluation revealed difficulties with bilateral coordination, motor planning, and VMI.	• Very shy, with a tendency to tear up or cry when confronted with a task she considers to be difficult. Her difficulty with motor planning and VMI affects her ability to initiate novel tasks in a timely manner. She has poor self-confidence. • Difficulty with shoe-tying and clothing fasteners. • Becomes anxious when she is in a busy environment (e.g., playground, cafeteria) with lots of movement. She is noted to "shut down," decreasing eye contact and not eating her lunch in the cafeteria. In the playground, she tends to sit by herself near the fence. She is also unwilling to try novel tasks.	• During the evaluation, Abby tells the OT that she feels "stupid" because she cannot tie her shoes. When asked about playing with her friends, Abby begins to cry and says she has no friends to play with. Abby wants to be an artist and an illustrator when she grows up. • The OT educates Abby and her family in techniques (e.g., deep pressure, heavy work activities, visual supports/schedules) to decrease anxiety and promote a feeling of calm and organization of self. • Activities and games promoting bilateral coordination, rhythm, sequencing, and problem-solving result in improved independence with clothing fasteners, handwriting, and VMI skills, as well as increased feelings of self-control and self-esteem. • As Abby becomes more successful in her academic and self-care tasks, she exhibits less anxiety when confronted with novel environments and tasks. When her anxiety increases, she is able to use learned techniques to calm herself and participate in the novel tasks (Ayres, 2005; Ben-Sasson, Carter, & Briggs-Gowan, 2009; Miller, 2006).
Donna, age 56, was initially referred for outpatient occupational therapy due to pain in both hands. Since being laid off 3 years ago from a clerical job, Donna has been relying on social assistance and receives routine medical care through a free health clinic to help manage her hypertension, thyroid disorder, and adult-onset diabetes. She also receives prescriptions for depression and anxiety. The clinic is designated as an FQHC. Donna has her own apartment but has been staying with her daughter to help care for her 2 grandchildren. Her daughter recently separated from her husband and had to take employment at minimum-wage jobs to support the family. Donna has also assumed many of her daughter's household management roles.	• Although Donna's reason for referral was to address the pain in her hands, it became apparent that many of the confounding factors that led to her referral were due to poor self-management and health maintenance. • During the initial evaluation, it is revealed that Donna has difficulties maintaining a steady routine for herself and her family. Donna often forgets to take her medications, and multiple days will elapse before she refills her medications. Her eating schedule is irregular, and her diet is generally unhealthy (e.g., high salt and sugar content) considering her medical diagnoses. In addition, Donna is mostly sedentary, fatigues easily, and has gained weight in the past 3 years, with a BMI increasing from 26 to 38. • Donna worries about her health and does not feel she is in control of her situation. She has been anxious about not being able to manage her roles well as caregiver/grandmother, a homemaker, and a caretaker.	• The OT and Donna, in collaboration with a Certified Diabetes Educator, discuss several self-management strategies (HHS, 2015), along with developing a routine for Donna and her grandchildren. Initial emphasis is on medication management and healthy eating patterns for herself and grandchildren to better manage her sugar and fatigue levels. Through social services, Donna is able to obtain free day care for her grandchildren to give her respite. • In collaboration with Donna's primary health care provider at the FQHC, a referral for EMG is made, which rules out CTS. Instead, Donna discovers she has diabetic neuropathy and realizes the link between managing her diabetes and hand pain. • Additional strategies include self-monitoring of blood sugar and pain levels throughout the day and implementing cardiovascular and flexibility exercises (Colberg et al., 2010) and pain management techniques to give Donna a better sense of control of her own health. • With better eating habits, activity patterns, and routinized medication management, Donna notices improved sleep and better pain control. Donna also reports feeling less anxious and has heightened energy levels to engage with her grandchildren and complete her daily household and self-care routines efficiently.

(Continued)

Table 1. Case Examples of Occupational Therapy Interventions With a Focus on Mental Health *(cont.)*

Case Example	Challenges to Occupational Performance and Mental Health	Occupational Therapy Interventions, With a Focus on Mental Health
Marta, age 25, has schizoaffective disorder. She lives with her mother, who is supportive but works 2 jobs to care for the family and is not able to spend much time with Marta. She has been going to the community mental health center once a month to see her psychiatrist.	• The OT uses the COPM (Law et al., 2014) to identify Marta's priorities in occupational performance. Marta is dissatisfied with her lack of productive and leisure occupations and feels isolated, bored, and lonely at home. • One of Marta's desired roles is to get a GED so that she can find a part-time job to help with home expenses. She feels responsible for her mother working so hard. She also wants to develop friendships and spend leisure time with people her own age. • Marta lacks self-confidence, stating she feels "stupid" and is unsure if she can accomplish her goals. She is anxious that other students will ask why she still lives with her mother and, because of the social stigma, is fearful of people finding out she has an SMI. She is sad at how her illness has taken away the life she planned (e.g., college, career, family). She expresses anxiety about navigating the college campus as well as signing up for classes. She is unsure what is involved in getting a GED and is worried she won't be able to do the homework, because concentrating is difficult, and medications make it hard for her to get up in the morning. Although she is interested in meeting people her own age, she doesn't know what to talk about with people she doesn't know. • Despite these fears, Marta has a positive attitude and is motivated to work toward her goals. She also has learned some coping strategies she has found to be helpful in dealing with stressful situations.	• Using active listening skills, the OT spends time talking to a tearful Marta about her fears and goals. To assist her as she works toward managing and adjusting to these chronic health issues, Marta is asked to complete a list of what she does well and what is difficult. Marta and the OT collaborate on setting priorities and weekly goals. The OT talks with Marta about how she has handled stressful situations in the past and asks her to identify successful strategies. • The OT facilitates involvement with the Disabilities Office at the community college, where she meets a peer specialist who shows her around the college and answers questions about the GED class. The OT and Marta obtain a copy of the course curriculum and work together to plan how Marta can structure her time at home to complete homework. They discuss her fears about meeting new people and identify conversational strategies she can use when in the classroom and on campus. They identify possible questions about her life that she might get from classmates and practice responses (Arbesman & Logsdon, 2011). • The OT advises Marta about how to connect with a NAMI group for young adults for further support. The OT continues to use the COPM on an ongoing basis to identify Marta's areas of improved performance and satisfaction and identify new goals.
Daniel, age 32, enlisted in the U.S. Marine Corps after graduating from college with a degree in mechanical engineering. His father is a retired colonel, and his brother is currently serving and is a first lieutenant. Daniel is assigned to the tank division and has had 2 deployments to Afghanistan and 1 to Iraq. During his last deployment, his group went under fire, tanks crossed land mines, and 35 lives were lost. Daniel suffered leg and pelvic fractures and amputation of his right arm and returned to the United States for rehabilitation. Daniel was committed to return to combat with his group.	• The OT gathers information about Daniel's past, present, and future perceptions of occupational performance related to roles and routines through the development of the occupational profile and occupational history. Also, the OT conducts biomechanical assessment of BUE strength, ROM, and dexterity of the LUE. Pain is assessed using a 10-point Likert scale. A physical inspection of the residual limb is performed. The OT completes the Epworth Sleepiness Scale (Johns, 1991). According to the results, Daniel is ambivalent about therapy and receiving a prosthetic limb. He relates that he is a disappointment to his family and to the Marines. He expresses guilt about surviving, stating that those who died had wives and children but he has nothing. He is unable to address the future, stating there are too many uncertainties.	• The OT and Daniel collaborate to identify goals, which include addressing sleep, routines, and participation in work exploration and social activities. The OT uses the collaborative mode of interaction to encourage Daniel to discuss his concerns. • The OT must first develop trust for Daniel to participate and share in rehabilitation. Because of Daniel's interest in physical fitness, the OT uses exercise as a means of building collaboration with him. Daniel provides input into his UE exercises and shares his prior knowledge and workouts with the OT. Daniel agrees to participate in a group with other persons with PTSD. The OT educates Daniel about evidence around sleep and rest. They discuss his sleep routines and strategies to promote healthy rest and sleep.

Table 1. Case Examples of Occupational Therapy Interventions With a Focus on Mental Health *(cont.)*

Case Example	Challenges to Occupational Performance and Mental Health	Occupational Therapy Interventions, With a Focus on Mental Health
During his treatment, Daniel begins drinking more and has increased thoughts of suicide. He drinks even more and tries to suppress feelings of guilt and fear, difficulty sleeping, loss of concentration, and irritability. He expresses feelings of deserting and of being a failure. Daniel is referred for psychiatric evaluation and is diagnosed with PTSD. He is currently a patient at the VA hospital and is undergoing UE prosthetic evaluation and training.	• The results of the biomechanical assessment are positive, and based on the biomechanical findings, Daniel has a good prognosis for functional use of the prosthetic limb. • Occupational areas presenting challenges are loss of worker role; rest and sleep; and social participation with family, friends, and community. Contributing client factors are his value of service and, decreased mental functions. Strengths that Daniel has are a good intellect, family and military family support, and a history of successful roles and routines.	• Using client-centered treatment, the OT and Daniel together plan each treatment session, addressing desensitizing his residual limb, residual limb dressing, exercises, rest and sleep, and planning for future work. • In rehabilitation, the OT suggests Daniel volunteer at a local children's hospital, sharing his mechanical skills teaching others about his passion of building with Legos®. He is now spending 2 days a week working with children at the Lego room.
Qasim, age 29, sustained an SCI in a diving accident 5 months ago. Qasim works as a carpenter specializing in roofing. He is a husband and the father of 2 young children. He has recently returned home after spending 3 months in a spinal cord rehabilitation facility.	• The OT gathers information about Qasim's psychosocial adjustment to his disability through the development of the occupational profile and occupational history. Additionally, the Moorong Self Efficacy Scale (Miller, 2009) is used to obtain information about self-efficacy. The Ways of Coping Questionnaire (Folkman & Lazarus, 1987) was also administered. • According to the results, Qasim is resentful about his disability status and fearful that the will not be able to function in his roles as father and husband. He is unsure of how, as a person with a disability, he will support himself and his family financially. • Qasim is experiencing feelings and concerns that are typical in individuals who are facing a permanent change in function due to a major injury (Pendleton & Schultz-Krohn, 2013). Because of his loss of body functions and roles as family supporter and worker, Qasim acknowledges that he is experiencing a diminished sense of self-concept and -confidence and a depressed and anxious mood. He does not desire to engage with others in social situations and expresses a sense of helplessness and hopelessness about the future. He is having difficulty communicating these concerns to family members or other health care professionals.	• The OT and Qasim collaborate to identify goals, which include addressing the areas of coping skills and stress management, social participation, sexuality, child care, and work. The OT offers Qasim the opportunity to express his concerns for his future roles and invites him to join a peer-run SCI support group. • The OT works with Qasim to explore previously successful strategies for coping with change and to modify them to meet the challenges of his new physical situation. Other activities such as making adaptations to his environment, setting realistic future goals, and planning and carrying out activities to rebuild his sense of self-efficacy and reshape his self-concept will be explored. One such activity might include planning and executing an afternoon outing with his 6-year-old daughter and wife. • The OT also works with Qasim to explore program offerings at the local community college and to set up appointments with the local vocational rehabilitation office and college disabilities counselors.
Ann, age 78 and a resident of the Parkside Manor congregate care facility, was transferred from the apartment where she had been living with assistance from her husband to the rehab floor for occupational therapy and physical therapy services following knee surgery. She was progressing well until her performance declined over the course of a couple of weeks.	• Markedly slowed movement with all functional mobility and ADL tasks. • Decreased engagement with her children and grandchildren when they visited. • Speech limited to monosyllabic responses to direct questions. • Flattened affect.	• In response to staff concerns that Ann might be showing early signs of some type of neurocognitive disorder, the OT administers the Montreal Cognitive Assessment (Nasreddine et al., 2005; Trzepacz, Hochstetler, Wang, Walker, & Saykin, 2015). Ann either does not respond or gives incomplete responses to all of the subtests until asked her location. Her prompt response is "the Parkside House of Terror and Tribulation."

(Continued)

Table 1. Case Examples of Occupational Therapy Interventions With a Focus on Mental Health *(cont.)*

Case Example	Challenges to Occupational Performance and Mental Health	Occupational Therapy Interventions, With a Focus on Mental Health
		• Given the speed and content of her answer, the OT suspects that depression, rather than dementia, might be underlying Ann's decline. Using empathy and active listening skills, the OT asks Ann about her mood, her understanding of her recovery from the surgery, and activities that were of particular importance to her. The OT determines that Ann believes she is not recovering well or quickly enough from the surgery and will never be allowed to return to live with her husband in their apartment. She describes mourning the loss of the activities they had done together and feeling sad that she would never be able to cook again for her family. She says that she has "given up." • The OT shares the assessment results with the rest of the team. A team meeting is held with the client and husband, at which it is clearly identified what would need to happen for Ann to go home, along with an anticipated discharge date. The OT incorporates cooking activities with foods that can be served to family members when they visit Ann's therapy sessions. Ann participates well in occupational and physical therapy, progresses as per the expected timeline, engages well in socialization activities on the unit with improved mood, and is discharged back to her apartment.
The **Positive Behavioral Support (PBS) Team at Weston Elementary School** received a high number of behavior referrals during the month of November. In reviewing the referral data, the team identifies a problem with aggressive behaviors occurring on the playground during lunch recess, especially among second- and third-grade students. The school OT volunteers to evaluate the recess environment by observing the second and third graders during lunch recess. Based on her observation, she identifies the following problems: limited playground equipment and activity options, unclear playground rules, and negative interactions between recess supervisors and students that focus on rule enforcement.	• The children who are engaging in aggressive behaviors have difficulty making and keeping friends; the friendships they have are often poor quality. • Several children have expressed being fearful about going to recess. • Some children limit their recess activities to avoid the aggressive children. • Teachers have noticed that students have been having difficulty calming down and focusing on classwork when returning to the classroom after recess.	• The OT works with the PBS Team to implement a schoolwide plan to address recess behaviors. The PBS Team schedules a staff meeting to review and revise the playground rules. The OT provides input on how to simplify the rules, use picture supports, and teach the rules using examples of appropriate playground behavior as well as examples of what would be considered inappropriate playground behavior (Upah, 2008). • The OT takes the lead in promoting and implementing "Refreshing Recess," a 6-week program designed to help staff create a positive recess environment (Mohler, Kearns, & Bazyk, 2014). The program is targeted at the second- and third-grade students during their recess time and includes weekly activities that foster inclusion and positive peer interactions as well as coaching for recess supervisors on how to support behavior and engage positively with students.

Table 1. Case Examples of Occupational Therapy Interventions With a Focus on Mental Health *(cont.)*

Case Example	Challenges to Occupational Performance and Mental Health	Occupational Therapy Interventions, With a Focus on Mental Health
Ronda, age 60, is a semiretired bookkeeper. She lives alone and cares for three cats. Ronda was admitted to the hospital as a result of worsening respiratory tract infection that did not respond to antibiotics. She was found to have emphysema and underwent abscess removal, but her condition worsened with multiorgan failure due to sepsis. She is transferred to critical care where she receives broad spectrum therapy and mechanical ventilation. Ronda is referred for rehabilitation as part of the early mobilization protocol.	• Throughout her hospital course, Ronda is made aware of her medical status to the extent she is cognitively able. It is noted that while in critical care, Ronda has had episodes of delirium. Upon her initial occupational therapy session, Ronda complains of feeling generally fatigued, sore and achy, and restrained by lines and tubes connected to her body. • Ronda experiences frequent disruption in her sleep due to routine medical and nursing procedures. Although she is oriented to her situation, she complains of being disoriented to time and has difficulties with short-term recall and sustained attention. She has had frequent thoughts of near-death experience and expresses feelings of uncertainty over her future.	• The OT initiates an orientation program, which includes visual reminders of the date, medication schedule, and the names of her providers. The OT also collaborates with the nursing staff to reinforce this approach and to provide timely information on expected medical procedures before discharge. • The OT and PT collaborate on establishing a routine for early active mobilization (Pohlman et al., 2010) as Ronda is weaned from mechanical ventilation. • During rounds, the OT advocates for mental health assessment. Results on the Intensive Care Psychological Assessment Tool (Wade et al., 2014) indicate that Ronda has had episodes of psychological distress. • To provide Ronda opportunities for engagement, the OT introduces the use of a tablet computer with apps for Ronda's favorite magazines, card games, and social media (e.g., Facebook, Instagram) featuring stories about and images of cats.

Note. ADLs = activities of daily living; BUE = bilateral upper extremity ; COPM = Canadian Occupational Performance Measure; CTS = carpal tunnel syndrome; EMG = electromyogram; FQHC = Federally Qualified Health Center; GED = general equivalency diploma; LUE = left upper extremity; NAMI = National Alliance on Mental Illness; OCD = obsessive–compulsive disorder; OT = occupational therapist; PBS = positive behavior support; PT = physical therapist; PTSD = posttraumatic stress disorder; ROM = range of motion; SCI = spinal cord injury; SMI = serious mental illness; UE = upper extremity; VA = Veterans Affairs; VMI = visual–motor impairment.

References

Accreditation Council for Occupational Therapy Education. (2012). 2011 Accreditation Council for Occupational Therapy Education (ACOTE®) standards. *American Journal of Occupational Therapy, 66,* S6–S74. http://dx.doi.org/10.5014/ajot.2012.66S6

American Occupational Therapy Association. (1997). The psychosocial core of occupational therapy position paper. *American Journal of Occupational Therapy, 51,* 868–869. http://dx.doi.org/10.5014/ajot.51.10.868

American Occupational Therapy Association. (2014a). Guidelines for supervision, roles, and responsibilities during the delivery of occupational therapy services. *American Journal of Occupational Therapy, 68*(Suppl. 3), S16–S22. http://dx.doi.org/10.5014/ajot.2014.686S03

American Occupational Therapy Association. (2014b). Occupational therapy practice framework: Domain and process (3rd ed.). *American Journal of Occupational Therapy, 68*(Suppl. 1), S1–S48. http://dx.doi.org/10.5014/ajot.2014.682006

American Occupational Therapy Association. (2015). Policy A.23. Categories of occupational therapy personnel. In *Policy Manual* (pp. 25–26). Bethesda, MD: Author.

Arbesman, M., & Logsdon, D. W. (2011). Occupational therapy interventions for employment and education for adults with serious mental illness: A systematic review. *American Journal of Occupational Therapy, 65,* 238–246. http://dx.doi.org/10.5014/ajot.2011.001289

Ayres, A. J. (2005). *Sensory integration and the child: Understanding hidden sensory challenges* (25th anniversary ed.). Los Angeles: Western Psychological Services.

Bandura, A. (1994). Self-efficacy. In V. S. Ramachaudran (Ed.), *Encyclopedia of human behavior* (Vol. 4, pp. 71–81). New York: Academic Press. (Reprinted in H. Friedman [Ed.], 1998, *Encyclopedia of mental health.* San Diego: Academic Press)

Ben-Sasson, A., Carter, A. S., & Briggs-Gowan, M. J. (2009). Prevalence and correlates of sensory overresponsivity from infancy to elementary school. *Journal of Abnormal Child Psychology, 37,* 705–716. http://dx.doi.org/10.1007/s10802-008-9295-8

Bonder, B. R. (1993). Issues in assessment of psychosocial components of function. *American Journal of Occupational Therapy, 47,* 211–216. http://dx.doi.org/10.5014/ajot.47.3.211

Bonder, B. (1997). Coping with psychological and emotional challenges. In C. Christiansen & C. Baum (Eds.), *Occupational therapy: Enabling function* (pp. 313–334). Thorofare, NJ: Slack.

Burnett, S. E. (2013). Personal and social contexts of disability: Implications for occupational therapists. In H. M. Pendleton & W. Schultz-Krohn (Eds.), *Pedretti's occupational therapy: Practice skills for physical dysfunction* (pp. 83–106). St. Louis, MO: Elsevier.

Christiansen, C., & Townsend, E. (2010). An introduction to occupation. In *Introduction to occupation: The art and science of living* (2nd ed., pp. 1–34). Upper Saddle River, NJ: Pearson.

Colberg, S. R., Sigal, R. J., Fernhall, B., Regensteiner, J. G., Blissmer, B. J., Rubin, R. R., . . . Braun, B.; American College of Sports Medicine; American Diabetes Association. (2010). Exercise and type 2 diabetes: The American College of Sports Medicine and the American Diabetes Association: Joint position statement. *Diabetes Care, 33,* e147–e167. http://dx.doi.org/10.2337/dc10-9990

Crist, P. (2011). Psychosocial concerns with disability. In C. Brown & V. C. Stoffel (Eds.), *Occupational therapy in mental health: A vision for participation* (pp. 47–56). Philadelphia: F. A. Davis.

Drench, M., Noonan, A., Sharby, N., & Ventura, S. (2011). *Psychosocial aspects of health care* (3rd ed.). Upper Saddle River, NJ: Pearson.

Egan, M., & Dubouloz, C. J. (2014). Practical foundations for practice: Planning, guiding, documenting, and reflecting. In M. V. Radomski & C. A. Trombly Latham (Eds.), *Occupational therapy for physical dysfunction* (7th ed., pp. 25–49). Baltimore: Lippincott Williams & Wilkins.

Folkman, S., & Lazarus, R. (1987). *The Ways of Coping Questionnaire.* Palo Alto, CA: Consulting Psychologists Press.

Graff, M. J., Vernooij-Dassen, M. J., Thijssen, M., Dekker, J., Hoefnagels, W. H., & Rikkert, M. G. (2006). Community based occupational therapy for patients with dementia and their care givers: Randomised controlled trial. *BMJ, 333,* 1196–1202. http://dx.doi.org/10.1136/bmj.39001.688843.BE

Hocking, C. (2014). Contributions of occupation to health and well-being. In B. A. B. Schell, G. Gillen, M. Scaffa, & E. S. Cohn (Eds.), *Willard and Spackman's occupational therapy* (12th ed., pp. 72–81). Baltimore: Lippincott Williams & Wilkins.

Johns, M. W. (1991). A new method for measuring daytime sleepiness: The Epworth Sleepiness Scale. *Sleep, 14,* 540–545.

Keyes, C. L. (2009). Toward a science of mental health. In C. R. Snyder & S. J. Lopez (Eds.), *Handbook of positive psychology* (2nd ed., pp. 89–96). New York: Oxford University Press.

Kielhofner, G. (Ed.). (2009). *Conceptual foundations of occupational therapy* (4th ed.). Philadelphia: F. A. Davis.

Law, M., Baptiste, S., Carswell, A., McColl, M. A., Polatajko, H., & Pollock, N. (2014). *Canadian Occupational Performance Measure* (5th ed.). Ottawa: CAOT Publications.

Livneh, H., & Antonak, R. (2005). Psychosocial adaptation to chronic illness and disability: A primer for counselors. *Journal of Counseling and Development, 83,* 12–20. http://dx.doi.org/10.1002/j.1556-6678.2005.tb00575.x

Meyer, A. (1922). The philosophy of occupational therapy. *Archives of Occupational Therapy, 1,* 1–10.

Miller, L. J. (2006). *Sensational kids: Hope and help for children with sensory processing disorder (SPD).* New York: Penguin Books.

Miller, S. M. (2009). The measurement of self-efficacy in persons with spinal cord injury: Psychometric validation of the Moorong Self-Efficacy Scale. *Disability and Rehabilitation, 31,* 988–993. http://dx.doi.org/10.1080/09638280802378025

Mohler, R., Kearns, S., & Bazyk, S. (2014). *Refreshing Recess Program: A model program for Every Moment Counts.* Washington, DC: U.S. Department of Education, Office of Special Education Programs.

Mosey, A. (1996). *Psychosocial components of occupational therapy.* Philadelphia: Lippincott-Raven.

Nasreddine, Z. S., Phillips, N. A., Bédirian, V., Charbonneau, S., Whitehead, V., Collin, I., . . . Chertkow, H. (2005). The Montreal Cognitive Assessment, MoCA: A brief screening tool for mild cognitive impairment. *Journal of the American Geriatrics Society, 53,* 695–699. http://dx.doi.org/10.1111/j.1532-5415.2005.53221.x

Nilsson, I., & Townsend, E. (2010). Occupational justice—Bridging theory and practice. *Scandinavian Journal of Occupational Therapy, 17,* 57–63. http://dx.doi.org/10.3109/11038120903287182

Pendleton, H. M., & Schultz-Krohn, W. (2013). Psychosocial issues in physical disability. In E. Cara & A. MacRae (Eds.), *Psychosocial occupational therapy: An evolving practice* (3rd ed., pp. 501–540). Clifton Park, NY: Delmar Cengage Learning.

Pohlman, M. C., Schweickert, W. D., Pohlman, A. S., Nigos, C., Pawlik, A. J., Esbrook, C. L., . . . Kress, J. P. (2010). Feasibility of physical and occupational therapy beginning from initiation of mechanical ventilation. *Critical Care Medicine, 38,* 2089–2094. http://dx.doi.org/10.1097/ccm.0b013e3181f270c3

Reilly, M. (1962). Occupational therapy can be one of the great ideas of 20th century medicine. *American Journal of Occupational Therapy, 16,* 1–9.

Schell, B. A., & Schell, J. W. (Eds.). (2008). *Clinical and professional reasoning in occupational therapy.* Baltimore: Lippincott Williams & Wilkins.

Slagle, E. C. (1924). A year's development of occupational therapy in New York state hospitals. *Modern Hospital, 11,* 98–104.

Taylor, R. (2008). *The intentional relationship: Occupational therapy and use of self.* Philadelphia: F. A. Davis.

Taylor, R. R., & Van Puymbroeck, L. (2013). Therapeutic use of self: Applying the intentional relationship model in group therapy. In J. C. O'Brien & J. W. Solomon (Eds.), *Occupational analysis and group process* (pp. 36–52). St. Louis, MO: Elsevier.

Trzepacz, P. T., Hochstetler, H., Wang, S., Walker, B., & Saykin, A. J.; Alzheimer's Disease Neuroimaging Initiative. (2015). Relationship between the Montreal Cognitive Assessment and Mini-Mental State Examination for assessment of mild cognitive impairment in older adults. *BMC Geriatrics, 15,* 107. http://dx.doi.org/10.1186/s12877-015-0103-3

U.S. Department of Health and Human Services. (2015). *AoA diabetes self management (DSMT) toolkit.* Retrieved June 1, 2015, from http://www.aoa.acl.gov/AoA_Programs/HPW/Diabetes/docs/AoA-DSMT-Toolkit-2015.pdf

U.S. Department of Health and Human Services. (2016). Mental health. In *Healthy people 2020.* Washington, DC: Author. Retrieved from https://www.healthypeople.gov/2020/topics-objectives/topic/mental-health-and-mental-disorders

Upah, K. R. F. (2008). Best practices in designing, implementing, and evaluating quality interventions. In A. Thomas & J. Grimes (Eds.), *Best practices in school psychology* (Vol. V, pp. 209–223). Bethesda, MD: National Association of School Psychologists.

Wade, D. M., Hankins, M., Smyth, D. A., Rhone, E. E., Mythen, M. G., Howell, D. C., & Weinman, J. A. (2014). Detecting acute distress and risk of future psychological morbidity in critically ill patients: Validation of the Intensive Care Psychological Assessment Tool. *Critical Care, 18,* 519–527. http://dx.doi.org/10.1186/s13054-014-0519-8

World Health Organization. (2001). *International classification of functioning, disability and health.* Geneva: Author.

World Health Organization. (2004). *Promoting mental health: Concepts, emerging evidence, practice* [Summary report]. Geneva: Author.

Yerxa, E. (1967). Authentic occupational therapy (Eleanor Clarke Slagle Lecture). *American Journal of Occupational Therapy, 21,* 1–9.

Additional Resources

American Occupational Therapy Association. (n.d.). *Children and youth mental health.* Retrieved from http://www.aota.org/Practice/Children-Youth/Mental%20Health.aspx

American Psychiatric Association. (2013). *Diagnostic and statistical manual of mental disorders* (5th ed.). Washington, DC: Author.

Authors

Kathleen Kannenberg, MA, OTR/L, CCM
Deborah Amini, EdD, OTR/L, CHT
Kimberly Hartmann, PhD, OTR/L, FAOTA

for

The Commission on Practice
Janet DeLany, DEd, OTR/L, FAOTA, *Chairperson, 2008–2011*

Revised by the Commission on Practice, 2015

Kathleen Kannenberg, MA, OTR/L, CCM, *Chairperson*

Adopted by the Representative Assembly Coordinating Council (RACC) for the Representative Assembly 2015

The Philosophical Base of Occupational Therapy

Occupations are activities that bring meaning to the daily lives of individuals, families, and communities and enable them to participate in society. All individuals have an innate need and right to engage in meaningful occupations throughout their lives. Participation in these occupations influences their development, health, and well-being across the lifespan. As such, participation in meaningful occupation is a determinant of health.

Occupations occur within diverse social, physical, cultural, personal, temporal, or virtual contexts. The quality of occupational performance and the experience of each occupation are unique in each situation due to the dynamic relationship between factors intrinsic to the individual, the contexts in which the occupation occurs, and the characteristics of the activity.

The focus and outcome of occupational therapy are individuals' engagement in meaningful occupations that support their participation in life situations. Occupational therapy practitioners conceptualize occupations as both a means and an end to therapy. That is, there is therapeutic value in occupational engagement as a change agent, and engagement in occupations is also the ultimate goal of therapy.

Occupational therapy is based on the belief that occupations may be used for health promotion and wellness, remediation or restoration, health maintenance, disease and injury prevention, and compensation/adaptation. The use of occupation to promote individual, community, and population health is the core of occupational therapy practice, education, research, and advocacy.

Authors

The Commission on Education:

Jyothi Gupta, PhD, OTR/L, OT(C), *Chairperson*
Andrea R. Bilics, PhD, OTR/L, FAOTA
Donna M. Costa, DHS, OTR/L, FAOTA
Debra J. Hanson, PhD, OTR
Mallory Duncan, *ASD Liaison* (ASD)
Susan M. Higgins, MA, OTR/L
Linda Orr, MPA, OTR/L
Diane Parham, PhD, OTR/L, FAOTA
Jeff Snodgrass, PhD, MPH, OTR, CWCE
Neil Harvison, PhD, OTR/L, FAOTA, *AOTA Staff Liaison*

Adopted by the Representative Assembly

Revised by the Commission on Education 2011

Reviewed by the Commission on Education and the Commission on Practice 2004

Note. This revision replaces the 1979 document *The Philosophical Base of Occupational Therapy,* previously published and copyrighted in 1995 by the American Occupational Therapy Association in the *American Journal of Occupational Therapy, 49,* 1026.

Philosophy of Occupational Therapy Education

Preamble

Occupational therapy education prepares occupational therapy practitioners to address the occupational needs of individuals, groups, communities, and populations. The education process includes academic and fieldwork components. The philosophy of occupational therapy education parallels the philosophy of occupational therapy yet remains distinctly concerned with beliefs about knowledge, learning, and teaching.

What are the fundamental beliefs of occupational therapy education?

Students are viewed as occupational beings who are in dynamic transaction with the learning context and the teaching–learning process. The learning context includes the curriculum and pedagogy and conveys a perspective and belief system that includes a view of humans as occupational beings, occupation as a health determinant, and participation as a fundamental right. Education promotes clinical reasoning and the integration of professional values, theories, evidence, ethics, and skills. This approach will prepare practitioners to collaborate with clients to achieve health, well-being, and participation in life through engagement in occupation (American Occupational Therapy Association, 2014). Occupational therapy education is the process by which practitioners acquire their professional identity.

What are the values within occupational therapy education?

Enacting the above beliefs to facilitate the development of a sound reasoning process that is client centered, occupation based, and theory driven while encouraging the use of best evidence and outcomes data to inform the teaching learning experience may include supporting

- Active and diverse learning within and beyond the classroom environment;

- A collaborative process that builds on prior knowledge and experience;

- Continuous professional judgment, evaluation, and self-reflection; and

- Lifelong learning.

Reference

American Occupational Therapy Association. (2014). Occupational therapy practice framework: Domain and process (3rd ed.). *American Journal of Occupational Therapy, 68*(Suppl. 1), S1–S48. http://dx.doi.org/10.5014/ajot.2014.682006

The Commission on Education
Andrea Bilics, PhD, OTR/L, FAOTA, *Chairperson*
Tina DeAngelis, EdD, OTR/L
Jamie Geraci, MS, OTR/L
Julie McLaughlin Gray, PhD, OTR/L

Michael Iwama, PhD, OT(c)
Julie Kugel, OTD, MOT, OTR/L
Kate McWilliams
Maureen S. Nardella, MS, OTR/L
Renee Ortega, MA, COTA
Kim Qualls, MS, OTR/L
Tamra Trenary, OTD, OTR/L, BCPR
Neil Harvison, PhD, OTR/L, FAOTA, *AOTA Headquarters Liaison*

Adopted by the Representative Assembly 2014NovCO49

Note. This revision replaces the 2007 document *Philosophy of Occupational Therapy Education,* previously published and copyrighted in 2007 by the American Occupational Therapy Association in the *American Journal of Occupational Therapy, 61,* 678. http://dx.doi.org/10.5014/ajot.61.6.678

Citation. American Occupational Therapy Association. (2015). Philosophy of occupational therapy education. *American Journal of Occupational Therapy, 69*(Suppl. 3), 6913410052. http://dx.doi.org/10.5014/ajot.2015.696S17

The Role of Occupational Therapy in End-of-Life Care

The purpose of this statement is to describe the role of occupational therapists and occupational therapy assistants in providing services to clients who are living with chronic or terminal conditions and are at the end of life. It also serves as a resource for occupational therapy practitioners,[1] hospice and palliative care programs, policymakers, funding sources, and clients and caregivers who receive hospice and palliative care services. Occupational therapy practitioners provide skilled intervention to improve quality of life by facilitating engagement in daily life occupations throughout the entire life course. Participation in meaningful life occupations continues to be as important at the end of life as it is at earlier stages. The term *end-of life care* has replaced the term *terminal care* and encompasses both hospice and palliative care that can occur during the final stages of life.

Hospice

The contemporary definition of *hospice* encompasses a philosophy of care for individuals of any age with life-limiting illnesses for whom further curative measures are no longer desired or appropriate. Hospice referrals require that the client have a life expectancy of 6 months or less with the usual course of the diagnosis (Centers for Medicare and Medicaid Services, 2010). Hospice care focuses on symptom control and meeting the emotional, social, spiritual, and functional needs of the client and family. As an example, the *Medicare Benefit Policy Manual* states that "Physical therapy, occupational therapy, and speech–language pathology services may be provided for purposes of symptom control or to enable the individual to maintain activities of daily living and basic functional skills."

Reimbursement for hospice care may be provided by a variety of medical insurers, including Medicare, Medicaid, and private insurance. Some hospice organizations receive funds from grants and private donations that are used to cover services. Local civic, charitable, or religious organizations also may provide funding to help patients and their families with hospice expenses.

The basic philosophy of hospice is described in the *Standards of Practice for Hospice Programs* (National Hospice and Palliative Care Organization, 2002):

> Hospice provides support and care for persons in the last phases of incurable disease so that they may live as fully and as comfortably as possible. Hospice recognizes that the dying process is a part of the normal process of living and focuses on enhancing the quality of remaining life. Hospice affirms life and neither hastens nor postpones death. Hospice exists in the hope and belief that, through appropriate care and the promotion of a caring community sensitive to their needs, individuals and their families may be free to attain a degree of satisfaction in preparation for death. Hospice recognizes that human growth and development can be a lifelong process. Hospice seeks to preserve and promote the inherent potential for growth within individuals and families without regard to age, gender, nationality, race, creed, sexual orientation, disability, diagnosis, availability of a primary caregiver, or ability to pay. (p. ii)

---

[1]When the term *occupational therapy practitioner* is used in this document, it refers to both occupational therapists and occupational therapy assistants (AOTA, 2006). *Occupational therapists* are responsible for all aspects of occupational therapy service delivery and are accountable for the safety and effectiveness of the occupational therapy service delivery process. *Occupational therapy assistants* deliver occupational therapy services under the supervision of and in partnership with an occupational therapist (AOTA, 2009).

Palliative Care

Hospice and palliative care are closely related. Both approaches are directed toward providing intervention services to those with life-threatening illnesses. Palliative care differs from hospice care in that it can be initiated at any point in the course of the client's illness. Curative care interventions also may be used within the context of palliative approach, whereas curative services are not provided when a client is receiving hospice care. A client receiving palliative and curative services simultaneously may transition to a hospice service when curative therapies are no longer appropriate or desired and the end of life is more imminent. The World Health Organization (2002) defines *palliative care* as

> An approach that improves the quality of life of patients and their families facing the problem associated with life-threatening illness, through the prevention and relief of suffering by means of early identification and impeccable assessment and treatment of pain and other problems, physical, psychosocial, and spiritual.

Care Settings

End-of-life care may take place in a variety of settings, depending on the client's need and situation. Many individuals served by hospice organizations are seen in their homes (Marrelli, 2005). Hospice care also may be provided in freestanding community in-patient facilities and in specified units or beds within a skilled nursing facility or hospital. Some home health care agencies also provide hospice services staffed by designated hospice care providers.

Hospice teams are interdisciplinary. In addition to occupational therapy practitioners, teams include counselors, clergypersons, and volunteers, as well as physicians, nurses, social workers, dieticians, physical therapists, and speech–language pathologists.

Role of Occupational Therapy

Individuals with life-threatening and life-limiting illness often have difficulty participating in daily occupations because of decline in their motor, sensory, emotional, cognitive, or communication skills. Occupational therapy practitioners help clients find relief from pain and suffering and improve their quality of life by supporting their engagement in daily life occupations that clients find meaningful and purposeful. The occupational therapy practitioner considers environmental and contextual factors (e.g., caregiver training, accessibility of objects or places in the environment, social contacts available to prevent isolation), as well as personal factors (e.g., decreased endurance, increased anxiety) that may be limiting a client's abilities and satisfaction when performing desired occupations. The occupational therapy practitioner collaborates with the client and family members throughout the occupational therapy process to identify occupations that are especially meaningful and to incorporate strategies that support occupational engagement. As Kaye (2006) points out in *Notes on Symptom Control in Hospice and Palliative Care*, "Loss of independence and role can result in social death prior to biological death. Occupational therapy can help a person to adopt new and appropriate functions and roles and to maintain self-esteem" (p. 214).

Quality of Life at the End of Life

Improved quality of life is a primary outcome of all occupational therapy interventions (AOTA, 2008). Occupational therapy practitioners believe that engaging in occupations underlies health and quality of life. At the end of life when clients often face loss of previously established occupational roles, occupations, and performance abilities, their need to identify and sustain meaningful engagement is heightened. Family members and professionals alike may find it difficult to comprehend the diminution of life quality when illness interferes with abilities to carry out familiar occupations. The pleasure and sense of self-worth inherent in participating in familiar occupations, even those as basic as making a cup of coffee at the time one wants to have a cup of coffee, is immeasurable. The value lies not so much in the cup of coffee, which can be provided by someone else, but in having control over choosing when to have the coffee and perhaps making the coffee when desired.

Numerous researchers have examined how persons at the end of life view their quality of life and quality of care. Many of these research studies have identified factors that affect quality of life and quality of care that are similar to the factors that occupational therapy practitioners address during their interventions (see Table 1).

Research to Support Practice

Although occupational therapy practice with clients at the end of life is not new, evidence that supports this area of practice is less well developed. Since the 1970s, occupational therapists have investigated and described how occupational therapy practitioners provide services to clients at this life stage (Bye, 1998; Picard & Magno, 1982; Pizzi, 1984; Pizzi & Briggs, 2004; Rahman, 2000; Tiggs & Sherman, 1983). These studies have pointed out occupational therapy's role in supporting the individual's quality of life by facilitating role performance and function in desired occupations, competence, control, and coping

Table 1. Factors Influencing Quality of Life and Quality of Care at the End of Life

Factor	Relationship to Occupational Therapy	References
Maintaining functioning and involvement in desired life activities contributes to quality of life.	Occupational therapy practitioners believe that continuing to engage in occupations allows a person to continue his or her life—and is central to health and quality of life. Modifying previous occupations so that they can still be performed and adding new occupations to replace lost ones prevents isolation, a common experience at the end of life, and contributes to the sustainment of self-worth.	Arnold, Artin, Griffith, Person, & Graham, 2006; Egan & DeLaat, 1997; Gourdjii, McVey, & Purden, 2009; Jacques & Hasselkus, 2004; Lyons, Orozovic, Davis, & Newman, 2002; Ryan, 2005
Maintaining a sense of control contributes to quality of life.	By participating in daily life occupations that they value as purposeful and meaningful, individuals make choices that give them a sense of control, identity, and competence.	Christiansen, 1999; Egan & DeLaat, 1997; Singer, Martin, & Kelner, 1999; Vrkljan & Miller-Polgar, 2001
Continuing to contribute to others and staying connected to important relationships contributes to quality of life.	Engaging individuals in tasks and activities is a central focus of the occupational therapy intervention process. Completing tasks such as writing letters to grandchildren or recording favorite recipes within an individual's social context allows a person to feel productive and to strengthen social relationships.	Enes, 2003; Gourdji et al., 2009; Hunter, 2008; Lyons et al., 2002; Singer et al., 1999; Steinhauser et al., 2000
Continuing to search for meaning and purpose in life and one's relationship to a higher being also is referred to as *spirituality*.	Occupational therapy practitioners recognize spirituality as an important client factor. They believe that the process of engaging in occupations helps the person connect to the meaning and purpose in life, which enhances spiritual well-being, quality of life, and ability to cope. Engaging in occupations can counteract feelings of hopelessness, helplessness, and uselessness that may develop during the end of life. Occupational therapy practitioners help individuals identify meaningful occupations in which they want to engage and teach coping strategies that allow continued participation.	AOTA, 2008; Chochinov & Cann, 2005; Egan & DeLaat, 1997; Lin & Bauer-Wu, 2003; Pizzi & Briggs, 2004; Prince-Paul, 2008; Unruh, Smith, & Scammell, 2000

to assist the person in bringing closure to his or her life. Several phenomenological studies conducted by occupational therapists have elucidated how occupations contribute to living at the end of life and how individuals at the end of life describe the benefits of engaging in daily life occupations (Lyons et al., 2002; Unruh et al., 2000).

The validity of specific interventions that occupational therapy practitioners may use is beginning to be investigated. La Cour, Josephsson, and Luborsky (2005) and La Cour, Josephsson, Tishelman, and Nygård (2007) have explored the effects of using creative activities with clients who have life-threatening illnesses. In both studies, the researchers found that participation in creative activities allowed clients to cope with declining abilities and to create connections to life. Clients reported an improved existential awareness of their past, their present, and possible future.

Hunter (2008) further explored the ideas of existential meaning, which people at the end of life confront. She explored the responses of 38 women to understand how they defined legacy and its importance in their lives. She found that legacy is closely related to transmitting one's sense of who they are to others. Legacy transmission can be effected by transmitting actions (behaviors) as well as artifacts (concrete items). In either case, these legacies are closely connected to the occupations and occupational identities that people develop throughout their life. Occupational therapy practitioners who are sensitive to the client's occupational profile and identity can facilitate the client's ability to identify and transmit purposeful legacies.

Effectiveness of palliative care programs also is beginning to be documented. Several studies have reported on how outpatient palliative rehabilitation programs, palliative day care programs, and inpatient palliative care units have improved patient satisfaction, functional performance, emotional well-being, and symptoms (Cohen, Boston, Mount, & Porterfield, 2001; Hospital Case Management, 2003; Strasser et al., 2004; Svidön, Fürst, von Koch, & Borell, 2009). In two of these studies (Hospital Case Management, 2003; Strasser et al., 2004), an occupational therapist was specifically mentioned as a member of the team.

Saarik and Hartley (2010) reported on a 4-week fatigue management program in Britain carried out by an occupational therapist and a physiotherapist specializing in palliative care. The program was delivered in a hospice day care program with patients with cancer. Clients who completed the program reported decreased fatigue levels, overall improved functioning, and enhanced ability to cope.

Occupational therapy practitioners have recognized the need to provide evidence that supports the profession's contribution to quality of life at the end of life. Pearson, Todd, and Futcher (2007) have proposed that occupational therapy practitioners use a quality of life measure during their evaluations to measure the effectiveness of occupational therapy interventions in palliative care practice. They identified 24 possible tools and plan to evaluate them further for application by occupational therapists.

Occupational Therapy Process

Evaluation

A client may be referred for occupational therapy at any point during the end-of-life process. Any health care provider may identify the need for occupational therapy.

The occupational therapist begins the evaluation process by conducting an occupational profile. The occupational therapist gathers information for the profile by talking to the client to gain an understanding of meaningful and relevant occupations, daily routines, interests, values, and priorities, as well as the client's view of life and expectations of dying. Interviewing caregivers, including family or significant others, to determine their priorities and concerns is important, especially when the client is unable to express his or her desires and wishes pertaining to end-of-life care. The interview also examines cultural, spiritual, and social factors that influence a client's expectations for the end of life.

This client-centered approach enables the occupational therapy practitioner to establish a relationship that facilitates discussion of important occupational areas. For example, the client may prefer to be dressed by the caregiver to save energy to tape stories to share with his or her grandchild.

On the basis of these priorities and concerns, the occupational therapist may specifically assess and analyze the client's or caregivers' performance skills in the desired activities and roles. Although clients receiving hospice or palliative care services may have declining performance skills, the occupational therapist assesses strengths and capacities that can support continued performance of desired occupations. The occupational therapist analyzes the demands of activities important to the client and the supports and barriers of the context or environment as they affect outcomes. The evaluation also may include assessment of caregivers' skills and need for skill training and support, as well as identification of the adaptive or compensatory strategies needed to carry out task performance and/or the environmental modifications that need to be implemented to support the client's skills and capabilities. Identification of the client's needs and wishes, combined with analysis of the client's performance capacities, allows the occupational therapist to identify effective and client-centered occupational therapy interventions, which are then incorporated into the interdisciplinary plan of care.

Intervention

The occupational therapist develops an intervention plan in collaboration with the client and the caregivers. The intervention plan identifies the outcomes of intervention and the approaches to be used. Occupational therapy interventions are targeted toward creating a fit between the client's and caregivers' capabilities and the demands of the activities that are important to the client and caregivers. Intervention may be provided directly to the client or the caregivers or family members. Intervention directed toward caregivers frequently consists of education and consultation to support efficacy and satisfaction with the care they provide. Interventions chosen will depend on the client's needs and desires and medical status at the time of referral. For example, a client with cancer who is alert and aware of his or her surroundings but dealing with issues of pain management, symptom control, and loss of occupational roles and relationships will face different challenges than a client who is referred in the later stages of Alzheimer's disease who is cognitively disoriented but is experiencing little pain. In the latter situation, intervention may more appropriately be directed at numerous challenges facing caregivers, such as instruction in managing behaviors and safety precautions.

Interventions for the client may focus on relieving symptoms that interfere with function. For example, if pain or shortness of breath is limiting function, repositioning to a supported sitting position in bed may relieve pain and improve breathing, enabling the client to write letters. Engaging in meaningful occupations not only improves quality of life but also can serve as an important tool for symptom management. Clients whose attention is focused on meaningful occupations pay less attention to physical symptoms.

Approaches most commonly used by occupational therapy at the end of life are compensation, adaptation, and preservation of existing capacities. Occupational therapy practitioners focus on modifying the demands of activities or the habits and routines associated with the occupations to match the client's or caregiver's performance skills, tolerances, and capacities. Occupational therapy practitioners also use interventions targeted toward minimizing barriers to performance.

Ongoing review of occupational therapy interventions is critical in evaluating effectiveness and progress toward targeted outcomes. Because clients may experience sudden and sometimes unexpected changes, interventions may have to be modified significantly as the client's status changes. Progress also is defined by the nature of care. Acceptance and improved quality of life is progress, even as a client's body systems and performance skills decline. Occupational therapy services may be appropriate at different points during the course of hospice and palliative care for a given client as that client's needs, priorities, and abilities change over time.

Outcomes

The ultimate outcome of end-of-life care is supporting or improving the client's and family's quality of life. The following case examples (Table 2) illustrate how occupational therapy intervention may be provided to address different needs and priorities for clients, caregivers, and families that contribute to quality of life.

Table 2. Case Examples

Case Description	Occupational Therapy Interventions	Outcomes
Gertrude, an 80-year-old grandmother with 11 supportive grandchildren, moved into a hospice facility after a significant decline in her physical status. The hospice team was concerned about her refusal to follow the pain medication regime and requested an occupational therapy referral to address strategies for pain management.	After talking to Gertrude, the occupational therapist determined that Gertrude avoided taking her pain medication because she was afraid of having slurred speech and being confused and lethargic, symptoms that might frighten her grandchildren when they visited. Although without pain medications she was alert when her grandchildren visited, her pain limited her ability to enjoy these visits or to participate in other activities that were important to her. The occupational therapist recommended changes in Gertrude's daily routines to accommodate her desired roles, meaningful occupations, and pain management needs. The occupational therapist facilitated the collaboration of the hospice team. Together, they worked with Gertrude and her family to develop a modified visitation and medication schedule so that family visits were not occurring at times when the medication's effects on Gertrude's alertness were most intense.	With her anxiety about frightening her grandchildren lessened, Gertrude was more agreeable to taking her medications regularly. The resulting effective management of her pain allowed her to increase involvement in valued occupations and to maintain her role as a loving grandmother.
Gustavo, a man in his 50s, had several metastatic tumors, including one recently removed from his right shoulder. Gustavo was ambulatory, and although he did not have any active right shoulder movement, he was able to complete basic self-care and was to be discharged to his home with hospice care. Gustavo expressed discouragement at his inability to complete two meaningful projects at home: a mural on the living room wall and a wooden boat he was building.	The occupational therapist worked with Gustavo on fatigue management, ergonomics, pacing, and setting priorities for activities. Strategies included positioning his right arm on a leaning pole to act as a support while completing the mural. Adaptive techniques for building the boat included having his nephew work as an apprentice to help with the heavy tasks while Gustavo passed on his boat-building skills.	Gustavo now looked forward to going home, "because I'm not going home to die, I'm going back to my art."
Asuka, a 60-year-old woman from Japan, had difficulty expressing her desires even with the support of an interpreter. She appeared depressed and usually stayed in her room sleeping with the lights off rather than visiting with her daughters when they arrived at the facility.	The occupational therapist met with Asuka's daughters to identify any meaningful activities that she had done in the past. Her daughters identified origami as a valued family activity that their mother used to enjoy. The occupational therapist encouraged the daughters to bring in origami supplies and to work on this activity even though their mother did not respond. As the daughters struggled to remember how to fold the paper to look like a crane, they began laughing. Their laughter woke Asuka, who sat up, asked to have the lights turned on, took the paper from them, and demonstrated how to create an origami crane.	Engagement in this activity allowed Asuka to resume the role of mother and teacher of activities that she valued as culturally significant. She went on to draw each child's name in Japanese calligraphy. This generated increased family interactions and provided meaningful time together.

Table 2. Case Examples *(cont.)*

Case Description	Occupational Therapy Interventions	Outcomes
Dmitri resided in an assisted living facility (ALF) with his wife of 52 years. When Dmitri's health condition was considered terminal, he elected to receive hospice care. Dmitri, his wife, and the hospice team were concerned that, as his abilities declined, his need for assistance might exceed the level permitted for him to remain in the ALF. Care provided by professionals or paraprofessionals was limited to a specific number of hours per week for Dmitri to remain in the ALF, but care provided by his wife was not included in this limit. During the initial occupational therapy encounter, it became evident that Dmitri's concern was not to burden his wife with his increasing needs for assistance.	The occupational therapy practitioner implemented an intervention plan that involved both Dmitri and his wife. Instructions were provided regarding techniques for completing activities of daily living—bathing, dressing, and toileting—as well as assuring both Dmitri and his wife's safety. Planning with his family to address his continued physical decline included introducing adaptive equipment and modifications to the home, which reduced the demands of important activities and made them manageable for Dmitri and his wife. His environment was adapted to allow him to continue to participate in his long-standing weekly poker party and to maintain his role as a vital and active member in the ALF.	Dmitri was able to stay in his ALF home environment without the need of additional staff time. His wife was able to care for him effectively, and he was able to maintain his roles as husband and community member during his last days as a result of these interventions.
Fatima wanted to maintain her role as a mother despite being diagnosed with terminal cancer. Because Fatima had two small children, a referral was made to occupational therapy to identify strategies for her to participate in caring for her children and engaging in other occupations related to being a mother.	The occupational therapist provided services to both Fatima and her husband. The occupational therapist recommended positioning techniques to allow Fatima to hold and feed her toddler. Other interventions focused on strategies so that she could bathe her toddler, assist her older daughter with picking out clothes for school, and participate in family outings. The occupational therapy assistant worked with Fatima to write letters and make video recordings and other remembrances so that she would be able to leave something for each of her children as they went through milestones of life, such as high school graduation, entering college, marriage, and the birth of a child.	This occupational therapy intervention supported Fatima's desire to maintain her role as mother until her death and then to leave something behind so that she would still be a presence in the lives of her children.
Peter was a 5-year-old boy who received hospice care. Both of his parents and two older siblings lived with Peter and were involved in his care. Occupational therapy was included in the hospice plan of care to maintain Peter's ability to play and engage socially with his family despite declining physical and cognitive abilities.	The occupational therapy practitioner involved both Peter and his family in interventions, which included modifications for current games and activities that Peter enjoyed and appropriate positioning strategies to support his participation.	Peter was able to successfully maintain his ability to engage in play and family interaction even as his condition deteriorated.
Ethel, an older woman with cancer, lived with her husband. When her cancer metastasized, Ethel made the decision to terminate planned interventions and to elect hospice care. Initially, Ethel's ability to engage in daily routines and roles was unchanged, but she gradually experienced significant fatigue and had difficulty performing valued activities, such as cooking and cleaning her house.	The occupational therapy practitioner taught Ethel how to use energy conservation strategies to reduce fatigue and accommodate her limited tolerance while continuing to perform household tasks. As Ethel's disease progressed and her ability to perform these occupations declined, interventions focused on interdependence by using modifications to activities that she and her husband could do together.	Ethel still could participate actively in valued activities such as planning meals and helping her husband prepare a grocery list, while her husband completed components of the activities to reduce stress and fatigue. At all stages the occupational therapist worked with Ethel to help her to begin to plan for her death. Occupational therapy interventions involved occupations such as passing on recipes to family members, teaching family members how to make specific foods and recipes, and bequeathing a favorite cooking utensil to a particular family member.

Summary

Occupational therapy practitioners are an important part of hospice and palliative care teams as direct care providers and consultants. Occupational therapy practitioners educate other team members on the meaning and importance of occupation in a person's life and in the dying process. An occupational therapy practitioner's deep understanding of the meaning of occupation makes a powerful contribution to the process of caring for the dying person.

To this end, occupational therapy practitioners function across the continuum of end-of-life care to help support the roles of the client with terminal illness. Although a client's body systems and skills may deteriorate, occupational therapy interventions can support the client's ability to maintain important roles and relationships and to engage in the occupations related to those roles. Having choices and being able to participate in daily activities of self-care can support a sense of self-efficacy and control during the dying process. Continuation of important rituals of everyday activity can support meaningfulness in the dying person's final days (Thompson, 1991).

References

American Occupational Therapy Association. (2006). Policy 1.44: Categories of occupational therapy personnel. In *Policy manual* (2009 ed.). Bethesda, MD: Author.

American Occupational Therapy Association. (2008). Occupational therapy practice framework: Domain and process (2nd ed.). *American Journal of Occupational Therapy, 62*(6), 625–683.

American Occupational Therapy Association. (2009). Guidelines for supervision, roles, and responsibilities during the delivery of occupational therapy services. *American Journal of Occupational Therapy, 63*(6), 797–803.

Arnold, E. M., Artin, K. A., Griffith, D., Person, J. L., & Graham, K. G. (2006). Unmet needs at the end of life: Perceptions of hospice social workers. *Journal of Social Work End-of-Life Palliative Care, 2*(4), 61–83.

Bye, R. A. (1998). When clients are dying: Occupational therapists' perspectives. *Occupational Therapy Journal of Research, 18*(1), 3–24.

Centers for Medicare and Medicaid Services. (2010). Coverage of hospice services under hospital insurance. *Medicare benefit policy manual* (rev. 121). Available online at https://www.cms.gov/manuals/Down loads/bp102c09.pdf

Chochinov, H. M., & Cann, B. J. (2005). Intervention to enhance the spiritual aspects of dying. *Journal of Palliative Medicine, 8*(Suppl. 1), 103–115.

Christiansen, C. H. (1999). Defining lives: Occupation as identity: An essay on competence, coherence, and the creation of meaning (1999 Eleanor Clarke Slagle Lecture). *American Journal of Occupational Therapy, 53*(6), 547–558.

Cohen, S. R., Boston, P., Mount, B. M., & Porterfield, P. (2001). Changes in quality of life following admission to palliative care units. *Palliative Medicine, 15*(5), 363–371.

Egan, M., & DeLaat, M. D. (1997). The implicit spirituality of occupational therapy practice. *Canadian Journal of Occupational Therapy, 64*(3), 115–121.

Enes, S. P. (2003). An exploration of dignity in palliative care. *Palliative Medicine, 17*, 263–269.

Gourdji, I., McVey, L., & Purden, M. (2009). A quality end of life from a palliative care patient's perspective. *Journal of Palliative Care, 25*(1), 40–50.

Hospital Case Management. (2003, October). Critical path network—Cancer rehab improves function, quality of life. *Hospital Case Management*, pp. 151–152.

Hunter, E. G. (2008). Legacy: The occupational transmission of self through actions and artifacts. *Journal of Occupational Science, 15*(1), 48–54.

Jacques, N. D., & Hasselkus, B. R. (2004). The nature of occupation surrounding dying and death. *OTJR: Occupation, Participation and Health, 24*, 44–53.

Kaye, P. (2006). *Notes on symptom control in hospice and palliative care.* Machiasport, ME: Hospice Education Institute.

La Cour, K., Josephsson, S., & Luborsky, M. (2005). Creating connections to life during life-threatening illness: Creative activity experienced by elderly people and occupational therapists. *Scandinavian Journal of Occupational Therapy, 12*, 98–109.

La Cour, K., Josephsson, S., Tishelman, C., & Nygård, L. (2007). Experiences of engagement in creative activity at a palliative care facility. *Palliative and Supportive Care, 5*(3), 241–250.

Lin, H. R., & Bauer-Wu, S. M. (2003). Psycho-spiritual well-being in patients with advanced cancer: An integrative review of the literature. *Journal of Advanced Nursing, 44*(1), 69–80.

Lyons, M., Orozovic, N., Davis, J., & Newman, J. (2002). Doing–being–becoming: Occupational experiences of persons with life-threatening illnesses. *American Journal of Occupational Therapy, 56*(3), 285–295.

Marrelli, T. M. (2005). *Hospice and palliative care handbook: Quality, compliance, and reimbursement* (2nd ed.). St. Louis, MO: Elsevier/Mosby.

National Hospice and Palliative Care Organization. (2002). *Standards of practice for hospice programs.* Arlington, VA: Author.

Pearson, E. J., Todd, J. G., & Futcher, J. M. (2007). How can occupational therapists measure outcomes in palliative care? *Palliative Medicine, 21*(6), 477–485.

Picard, H., & Magno, J. (1982). The role of occupational therapy in hospice care. *American Journal of Occupational Therapy, 36*(9), 597–598.

Pizzi, M. (1984). Occupational therapy in hospice care. *American Journal of Occupational Therapy, 38*(4), 252–257.

Pizzi, M., & Briggs, R. (2004). Occupational and physical therapy in hospice—The facilitation of meaning, quality of life, and well-being. *Topics in Geriatric Rehabilitation, 29*(2), 120–130.

Prince-Paul, M. (2008). Relationship among communicative acts, social well-being, and spiritual well-being on the quality of life at the end of life in patients with cancer enrolled in hospice. *Journal of Palliative Medicine, 11*(1), 20–25.

Rahman, H. (2000). Journey of providing care in hospice: Perspectives of occupational therapists. *Qualitative Health Research, 10*, 806–818.

Ryan, P. Y. (2005). Approaching death: A phenomenologic study of five older adults with advanced cancer. *Oncology Nursing Forum, 32*(6), 1101–1108.

Saarik, J., & Hartley, J. (2010). Living with cancer-related fatigue: Developing an effective management programme. *International Journal of Palliative Nursing, 16*(1), 8–12.

Singer, P. A., Martin, D. K., & Kelner, M. (1999). Quality end-of-life care: Patient's perspective. *Journal of the American Medical Association, 13*(2), 163–168.

Steinhauser, K. E., Clipp, E. C., McNeilly, M., Christakis, N. A., Mcintyre, L. M., & Tulsky, J. A. (2000). In search of a good death: Observations of patients, families, and providers. *Annals of Internal Medicine, 132*(10), 825–832.

Strasser, F., Sweeney, C., Willey J., Benisch-Tolley, S., Palmer, J. L., & Bruera, E. (2004). Impact of a half-day multidisciplinary symptoms control and palliative care outpatient clinic in a comprehensive cancer center on recommendations, symptoms intensity, and patient satisfactions: A retrospective descriptive study. *Journal of Pain Symptom Management, 27*(6), 481–491.

Svidòn, G. A., Fürst, C. J., von Koch, L., & Borell, L. (2009). Palliative day care—A study of well-being and health-related quality of life. *Palliative Medicine, 23*(5), 441–447.

Tiggs, K., & Sherman, L. (1983). The treatment of the hospice patient: From occupational history to occupational role. *American Journal of Occupational Therapy, 37*(4), 235–238.

Thompson, B. (1991). Occupational therapy with the terminally ill. In J. Kiernat (Ed.), *Occupational therapy and the older adult* (pp. 324–337). Gaithersburg, MD: Aspen.

Unruh, A. M., Smith N., & Scammell, C. (2000). The occupation of gardening in a life-threatening illness: A qualitative pilot project. *Canadian Journal of Occupational Therapy, 67*(1), 70–77.

Vrkljan, B. H., & Miller-Polgar, J. (2001). Meaning of occupational engagement in life-threatening illness: A qualitative pilot project. *Canadian Journal of Occupational Therapy, 68*(4), 237–246.

World Health Organization. (2002). *National cancer control programmes: Polices and managerial guidelines* (2nd ed.). Geneva: Author.

Related Readings

Albom, M. (1997). *Tuesdays with Morrie.* New York: Doubleday.

Byock, I. (1997). *Dying well: The prospect for growth at the end of life.* New York: Riverhead.

Callahan, M., & Kelley, P. (1992). *Final gifts.* New York: Bantam.

Jacques, N. D., & Thompson, B. (2001). Occupational therapy. In *Complementary therapies in end-of-life care* (pp. 69–82). Arlington, VA: National Hospice and Palliative Care Organization.

Levine, S. (1982). *Who dies?* Garden City, NY: Anchor Press/Doubleday.

Nuland, S. (1993). *How we die.* New York: Random.

Trump, S. M. (2000). The role of occupational therapy in hospice. *Home and Community Health Special Interest Section Quarterly, 7*(2), 1–4.

Trump, S. M. (2001). Occupational therapy and hospice: A natural fit. *OT Practice, 6*(20).

Authors
Ann Burkhardt, OTD, OTR/L, BCN, FAOTA
Mack Ivy, MOT, OTR
Kathleen R. Kannenberg, MS, OTR/L, CCN
Jaclyn F. Low, PhD, LOT
James Marc-Aurele, MBA, OTR/L
Mary Jane Youngstrom, MS, OTR, FAOTA

for

The Commission on Practice
Janet DeLany, DEd, OTR/L, FAOTA, *Chairperson*

Adopted by the Representative Assembly 2011AprC14

Scope of Occupational Therapy Services for Individuals With Autism Spectrum Disorder Across the Life Course

The primary purpose of this paper is to define the role of occupational therapy and the scope of occupational therapy services available for individuals with autism spectrum disorder (ASD) to persons outside of the occupational therapy profession. In addition, this document is intended to clarify the role of occupational therapy with this population for occupational therapists and occupational therapy assistants.

Background

The American Occupational Therapy Association (AOTA; 2014c) strongly supports the right of all individuals to "have the same opportunities to participate in the naturally occurring activities of society" (p. S23). Occupational therapy practitioners[1] work collaboratively with individuals on the autism spectrum, their families, other professionals, organizations, and community members in multiple contexts to advocate for and provide a range of needed resources and services that support the individuals' ability to participate fully in life (Case-Smith & Arbesman, 2008; Kuhaneck, Madonna, Novak, & Pearson, 2015; Tanner, Hand, O'Toole, & Lane, 2015; Watling & Hauer, 2015a; Weaver, 2015). According to a study conducted by the Interactive Autism Network (2011), occupational therapy ranks second to speech–language pathology as the most frequently provided services for individuals with autism throughout the United States.

Prevalence data suggest that ASD currently affects approximately 1 in 68 children (Centers for Disease Control and Prevention, 2014), and the World Health Organization (WHO; 2013) estimates the prevalence of ASD to be 1 in 160 individuals worldwide. Other estimates of ASD diagnoses in the United States have suggested that these rates might be higher, with as many as 2% of children ages 6–17 years having a parent-reported diagnosis (Blumberg et al., 2013). These figures reflect a dramatic increase in the number of individuals living with ASD in the United States over the past 20 years.

ASD is the diagnosis used in the *Diagnostic and Statistical Manual of Mental Disorders* (*DSM;* 5th ed., American Psychiatric Association [APA], 2013) to describe a cluster of symptoms that range in type and severity and include (1) "persistent deficits in social communication and social interaction" and (2) "restricted, repetitive patterns of behavior, interests or activities" (p. 31). This diagnostic category combines a range of disorders, including autistic disorder, Asperger disorder, and pervasive developmental disorder–not otherwise specified, which were identified as separate diagnoses in the previous edition of the *DSM* (4th ed., text rev., APA, 2000).

Rather than using the term *autism spectrum disorder,* the Individuals With Disabilities Education Improvement Act of 2004 (IDEA; Pub. L. 108–446) uses the term *autism* as a disability category under which children might be eligible for special education and related services. IDEA regulations define *autism* as "a developmental disability significantly affecting verbal and nonverbal communication and social interaction generally evident before age 3 that adversely affects a child's educational performance." Other charac-

---

[1]The term *occupational therapy practitioner* refers to both occupational therapists and occupational therapy assistants (AOTA, 2013a) *Occupational therapists* are responsible for all aspects of occupational therapy service delivery and are accountable for the safety and effectiveness of the occupational therapy service delivery process. *Occupational therapy assistants* deliver occupational therapy services under the supervision of and in partnership with an occupational therapist (AOTA, 2014a).

teristics often associated with autism are engagement in repetitive activities and stereotyped movements, resistance to environmental change or change in daily routines, and unusual responses to sensory experiences (§300.8[c][1][i]).

Under Part B of IDEA, occupational therapy is a related service; under Part C, occupational therapy is a primary service. Thus, occupational therapy must be provided to children with autism if those services will help the child benefit from special education (§602[26][A]). Because educational classification and identification criteria vary considerably from state to state, readers are referred to specific state policies and requirements.

Occupational Therapy Domain and Process

Occupations are daily life activities that are "central to a client's . . . identity and sense of competence and have a particular meaning and value to that client" (AOTA, 2014b, p. S5). Occupational therapy services focus on "achieving health, well-being, and participation in life through engagement in occupation" (AOTA, 2014b, p. S4). Occupations are categorized into activities of daily living, instrumental activities of daily living (IADLs), rest and sleep, education, work, play, leisure, and social participation within their natural and daily contexts. Consistent with all occupational therapy intervention, the focus of services for individuals with ASD is determined by the client's specific goals and priorities for participation. Given that individuals with ASD may experience complex challenges, including social–communication difficulties, collaboration with key individuals such as family members, caregivers, and educators is important for determining goals and priorities. Some examples of occupations (daily life activities) that may be challenging for individuals with ASD and that can be addressed by occupational therapy practitioners are included in Table 1.

The process of client-centered occupational therapy service delivery includes evaluation and intervention to achieve targeted outcomes using occupations to promote health, well-being, and participation in life (AOTA, 2014b). Services can be provided to the client at the person, group, and population levels and may include direct service, consultation, education, and advocacy to support the person, family members, health professionals, educational staff, and community agencies.

At the person and group levels, collaboration with family, caregivers, educators, and other team members is essential for understanding the daily life experiences of individuals with ASD and those with whom they interact. At the systems level, services may focus on educating staff and designing programs and environments for individuals or groups that are served by an organization to be more socially inclusive for persons on the autism spectrum. At the population level, occupational therapy practitioners may engage in education, consultation, and advocacy initiatives with communities or ASD consumer groups.

Evaluation

The evaluation process is designed to provide an understanding of the client's occupational profile and performance. This process includes an analysis of the client's strengths and challenges related to occupations, performance skills, performance patterns, body functions and body structures, and activity demands. Evaluation is comprehensive and tailored to the concerns of the specific client, organization, or population. Information collected through interviews, structured observations, and standardized assessments guides occupational therapy services.

Because the literature shows that individuals with ASD may have difficulties in areas of occupation such as self-care; IADLs; sleep; functional and pretend play; leisure pursuits; social participation; education and work performance; and performance skills, performance patterns, and client factors such as sensory integration and modulation, self-regulation, praxis, and motor imitation, occupational therapy evaluations conducted at the individual level should assess these areas (Baranek, 2002; Case-Smith & Bryan, 1999;

Foster & Cox, 2013; Johnson & Myers, 2007; Kientz & Dunn, 1997; Libby, Powell, Messer, & Jordan, 1998; Rutherford & Rogers, 2003; Shattuck et al., 2007; Tomchek & Case-Smith, 2009; Watson, Baranek, & DiLavore, 2003; Zaks, 2006). At the group level, the evaluation process may focus on analyzing the program structure, resources, and services that support individuals on the autism spectrum to engage in desired occupations. At the population level, the evaluation process may focus on collaborating with ASD consumer groups to identify their capacities and needs to support societal participation. Recent book chapters and practice guidelines have been developed to inform the practice of occupational therapy related to ASD and include comprehensive chapters on the evaluation process (Boyt Schell, Gillen, & Scaffa, 2014; Case-Smith & O'Brien 2015; Foster & Cox, 2013; Tomchek & Case-Smith, 2009; Watling, 2010).

Intervention

Occupational therapy intervention is based on the results of the evaluation and is implemented to foster occupational engagement and social participation by attending to the transactions among the client, the activity, and the environment. The goal of intervention is to promote engagement in and performance of daily activities, personal satisfaction, adaptation, health and wellness, role competence, quality of life, and occupational justice for individuals with ASD within the contexts of their families and communities.

At the individual level, the intervention may emphasize social engagement and participation, include strategies to improve adaptive behaviors and occupational performance, and support family priorities. Some research has demonstrated the effectiveness of occupational therapy interventions for children and adolescents with ASD that lead to improvement in self-care and play (Tanner et al., 2015; Weaver, 2015). These interventions include the use of activities that promote social interaction, problem solving, and pivotal behaviors (e.g., joint attention, initiative, persistence, executive functioning, cooperation) and address specific skill acquisition (Tanner et al., 2015). Effective interventions also address contextual factors such as structure, consistency of routine, sensory environments that optimize attention and arousal, and caregiver skills that contribute to occupational performance.

Research indicates that the occupational therapy intervention process should be individualized, intensive, and comprehensive; include the family; and facilitate active engagement of the individual (see Tomchek & Case-Smith, 2009). The literature provides additional support for the use of developmental and behavioral approaches to intervention, particularly for young children (Callahan, Henson, & Cowan, 2008; Dawson et al., 2010; National Autism Center [NAC], 2015; Rogers & Vismara, 2008). Environmental modification to address problem behaviors also has been shown to be effective (Horner, Carr, Strain, Todd, & Reed, 2002), and emerging evidence shows that families of children with ASD can be supported through telehealth and other online communication technologies (AOTA, 2013b; Gibbs & Toth-Cohen, 2011; Vismara, McCormick, Young, Nadhan, & Monlux, 2013).

At the systems level, interventions could include recommendations for educational and policy initiatives, participation on a transition team, provision of staff education, and development of new programs. At the population level, emphasis may be on inclusion and advocacy initiatives.

Outcomes

Targeting outcomes of service is an integral part of the occupational therapy process. Outcomes describe what clients can achieve through occupational therapy intervention and are important for determining future actions. Targeting outcomes involves monitoring the client's responses to intervention, reevaluating and modifying the intervention plan, and measuring intervention success through outcomes that are important to the client within the dynamic physical and social environments and cultural contexts where functioning occurs. Progress is noted through improvement in the client's occupational performance, adaptation, participation in desired activities, satisfaction, role competence, health and wellness, and quality of life and through prevention of further difficulties and facilitation of effective transitions.

Occupational therapy practice for individuals with ASD is consistent with the WHO's (2013) action agenda for ASD and the National Research Council's (2001) recommended practices for educating individuals with ASD. Occupational therapy practitioners also use established interventions as identified by the NAC (2015). Table 2 provides case examples that reflect a range of occupational therapy evaluation and intervention services for individuals with ASD at the individual, group, and population levels across the lifespan.

References

American Occupational Therapy Association. (2013a). Policy 1.44: Categories of occupational therapy personnel. In *Policy manual* (2009 ed.). Bethesda, MD: Author.

American Occupational Therapy Association. (2013b). Telehealth. *American Journal of Occupational Therapy, 67*(Suppl. 6), S69–S90. http://dx.doi.org/10.5014/ajot.2013.67s69

American Occupational Therapy Association. (2014a). Guidelines for supervision, roles, and responsibilities during the delivery of occupational therapy services. *American Journal of Occupational Therapy, 68*(Suppl. 3), S16–S22. http://dx.doi.org/10.5014/ajot.2014.686S03

American Occupational Therapy Association. (2014b). Occupational therapy practice framework: Domain and process (3rd ed.). *American Journal of Occupational Therapy, 68*(Suppl. 1), S1–S48. http://dx.doi.org/10.5014/ajot.2014.682006

American Occupational Therapy Association. (2014c). Occupational therapy's commitment to nondiscrimination and inclusion. *American Journal of Occupational Therapy, 68*(Suppl. 3), S23–S24. http://dx.doi.org/10.5014/ajot.2014.686S05

American Psychiatric Association. (2000). *Diagnostic and statistical manual of mental disorders* (4th ed., text rev.). Washington, DC: Author.

American Psychiatric Association. (2013). *Diagnostic and statistical manual of mental disorders* (5th ed.). Arlington, VA: American Psychiatric Publishing.

Baranek, G. T. (2002). Efficacy of sensory and motor interventions for children with autism. *Journal of Autism and Developmental Disorders, 32,* 397–422. http://dx.doi.org/10.1023/A:1020541906063

Baron, K., Kielhofner, G., Iyenger, A., Goldhammer, V., & Wolenski, J. (2006). *Occupational Self Assessment (OSA)* (version 2.2). Chicago: MOHO Clearinghouse.

Bayley, N. (2006). *Bayley Scales of Infant and Toddler Development* (3rd ed.). San Antonio, TX: Psychological Corporation.

Bellini, S., & Akullian, J. (2007). A meta-analysis of video modeling and video self-modeling interventions for children and adolescents with autism spectrum disorders. *Exceptional Children, 73,* 264–287. http://dx.doi.org/10.1177/001440290707300301

Blumberg, S. J., Bramlett, M. D., Kogan, M. D., Schieve, L. A., Jones, J. R., & Lu, M. C. (2013). Changes in prevalence of parent-reported autism spectrum disorder in school-aged U.S. children: 2007 to 2011–2012. *National Health Statistics Reports, 65,* 1–11.

Borrero, C. S., & Borrero, J. C. (2008). Descriptive and experimental analyses of potential precursors to problem behavior. *Journal of Applied Behavior Analysis, 41,* 83–96. http://dx.doi.org/10.1901/jaba.2008.41-83

Boyt Schell, B. A., Gillen, G., & Scaffa, M. E. (Eds.). (2014). *Willard and Spackman's occupational therapy* (12th ed.). Philadelphia: Wolters Kluwer Health/Lippincott Williams & Wilkins.

Brown, C., & Dunn, W. (2002). *Adolescent/Adult Sensory Profile.* San Antonio, TX: Pearson.

Brown, C., Rempfer, M., & Hamera, E. (2009). *Test of Grocery Shopping Skills.* Bethesda, MD: AOTA Press.

Bruininks, R. H., Woodcock, R. W., Weatherman, R. F., & Hill, B. K. (1997). *Scales of Independent Behavior–Revised*. Rolling Meadows, IL: Riverside.

Callahan, K., Henson, R. K., & Cowan, A. K. (2008). Social validation of evidence-based practices in autism by parents, teachers, and administrators. *Journal of Autism and Developmental Disorders, 38*, 678–692. http://dx.doi.org/10.1007/s10803-007-0434-9

Case-Smith, J., & Arbesman, M. (2008). Evidence-based review of interventions for autism used in or of relevance to occupational therapy. *American Journal of Occupational Therapy, 62*, 416–429. http://dx.doi.org/10.5014/ajot.62.4.416

Case-Smith, J., & Bryan, T. (1999). The effects of occupational therapy with sensory integration emphasis on preschool-age children with autism. *American Journal of Occupational Therapy, 53*, 489–497. http://dx.doi.org/10.5014/ajot.53.5.489

Case-Smith, J., & O'Brien, J. (2015). *Occupational therapy for children and adolescents* (7th ed.). St. Louis, MO: Mosby/Elsevier.

Case-Smith, J., & Weaver, L. (2015a). *What is the evidence for the effectiveness of interventions within the scope of occupational therapy practice to improve performance in education for persons with autism spectrum disorder (ASD)?* [Critically Appraised Topic]. Bethesda, MD: American Occupational Therapy Association, Evidence-Based Practice Project. Retrieved from http://www.aota.org/-/media/Corporate/Files/Secure/Practice/CCL/Autism/Autism_Education_CAT.pdf

Case-Smith, J., & Weaver, L. (2015b). *What is the evidence for the effectiveness of interventions within the scope of occupational therapy practice to improve performance in work and vocational tasks for persons with autism spectrum disorder (ASD)?* [Critically Appraised Topic]. Bethesda, MD: American Occupational Therapy Association, Evidence-Based Practice Project. Retrieved from http://www.aota.org/-/media/Corporate/Files/Secure/Practice/CCL/Autism/Autism_Work_CAT.pdf

Centers for Disease Control and Prevention. (2014). Prevalence of autism spectrum disorders among children aged 8 years—Autism and Developmental Disabilities Monitoring Network, 11 sites, United States, 2010. *Morbidity and Mortality Weekly Report, 63*, 2–21. Retrieved from http://www.cdc.gov/mmwr/pdf/ss/ss6302.pdf

Classen, S., Monahan, M., & Wang, Y. (2013). Driving characteristics of teens with attention deficit hyperactivity and autism spectrum disorder. *American Journal of Occupational Therapy, 67*, 664–673. http://dx.doi.org/10.5014/ajot.2013.008821

Cohen, H., Amerine-Dickens, M., & Smith, T. (2006). Early intensive behavioral treatment: Replication of the UCLA model in a community setting. *Development and Behavioral Pediatrics, 27*(Suppl.), S145–S155. http://dx.doi.org/10.1097/00004703-200604002-00013

Coster, W., Deeney, T., Haltiwanger, J., & Haley, S. (1998). *School Function Assessment*. San Antonio, TX: Psychological Corporation.

Dawson, G., Rogers, S., Munson, J., Smith, M., Winter, J., Greenson, J., . . . Varley, J. (2010). Randomized, controlled trial of an intervention for toddlers with autism: The Early Start Denver Model. *Pediatrics, 125*, 17–23. http://dx.doi.org/10.1542/peds.2009-0958

Dunn, W. (2014). *Sensory Profile–2*. San Antonio, TX: Psychological Corporation.

Dunn, W., Cox, J., Foster, L., Mische-Lawson, L., & Tanquary, J. (2012). Impact of a contextual intervention on child participation and parent competence among children with autism spectrum disorders: A pretest–posttest repeated-measures design. *American Journal of Occupational Therapy, 66*, 520–528. http://dx.doi.org/10.5014/ajot.2012.004119

Foster, L., & Cox, J. (2013). Best practices in supporting students with autism. In G. Frolek Clark & B. E. Chandler (Eds.), *Best practices for occupational therapy in schools* (pp. 273–284). Bethesda, MD: AOTA Press.

Ganz, J. B. (2007). Classroom structuring methods and strategies for children and youth with autism spectrum disorders. *Exceptionality, 15,* 249–260. http://dx.doi.org/10.1080/09362830701655816

Gibbs, V., & Toth-Cohen, S. (2011). Family-centered occupational therapy and telerehabilitation for children with autism spectrum disorders. *Occupational Therapy in Health Care, 25,* 298–314. http://dx.doi.org/10.3109/07380577.2011.606460

Gray, C. (2010). *The new social story book.* Arlington, TX: Future Horizons.

Greenspan, S. I., & Wieder, S. (1997). Developmental patterns and outcomes in infants and children with disorders in relating and communicating: A chart review of 200 cases of children with autistic spectrum diagnoses. *Journal of Developmental and Learning Disorders, 1,* 87–141.

Haley, S. M., Coster, W. J., Ludlow, L. H., Haltiwanger, J. T., & Andrellos, P. J. (1992). *Pediatric Evaluation of Disability Inventory.* San Antonio, TX: Psychological Corporation.

Harper, C. B., Symon, J. B., & Frea, W. D. (2008). Recess is time-in: Using peers to improve social skills of children with autism. *Journal of Autism and Developmental Disorders, 38,* 815–826. http://dx.doi.org/10.1007/s10803-007-0449-2

Horner, R. H., Carr, E. G., Strain, P. S., Todd, A. W., & Reed, H. K. (2002). Problem behavior interventions for young children with autism: A research synthesis. *Journal of Autism and Developmental Disorders, 32,* 423–446. http://dx.doi.org/10.1023/A:1020593922901

Hwang, B., & Hughes, C. (2000). The effects of social interactive training on early social communicative skills of children with autism. *Journal of Autism and Developmental Disorders, 30,* 331–343. http://dx.doi.org/10.1023/A:1005579317085

Individuals With Disabilities Education Improvement Act of 2004, Pub. L. 108–446, 20 U.S.C. §§ 1400-1482.

Interactive Autism Network. (2011). *IAN research findings: Treatment series.* Retrieved from https://iancommunity.org/cs/ian_treatment_reports/overview

Johnson, C. P., & Myers, S. M.; American Academy of Pediatrics Council on Children With Disabilities. (2007). Identification and evaluation of children with autism spectrum disorders. *Pediatrics, 120,* 1183–1215. http://dx.doi.org/10.1542/peds.2007-2361

Kasari, C., Freeman, S., & Paparella, T. (2006). Joint attention and symbolic play in young children with autism: A randomized controlled intervention study. *Journal of Child Psychology and Psychiatry, and Allied Disciplines, 47,* 611–620. http://dx.doi.org/10.1111/j.1469-7610.2005.01567.x

Kientz, M. A., & Dunn, W. (1997). A comparison of the performance of children with and without autism on the Sensory Profile. *American Journal of Occupational Therapy, 51,* 530–537. http://dx.doi.org/10.5014/ajot.51.7.530

Kuhaneck, H. M., Madonna, S., Novak, A., & Pearson, E. (2015). Effectiveness of interventions for children with autism spectrum disorder and their parents: A systematic review of family outcomes. *American Journal of Occupational Therapy, 69,* 6905180040. http://dx.doi.org/10.5014/ajot.2015.017855

Law, M., Baptiste, S., Carswell, A., McColl, M., Polatajko, H., & Pollack, N. (2014). *Canadian Occupational Performance Measure* (5th ed.). Ottawa, ON: CAOT Publications.

Ledford, J. R., & Gast, D. L. (2006). Feeding problems in children with autism spectrum disorders: A review. *Focus on Autism and Other Developmental Disabilities, 21,* 153–166. http://dx.doi.org/10.1177/10883576060210030401

Libby, S., Powell, S., Messer, D., & Jordan, R. (1998). Spontaneous play in children with autism: A reappraisal. *Journal of Autism and Developmental Disorders, 28,* 487–497. http://dx.doi.org/10.1023/A:1026095910558

Mahoney, G., & Perales, F. (2005). Relationship-focused early intervention with children with pervasive developmental disorders and other disabilities: A comparative study. *Developmental and Behavioral Pediatrics, 26,* 77–85. http://dx.doi.org/10.1097/00004703-200504000-00002

Miller, L. J. (2006). *Miller Function and Participation Scales (M–FUN)*. San Antonio, TX: Psychological Corporation.

National Autism Center. (2015). *Findings and conclusions: National standards project, phase 2*. Randolph, MA: Author.

National Research Council. (2001). *Educating children with autism*. Washington, DC: National Academy Press.

Ozonoff, S., & Cathcart, K. (1998). Effectiveness of a home program intervention for young children with autism. *Journal of Autism and Developmental Disorders, 28*, 25–32. http://dx.doi.org/10.1023/A:1026006818310

Panerai, S., Ferrante, L., & Zingale, M. (2002). Benefits of the Treatment and Education of Autistic and Communication Handicapped Children (TEACCH) programme as compared with a non-specific approach. *Journal of Intellectual Disability Research, 46*, 318–327. http://dx.doi.org 10.1046/j.1365-2788.2002.00388.x

Reynhout, G., & Carter, M. (2006). Social Stories for children with disabilities. *Journal of Autism and Developmental Disorders, 36*, 445–469. http://dx.doi.org/10.1007/s10803-006-0086-1

Rogers, S. J., & Vismara, L. A. (2008). Evidence-based comprehensive treatments for early autism. *Journal of Clinical Child and Adolescent Psychology, 37*, 8–38. http://dx.doi.org/10.1080/15374410701817808

Rutherford, M. D., & Rogers, S. J. (2003). Cognitive underpinnings of pretend play in autism. *Journal of Autism and Developmental Disorders, 33*, 289–302. http://dx.doi.org/10.1023/A:1024406601334

Salt, J., Sellars, V., Shemilt, J., Boyd, S., Coulson, T., & McCool, S. (2001). The Scottish Centre for Autism preschool treatment programme. I: A developmental approach to early intervention. *Autism, 5*, 362–373. http://dx.doi.org/10.1177/1362361301005004003

Salt, J., Shemilt, J., Sellars, V., Boyd, S., Coulson, T., & McCool, S. (2002). The Scottish Centre for Autism preschool treatment programme. II: The results of a controlled treatment outcome study. *Autism, 6*, 33–46. http://dx.doi.org/10.1177/1362361302006001004

Shattuck, P. T., Seltzer, M. M., Greenberg, J. S., Orsmond, G. I., Bolt, D., Kring, S., . . . Lord, C. (2007). Change in autism symptoms and maladaptive behaviors in adolescents and adults with an autism spectrum disorder. *Journal of Autism and Developmental Disorders, 37*, 1735–1747. http://dx.doi.org/10.1007/s10803-006-0307-7

Smith, T., Groen, A. D., & Wynn, J. W. (2000). Randomized trial of intensive early intervention for children with pervasive developmental disorder. *American Journal of Mental Retardation, 105*, 269–285. http://dx.doi.org/10.1352/0895-8017(2000)105<0269:RTOIEI>2.0.CO;2

Tanner, K., Hand, B. N., O'Toole, G., & Lane, A. E. (2015). Effectiveness of interventions to improve social participation, play, leisure, and restricted and repetitive behaviors in people with autism spectrum disorder: A systematic review. *American Journal of Occupational Therapy, 69*, 6905180010. http://dx.doi.org/10.5014/ajot.2015.017806

Tomchek, S. D., & Case-Smith, J. (2009). *Occupational therapy practice guidelines for children and adolescents with autism*. Bethesda, MD: AOTA Press.

Vismara, L. A., McCormick, C., Young, G. S., Nadhan, A., & Monlux, K. (2013). Preliminary findings of a telehealth approach to parent training in autism. *Journal of Autism and Developmental Disorders, 43*, 2953–2969. http://dx.doi.org/10.1007/s10803-013-1841-8

Watling, R. (2010). Occupational therapy evaluation for individuals with an autism spectrum disorder. In H. Miller Kuhanek & R. Watling (Eds.), *Autism: A comprehensive occupational therapy approach* (3rd ed., pp. 285–303). Bethesda, MD: AOTA Press.

Watling, R., & Hauer, S. (2015a). Effectiveness of Ayres Sensory Integration® and sensory-based interventions for people with autism spectrum disorder: A systematic review. *American Journal of Occupational Therapy, 69*, 6905180030. http://dx.doi.org/10.5014/ajot.2015.018051

Watling, R., & Hauer, S. (2015b). *What is the evidence for non-Ayres Sensory Integration® (ASI®) sensory-based interventions within the scope of occupational therapy practice to improve performance in daily life activities and occupations for children with autism spectrum disorder (ASD)?* [Critically Appraised Topic]. Bethesda, MD: American Occupational Therapy Association, Evidence-Based Practice Project. Retrieved from http://www.aota.org/-/media/Corporate/Files/Secure/Practice/CCL/Autism/Autism_Sensory_Non-Ayres_%20SI_CAT.pdf

Watling, R., & Hauer, S. (2015c). *What is the evidence for using Ayres Sensory Integration® (ASI®) intervention to improve performance in daily life activities and occupations for children with autism spectrum disorder (ASD)?* [Critically Appraised Topic]. Bethesda, MD: American Occupational Therapy Association, Evidence-Based Practice Project. Retrieved from http://www.aota.org/-/media/Corporate/Files/Secure/Practice/CCL/Autism/Autism_Sensory_Ayres_SI_CAT.pdf

Watson, L. R., Baranek, G. T., & DiLavore, P. C. (2003). Toddlers with autism: Developmental perspectives. *Infants and Young Children, 16,* 201–214. http://dx.doi.org/10.1097/00001163-200307000-00003

Weaver, L. L. (2015). Effectiveness of work, activities of daily living, education, and sleep interventions for people with autism spectrum disorder: A systematic review. *American Journal of Occupational Therapy, 69,* 6905180020. http://dx.doi.org/10.5014/ajot.2015.017962

Williams, M. S., & Shellenberger, S. (1996). *How does your engine run? A leader's guide to the Alert Program for Self-Regulation.* Albuquerque, NM: Therapy Works.

World Health Organization. (2013). *Meeting Report—Autism spectrum disorders and other developmental disorders: From raising awareness to building capacity.* Geneva: Author. Retrieved July 2014 from http://apps.who.int/iris/bitstream/10665/103312/1/9789241506618_eng.pdf?ua=1

Zaks, Z. (2006). *Life and love: Positive strategies for autistic adults.* Shawnee Mission, KS: Autism Asperger Publishing.

Authors

Scott Tomchek, PhD, OTR/L, FAOTA

Patti LaVesser, PhD, OTR/L

Renee Watling, PhD, OTR/L

for

The Commission on Practice

Janet DeLany, DEd, OTR/L, FAOTA, *Chairperson (2008–2011)*

Revised by the Commission on Practice, 2015

Kathleen Kannenberg, MA, OTR/L, CCM, *Chairperson*

Adopted by the Representative Assembly Coordinating Council for the Representative Assembly (2015)

Note. This revision replaces the 2010 document *The Scope of Occupational Therapy Services for Individuals With an Autism Spectrum Disorder Across the Life Course,* previously published and copyrighted in 2010 by the American Occupational Therapy Association in the *American Journal of Occupational Therapy, 64*(6, Suppl.), S125–S136. http://dx.doi.org/10.5014/ajot.2010.64S125-64S136

Citation. American Occupational Therapy Association. (2015). Scope of occupational therapy services for individuals with autism spectrum disorder across the life course. *American Journal of Occupational Therapy, 69*(Suppl. 3), 6913410054. http://dx.doi.org/10.5014/ajot.2015.696S18

Table 1. Examples of Potentially Challenging Areas of Occupation for Individuals With ASD

Occupation	Example
ADLs	Participating in daily self-care routines such as showering, toileting, and dressing; accepting a healthy variety of foods during mealtime; tolerating the sensory aspects of grooming activities
IADLs	Accessing the community by driving or using public transportation; managing finances; running a household; planning and preparing healthful, balanced meals
Rest and sleep	Achieving a calm state to rest, preparing for sleep, developing routines and rituals that support sleep, participating in and achieving restful sleep
Education	Engaging in formal education activities such as reading, writing, and math; accessing academic curricula; organizing and using school tools and materials; participating in various school environments and activities such as cafeteria, playground, and gym; identifying and pursuing informal educational interests and needs
Work	Identifying and pursuing employment options, seeking and acquiring employment, sequencing job tasks, developing effective job performance and interaction skills, exploring and participating in volunteer work
Play	Identifying a range of play interests, exploring and participating in a variety of play activities, developing interactive play skills
Leisure	Exploring and participating in community recreational leisure activities, developing leisure skills and interests
Social participation	Developing peer friendships, interacting appropriately with others, engaging in community-based social activities and outings, understanding social nuances and maintaining appropriate behavior, participating in family gatherings and rituals

Note. ADLs = activities of daily living; ASD = autism spectrum disorder; IADLs = instrumental activities of daily living.

Table 2. Case Examples of Occupational Therapy Evaluation and Intervention Services for Individuals With ASD

Client Description	Evaluation	Intervention
Kamau, age 2 1/2 years, has autism. His language consists of single-word utterances. He has an intense interest in a few objects such as wheels and mobiles. His mother's primary concerns are his limited social interaction, delayed pretend play, hyperactive behaviors, and picky eating. Kamau also is receiving speech therapy services and an applied behavioral analysis program at home through the state early intervention program.	Develop occupational profile of play behaviors, family interactions, and food preferences through parent interview. Gather clinical observations of behavior, self-regulation, and parent–child interaction during free play and interactive parent–child play. Conduct structured observation of parent–child interaction during play and while Kamau is eating. Administer Toddler Sensory Profile–2 (Dunn, 2014); Bayley Scales of Infant and Toddler Development (Bayley, 2006); and Pediatric Evaluation of Disability Inventory, Self-Care Scale (Haley, Coster, Ludlow, Haltiwanger, & Andrellos, 1992).	Provide weekly occupational therapy in the home setting with mother present to help Kamau establish self-regulation, social engagement, and pretend play skills (Greenspan & Wieder, 1997; Kasari, Freeman, & Paparella, 2006; Mahoney & Perales, 2005; Salt et al., 2001). Use sensory integration methods (Watling & Hauer, 2015c); behavioral strategies, including positive reinforcement; and reciprocal play to improve social interaction. Collaborate with the SLP regarding Kamau's intervention program, and arrange cotreatment sessions to promote social interaction. Collaborate with the behavioral therapist (Cohen, Amerine-Dickens, & Smith, 2006; Smith, Groen, & Wynn, 2000) to integrate sensory and behavioral strategies helpful in modulating Kamau's behavior. Provide parent training related to sensory processing and behavior management strategies and social participation (NAC, 2015). Provide parent consultation to improve the family's mealtime routine and the variety of foods Kamau eats (Horner et al., 2002; Ledford & Gast, 2006).

(Continued)

Table 2. Case Examples of Occupational Therapy Evaluation and Intervention Services for Individuals With ASD *(cont.)*

Client Description	Evaluation	Intervention
Heang, age 4 years, has autism and attends an inclusive preschool through her school district. Her parents have sought individualized occupational therapy services from an outpatient clinic. Heang uses only a few basic gestures to communicate. She primarily engages in solitary sensory–motor exploration of her environment and does not yet spontaneously play beside other children or with toys. She has frequent tantrums and screams particularly when there are changes in the environment or when she is being directed toward a specific task.	Develop an occupational profile of behavior and self-regulation in play through parent and teacher interview. Conduct clinical observations of behavior, self-regulation, parent–child and teacher–child interaction, and play skills. Administer the Sensory Profile–2 (Dunn, 2014) and the Miller Function and Participation Scales (Miller, 2006).	Provide weekly occupational therapy in a clinical setting with the parent present. Consult with preschool team, including teacher and SLP. Provide interventions to improve self-regulation to allow for socially appropriate behavior (Greenspan & Wieder, 1997; Kasari et al., 2006; Mahoney & Perales, 2005; NAC, 2015; Salt et al., 2001, 2002). Incorporate sensory integration techniques (Baranek, 2002; Watling & Hauer, 2015a, 2015b, 2015c); visual supports for structure (NAC, 2015; Ozonoff & Cathcart, 1998) and communication; and behavioral strategies, including positive reinforcement, redirection, elimination of antecedents to her tantrums, and reinforcement of her positive behaviors (Horner et al., 2002; NAC, 2015; Rogers & Vismara, 2008). Educate parents on how to recognize when Heang is becoming overaroused, and implement both positive behavior (Horner et al., 2002) and sensory-based strategies to help her modulate her arousal (Baranek, 2002; Watling & Hauer, 2015a).
Jorge, age 6 years, is a kindergartener with a diagnosis of PDD–NOS. He demonstrates minimal social initiation with peers, although he interacts better with adults. When peers initiate interaction, Jorge withdraws or responds aggressively. He needs direct adult supervision to manage his school materials and complete school tasks.	Develop an occupational profile of play, work–reward routine, and behavior regulation through parent and teacher interview. Conduct structured clinical observations of classroom behavior, social–communication skills, parent–child interaction, and play skills. Administer Sensory Profile–2 (Dunn, 2014) and School Function Assessment (Cognitive/Behavior Scales; Coster, Deeney, Haltiwanger, & Haley, 1998). Conduct formal functional behavior analysis of aggressive behaviors.	Provide occupational therapy services within the school setting (Case-Smith & Weaver, 2015a; Weaver, 2015). Collaborate with teacher to implement structured teaching methods based on TEACCH (Ozonoff & Cathcart, 1998; Panerai, Ferrante, & Zingale, 2002) and a visual schedule in the classroom (Ganz, 2007). Implement positive behavior supports (Horner et al., 2002; NAC, 2015) and a sensory diet, including strategies for self-regulation based on the functional analysis of aggressive behaviors (Borrero & Borrero, 2008). Develop and implement Social Stories (NAC, 2015; Reynhout & Carter, 2006) before challenging school situations (e.g., standing in line, assemblies, fire drills) to encourage appropriate behavior. Develop peer buddies and modeling program to build social–communication skills during naturally occurring play activities (Harper, Symon, & Frea, 2008; NAC, 2015). Consult with the classroom teacher and family to promote generalization of strategies across home and school settings.
The local **museum of science** is interested in making the museum more accessible to individuals with ASD. The museum hosts school classes daily and specialized weekend learning programs.	Develop an occupational profile of supports and inhibitors to engagement in museum activities through observation of museum patrons of various ages interacting with museum exhibits. Complete structured observation of behavioral, sensory, and social demands of the museum, including structure, timing, and transitions of docent-led groups; signage; "way-finding" materials; and universal design features of physical space.	Provide an educational presentation to museum education staff about the characteristics associated with ASD and strategies for supporting informal learning. Consult with museum staff to develop a Social Story (Gray, 2010) to be placed on the museum website for families to use before visiting the museum. Consult with museum staff to develop an after-school program for adolescents with ASD.

(Continued)

Table 2. Case Examples of Occupational Therapy Evaluation and Intervention Services for Individuals With ASD *(cont.)*

Client Description	Evaluation	Intervention
	Conduct focus groups at the museum with parents who have children with ASD to elicit their recommendations for improving accessibility.	
T. J., age 21 years, is a young man with high-functioning autism. T. J. currently is enrolled in a junior college and is having difficulty finding a needed part-time job. He lives independently in an apartment. T. J. presents with poor grooming and hygiene skills and pragmatic language deficits. He has several interests but spends most of his free time reading about antique cars. His interest in cars has led to distractibility during driving and resulted in a minor auto accident and a traffic citation for failing to stop at a stop sign.	Develop an occupational profile of ADL and IADL performance, leisure activities, and driving behaviors through personal interview about his concerns and his interests. Conduct structured observation of role playing a job interview. Administer the Scales of Independent Behavior–Revised (Bruininks, Woodcock, Weatherman, & Hill, 1997) and Occupational Self Assessment (Baron, Kielhofner, Iyenger, Goldhammer, & Wolenski, 2006). Develop an occupational profile for behavior regulation and interpersonal relatedness through interview.	Initially provide occupational therapy weekly in the clinic, then in the community (Case-Smith & Weaver, 2015a; Weaver, 2015). Provide direct intervention to address grooming and hygiene needs through the use of a step-by-step self-monitoring system. Consult with the Division of Vocational Rehabilitation to assist in the employment search. Use role playing, video self-modeling, and collaborative problem solving to address social communication and pragmatic language needs related to the interview process and interaction with coworkers (Case-Smith & Weaver, 2015b; Weaver, 2015). Initiate job coaching to allow T. J. to learn and master job functions and to problem solve when needed. Refer to an occupational therapy DRS to assess driving safety and provide interventions to improve executive functioning and focused attention during driving (Classen, Monahan, & Wang, 2013). Facilitate T. J.'s enrollment in an existing on-campus support group of other college students with Asperger disorder.
Sanjaya, age 34 years, has Asperger disorder. He lives in an apartment with his wife and contributes to the family income through an online business. Sanjaya has challenges with arousal regulation and coping skills, difficulty with body space awareness, and difficulty reading and sending body language signals that affect his social participation. Sanjaya has tactile defensiveness, which leads to difficulties with intimacy.	Administer the Adolescent/Adult Sensory Profile (Brown & Dunn, 2002) and the COPM (Law et al., 2014).	Initially provide occupational therapy services in the OT's office to address Sanjaya's poor processing of tactile, vestibular, and proprioceptive input. Develop a sensory diet for Sanjaya to implement daily in his natural environment (Dunn, Cox, Foster, Mische-Lawson, & Tanquary, 2012; Watling & Hauer, 2015a). Consult with and train Sanjaya and his wife in the Alert Program (Williams & Shellenberger, 1996) to recognize when his arousal level is high and to provide a language to aid in their communication. Perform video analysis (Bellini & Akullian, 2007) and role playing to help develop an awareness of nonverbal communication through facial expression and body language and to practice pragmatic skills. Train Sanjaya and his wife in the use of massage to provide deep tactile pressure and proprioceptive input to diminish tactile defensiveness.

(Continued)

Table 2. Case Examples of Occupational Therapy Evaluation and Intervention Services for Individuals With ASD *(cont.)*

Client Description	Evaluation	Intervention
Martina, age 47 years, has autism and has recently transitioned from her parent's home to a group home with 24-hour supervision due to her parents' declining ability to care for her. Martina works at a local library where she sorts and reshelves books. She has funding for services through the Department of Developmental Disabilities and a small amount of private resources. Martina becomes anxious when her routine is disturbed, demands are placed on her, or her desires are not granted. She enjoys leisure activities with her parents, but her parents are worried about her making friends and joining activities with peers at the group home. Her parents have arranged for contract occupational therapy services to facilitate her transition to the group home, with a focus on establishing routines for self-care and household chores, understanding and using transportation services to and from work, and participation in leisure activities with peers at the group home.	Develop an occupational profile through observation of and interview with Martina and her parents. Administer the COPM (Law et al., 2014), Adolescent/Adult Sensory Profile (Brown & Dunn, 2002), and Test of Grocery Shopping Skills (Brown, Rempfer, & Hamera, 2009). Conduct clinical observations of behavior during leisure, self-care, cooking, laundry, and cleaning tasks and of path finding and skills for using public transportation.	Provide occupational therapy services in the group home to help Martina organize her belongings; establish a routine for daily self-care and weekly household tasks; and ensure her success in using the available microwave oven, washer, dryer, and vacuum (Weaver, 2015). Work with Martina in using public transportation to get to and from work each day. Coach Martina in how to follow a picture sequence on her smart phone to help her follow her walking route, identify where to get off the bus, and know what to do if the bus is late. Teach residential program staff to implement educational strategies, such as forward and backward chaining, visual supports, and environmental structure to support success during intervention (Horner et al., 2002; Hwang & Hughes, 2000; NAC, 2015) and during everyday activities. Conduct staff training regarding environmental accommodations and environmental supports. Collaborate with group home staff to identify leisure activity choices that match the interests Martina and her parents identified during the occupational profile. Coach Martina in how to engage with peers during leisure activities and provide Social Stories, scripts, and role-playing opportunities to help her learn new routines and what to do and say (Tanner et al., 2015).

Note. ADL = activity of daily living; ASD = autism spectrum disorder; COPM = Canadian Occupational Performance Measure; DRS = driving rehabilitation specialist; IADL = instrumental activity of daily living; NAC = National Autism Center; OT = occupational therapist; PDD–NOS = pervasive developmental disorder, not otherwise specified; SLP = speech–language pathologist; TEACCH = Treatment and Education of Autistic and Related Communication Handicapped Children.

PART II

Societal Statements

AOTA's Societal Statement on Combat-Related Posttraumatic Stress

Self-report of symptoms of post-traumatic stress disorder (PTSD) have tripled among combat-exposed military personnel, compared to those who have not deployed, since 2001 (Smith et al., 2008). Tanielian and Jaycox (2008) have estimated that approximately 300,000 military personnel previously deployed to Iraq or Afghanistan currently experience PTSD or major depression. Military personnel are returning home and demonstrating signs and symptoms of combat-related PTSD, such as nightmares, flashbacks, memory loss, insomnia, depression, avoidance of social interaction, fear, decreased energy, drug and alcohol use, and the inability to concentrate. These signs and symptoms could affect these individuals' ability to effectively negotiate their personal lives and work roles. Specifically during work, the avoidance of social interactions and avoidance of situations that resemble the traumatic event may interfere with coworker relationships or may be perceived as the lack of motivation or ability to be successful in a work setting (Penk, Drebing, & Schutt, 2002).

Combat-related PTSD not only affects military personnel but also the family and the community in which military personnel interact. If unidentified and untreated, the effects of combat-related PTSD may have a delayed onset and cause problems such as depression, social alienation, marital communication problems, difficulty with parenting, and alcohol and drug abuse, and each can cause a disruption in military personnel's personal lives, professional abilities, and overall physical and mental health (Baum, 2008). It is vital for military personnel and health care providers to be educated on these signs and symptoms and detect them early to ensure that military personnel receive adequate opportunities for prompt intervention services and to access support. This is something that occupational therapists and occupational therapy assistants can do.

The overarching goal of occupational therapy for military personnel coping with combat-related PTSD is to use strategies to help them recover, compensate, or adapt so they can reengage with activities that are necessary for their daily life. Occupational therapists and occupational therapy assistants also help military personnel coping with combated-related PTSD to develop strategies to self-manage the long-term consequences of the condition. These strategies are important to promote their health and participation in family, community, and military life because these strategies support their ability to engage or re-engage in daily life activities and occupations that are necessary and meaningful to them. Because of their knowledge and skills in addressing the physical, cognitive, and psychosocial factors associated with combat-related PTSD, occupational therapists and occupational therapy assistants bring broad expertise to help personnel identify the barriers that are limiting their recovery and participation in meaningful activities (American Occupational Therapy Association [AOTA], 2005). AOTA supports recognition of and intervention services for military personnel coping with combat-related PTSD, including research, advocacy, education, and resource allocation consistent with professional standards and ethics.

References

American Occupational Therapy Association. (2005). Occupational therapy code of ethics (2005). *American Journal of Occupational Therapy, 59,* 639–642.

Baum, C. M. (2008, April 1). *Post traumatic stress disorder treatment and research: Moving ahead toward recovery.* Statement of Carolyn M. Baum, PhD, OTR/L, FAOTA, before the House Committee on Veterans' Affairs. Available online at http://veterans.house.gov/hearings/Testimony.aspx?TID=26235& Newsid=188 &Name=%20Carolyn%20M.%20Baum,%20Ph.D,%20OTR/L,%20FAOTA

Penk, W., Drebing, C., & Schutt, R. (2002). PTSD in the workplace. In J. C. Thomas & M. Hersen (Eds.), *Handbook of mental health in the workplace* (pp. 215–248). Thousand Oaks, CA: Sage.

Smith, T. C., Ryan, M. A., Wingard, D. L., Slymen, D. J., Sallis, J. F., & Kritz-Sivlerstein, D. (2008). New onset and persistent symptoms of post-traumatic stress disorder self-reported after deployment and combat exposures: prospective population-based US military cohort study. *British Medical Journal, 336,* 336–371.

Tanielian, T. L., & Jaycox, L. H. (Eds. 2008). *Invisible wounds of war: Psychological and cognitive injuries, their consequences, and services to assist recovery.* Santa Monica, CA: Rand Corporation. Available online at http://www.rand.org/pubs/monographs/2008/RAND_MG720.pdf

Authors

Robinette J., Amaker, PhD, OTR/L, CHT, FAOTA
Yvette Woods, PhD, OTR/L
Steven M. Gerardi, MS, OTR/L, CHT

The views expressed in this article are those of the authors and do not reflect the official policy or position of the Department of the Army, Department of Defense, or the U.S. Government.

for

The Representative Assembly Coordinating Council (RACC):
Deborah Murphy-Fischer, MBA, OTR, BCP, IMT, *Chairperson*
Brent Braveman, PhD, OTR/L, FAOTA
Coralie Glantz, OTR/L, BCG, FAOTA
René Padilla, PhD, OTR/L, FAOTA
Kathlyn Reed, PhD, OTR, FAOTA, MLIS
Barbara Schell, PhD, OTR/L, FAOTA
Pam Toto, MS, OTR/L, BCG, FAOTA
Carol H. Gwin, OT/L, *AOTA Staff Liaison*

Adopted by the Representative Assembly 2008CS84

AOTA's Societal Statement on Health Disparities

It is widely recognized that disparities in health status and the availability of or access to health and social services exist in the United States. The Trans–National Institutes of Health (NIH) Work Group on Health Disparities defined the term health disparities as "differences in incidence, prevalence, morbidity, mortality, and burden of diseases and other adverse health conditions that exist among specific population groups" (NIH, 2002).

Health disparities result from the complex interactions among biological factors (e.g., genetics, family history), the environment (e.g., social discrimination; availability, access, and quality of health care), and specific health behaviors (e.g., smoking, alcohol abuse). Health disparities can affect population groups on the basis of gender, age, ethnicity, socioeconomic and educational status, geography, sexual orientation, and disability. Inequities in health exist when the disparities in factors are avoidable and unfair (United Nations Committee for Development Policy, 2009). Groups who have persistently experienced historical trauma, social disadvantage, or discrimination systematically experience worse health or greater health risks than more advantaged social groups (Williams, 2010).

Occupational therapy practitioners have the responsibility to intervene with individuals and communities to limit the effects of inequities that result in health disparities. Practitioners have knowledge and skills in evaluating and intervening with individuals and groups who face physical, social, emotional, or cultural challenges to participation. Further, the American Occupational Therapy Association (AOTA) supports advocacy to increase access to health services for persons in need, and efforts to lessen or eliminate health disparities are consistent with the *Occupational Therapy Code of Ethics and Ethics Standards (2010)* (AOTA, 2010).

References

American Occupational Therapy Association. (2010). Occupational therapy code of ethics and ethics standards (2010). *American Journal of Occupational Therapy, 64*(6 Suppl.), S17–S26. http://dx.doi.org/10.5014/ajot.2010.64S17

National Institutes of Health. (2002). *Strategic research plan and budget to reduce and ultimately eliminate health disparities, Vol. 1, Fiscal years 2000–2006.* Washington, DC: U.S. Department of Health and Human Services. Retrieved June 23, 2011, from www.nimhd.nih.gov/our_programs/strategic/pubs/VolumeI_031003EDrev.pdf

United Nations Committee for Development Policy. (2009). *Policy note: Implementing the Millenium Development Goals: Health inequality and the role of global health partnerships.* New York: Author. Retrieved January 14, 2011, from www.un.org/esa/policy/devplan/cdppublications/2009cdp_mdg health.pdf

Williams, R. A. (2010). Historical perspectives on healthcare disparities: Is the past prologue? In R. A. Williams (Ed.), *Eliminating healthcare disparities in America: Beyond the IOM report* (pp. 3–20). Totowa, NJ: Humana Press.

Authors
Brent Braveman, PhD, OTR/L, FAOTA
Jyothi Gupta, PhD, OTR/L
René Padilla, PhD, OTR/L, FAOTA

The Representative Assembly Coordinating Council (RACC):
Denise Chisholm, PhD, OTR/L, FAOTA, *Chairperson*
Yvonne Randall, EdD, OTR/L, FAOTA
Jyothi Gupta, PhD, OTR/L
Andrea Bilics, PhD, OTR/L
Barbara Hemphill, DMin, OTR, FAOTA, FMOTA
Yvette Hachtel, JD, MEd, OTR/L
Debbie Amini, EdD, OTR/L, CHT
Mary Kay Currie, OT, BCPR
Kimberly Hartmann, PhD, OTR/L, FAOTA
Laurel Cargill Radley, MS, OTR/L, *AOTA Staff Liaison*

Adopted by the Representative Assembly 2006C360; revised 2011 by the RACC; revised 2013 by the RACC

AOTA's Societal Statement on Health Literacy

Health literacy, or the ability of individuals to gather, interpret, and use information to make suitable health-related decisions (Institute of Medicine, 2004), promotes participation, empowerment, and control over daily life (Nutbeam, 2008). Persons with inadequate health literacy are more likely to experience adverse health outcomes (DeWalt, Berkman, Sheridan, Lohr, & Pignone, 2004). Although those who possess adequate health literacy achieve better health outcomes, an estimated 90 million people in the United States have limited reading literacy, which also affects their ability to access services and achieve optimal health (Kirsch, Jungeblut, Jenkins, & Kolstat, 2002). Inadequate health literacy disproportionately affects people living at or below the poverty level, limiting their ability to sufficiently participate in health-related activities (Greenfield, Sugarman, Nargiso, & Weiss, 2005).

Occupational therapy can promote health through the development and use of health education approaches and materials that are understandable, accessible, and usable by the full spectrum of consumers. Occupational therapy practitioners can assist in ensuring that all health-related information and education provided to recipients of occupational therapy or other health related services match that person's literacy abilities; cultural sensitivities; and verbal, cognitive, and social skills.

In line with the health communication objectives (U.S. Department of Health and Human Services, 2010), the American Occupational Therapy Association strives to ensure that occupational therapy practitioners possess appropriate communication and education skills that can help enable all people to gain access to, understand, and use occupational therapy and other health-related services, information, and education to promote self-management for optimum health and participation.

References

DeWalt, D. A., Berkman, N. D., Sheridan, S., Lohr, K. N., & Pignone, M. P. (2004). Literacy and health outcomes: A systematic review of the literature. *Journal of General Internal Medicine, 19,* 1228–1239.

Greenfield, S., Sugarman, D., Nargiso, J., & Weiss, R. (2005). Readability of patient handout materials in a nationwide sample of alcohol and drug abuse treatment programs. *American Journal on Addictions, 14,* 339–345.

Institute of Medicine. (2004). *Health literacy: A prescription to end confusion.* Washington, DC: National Academies Press.

Kirsch, I., Jungeblut, A., Jenkins, L., & Kolstat, A. (2002). *Adult literacy in America: A first look at the findings of the National Adult Literacy Survey* (3rd ed.). Washington, DC: National Center for Education, U.S. Department of Education.

Nutbeam, D. (2008). The evolving concept of health literacy. *Social Science and Medicine, 67,* 2072–2078.

U.S. Department of Health and Human Services. (2010). *Public comment on healthy people 2020.* Retrieved November 16, 2010, from http://www.healthypeople.gov/HP2020/Objectives/TopicArea.aspx?id=25&TopicArea=Health+Communication+and+Health+IT

Authors

Kris Pizur-Barnekow, PhD, OTR/L

Amy Darragh, PhD, OTR/L

for

The Representative Assembly Coordinating Council (RACC):

Mary F. Baxter, PhD, LOT, FAOTA, *Chairperson*

Janet V. DeLany, DEd, OTR/L, FAOTA

Barbara Hemphill, DMin, OTR, FAOTA, FMOTA

Yvonne Randall, EdD, OTR/L, FAOTA

Barbara Schell, PhD, OT/L, FAOTA

Pam Toto, PhD, OTR/L, BCG, FAOTA

Laurel Cargill Radley, MS, OTR/L, *AOTA Staff Liaison*

Adopted by the Representative Assembly 2011AprC21

AOTA's Societal Statement on Livable Communities

Livability has been defined as "the sum of the factors that add up to a community's quality of life—including the built and natural environments, economic prosperity, social stability and equity, educational opportunity, and cultural, entertainment and recreation possibilities" (Partners for Livable Communities, n.d., para. 1). Livable communities support quality of life for older adults (Kochera & Bright, 2005; Kochera, Straight, & Guterbock, 2005), health for disadvantaged populations (Miller, Pollack, & Williams, 2011), youth development (Miller et al., 2011), and participation of people with disabilities (Oberlink, 2005). The National Council on Disability's report on *Livable Communities for Adults with Disabilities* (2004) states that a *livable community*

- Provides affordable, appropriate, accessible housing;

- Ensures accessible, affordable, reliable, safe transportation;

- Adjusts the physical environment for inclusiveness and accessibility;

- Provides work, volunteer, and education opportunities;

- Ensures access to key health and support services; and

- Encourages participation in civic, cultural, social, and recreational activities. (p. 8)

Healthy People 2020 emphasizes the importance of livable communities in its goals for social determinants of health to "create social and physical environments that promote good health for all," physical activity to "improve health, fitness, and quality of life through daily physical activity," and disability and health to "promote the health and well-being of people with disabilities" (U.S. Department of Health and Human Services, 2012). The proposed characteristics of livable communities are also similar to the World Health Organization's (WHO's; 2007) age-friendly cities and the Centers for Disease Control and Prevention's (CDC's; 2015) healthy communities. *Age-friendly cities* are characterized by features of the physical and social environment (Lui, Everingham,Warburton, Cuthill, & Bartlett, 2009), including outdoor spaces and buildings, transportation systems, housing, social participation activities, respect and social inclusion, civic participation and employment, communication and information, and community and health services (AARP, n.d.; Menec, Means, Keating, Parkhurst, & Eales, 2011; Plouffe, & Kalache, 2010; WHO, 2007). *Healthy communities* are designed to promote physical activity, safety, good nutrition, social connectedness, and environmental health (CDC, 2015).

Occupational therapy practitioners are committed to creating livable communities that support full participation in everyday life by people of all ages and ability levels. The development of livable communities requires involvement of community members; health, social services, and education professionals; policymakers and planners; designers and architects; and contractors. Occupational therapy practitioners have extensive knowledge of aging, health conditions, disabilities, and at-risk populations, as well as the features of the physical and social environment that support or limit full participation. Occupational therapy practitioners work with individuals and organizations to evaluate barriers in the environment that contribute to health inequities and diminished quality of life; design and modify home and community environments; and create opportunities for engagement in meaningful physical, social, vocational, and cultural activities.

References

AARP. (n.d.). *AARP livable communities.* Retrieved from http://www.aarp.org/livable-communities/

Centers for Disease Control and Prevention. (2015, June 9). *Healthy community design.* Retrieved from http://www.cdc.gov/healthyplaces/healthy_comm_design.htm

Kochera, A., & Bright, K. (2005). Livable communities for older people. *Generations, 29*(4), 32–36.

Kochera, A., Straight, A., & Guterbock, T. (2005). *Beyond 50.05: A report to the nation on livable communities—Creating environments for successful aging.* Washington, DC: AARP. Retrieved from http://assets.aarp.org/rgcenter/il/beyond_50_communities.pdf

Lui, C. W., Everingham, J. A., Warburton, J., Cuthill, M., & Bartlett, H. (2009). What makes a community age-friendly: A review of international literature. *Australasian Journal on Ageing, 28,* 116–121. http://dx.doi.org/10.1111/j.1741-6612.2009.00355.x

Menec, V. H., Means, R., Keating, N., Parkhurst, G., & Eales, J. (2011). Conceptualizing age-friendly communities. *Canadian Journal on Aging, 30,* 479–493. http://dx.doi.org/10.1017/S0714980811000237

Miller, W. D., Pollack, C. E., & Williams, D. R. (2011). Healthy homes and communities: Putting the pieces together. *American Journal of Preventive Medicine, 40*(Suppl. 1), S48–S57. http://dx.doi.org/10.1016/j.amepre.2010.09.024

National Council on Disability. (2004). *Livable communities for adults with disabilities.* Retrieved from http://www.ncd.gov/publications/2004/12022004

Oberlink, M. (2005). Livable communities for adults with disabilities. *Policy Brief (Center for Home Care Policy and Research [US]), 29,* 1–6.

Partners for Livable Communities. (n.d.). *What is livability?* Retrieved from http://livable.org/about-us/what-is-livability

Plouffe, L., & Kalache, A. (2010). Towards global age-friendly cities: determining urban features that promote active aging. *Journal of Urban Health, 87,* 733–739. http://dx.doi.org/10.1007/s11524-010-9466-0

U.S. Department of Health and Human Services, Office of Disease Prevention and Health Promotion. (2012). *Healthy people 2020.* Washington, DC: Author. Retrieved from http://www.healthypeople.gov

World Health Organization. (2007). *Ageing and life-course: Global age-friendly cities: A guide.* Retrieved from http://www.who.int/ageing/publications/age_friendly_cities_guide/en

Author

Julie D. Bass, PhD, OTR/L, FAOTA

for

The Representative Assembly Coordinating Committee:
Sara-Jane Crowley, Adv. Dip.OT, OTR/L, *Vice Speaker/Chair*
Deborah Slater, MS, OT/L, FAOTA, *AOTA Staff Liaison*

Adopted by the Representative Assembly Coordinating Committee 2016

Note. This document replaces the 2009 document *AOTA's Societal Statement on Livable Communities,* previously published and copyrighted in 2009 by the American Occupational Therapy Association in the *American Journal of Occupational Therapy, 63,* 847–848. http://dx.doi.org/10.5014/ajot.2009.63.6.847

Citation. American Occupational Therapy Association. (2016). AOTA's societal statement on livable communities. *American Journal of Occupational Therapy, 70*(Suppl. 2), 7012410020. http://dx.doi.org/10.5014/ajot.2016.706S01

AOTA's Societal Statement on Stress and Stress Disorders

Stress is a pervasive societal challenge that affects the social participation of people of varying ages, ethnicity, gender, and socioeconomic status (U.S. Department of Health and Human Services [USDHHS], 2000). It is a significant risk factor in a number of health problems, including mental illness, cognitive decline, cardiovascular disease, musculoskeletal disorders, and workplace injuries. Individuals with disabilities are disproportionately affected, with 49 percent of these people reporting adverse health effects from stress, compared with 34 percent of the general population (USDHHS, 2000).

Individuals, families, organizations, and communities differ significantly in their perceptions of and vulnerability to stressful events, as well as in their coping strategies. Organizational stressors, such as relocation or restructuring, may result in financial strain and loss of personnel. Community or population catastrophes, such as natural disasters or wars, result in stress from overwhelming personal loss, forced displacement, and a disruption of massive proportions in familiar daily routines and occupations (Wein, 2000).

The occupational therapy profession promotes the establishment of healthy habit patterns; familiar, predictable routines; and increased engagement in meaningful occupations that serve both as protective and healing factors in combating the negative effects of stress. Occupational therapy practitioners[1] develop evidence-based interventions based on this philosophy, and conduct research to establish their efficacy for coping with stress (Jackson, Carlson, Mandel, Zemke, & Clark, 1998; Nelson, 1996; Oaten & Chen, 2006; Wein, 2000).

References

American Occupational Therapy Association. (2006). Policy 1.44: Categories of occupational therapy personnel. *American Journal of Occupational Therapy, 60,* 683–684.

Hinojosa, J., & Kramer, P. (1997). Statement—Fundamental concepts of occupational therapy: Occupation, purposeful activity, and function. *American Journal of Occupational Therapy, 51,* 864–866.

Jackson, J., Carlson, M., Mandel, D., Zemke, R., & Clark, F. (1998). Occupation in lifestyle redesign: The Well Elderly Study Occupational Therapy Program. *American Journal of Occupational Therapy, 52,* 326–336.

Nelson, D. L. (1996). Therapeutic occupation: A definition. *American Journal of Occupational Therapy, 50,* 775–782.

Oaten, M., & Chen, K. (2006). Longitudinal gains in self-regulation from regular physical exercise. *British Journal of Health Psychology, 11,* 717–733.

U.S. Department of Health and Human Services. (2000). *Healthy people 2010: Understanding and improving health* (2nd ed.). Washington, DC: U.S. Government Printing Office.

---

[1]When the term *occupational therapy practitioner* is used in this document, it refers to both occupational therapists and occupational therapy assistants (AOTA, 2006).

Wein, H. (2000). *Stress and disease: New perspectives* [NIH Word on Health]. Retrieved October 20, 2006, from http://www.nih.gov/news/WordonHealth/oct2000/story01.htm

Related Reading

Selye, H. (1975). Stress and distress. *Comprehensive Therapy, 1*(8), 9–13.

Author
Susan Stallings-Sahler, PhD, OTR/L, FAOTA

for

The Representative Assembly Coordinating Council (RACC):
Deborah Murphy-Fischer, MBA, OTR, BCP, IMT, *Chairperson*
Brent Braveman, PhD, OTR/L, FAOTA
Linda Fazio, PhD, OTR/L, LPC, FAOTA
Coralie Glantz, OTR/L, BCG, FAOTA
Wendy C. Hildenbrand, MPH, OTR/L, FAOTA
Kathlyn L. Reed, PhD, OTR, FAOTA, MLIS
S. Maggie Reitz, PhD, OTR/L, FAOTA
Susanne Smith Roley, MS, OTR/L, FAOTA
Carol H. Gwin, OT/L, *AOTA Staff Liaison*

Adopted by the Representative Assembly 2007C82

AOTA's Societal Statement on Youth Violence

A nationwide crisis related to youth violence has resulted in this being the second-leading cause of death among all youth aged 15 to 24 years and the leading cause of death among African American youth of the same age (U.S. Department of Health and Human Services, 2000). Acts of violence include bullying, verbal threats, physical assault, domestic abuse, and gunfire. Premature death, disability, and academic failure occur due to violent activity that surrounds youth. Risk factors that lead to youth violence include history of being abused or abusing others, school truancy, poor time use, exposure to crime, mental illness, drug and alcohol use, gang involvement, access to guns, and absence of familial and social support structures. Rising health care costs, decreased property values, and social services disruption are indicators of the impact that violence has on the health of communities, as well as on individual participation in society (Centers for Disease Control & Prevention, 2006). Individual participation can be limited by reduced access to services, fear of harm to self or others, and the inability to perform valued roles. The severity of this issue has forced policymakers, health care providers, teachers, parents, and students to recognize, examine, and alter social conditions, cultural influences, and relationships.

The profession of occupational therapy has the societal duty and expertise to respond to youth violence by promoting overall health and well-being among youth (American Occupational Therapy Association, 2006). Occupational therapy practitioners work toward understanding the occupational nature of violence, researching effective interventions, creating collaborations, and advocating for public health and social services for youth. Violence and its antecedents can deprive this growing segment of youth of necessary and meaningful occupations (Whiteford, 2000), leaving them insufficiently prepared for their future. Positive change can occur by providing youth with opportunities to replace poor occupational choices with healthy, safe, productive, and socially acceptable activities (Snyder, Clark, Masunaka-Noriego, & Young, 1998). Ultimately, occupational therapy practitioners provide services that support a vision of social justice, dignity, and social action throughout the life span by addressing the engagement patterns and lifestyle choices of at-risk youth through methods such as effective transition services and life skills remediation.

References

American Occupational Therapy Association. (2006). *Centennial Vision: Ad hoc report on children and youth.* Retrieved August 7, 2007, from http://www.aota.org/News/Centennial/Updates/AdHoc.aspx

Centers for Disease Control and Prevention. (2006). *Understanding youth violence* [Fact Sheet]. Retrieved August 9, 2007, from http://www.cdc.gov/ncipc/pub-res/YVFactSheet.pdf

Snyder, C., Clark, F., Masunaka-Noriega, M., & Young, B. (1998). Los Angeles street kids: New occupations for life program. *Journal of Occupational Science, 5,* 133–139.

U.S. Department of Health and Human Services. (2000). *Healthy People 2010: Injury and violence prevention.* Retrieved November 17, 2006, from http://www.healthypeople.gov/docuament/html/volume1/07ed.htm

Whiteford, G. (2000). Occupational deprivation: Global challenge in the new millennium. *British Journal of Occupational Therapy, 63,* 200–204.

Author
Heather D. Goertz, OTD, OTR/L

Author
Creighton University Class of 2007 occupational therapy doctoral students:
  Bryan Benedict, Oanh Bui, Stacy Peitz, Rose Ryba
Susan Cahill, MAEA, OTR/L, Clinical Instructor, University of Illinois at Chicago

for

The Representative Assembly Coordinating Council (RACC):
Deborah Murphy-Fischer, MBA, OTR, BCP, IMT, *Chairperson*
Brent Braveman, PhD, OTR/L, FAOTA
Janet V. Delany, DEd, OTR/L, FAOTA
Coralie Glantz, OTR/L, BCG, FAOTA
René Padilla, PhD, OTR/L, FAOTA
Kathlyn L. Reed, PhD, OTR, FAOTA, MLIS
Barbara Schell, PhD, OTR/L, FAOTA
Susanne Smith Roley, MS, OTR/L, FAOTA
Carol H. Gwin, OT/L, *AOTA Staff Liaison*

Adopted by the Representative Assembly 2007CO144

PART III

Rescissions, Revisions, and Changes

Rescissions, Revisions, and Changes

The following rescissions, revisions, and changes have been made since the publication of previous editions of the *Reference Manual of the Official Documents of the American Occupational Therapy Association, Inc.* The final version (for rescinded or replaced documents) or most recent version (for documents still in force) is in the "Document" column. The document's history is in the next column. Documents that have been revised or incorporated into new documents are listed in the "History" column.

Summary of Official Document Rescissions, Revisions, and Changes

Document (Final or Most Recent Version)	History
Bylaws	
• Bylaws (2016). • Incorporation Papers (2013). • Glossary (2014).	• Incorporation Papers and Bylaws (1991, 1996, 1999, 2002, 2003, 2005). Bylaws and Glossary **revised** and **replaced** 2007. Bylaws, Glossary, and Incorporation Papers **revised** and **replaced** 2010. • Incorporation Papers and Bylaws **revised** and **replaced** 2013. • Bylaws **edited** 2014. **Revised** 2016. • Glossary **revised** 2014.
Accreditation	
2011 Accreditation Council for Occupational Therapy Education (ACOTE®) Standards (2012).	• Accreditation Standards for a Doctoral-Degree-Level Educational Program for the Occupational Therapist (2007), Accreditation Standards for a Master's-Degree-Level Educational Program for the Occupational Therapist (2007), and Accreditation Standards for an Educational Program for the Occupational Therapy Assistant (2007). **Replaced** by 2011 Accreditation Council for Occupational Therapy Education (ACOTE®) Standards (2012). • Essentials and Guidelines for an Accredited Educational Program for the Occupational Therapist (1935, 1943, 1949, 1965, 1973, 1983, 1991, 1995, 1998). **Rescinded** 2007. **Replaced** by Accreditation Standards for a Doctoral-Degree-Level Educational Program for the Occupational Therapist (2007) and Accreditation Standards for a Master's-Degree-Level Educational Program for the Occupational Therapist (2007). **Replaced** by 2011 Accreditation Council for Occupational Therapy Education (ACOTE®) Standards (2012). • Essentials and Guidelines for an Accredited Educational Program for the Occupational Therapy Assistant (1958, 1962, 1967, 1970, 1975, 1983, 1991, 1995, 1998). **Rescinded** 2007. **Replaced** by Accreditation Standards for an Educational Program for the Occupational Therapy Assistant (2007). **Replaced** by 2011 Accreditation Council for Occupational Therapy Education (ACOTE®) Standards (2012).
Concept Papers	
Cross-Training Concept Paper (1997).	**Rescinded** 2002.

(Continued)

Summary of Official Document Rescissions, Revisions, and Changes *(cont.)*

Document (Final or Most Recent Version)	History
Concept Papers *(cont.)*	
The Role of Occupational Therapy in Disaster Preparedness, Response, and Recovery: A Concept Paper (2011).	The Role of Occupational Therapy in Disaster Preparedness, Response, and Recovery: A Concept Paper (2006). **Revised** 2011.
Scholarship in Occupational Therapy (2009).	Scholarship and Occupational Therapy (2003). **Revised** 2009, 2016.
Service Delivery in Occupational Therapy (1995).	**Rescinded** 2004.
Education	
Academic Terminal Degree (2008).	Academic Terminal Degree (2003). **Replaced** by Academic Terminal Degree (2008).
Occupational Therapy Fieldwork Education: Value and Purpose (2009).	Purpose and Value of Occupational Therapy Fieldwork Education (1996). **Replaced** by The Purpose and Value of Occupational Therapy Fieldwork Education (2003). **Replaced** by Occupational Therapy Fieldwork Education: Value and Purpose (2009).
Philosophy of Occupational Therapy Education (2014).	Philosophy of Professional Education (1997, 2003). **Replaced** by Philosophy of Occupational Therapy Education (2007). **Replaced** by Philosophy of Occupational Therapy Education (2014).
Standards and Guidelines for an Occupational Therapy Affiliation Program (1970).	**Rescinded** 1983.
Value of Occupational Therapy Assistant Education to the Profession (2015).	The Viability of Occupational Therapy Assistant Education (2002). **Replaced** by the Importance of Occupational Therapy Assistant Education (2008). **Replaced** by Value of Occupational Therapy Assistant Education to the Profession (2015).
Ethics	
Core Values and Attitudes of Occupational Therapy Practice (1993).	**Rescinded** 2010.
Enforcement Procedures for the Occupational Therapy Code of Ethics and Ethics Standards (2014).	Enforcement Procedures for Occupational Therapy Code of Ethics (1994, 1996, 1998, 2000, 2002, 2004, 2005, **edited** 2006). **Replaced** by Enforcement Procedures for Occupational Therapy Code of Ethics (2007). **Replaced** by Enforcement Procedures for Occupational Therapy Code of Ethics and Ethics Standards (2010). **Replaced** by Enforcement Procedures for the Occupational Therapy Code of Ethics and Ethics Standards (2014).
Guidelines to the Occupational Therapy Code of Ethics (2006).	Guidelines to the Occupational Therapy Code of Ethics (1998). **Replaced** by the Guidelines to the Occupational Therapy Code of Ethics (2006). **Rescinded** 2010.
Occupational Therapy Code of Ethics (2015).	Occupational Therapy Code of Ethics (1988, 1994, 2000). **Replaced** by Occupational Therapy Code of Ethics (2005, **edited** 2006). **Replaced** by Occupational Therapy Code of Ethics and Ethics Standards (2010). **Replaced** by Occupational Therapy Code of Ethics (2015).
Guidelines	
Guidelines for Documentation of Occupational Therapy (2013).	Guidelines for Occupational Therapy Documentation (1986). **Replaced** by Elements of Clinical Documentation (1994). **Rescinded** 2003. **Replaced** by Guidelines for Documentation of Occupational Therapy (2003, **edited** 2007). **Replaced by** Guidelines for Documentation of Occupational Therapy (2013).
Guidelines for Reentry Into the Field of Occupational Therapy (2015).	Guidelines for Reentry Into the Field of Occupational Therapy (2010). **Replaced** by Guidelines for Reentry Into the Field of Occupational Therapy (2015).

(Continued)

Summary of Official Document Rescissions, Revisions, and Changes *(cont.)*

Document (Final or Most Recent Version)	History
Guidelines *(cont.)*	
Guidelines for Supervision, Roles, and Responsibilities During the Delivery of Occupational Therapy Services (2014).	The following documents have been superseded by the Guidelines for Supervision, Roles, and Responsibilities During the Delivery of Occupational Therapy Services (2004, **edited** 2009, 2014): • Statement of Occupational Therapy Referral (1969, 1980, 1994). **Rescinded** 2004. (Also **replaced** by Scope of Practice [2004; **edited** 2005]). • Supervision Guidelines (1986). **Rescinded** 1992. • Use of Occupational Therapy Aides in Occupational Therapy Practice (1995, **edited** 1996). **Rescinded** 1999. **Replaced** by Guidelines for the Use of Aides in Occupational Therapy Practice (1996, 1999 [correction, *AJOT, 54,* 235]). **Rescinded** 2004. (Also **replaced** by Scope of Practice [2004; **edited** 2005]). • Occupational Therapy Roles (1993) and Career Exploration and Development: A Companion Guide to the Occupational Therapy Roles Document (1994). **Rescinded** 2004. (Also **replaced** by Scope of Practice [2004; **edited** 2005]). • Guide for Supervision of Occupational Therapy Personnel (1994). **Rescinded** 1999. **Replaced** by Guide for Supervision of Occupational Therapy Personnel in the Delivery of Occupational Therapy Services (1999 [correction, *AJOT, 54,* 235]). **Rescinded** 2004.
Hierarchy of Competencies Relating to the Use of Standardized Instruments and Evaluation Techniques by Occupational Therapists (1984).	**Rescinded** 1992.
Occupational Therapy Practice Framework: Domain and Process, 3rd Edition (2014).	Occupational Therapy Practice Framework: Domain and Process (2002). **Replaced** by Occupational Therapy Practice Framework: Domain and Process, 2nd Edition (2008). **Replaced** by Occupational Therapy Practice Framework: Domain and Process, 3rd Edition (2014).
Occupational Therapy Product Output Reporting System (1979).	**Rescinded** 1994.
Supervision Guidelines for Certified Occupational Therapy Assistants (1990).	**Rescinded** 1993.
Uniform Occupational Therapy Evaluation Checklist (1981).	**Rescinded** 1994.
Uniform Terminology for Occupational Therapy (Third Edition) and Application to Practice (1994).	Uniform Terminology for Reporting Occupational Therapy Services—First Edition (1979). **Replaced** by Uniform Terminology for Occupational Therapy (Second Edition) and the Application of Uniform Terminology to Practice (1989). **Replaced** by Uniform Terminology for Occupational Therapy (Third Edition) and Application to Practice (1994). **Rescinded** 2002. **Replaced** by Occupational Therapy Practice Framework: Domain and Process (2002).
Specialized Knowledge and Skills Papers	
Specialized Knowledge and Skills for Occupational Therapy Practice in the Neonatal Intensive Care Unit (2006).	Specialized Knowledge and Skills for Occupational Therapy Practice in the Neonatal Intensive Care Unit (1993, 2000). **Replaced** by Specialized Knowledge and Skills for Occupational Therapy Practice in the Neonatal Intensive Care Unit (2006).
Specialized Knowledge and Skills in Adult Vestibular Rehabilitation for Occupational Therapy Practice (2006).	Specialized Knowledge and Skills in Adult Vestibular Rehabilitation for Occupational Therapy Practice (2000). **Replaced** by Specialized Knowledge and Skills in Adult Vestibular Rehabilitation for Occupational Therapy Practice (2006).

(Continued)

Summary of Official Document Rescissions, Revisions, and Changes *(cont.)*

Document (Final or Most Recent Version)	History
Specialized Knowledge and Skills Papers *(cont.)*	
Specialized Knowledge and Skills in Feeding, Eating, and Swallowing for Occupational Therapy Practice (2007).	Occupational Therapy and Eating Dysfunction (1989). **Replaced** by Eating Dysfunction Position Paper (1996). **Replaced** by Specialized Knowledge and Skills in Eating and Feeding in Occupational Therapy Practice (2000). **Replaced** by Specialized Knowledge and Skills in Feeding, Eating, and Swallowing for Occupational Therapy Practice (2007).
Specialized Knowledge and Skills of Occupational Therapy Educators of the Future (2009).	Role Competencies for an Academic Fieldwork Coordinator (2003), Role Competencies for a Faculty Member in an OTA Academic Setting (2005), Role Competencies for a Fieldwork Educator (2005), Role Competencies for a Professional-Level OT Faculty Member in an Academic Setting (2005), Role Competencies for a Professional-Level Program Director in an Academic Setting (2009), and Role Competencies for a Program Director in an OTA Academic Setting (2003) all **rescinded** 2009 and **replaced** by Specialized Knowledge and Skills of Occupational Therapy Educators of the Future (2009).
Specialized Knowledge and Skills in Technology and Environmental Interventions for Occupational Therapy Practice (2009)	The Use of General Information and Assistive Technology Within Occupational Therapy Practice (1991, 1998). **Rescinded** 2004. **Replaced** by Assistive Technology Within Occupational Therapy Practice [Position Paper] (2004). **Rescinded** 2009. **Replaced** by Specialized Knowledge and Skills in Technology and Environmental Interventions for Occupational Therapy Practice (2009). **Rescinded** 2016. Replaced by Assistive Technology and Occupational Performance [Statement], 2016.
Position Papers	
Broadening the Construct of Independence (1995, 2002).	**Rescinded** 2007.
Complementary and Alternative Medicine (2011).	Complementary and Alternative Medicine Position Paper (CAM) (2005). **Revised** 2011.
Complex Environmental Modifications (2015).	New in 2015.
Importance of Interprofessional Education in Occupational Therapy Curricula (2015).	New in 2015.
Obesity and Occupational Therapy (2013).	Obesity and Occupational Therapy (2007). **Revised** 2013.
Occupation: A Position Paper (1995).	**Rescinded** 2004.
Occupational Performance: Occupational Therapy's Definition of Function (1995).	**Rescinded** 2002.
Occupational Therapy and Long-Term Services and Supports (1994).	**Rescinded** 2002.
Occupational Therapy and the Americans With Disabilities Act (ADA) (1993, 2000).	**Rescinded** 2005.
Occupational Therapy as an Education-Related Service (1981).	**Rescinded** 1987.
Occupational Therapy for Sensory Integrative Dysfunction (1982).	**Rescinded** 1991.
Occupational Therapy in Adult Day-Care (1986).	**Rescinded** 1992.
Occupational Therapy Services for Persons With Alzheimer's Disease and Other Dementias (Statement [1994]).	Occupational Therapy Services for Alzheimer's Disease and Related Disorders Position Paper (1986). **Replaced** by Occupational Therapy Services for Persons With Alzheimer's Disease and Other Dementias (Statement [1994]). **Rescinded** 2000.

(Continued)

Summary of Official Document Rescissions, Revisions, and Changes *(cont.)*

Document (Final or Most Recent Version)	History
Position Papers *(cont.)*	
Occupational Therapy's Commitment to Nondiscrimination and Inclusion (2014).	Occupational Therapy: A Profession in Support of Full Inclusion (1995) with White Paper: The Role of the Occupational Therapy Practitioner in the Implementation of Full Inclusion (1996). Position Paper and White Paper **rescinded** 1999. **Replaced** by Occupational Therapy's Commitment to Nondiscrimination and Inclusion (1999, *AJOT, 53,* 598 [correction, *54*(2), 235]). **Edited** 2009, 2014.
Occupational Therapy's Perspective on the Use of Environments and Contexts to Facilitate Health, Well-Being, and Participation in Occupations (2015).	Occupational Therapy's Perspective on the Use of Environments and Contexts to Support Health and Participation in Occupations (2010). **Replaced** by Occupational Therapy's Perspective on the Use of Environments and Contexts to Facilitate Health, Well-Being, and Participation in Occupations (2015).
Physical Agent Modalities (2012).	Physical Agent Modalities: A Position Paper (1992). **Replaced** by Physical Agent Modalities Position Paper (**edited** 1997). **Rescinded** 2003. **Replaced** by Physical Agent Modalities: A Position Paper (2003, **edited** 2007). **Replaced** by Physical Agent Modalities (2012).
Position Paper: Purposeful Activity (1993).	Purposeful Activities (1983). **Replaced** by Position Paper: Purposeful Activity (1993). **Rescinded** 2002.
Providing Services for Persons With HIV/AIDS and Their Caregivers (1996).	Human Immunodeficiency Virus (1984). **Replaced** by Providing Services for Persons with HIV/AIDS and Their Caregivers (1996). **Rescinded** 2002.
Scope of Practice (2014).	Scope of Practice (2004). **Replaced** by Scope of Practice (2009). **Replaced** by Scope of Practice (2014).
Telehealth (2013).	Telerehabilitation (2005). **Revised** (2010). **Replaced** by Telehealth (2013).
Roles Papers	
Definitions (1981).	Occupational Therapy: Its Definitions and Functions (1972). **Replaced** by Definitions (1981). **Rescinded** 1992.
Occupational Therapy and Long-Term Services and Supports (Position Paper [1994]).	Roles and Functions of Occupational Therapy in Long-Term Care: Occupational Therapy and Activity Programs (1983). **Rescinded** 1992. **Replaced** by Occupational Therapy and Long-Term Services and Supports (Position Paper [1994]).
Occupational Therapy Roles (1993) and Companion Guide (1994).	Minimal Occupational Therapy Classification Standards (1971). **Revised** 1997. **Replaced by** Guide to Classification of Occupational Therapy Personnel (1987). **Rescinded** 1991. **Replaced** by Occupational Therapy Roles (1993) and Companion Guide (1994).
	Entry-Level Role Delineation for OTRs and COTAs (1981). **Revised** 1990. **Rescinded** 1994. **Replaced** by Occupational Therapy Roles (1993) and Companion Guide (1994).
The Role of Occupational Therapy in End-of-Life Care (2011).	Occupational Therapy and Hospice (1986, 1991). **Replaced** by Statement, Occupational Therapy and Hospice (1998). **Replaced** by Occupational Therapy and Hospice (2004). **Replaced** by The Role of Occupational Therapy in End-of-Life Care (2011).
The Role of Occupational Therapy in the Independent Living Movement (Statement [1993]).	Occupational Therapy's Role in Independent or Alternative Living Situations (1981). **Rescinded** 1991. **Replaced** by The Role of Occupational Therapy in the Independent Living Movement (Statement [1993]). **Rescinded** 1999.
The Role of Occupational Therapy in the Vocational Rehabilitation Process (1980).	**Rescinded** 1991.
Roles and Functions of Occupational Therapy in Adult Day-Care (1986).	**Rescinded** 1992.
Roles and Functions of Occupational Therapy in Burn Care Delivery (1985).	**Rescinded** 1991.

(Continued)

Summary of Official Document Rescissions, Revisions, and Changes *(cont.)*

Document (Final or Most Recent Version)	History
Roles Papers *(cont.)*	
Roles and Functions of Occupational Therapy in Hand Rehabilitation (1985).	**Rescinded** 1991.
Roles and Functions of Occupational Therapy in Mental Health (1986).	**Rescinded** 1991.
Roles and Functions of Occupational Therapy in the Management of Patients With Rheumatic Diseases (1986).	**Rescinded** 1992.
Roles and Functions of Occupational Therapy Services for the Severely Disabled (1983).	**Rescinded** 1992.
Roles and Functions of the Occupational Therapist in the Treatment of Sensory Integrative Dysfunction (1982).	**Rescinded** 1991.
Roles of Occupational Therapists and Occupational Therapy Assistants in Schools (1987).	**Rescinded** 1997.
Standards	
Glossary of Terms Used in the Standards of Practice (1985).	**Rescinded** 1991.
Standards for Continuing Competence (2015).	Standards for Continuing Competence (1999). **Replaced** by Standards for Continuing Competence (2005). **Edited** 2006. **Revised** 2010, 2015.
Standards of Practice: Developmental Disabilities (1979, 1988).	**Rescinded** 1991.
Standards of Practice: Home Health (1979, 1988).	**Rescinded** 1991.
Standards of Practice: Mental Health (1979, 1988).	**Rescinded** 1991.
Standards of Practice: Physical Disabilities (1979, 1988).	**Rescinded** 1991.
Standards of Practice for Occupational Therapy (2015).	Standards of Practice for Occupational Therapy (1983, 1992, 1994, 1998). **Replaced** by Standards of Practice for Occupational Therapy (2005). **Revised** 2010, 2015.
Standards of Practice for Occupational Therapy Services in Schools (1987).	**Rescinded** 1994.
Statements	
AOTA Statement of Physical Agent Modalities (1991).	**Rescinded** 1997.
Assistive Technology and Occupational Performance (2016).	The Use of General Information and Assistive Technology Within Occupational Therapy Practice (1991, 1998). **Rescinded** 2004. **Replaced** by Assistive Technology Within Occupational Therapy Practice [Position Paper] (2004). **Rescinded** 2009. **Replaced** by Specialized Knowledge and Skills in Technology and Environmental Interventions for Occupational Therapy Practice (2009). Rescinded 2016. Replaced by Assistive Technology and Occupational Performance (2016).
Driving and Community Mobility (2015).	Driving and Community Mobility (2005). **Replaced by** Driving and Community Mobility (2010). **Revised** 2015.
Fundamental Concepts of Occupational Therapy: Occupation, Purposeful Activity, Function (1997).	**Rescinded** 2005.

(Continued)

Summary of Official Document Rescissions, Revisions, and Changes *(cont.)*

Document (Final or Most Recent Version)	History
Statements *(cont.)*	
Management of Occupational Therapy Services for Persons With Cognitive Impairments (1999).	Occupational Therapy Services Management of Persons With Cognitive Impairments (1991). **Rescinded** 1999. **Replaced** by Management of Occupational Therapy Services for Persons With Cognitive Impairments (1999). **Rescinded** 2003.
Nondiscrimination and Inclusion Regarding Members of the Occupational Therapy Professional Community (1995).	**Rescinded** 2005.
The Occupational Therapist as Case Manager (1991).	**Rescinded** 2002.
Occupational Therapy in the Promotion of Health and Well-Being (2013).	The Role of the Occupational Therapist in the Promotion of Health and Prevention of Disabilities (1976). **Replaced** by Occupational Therapy in the Promotion of Health and the Prevention of Disease and Disabilities (1976). **Replaced** by Occupational Therapy in the Promotion of Health and the Prevention of Disease and Disability (1989). **Rescinded** 2000. **Replaced** by Occupational Therapy in the Promotion of Health and the Prevention of Disease and Disability (2000). **Replaced** by Occupational Therapy in the Promotion of Health and the Prevention of Disease and Disability (2007). **Replaced** by Occupational Therapy in the Promotion of Health and Well-Being (2013).
Occupational Therapy Services in the Promotion of Psychological and Social Aspects of Mental Health (2010).	The Psychosocial Core of Occupational Therapy (1995, **edited** 1997). **Rescinded** 2004. **Replaced** by Psychosocial Aspects of Occupational Therapy (2004). **Replaced** by Occupational Therapy Services in the Promotion of Psychological and Social Aspects of Mental Health (2010). **Revised** 2015.
Occupational Therapy Services for Individuals Who Have Experienced Domestic Violence (2011).	Occupational Therapy Services for Individuals Who Have Experienced Domestic Violence (2006). **Revised** 2011.
Occupational Therapy Services for Persons With Alzheimer's Disease and Other Dementias (1994).	**Rescinded** 2000.
Occupational Therapy Services in Early Childhood and School-Based Settings (2011).	Occupational Therapy Provision for Children With Learning Disabilities and/or Mild to Moderate Perceptual and Motor Deficits (1991). **Replaced** by Occupational Therapy for Individuals With Learning Disabilities (1998). **Rescinded** 2004. **Replaced** by Occupational Therapy Services in Early Intervention and School-Based Programs (2004). **Replaced** by Occupational Therapy Services in Early Childhood and School-Based Settings (2011).
Occupational Therapy Services in Facilitating Work Performance (2011).	Work Hardening Guidelines (1986). **Replaced** by Occupational Therapy Services in Work Practice (1992). **Replaced** by Occupational Therapy Services in Facilitating Work Performance (2000). **Replaced** by Occupational Therapy Services in Facilitating Work Performance (2005). **Revised** 2011.
The Philosophical Base of Occupational Therapy (2011).	The Philosophical Base of Occupational Therapy (1979, 1995, 2004). **Replaced** by The Philosophical Base of Occupational Therapy (2011).
Psychosocial Concerns Within Occupational Therapy Practice (1995).	**Rescinded** 2004.
The Scope of Occupational Therapy Services for Individuals With an Autism Spectrum Disorder Across the Life Course (2010).	The Scope of Occupational Therapy Services for Individuals With an Autism Spectrum Disorder Across the Life Span (2005). **Replaced** by The Scope of Occupational Therapy Services for Individuals With an Autism Spectrum Disorder Across the Life Course (2010). **Revised** 2015.
The Role of Occupational Therapy in the Independent Living Movement (1993).	**Rescinded** 1999.

(Continued)

Summary of Official Document Rescissions, Revisions, and Changes *(cont.)*

Document (Final or Most Recent Version)	History
Societal Statements	
AOTA's Societal Statement on Autism Spectrum Disorders (2009).	**Rescinded** 2013.
AOTA's Societal Statement on Family Caregivers (2007).	**Rescinded** 2013.
AOTA's Societal Statement on Health Disparities (2013).	AOTA's Societal Statement on Health Disparities (2011). **Revised** 2013.
AOTA's Societal Statement on Obesity (2012).	AOTA's Societal Statement on Obesity (2006). **Revised** 2012. **Rescinded** 2013.
AOTA's Societal Statement on Play (2007).	**Rescinded** 2013.
Certification Document Changes	
The following certification documents have been removed from earlier editions of this manual:	
AOTA Certification Requirements.	**Rendered moot** by the formation of the American Occupational Therapy Certification Board.
Policy Governing Lapsed Certification of Occupational Therapists and Occupational Therapy Assistants.	**Rescinded** 1986.
Requirements for Graduates From Foreign Schools to Become OTRs.	**Rendered moot** by the formation of the American Occupational Therapy Certification Board.

Index

Note: Page references in *italic* refer to figures and tables.